Handbook of chronic pain management

edited by

GRAHAM D. BURROWS

Department of Psychiatry, University of Melbourne, Melbourne, Australia

DIANA ELTON

and

GORDON V. STANLEY

Department of Psychology, University of Melbourne, Melbourne, Australia

1987

Elsevier
Amsterdam · New York · Oxford

ISBN 0-444-80446-3

Published by:

Elsevier Science Publishers B.V. (Biomedical Division)
P.O. Box 211
1000 AE Amsterdam
The Netherlands

Sole distributors for the USA and Canada:
Elsevier Science Publishing Company, Inc.
52 Vanderbilt Avenue
New York, NY 10017
USA

Library of Congress Cataloging-in-Publication Data

Handbook of chronic pain management.

    Includes index.
    1. Intractable pain--Handbooks, manuals, etc.
I. Burrows, Graham D. II. Elton, Diana, 1933-
III. Stanley, Gordon. [DNLM: 1. Chronic Disease--therapy.
2. Pain--therapy. WL 704 H258]
RB127.H35 1987   616'.0472   87-13491
ISBN 0-444-80446-3 (U.S.)

Printed in The Netherlands

Handbook of chronic
pain management

Preface

This handbook attempts to provide the professional reader with an overview of the many and varied facets of the topic while at the same time having relevance for the health care practitioner who has to deal with pain in its clinical manifestations. The book is divided into two parts, the first dealing with reviewing the theoretical and experimental knowledge of pain, the second dealing with management of pain from the perspective of a number of different professions in the field of health care.

The last decade or so has seen a tremendous growth of knowledge in the area. The discovery of the endogenous analgesic system and the increasing knowledge about basic physiological systems represent important advances, yet there is still much to be discovered and understood.

At the psychological level there is an increasing understanding of the involvement of the social, cultural and cognitive variables in the individual patient's response to pain. While progress at this level has been made, it is clear that the interactions between many variables and systems indicate that the problem of pain, while addressable, is still far from being answered. The range of professional skills being applied to the study and relief of pain documented in this handbook does provide room for optimism that real progress is being made.

Graham Burrows
Diana Elton
Gordon Stanley

Foreword

This book deals with the most important and pressing issue of the health care system of most developed countries. This importance stems from the fact that chronic pain afflicts millions and millions of people worldwide, and in many patients it is inadequately managed. Consequently, chronic pain is the most frequent cause of suffering and disability which seriously impairs the quality of life of millions of people throughout the world. Moreover, it is a major economic problem for the population of the aforementioned countries. Because national epidemiologic studies on pain have not been done in any of the countries, for the past 20 years at intervals of 2 – 3 years, I have estimated the prevalence of chronic pain in the United States and other countries, by reviewing published reports of numerous local and regional surveys on back pain, headache, arthritis and other musculoskeletal disorders, cancer, heart disease and many other conditions carried out in the United States, the United Kingdom, Scandinavia, Germany, Italy, Israel, Australia, New Zealand and a number of other countries. I have also studied data published by federal health agencies and foundations concerned with such major chronic problems as arthritis, cancer and heart disease. These data were then extrapolated to the population of the United States and of a number of other countries and they consistently revealed that about 25 – 30% of the population suffer chronic pain, and of these, half to two thirds were either partially or totally disabled for periods ranging from a few days (e.g. recurrent headaches) to weeks, months and years (e.g. back pain, neuropathies), and some were permanently disabled (e.g. arthritis, low back pain, cancer). I also estimated the cost of these various chronic pain syndromes by estimating the number of work days lost and the cost of health care, payments for compensation, litigation and quackery. For example, recent estimates for the United States suggest that chronic pain cost the American people nearly $70 billion in 1983.

Even more important is the cost in terms of human suffering. It is the distressing fact that in this age of marvelous scientific and technologic advances which permit us to send people to the moon, there are millions of suffering patients who do not get the relief they deserve. Many of these patients are exposed to a high risk of iatrogenic complications from improper therapy including drug toxicity, narcotic dependence (and occasionally addiction), or have been subjected to multiple, often useless and at times, mutilating operations. A significant number of these patients give up medical care and consult quacks who not only deplete the patient's financial resources, but often do harm; some patients with severe intractable pain become so desperate as to contemplate or actually commit suicide.

Over the past 35 years I have also assessed the status of pain research and therapy at frequent intervals and the reasons for the deficiencies in the care of patients and found them to remain the same until a decade or so ago. These could be grouped into three major categories: a) great voids in knowledge about pain and its mechanisms due to insufficient and indeed total neglect of pain research by basic and clinical scientists; b) inadequate or improper application of the available knowledge and therapies due to total lack of educational programs for students and practitioners; and c) problems with transfer of information and communication.

Fortunately, during the past decade or so several changes have taken place which, if sustained and expanded, hold the promise of helping to rectify some of the past deficiencies and increase the capability of physicians and other health professionals to better cope with this serious problem. For one thing, there has been an impressive surge of interest among an increasing number of scientists in pain research and in collaborating with practitioners to begin to solve some of the major pain problems. Consequently, we have acquired a great deal of new information on the neurophysiologic, biochemical and psychologic substrates of acute pain and a significant amount of new information on the mechanisms of some chronic pain syndromes. This new knowledge has markedly enhanced our knowledge of sensory coding and sensory modulation, and has brought about a change in our conceptualization of clinical pain and pain therapy.

During this period there has also been improvement in the care of patients with acute, chronic and cancer pain. The recent worldwide movement in pain has prompted a significant number of physicians, psychologists and other health professionals to acquire more knowledge about pain and its treatment and an increasing number have taken training in pain diagnosis and therapy. Appreciation that pain is a very complex, multidimensional phenomenon composed of a vast array of sensory, perceptual, emotional, affective and interpersonal factors, and environmental influences has prompted development of an increasing number of multidisciplinary pain clinics/centers. Finally, there has been marked improvement in the diffusion of information through the activities of the International Association for the Study of Pain and its 16 chapters, publication of the journal *Pain* and the proceedings of the four World Congresses and a number of monographs.

The book edited by Drs. Burrows, Elton and Stanley, represents a very important event in the recent encouraging trends because it contains a comprehensive overview of the most important knowledge of the fundamental aspects of chronic pain and its management. The book is divided into two parts: a) Theoretical and Experimental, which includes 17 chapters; and b) Management, which includes 19 chapters. The first part includes chapters on anatomy, physiology, biochemistry, the scientific basis of acupuncture; on pain perception, cognition, and affect, pain measurement and on such relevant subjects as behavior modification, cultural factors, abnormal illness behavior and psychosomatic aspects, all written by world renowned authorities of each specific field. The second part dealing with management is presented in a manner which is different than the usual, traditional format of discussing therapy. Instead of discussing specific procedures in the therapy of chronic pain, each of the 19 chapters considers the management of chronic pain in general practice, dentistry, and the various specialties, also written by persons who are well known for their interest and work in pain. It is most refreshing to note inclusion of chapters on the role of nurses, social workers, and physiotherapists because these health professionals play very important roles in managing patients with chronic pain. There are also chapters on the management of cancer pain, the use of analgesics, and the use of hypnosis. Finally, there is an extensive chapter on the evolution and current status of pain clinics with emphasis on the multidisciplinary programs.

It is apparent that Drs. Burrows, Elton and Stanley have discharged their responsibility as editors of this volume in an exemplary manner with regard to the selection of topics and the authors of each of these topics. This book should be of great interest to practicing physicians and other health professionals who are involved in managing patients with chronic pain in their practice. It should also prove useful to medical students and registrars (residents) in training for specialization in the various fields considered in the volume. For all clinicians, the book should prove a highly effective source for the better understanding and treatment of chronic pain. I am therefore very pleased to highly recommend the volume and predict that it will help to improve the care of these patients which, after all, is an important *raison d'etre* of clinicians.

John J. Bonica

Chairman Emeritus and Professor, Anesthesiology
Director Emeritus, Multidisciplinary Pain Clinic
University of Washington, Seattle, Washington

List of contributors

Jo Clelland   243
  Division of Physical Therapy, School of Community and Allied Health, The University of Alabama at Birmingham, Birmingham, Alabama, U.S.A.

Laurel Archer Copp   227
  Carrington Hall, University of North Carolina, Chapel Hill, North Carolina, U.S.A.

Michael J. Cousins   163
  Department of Anaesthesia and Intensive Care, Flinders Medical Centre, Bedford Park, South Australia, Australia

Kenneth D. Craig   99
  Department of Psychology, University of British Columbia, Vancouver, Canada

Minaly Csikszentmihalyi   69
  Department of Behavioral Sciences, University of Chicago, Chicago, Illinois, U.S.A.

Antoine Depaulis   41
  Department of Psychology, University of California, Los Angeles, California, U.S.A.

Diana Elton   91, 271
  Department of Psychology, University of Melbourne, Victoria, Australia

Frederick J. Evans   285
  Carrier Foundation and The University of Medicine and Dentistry of New Jersey, Robert Wood Johnson Medical School, Belle Mead, New Jersey, U.S.A.

J.A. Gerschman   321
  Oro-Facial Pain Clinic, Department of Dental Medicine and Surgery, University of Melbourne, Victoria, Australia

Geoffrey K. Gourlay   163
  Pain Management Unit, Flinders Medical Centre, Bedford Park, South Australia, Australia

Lianfang He   47
  Laboratory of Neurophysiology, Research Department of Acupuncture, Shanghai Medical University, People's Republic of China

Brendan J. Holwill   301
  Repatriation General Hospital, Heidelberg, Victoria, Australia

A. Iggo   7
  Department of Veterinary Physiology, Royal (Dick) School of Veterinary Studies, Summerhall, Edinburgh, U.K.

Paolo Inghilleri   69
Institute of Psychology, Faculty of Medicine, University of Milan, Milan, Italy

Fiona K. Judd   301
Department of Psychiatry, University of Melbourne, Austin Hospital, Heidelberg, Victoria, Australia

Arthur Kleinman   109
Department of Psychiatry and Department of Medical Anthropology, William James Hall, Harvard University, Cambridge, Massachusetts, U.S.A.

John C. Liebeskind   41
Department of Psychology, University of California, Los Angeles, California, U.S.A.

Olov Lindahl   127
Lambarö, Vallingby, Sweden

John J. LaFerla   371
Department of Obstetrics-Gynecology, Hutzel Hospital, The Detroit Medical Center, Wayne State University School of Medicine, Detroit, Michigan, U.S.A.

Toshihiko Maruta   315
Pain Management Center, Department of Psychiatry and Psychology, Mayo Clinic and Mayo Foundation, Rochester, Minnesota, U.S.A.

Fausto Massimini   69
Department of Psychology, University of Turin, Turin, Italy

Patricia A. McGrath   205
Department of Paediatrics and Pain Management Program, Faculty of Medicine, Children's Hospital of Western Ontario, The University of Western Ontario, London, Canada

F. McKenna   331
Rheumatology and Rehabilitation Research Unit, School of Medicine, The University of Leeds, Leeds, U.K.

Joan Merrilyn McMeeken   259
Lincoln Institute of Health Sciences, School of Physiotherapy, Carlton, Victoria, Australia

Mark Mehta   147
Pain Relief Centre, United Norwich Hospitals, Norwich, England, U.K.

Donald Meichenbaum   85
Department of Psychology, Faculty of Arts, University of Waterloo, Waterloo, Ontario, Canada

H. Merskey   137
Department of Psychiatry, University of Western Ontario, London Psychiatric Hospital, London, Ontario, Canada

Rita B. Messing   19
Department of Pharmacology, Medical School, University of Minnesota, Minneapolis, Minnesota, U.S.A.

B.S. Nashold, Jr.   383
Department of Surgery, Division of Neurosurgery, Duke University Medical Center, Durham, North Carolina, U.S.A.

Robert N. Pechnick   41
Department of Psychology, University of California, Los Angeles, California, U.S.A.

Issy Pilowsky   131
Department of Psychiatry, The University of Adelaide, Royal Adelaide Hospital, South Australia, Australia

P.C. Reade   321
Department of Dental Medicine and Surgery, University of Melbourne, Victoria, Australia

Ranjan Roy   217
School of Social Work and Faculty of Medicine, Headache Clinic, Psychological Services Centre, University of Manitoba, Winnipeg, Canada

Emily Savinar   243
Department of Physical Therapy, Kaiser Permanente Medical Center, Oakland, California, U.S.A.

Katherine F. Shepard   243
Department of Physical Therapy, College of Allied Health Professions, Temple University, Philadelphia, Pennsylvania, U.S.A.

Menno E. Sluijter   147
Lutherse Diakonessen Ziekenhuis, Amsterdam, The Netherlands

G.C. Smith   2
Department of Psychological Medicine, Monash University, Prince Henry's Hospital, Melbourne, Victoria, Australia

Gordon V. Stanley   121, 271
Department of Psychology, University of Melbourne, Victoria, Australia

Barry Charles Stillman   259
Lincoln Institute of Health Sciences, School of Physiotherapy, Carlton, Victoria, Australia

Lars Terenius   33
Department of Pharmacology, University of Uppsala, Uppsala, Sweden

Dennis C. Turk   85
Center for Pain Evaluation and Treatment, University of Pittsburgh School of Medicine, Pittsburgh, Pennsylvania, U.S.A.

Jeffrey M. Wagner   407
Boston Pain Center, Spaulding Rehabilitation Hospital, Boston, Massachusetts, U.S.A.

T.D. Walsh   347
Department of Developmental Chemotherapy, Memorial Sloane Kettering Cancer Center, New York, New York, U.S.A.

Matisyohu Weisenberg   77
Department of Psychology, Bar-Ilan University, Ramat-Gan, Israel

R. Peter Welsh   401
Sports Medicine Clinic, Orthopaedic and Arthritic Hospital, Toronto, Ontario, Canada

George L. Wilcox   19
Department of Pharmacology, Medical School, University of Minnesota, Minneapolis, Minnesota, U.S.A.

V. Wright   331
Rheumatology and Rehabilitation Research Unit, School of Medicine, The University of Leeds, Leeds, U.K.

Margo G. Wyckoff   99
Springbrook Professional Building, 4540 Sand Point Way N.E., Suite 340, Seattle, Washington, U.S.A.

Contents

Burrows/Elton/Stanley (eds.) Handbook of Chronic Pain Management
© *1987 Elsevier Science Publishers B.V. (Biomedical Division)*

The anatomy of pain

G.C. SMITH

Department of Psychological Medicine, Monash University, Melbourne, Victoria, Australia

The traditional anatomical view of pain was that it was subserved by a specific receptor and a chain of three specific neurons whose axons passed upward in the lateral spinothalamic tract (STT) to the thalamus and cerebral cortex of the opposite side where, somehow, the information so conveyed was perceived as pain. Whilst this simple view still has a certain validity, and is sufficient to enable localization of major neurological lesions, it cannot explain many of the enigmas of pain such as the phenomena of chronic pain. Advances in knowledge, contributed mainly by electrophysiological studies, later led to the understanding that information relevant to perception of pain travelled in other primary sensory neurons as well, and in ascending tracts other than the STT, and that in particular the input, integration and output of the reticular formation of the brainstem was important.

These emerging data were used by Melzack and Wall (1965) to propose a hypothetical explanation of the anatomy of pain perception which they called the Gate Control theory. In its early form it proposed that information about various modalities of sensation, including pain, interacted synaptically in the dorsal horn of the spinal cord, so that information about pain which emerged to ascend to the brain in the spinothalamic and other tracts was modified or gated (Fig. 1). The theory also allowed for descending influences on input; a revolutionary idea, for although it had been accepted that there were higher influences on pain perception it had been assumed that the anatomical basis for this was intracerebral.

We now know much more about the anatomy of pain, and Wall (1978, 1984) and others have continually updated their models to encompass new knowledge. Much of this knowledge has come from neurophysiological studies, but as with all other areas of neurobiology, most has come from the application of revolutionary techniques of histochemistry. These have enabled neurons to be identified according to the neurotransmitters and neuromodulators they contain. Thus the nervous system has been re-mapped, and the vast networks of amine-containing and peptide-containing neurons identified. In some cases neurons containing both amines and peptides have been described. Of particular interest with respect to the anatomy of pain has been the identification of noradrenaline, 5-hydroxytryptamine (5-HT), opioid (endorphin and enkephalin) and substance P-containing neurons. Furthermore, it has been possible to inject

2

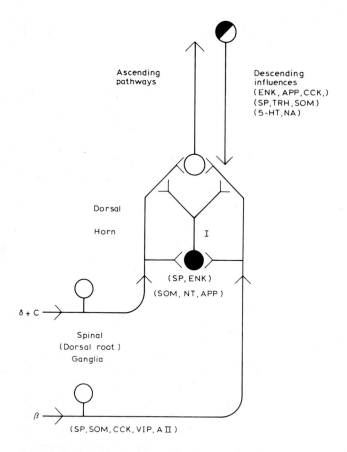

Fig. 1. Diagrammatic respresentation of the original Gate Control theory proposed by Melzack and Wall (1965), with subsequently identified amines and peptides indicated. δ and C refer to small myelinated and unmyelinated afferents. β refers to large myelinated afferents. I indicates inhibitory neuron. A II = angiotensin II; APP = avian polypeptide; CCK = cholecystokinin; ENK = enkephalin; 5-HT = 5-hydroxytryptamine; NA = noradrenaline; NT = neurotensin; SOM = somatostatin; SP = substance P; TRH = thyrotropin-releasing hormone; VIP = vasoactive intestinal polypeptide.

tracer substances into individual neurons and map the entire distribution of terminal fields of functionally identified neurons.

There are many functionally distinct classes of primary afferent neurons in cutaneous nerves, and each class has a specific type of anatomical termination pattern in the dorsal horn. Part of the problem of attempting to describe the anatomy of pain is that most of the information comes from animal experimentation where findings must be correlated with the application of noxious stimuli which are assumed to be perceived as pain. It is thus mainly about the anatomy of nociception. Furthermore, different tissues will have different responses to injury, and the phenomena occurring in neurons subsequent to injury are now known to include marked changes in neurotransmitter content and the development of noradrenergic receptors (Wall 1984). All of the classes of afferent neurons are likely to be activated and contribute to the perception of pain after injury, and some, in the A delta and C classes, respond only to injury (nociceptors).

The termination of primary afferent neurons in the spinal cord is now understood with such complexity that no single diagram could do justice to it. In summary, it can be said that there is evidence that nociceptors terminate in part in the superficial dorsal horn, and that a distinction between nociceptor and other neurons is maintained there, even though there is complex interaction. About one third of the primary sensory neurons contain a neuropeptide (Fig. 1). One of these is the opioid enkephalin, others include substance P, cholecystokinin (CCK), somatostatin (SOM) and vasoactive intestinal peptide (VIP) (Hökfelt et al. 1983). There is functional evidence to support a role for these substances in the phenomenon of pain. A population of enkephalin-containing interneurons in the dorsal horn shows capacity to modulate nociceptive input.

The major and essential ascending pathway with respect to transmission of noxious stimuli from the dorsal horn is the STT (Ralston 1984). It is now considered that there is only one such tract on each side, located in the anterolateral quadrant. However, another important ascending tract is the dorsal column postsynaptic system (DCPS). Other tracts may also be involved, and this diversity of ascending systems involved is one reason why it is difficult to predict how any one anatomical lesion, including one made for therapeutic purposes, will affect pain perception. Both noxious specific and non-noxious responding neurons project from the dorsal horn of the spinal cord in these tracts to the contralateral thalamus, particularly the ventroposterolateral (VPL) nucleus and intralaminar nucleus. The nociceptive fibres are mixed with fibres related to other modalities; there is much less localization than was previously thought. Spinoreticular tracts, which also convey information about noxious stimuli to the reticular formation, are also found in the anterolateral quadrant.

Cells in both the nucleus VPL and intralaminar nucleus of the thalamus respond to noxious stimuli. Stimulation of the VPL in man produces sharp, well localized pain, whilst stimulation of the intralaminar region produces burning and poorly localized pain. The VPL is a site of marked integrative activity, involving input from the thalamic reticular nuclei and the cerebral cortex, as well as interaction of the various modality specific inputs into the thalamus, via interneurons (Ralston 1984). However, the thalamus is no longer regarded as the highest centre of conscious elaboration of pain.

Frontal leucotomy including cingulotomy, severing of the cingulum bundle as it passes dorsal to the corpus callosum, has often been used for the relief of intractable pain, and it has been assumed that such operations sever connections between the frontal cortex and the limbic system. It is now known that there are neurons in the somatosensory cortex that are capable of responding to noxious stimuli. It has now been established that the nucleus submedius of the thalamus, which responds to noxious stimuli, projects to the orbitofrontal cortex.

The neurotransmitters involved in these second, third and higher order neurons of the spinal cord, thalamus and cortex are unknown.

Melzack and Wall (1965) allowed for descending influences on input to the spinal cord; enough is known about these now to be able to describe an endogenous analgesic system (Basbaum and Fields 1984). Reticular formation neurons containing noradrenaline or 5-hydroxytryptamine (5-HT) descend from the midbrain and medulla respectively to terminate in the dorsal horn (Fig. 2). 5-HT neurons provide a dense innervation particularly to the outer layer of the dorsal horn, on second order nociceptive neurons of both the STT and DCPS systems. Transection of these fibres or pharmacological blocking prevents morphine from having its analgesic effect. This may be a basis for the analgesic effect of neuroleptic and antidepressant drugs. Neurons containing the opioid β-endorphin, whose cell bodies are in the hypothalamus, terminate in the reticular formation and are considered to be part of this endogenous analgesic system, a possible site of integration of phenomena such as stress-induced analgesia (Lewis et al. 1984) (see also Chapter 5).

4

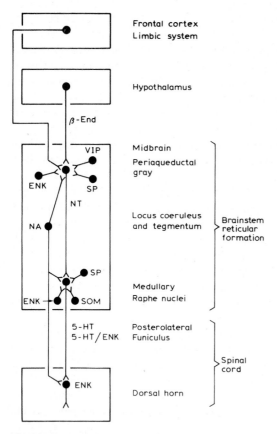

Fig. 2. Diagrammatic representation of the descending components of the postulated 'endogenous analgesic system'. The circuitry and number of neurotransmitters illustrated is not complete, but represents current concepts about neuronal organization and transmitters. β-End = β-endorphin; ENK = enkephalin; 5-HT = 5-hydroxytryptamine; NA = noradrenaline; NT = neurotensin; SOM = somatostatin; SP = substance P; VIP = vasoactive intestinal polypeptide.

Stimulation of the periaqueductal gray matter of the midbrain is now being used as an analgesic technique in cases of intractable pain (Young et al. 1984). Animal studies indicate that other areas of the reticular formation also need to be intact for periaqueductal stimulation to be analgesic. Although opioid levels in CSF are raised during such stimulation, it is not clear what role they play in this phenomenon, although enkephalin-containing neurons descending from the reticular formation to the dorsal horn are implicated.

Thus these advances in the knowledge of the anatomy of pain have already led to clinical application, as well as adding generally to our knowledge of the mechanisms of pain.

References

Basbaum, A. I. and Fields, H. L. (1984) Endogenous pain control systems: brainstem spinal pathways and endorphin circuitry. Ann. Rev. Neurosci. 7, 309–338.
Hökfelt, T., Skirboll, L., Lunberg, J. M., Dalsgaard, C-J., Johansson, O., Pernow, B. and Jansco,

G. (1983) Neuropeptides and pain pathways. In: J. J. Bonica, U. Linblom and A. Iggo (Eds.), Advances in Pain Research and Therapy, Vol. 5. Raven Press, New York, pp. 227 – 246.

Lewis, J. W., Terman, G. W., Shavit, Y., Nelson, L. R. and Liebeskind, J. C. (1984) Neural, neurochemical and hormonal bases of stress-induced analgesia. In: L. Kruger and J. C. Liebeskind (Eds.), Advances in Pain Research and Therapy, Vol. 6. Raven Press, New York, pp. 277 – 288.

Melzack, R. and Wall, P. D. (1965) Pain mechanisms: a new theory. Science 150, 971 – 979.

Ralston, H. J. (1984) Synaptic organisation of spinothalamic tract projections to the thalamus, with special reference to pain. In: L. Kruger and J. C. Liebeskind (Eds.), Advances in Pain Research and Therapy, Vol. 6. Raven Press, New York, pp. 183 – 195.

Wall, P. D. (1978) The gate control theory of pain mechanisms: a re-examination and re-statement. Brain 101, 1 – 18.

Wall, P. D. (1984) Mechanisms of acute and chronic pain. In: L. Kruger and J. C. Liebeskind (Eds.), Advances in Pain Research and Therapy, Vol. 6. Raven Press, New York, pp. 95 – 104.

Young, R. F., Feldman, R. A., Kroening, R., Fulton, W. and Morris, J. (1984) Electrical stimulation of the brain in the treatment of chronic pain in man. In: L. Kruger and J. C. Liebeskind (Eds.), Advances in Pain Research and Therapy, Vol. 6. Raven Press, New York, pp. 289 – 303.

Burrows/Elton/Stanley (eds.) Handbook of Chronic Pain Management
© *1987 Elsevier Science Publishers B.V. (Biomedical Division)*

2

Physiology of pain

A. IGGO

Department of Veterinary Physiology, Royal (Dick) School of Veterinary Studies,
University of Edinburgh, Edinburgh, U.K.

Introduction

A good starting point for a consideration of the physiological mechanisms that underlie pain is the definition of pain, and the qualifying notes, proposed by IASP in its 'Pain Terms' glossary (Pain (1979) 6, 250).

Pain is:

'An unpleasant sensory and emotional experience associated with actual or potential tissue damage, or described in terms of such damage. Pain is always subjective. Each individual learns the application of the word through experiences related to injury in early life. Biologists recognize that those stimuli which cause pain are liable to damage tissue. Accordingly, pain is that experience which we associate with actual or potential tissue damage. It is also always unpleasant and therefore also an emotional experience. Experiences which resemble pain., e.g. pricking, but are not unpleasant, should not be called pain. Unpleasant abnormal experiences (dysaesthesiae) may also be pain but are not necessarily so because, subjectively, they may not have the usual sensory qualities of pain.

Many people report pain in the absence of tissue damage or any likely pathophysiological cause; usually this happens for psychological reasons. There is no way to distinguish their experience from that due to tissue damage if we take the subjective report. If they regard their experience as pain and if they report it in the same ways as pain caused by tissue damage, it should be accepted as pain. This definition avoids tying pain to the stimulus. Activity induced in the nociceptor and nociceptive pathways by a noxious stimulus is not pain, which is always a psychological state, even though we may well appreciate that pain most often has a proximate physical cause.'

This definition stresses the fact that pain is a psychological experience and that it may be reported in the absence of tissue damage or any likely pathophysiological cause. It is reported only by conscious individuals and all the evidence points to the necessity of the cerebral cortex so that its full expression involves the highest levels of the central nervous system. The underlying physiological mechanisms of nociception, on the other hand, have been very extensively investigated at lower levels of the central nervous system during the last 20 years and a clear picture is now emerging of peripheral, spinal and brainstem mechanisms of nociception and analgesia.

Nociceptors

The primary detectors of noxious or potentially noxious stimuli applied to the peripheral tissues are the nociceptors. These sensory receptors are found in most tissues of the body and have the property of discharging impulses in the afferent fibres when mechanical, thermal or chemical stimuli exceed a threshold magnitude of intensity. They can be sharply distinguished from sensitive mechanoreceptors and thermoreceptors, that have much lower excitatory thresholds, and may indeed be driven to maximal activity at stimuli that are sub-threshold for the nociceptors (Iggo 1985). Some nociceptors in the skin are unable to discriminate between high intensity stimulation by mechanical, thermal or chemical stimuli and are therefore called 'polymodal nociceptors'. Many of these receptors have non-myelinated (C) afferent fibres. Other nociceptors are more selective, including the mechanical nociceptors with small myelinated (A delta) afferent fibres. This group of nociceptors is readily excited by pin-prick types of stimuli. These two broad categories of nociceptor, the A δ and the C, have very different conduction velocities, so that impulses started simultaneously from the respective receptors in each class would arrive at different times in the central nervous system – thus giving rise to two sensory responses, namely first and second pain (see Besson et al. 1982).

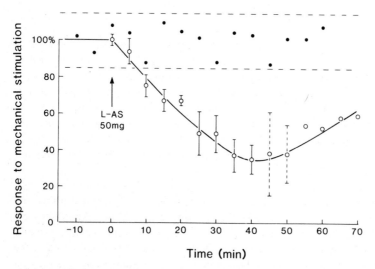

Fig. 1. Joint capsule nociceptors in normal and arthritic rats, and the effects of an NSAID (non-steroidal anti-inflammatory drug – acetylsalicylic acid). The control responses (expressed as 100%) of the receptors are shown at the left and the reduction in the responses of the arthritic receptor (-o-o-) following i.v. acetylsalicylate (L-AS) are clearly seen. In contrast, the receptors in normal rats (●●●) are unaffected. (From Guilbaud and Iggo, 1985.)

The threshold sensitivity of the nociceptors is not permanent and unalterable. Joint-capsule receptors in a normal rat, for example, have high thresholds and are difficult to excite except by noxious magnitudes of stimulation. In arthritic rats the receptors are very readily excited by light pressure (Guilbaud et al. 1985). This enhanced sensitivity of the nociceptors can be reversed by the i.v. administration of the analgesic, lysine acetylsalicylate (Fig. 1). The altered sensitivity of the receptors is almost certainly due to the continued formation in the inflamed joint capsule of a prostaglandin. The reversal by the aspirin is due to the inhibition of α-cyclooygenase (an enzyme that is essential early in the arachidonic cascade) leading to a rapid fall in tissue levels of prostaglandins (possibly prostacyclin or a thromboxane) with the consequent absence of the potentiating agent responsible for the enhanced sensitivity (see also Chapter 31). An interesting aspect of the action of these peripheral analgesics is that they do not appear to modify the sensitivity of the receptors in the absence of hyperalgesia, an effect in the case of the non-steroidal anti-inflammatory drugs (NSAIDs) that is accounted for by the indirect mechanism of action, viz. through the diminished production of the potentiating prostaglandin.

The sensitivity of the nociceptors can also be affected by opioids, and drugs such as morphine and the enkephalins can reduce stabilized hyperalgesia by an action on peripheral nociceptors. Such an action is additional to any central analgesic action of the opioids (Ferreira 1986) and may be supplemental to the action of non-steroidal analgesics (NSAIDs) such as aspirin.

Spinal mechanisms of nociception

The afferent fibres from the nociceptors all terminate in the spinal gray matter shortly after they enter the central nervous system, and their sensory effects are therefore mediated by other neurons (second order neurons) that project to the brainstem, thalamus and cortex by stages. These latter neurons in the spinal cord are in the dorsal (posterior) horn. Two major kinds of such neuron are present; those that are exclusively excited by an input from the nociceptors (nociceptor-specific neurons) (Fig. 2 F) and those excited by nociceptors and also by an input from sensitive mechanoreceptors (multireceptive neurons) (Fig. 2 A,E). The former are concentrated in the most superficial laminae of the horn, whereas the latter are common in deeper layers. Many nociceptor afferent fibres, especially the C-fibres, terminate in an intermediate layer, the substantia gelatinosa (Cervero and Iggo 1980), a region especially rich in neuropeptides. Some of these, such as substance P (SP) are in the terminals of the C-fibres, whereas others, such as the enkephalins, are in dorsal horn neurons. Great interest is at present concentrated on the physiology of these peptides, especially since their presence in neurons involved in nociception raises important questions concerning their roles in nociception and analgesia, but their exact functions are not yet established (Hökfelt et al. 1983).

The technique of epidural administration of drugs, from indwelling catheters in the intrathecal space (Yaksh and Reddy 1981) has proved that opioids such as morphine as well as catecholamines, such as noradrenaline and dopamine, can be analgesic by an action at the spinal level. Electrophysiological evidence establishes that the analgesia is probably due to a selective suppression of nociceptor-specific neurons. Both noradrenaline and dopamine when released locally in the dorsal horn can selectively suppress the responses of centrally-projecting multireceptive neurons to noxious stimuli (Fig. 3) as also can opioids such as β-endorphin. The antinociceptive action of the latter may indeed depend on the presence of noradrenaline in the spinal cord – an interesting and important discovery (Fleetwood-Walker et al. 1985).

An important feature of the dorsal horn neurons, in addition to their selectivity in relation

10

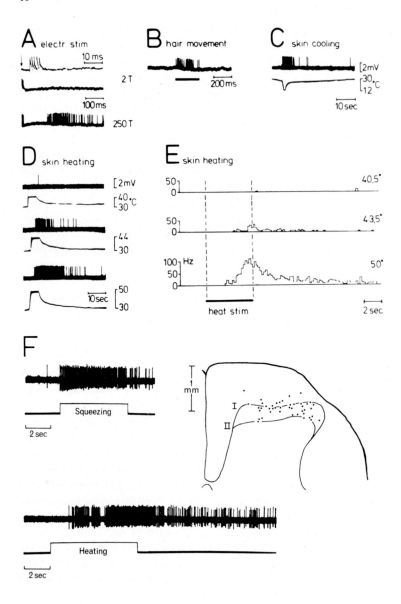

Fig. 2. Neuronal responses in the dorsal horn of the spinal cord of anaesthetised cats. (A – E) The discharges in a single multi-receptive neuron. (B) The brisk discharge when the hairs in the receptive field are stroked (afferent input in sensitive mechanoreceptors), (D) and (E) the responses when the same area of skin was heated to the temperatures shown (afferent input in nociceptors). (From Handwerker et al. 1975.) (F) The discharges of a nociceptor-specific neuron to noxious squeezing, upper records, and heating above 45°C of the skin, lower records. Note the very prolonged response of the neuron after the heat stimulus was removed in both (D), (E) and (F). The locations of the nociceptor specific neurons in lamina I are shown in the cross-sectional diagram of the spinal cord in (F). (From Cervero et al. 1979.)

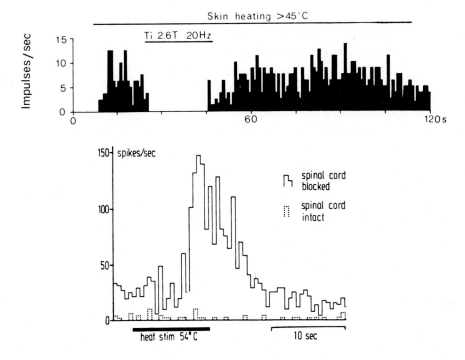

Fig. 3. Segmental and supraspinal inhibition. The upper histogram shows the discharge of a nociceptor-specific dorsal horn neuron before and during continuous heating of the skin above 45°C, the complete suppression of the response when mechanoreceptor afferent fibres in the tibial nerve are stimulated electrically at a frequency of 20/sec (Ti 2.6T 20 Hz bar) and the recovery of the response when the nerve stimulation is stopped. (From Cervero et al. 1976.)

to noxious peripheral stimuli, is their abilitiy to amplify to response. In general, a synchronous brief input in nociceptor afferents, causes a prolonged response from the neurons, lasting for many seconds. This means that there need not be a one-to-one temporal correspondence between a peripheral stimulus and the central neural activity and sensation evoked by it. Furthermore, the repeated application of an afferent input in C-fibres can lead to a progressive increase in response to successive stimuli (Mendell 1966) so that a nociceptive dorsal horn neuron may gradually be called into persistent high rates of discharge by repeated afferent input. The extent to which such effects are due to reverberatory circuits of neurons or to the accumulation of persistent transmitter (such as the neuropeptides) is not known.

Sensory pathways

The onward transmission of activity evoked in the dorsal spinal cord by nociceptor input is in 'second-order' neurons, not in the primary afferent fibres. Several pathways exist, that may operate in parallel. The classical pathway is the spinothalamic tract, in which the ascending fibres cross the spinal cord to ascend in the contralateral antero-lateral quadrant (forming the antero-lateral tract). Interruption of this tract is a classical surgical procedure for pain relief. These axons reach the thalamus in the medial lemniscus. There are two major regions of thalamic termination: 1) the ventro-basal complex, where they end on neurons thay may form a shell around other neurons that receive an exclusive input from the sensitive mechanoreceptors; 2) the intralaminar nuclei, a region devoid of neurons with an exclusive input from the sensitive mechanoreceptors. From the thalamus there are projections to the primary somato-sensory receiving area of the cerebral cortex. Knowledge of the cerebral projection of specific nociceptor-driven neurons has only recently become available (Andersson and Rydenhag 1985). This new information removes one obstacle to understanding the central mechanisms of pain, since it establishes that activity originating in nociceptors has direct access to the primary sensory processing areas in the brain. Beyond this point, however, the way in which such nociceptor-derived information is further processed by the conscious brain becomes conjectural. The role of the prefrontal cortex in the elaboration of 'pain-signals' is known from clinical evidence derived from surgical treatment of psychological disorders. Many of the emotional overtones of pain may be diminished if the interconnections of the frontal lobes with other parts of the cerebral cortex, or subcortical structures, are cut. In such patients there are reports that the sensory awareness of a pain may, after surgery, exist in the absence of a previously overwhelming emotional dominance by the pain (Bonner et al. 1952).

Antinociception and analgesia

The foregoing account of nociception can be misinterpreted as implying an unmodifiable pain pathway leading from the nociceptors to conscious awareness. Such is not the case. All sensory processing in the central nervous system is highly modifiable or plastic. At all levels in the sensory pathways, whenever a set of neurons is interposed, there is the possibility of plasticity due to the action of excitatory and inhibitory synaptic modification of the excitability of the output neuron. In addition, there may be convergence of different sensory receptor systems, so that previously 'specific' sets of neurons combine to generate a new 'non-specific' set. Processing of these kinds contributes to such phenomena as 'sensory acuity', 'attention', 'orientation-specificity' and so on. In part, this shaping of the sensory input depends on descending neural control, originating from higher levels in the nervous system, that often regulates the excitability of subordinate sets of neurons at a lower level – 'the integrative nature of the nervous system' in Sherrington's formulation.

All these processes operate in nociception, from the first synapses in the dorsal horn of the spinal cord, to those in the cerebral cortex. The existence of these mechanisms, some of which will now be briefly described, offers the opportunity for analgesia or anti-nociception. I shall deal with them systematically.

Nociceptors and analgesia

The way in which locally-produced chemicals can enhance the sensitivity of nociceptors has already been described. Analgesia at this level may be caused by preventing the formation of an algogenic agent, e.g. through the inhibition of α-cyclooxygenase by aspirin. In this case, the formation of the potentiating algogen has been prevented (Fig. 1) (Guilbaud and Iggo 1985). Alternatively, the action of the algogen may be prevented, as is possibly the case when opioids are used (Ferreira 1986), or the nociceptor may be inactivated by a local anaesthetic acting on the receptor or on the afferent fibre, a form of sensory paralysis. A therapeutic disadvantage of this last procedure is that other sensory receptors are also likely to be inactivated, with a consequent loss of all sensory input.

Various forms of hyperalgesia or disordered sensation (allodynia, Pain (1979) 6, 250) may result from damage to peripheral nerves, in part at least due to the formation of neuroma consequent on the imperfect repair or regeneration in the nerve trunk after traumatic injury. Such sensory disorders are not an inevitable consequence of injury, and when present may be due to central rather than peripheral consequences of the de-afferentation. In some circumstances where the pain is of peripheral origin it can be reduced or suppressed by treating the neuroma with an anti-sympathetic agent such as guanethidine (Wall et al. 1979). An explanation for such effects is that nerve axons in some neuromas become highly disorganized (Danielsen et al. 1986) and may develop unusual properties, such as sensitivity to catecholamines.

Spinal antinociception and analgesia

SEGMENTAL MECHANISMS

The modulation of sensory input in the dorsal horn provides an opportunity for the suppression of signals that result in pain. Since the neuronal circuitry of the dorsal horn is complex, including neural elements derived from afferent fibres, segmental interneurons, projection neurons and the terminals of supraspinal and long spinal neurons, it is not surprising that the onward transmission of nociceptive information can be modified (Cervero and Iggo 1980). At the simplest level, a nociceptive response can be suppressed by synaptic inhibition. This occurs, for example, when a multireceptive neuron responding to a noxious input has an additional input to it from sensitive mechanoreceptors. These latter, by a disynaptic path via an interneuron, cause a strong IPSP, that is sufficient to prevent the noxious input from causing the neuron to discharge. A more complex example would be where the inhibitory action was expressed on an internuncial neuron in the excitatory path from the nociceptor to the output neuron. What is clear is that an afferent input from sensitive cutaneous mechanoreceptors with large myelinated afferent fibres can suppress the excitation arising from nociceptors (Fig. 4). The detailed neuron circuits underlying these mechanisms are still under investigation, with particular attention being paid to the numerous small neurons in the substantia gelatinosa. This kind of anti-nociception, first recorded in laboratory experiments, probably underlies the relief from pain, in appropriate cases, afforded by transcutaneous nerve stimulation (TENS) a technique pioneered by Wall and Sweet (1967).

SUPRASPINAL MECHANISMS

The excitability of segmental nociresponsive neurons can be modified by supraspinal systems exerting an effect in the spinal cord. Some of these systems are tonically active, and may be exerting a continuous controlling action. An example is illustrated in Fig. 4. A vigorous response of a multi-receptive neuron when its cutaneous receptive field is heated to 54°C is present only when the spinal cord is blocked, so as to prevent descending impulses from reaching the spinal segment containing the neuron.

Mechanisms of this kind have aroused great interest because of their potential therapeutic value. Many systems are now under study, including those active when particular regions of the brainstem or cerebral cortex are stimulated electrically. These various brainstem systems have

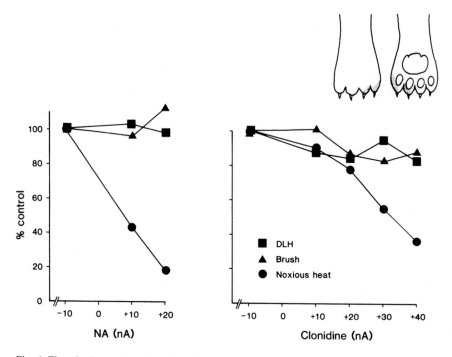

Fig. 4. The selective action of noradrenaline (NA) on the discharge of multi-receptive neurons in the dorsal horn of the cat. In both panels the responses of a neuron to light tactile stimuli (brush ▲), to a locally-applied cell excitant (dl-homocysteic acid, ■) and to noxious heat (> 45°C, ●) are shown. In the left-hand panel, the local application of NA by ionophoresis from a microelectrode, causes a selective depression of the response to the noxious stimulus. The right-hand panel shows that the effect is partially blocked by the α_2-adrenergic blocker, clonidine. The receptive fields on the toes are indicated by shading in the drawings. (Reproduced with permission from Fleetwood-Walker et al. 1985.)

already been used in human patients to provide pain relief by their electrical stimulation through implanted electrodes (Meyerson 1983), so-called stimulation-produced-analgesia (SPA) (see Chapter 5 for an account of stimulation-produced-analgesia).

Suprasegmental mechanisms also include those in which a noxious stimulus delivered anywhere in the body, can strongly inhibit the response of multi-receptive dorsal horn neurons to a local noxious stimulus. This effect is, in part, segmental, but supraspinal mechanisms are also involved. The effects may be prolonged. The 5-hydroxytryptamine (5-HT) containing n. raphe magnus neurons have been suggested as forming an essential component of the supraspinal efferent limb of this anti-nociceptive system (LeBars et al. 1983).

PHARMACOLOGY OF SPINAL AND SUPRASPINAL MECHANISMS

The intrathecal or epidural administration of opioids and catecholamines can cause behavioral analgesia in animals and pain relief in human patients. When the mechanisms are analysed electrophysiologically in animals it is seen that the drugs can depress, in a selective manner, the neural responses to noxious peripheral stimuli. The catecholamines in the spinal cord are contained in the terminals of axons that have cell bodies in the brainstem. Electrical stimulation of the cell bodies giving rise to these descending axons, using implanted electrodes, also suppresses selectively the neural responses to noxious stimuli (Fig. 5). Different cell groups are involved. If, for example, the A11 dopamine-containing cell group is stimulated, the anti-nociceptive effect can be blocked by local deposition in the spinal cord of a selective dopamine D_2-antagonist (Fleetwood-Walker et al. 1985). Another example is provided by 5-HT that is contained in neurons with cell bodies in the n. raphe magnus in the medulla oblongata. It too is anti-nociceptive at the spinal level. These supraspinal systems are only part of a surprisingly rich repertoire of descending control systems, all of which can modulate, by synaptic action, the onward transmission of information originating in nociceptors. It is not yet possible to assign to any of them a well-defined functional role but the mechanisms have the potential of future therapeutic application.

The opioids, such as morphine, are another group of anti-nociceptive agents, and aroused great interest when opiate receptors were discovered in the mid-brain in regions that caused analgesia on electrical stimulation (Basbaum and Fields 1978). Morphine microinjected into the same region (the periaqueductal gray, PAG) is analgesic (see also Chapter 3). Interest was still further heightened by the discovery of the endogenous opioids, Leu- and met-enkephalin (Kosterlitz 1983). These small neuropeptides act on the same opiate receptors as morphine and have raised hopes of their having a functional role as natural endogenous anti-nociceptive agents (see also Chapter 4). Their actual role is still being investigated, but they are present, for example, in the superficial dorsal horn regions of the spinal cord involved in regulating the responses to noxious stimuli.

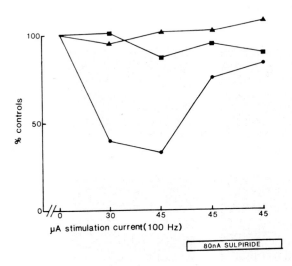

Fig. 5. Selective inhibition of the response of a multi-receptive dorsal horn neuron by electrical stimulation of the A11 dopamine-containing cell group in the brainstem. The response of the neuron to a noxious stimulus (●) is progressively reduced at increasing intensities of electrical stimulation (abscissa), while the response to tactile stimulation (▲) and to direct application of dl-homocysteic acid (■) is unaffected. The depressive effect of brainstem stimulation on the response to noxious stimulation was absent when the selective D_2-dopamine antagonist, sulpiride, was ionophoresed in the spinal cord. (Reproduced with permission from P. J. Hope.)

Deep and visceral pain

Nociceptors are present in the deeper somatic tissues, and those in muscles, tendons and joints share similar characteristics with the cutaneous C-nociceptors. The neural mechanisms in the spinal cord and higher levels of the nervous system are, however, much less well understood, although in general they share many characteristics. Localization of a noxious stimulation is much more poorly defined.

In the viscera, however, information is less exact and in particular the existence of a separate class of visceral nociceptors is still debated (Cervero and Morrison 1986). The visceral sensory innervation is more sparse than that of other structures, but there is no doubt about the intensity or potency of the pain that can be evoked. A new publication by Cervero and Morrison (1986) contains the latest review of the subject. One feature of the response to a noxious visceral stimulus is referred pain (e.g. angina pectoris). The probable explanation is convergence of visceral and somatic nociceptors on a common interneuron, the activity of which is normally associated with the more highly localizable cutaneous or muscle input.

Sensory receptors and pain

A long-debated issue is the role of sensory receptors in pain. Techniques are now available that allow the discharge of individual afferent fibres in conscious human subjects to be recorded. Systematic investigations applying rigorously controlled natural stimuli to the skin have confirmed the existence in humans of the various kinds of cutaneous receptors found in laboratory mammals (Vallbo et al. 1984). When combined in psychophysical studies, with the additional use of microstimulation, a convincing case has been established for attributing different sensation to

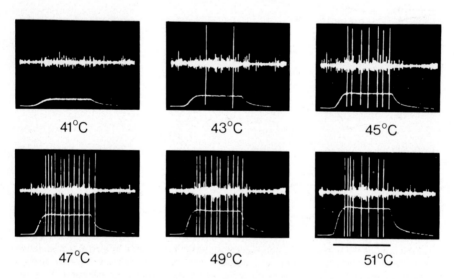

41°C   43°C   45°C

47°C   49°C   51°C

Fig. 6. Responses of a single C-nociceptive unit in the cutaneous nerve of a conscious human subject at the temperatures indicated, recorded with a microelectrode inserted through the skin and into the nerve fascicle. The response appeared at a temperature of 43°C, close to the threshold for perceived pain when the skin is heated. (From Torebjörk et al. 1984.)

activity in various classes of sensitive mechanoreceptor (Torebjörk et al. 1984; Vallbo et al. 1984). Although cutaneous nociceptors with C-fibres are present in human nerves (Fig. 6) their sensory role has been more difficult to establish because so many of the afferent fibres are non-myelinated. Pain induced by noxious thermal stimuli is, however, well-correlated with activity in thermal or polymodal nociceptors with afferent C-fibres (Handwerker et al. 1984), although the correlation for noxious mechanical stimuli is reported to be less clear-cut (Adriaensen et al. 1984).

These results relate to controlled laboratory trials, and need to be interpreted in relation to the definition of pain, given in the introduction to this chapter. The degree of correlation of primary receptor activity and pain then becomes astonishing, rather than the cause for scepticism.

References

Adriaensen, H., Gybels, J., Handwerker, H. O. and Van Hees, J. (1984) Nociceptor discharges and sensations due to prolonged noxious mechanical stimulation – a paradox. Hum. Neurobiol. 3, 53 – 58.

Andersson, S. A. and Rydenhag, B. (1985) Cortical nociceptive systems. Philos. Trans. R. Soc. London Ser. B: 308, 347 – 355.

Basbaum, A. I. and Fields, H. L. (1978) Endogenous pain control mechanisms. Review and hypothesis. Ann. Neurol. 7, 451 – 462.

Besson, J. M., Guilbaud, G., Abdelmoumene, M. and Chaoch, A. (1982) Physiologie de la nociception. J. Physiol. (Paris) 78, 7 – 107.

Bonner, F., Cobb, S., Sweet, W. H. and White, J. C. (1952) Frontal lobe surgery in the treatment of pain. Psychosomatic Med. 14, 383 – 405.

Cervero, F. and Iggo, A. (1980) Substantia gelatinosa of the spinal cord column: a critical review. Brain 103, 717 – 772.

Cervero, F. and Morrison, J. F. B. (Eds.) (1986) Visceral Sensation: Progress in Brain Research, Vol. 67. Elsevier Science Publ. B.V., Amsterdam.

Cervero, F., Iggo, A. and Ogawa, H. (1976) Nociceptor-driven dorsal horn neurones in the lumbar spinal cord of the cat. Pain 2, 5 – 24.

Cervero, F., Iggo, A. and Molony, A. (1979) Descending influences on neurones in the substantia gelatinosa Rolandi of the cat. J. Physiol. 292, 39 – 40P.

Danielsen, N., Shyu, B-C., Dahlin, L. B., Lundborg, G. and Andersson, S. A. (1986) Absence of ongoing activity in fibres arising from proximal nerve ends reinnervating into mesothelial chambers. Pain 26, 93 – 104.

Ferreira, S. H. (1986) Control of inflammatory pain. In: Advances in Inflammation Research. Raven Press, New York (in press).

Fleetwood-Walker, S. M., Mitchell, R., Hope, P. J. and Molony, V. (1985) Effects of opioid peptide agonists selective for μ, δ and $\varkappa$ receptors on identified dorsal horn neurons. In: A. Iggo, L. L. Iversen and F. Cervero (Eds.), Nociception and Pain. Royal Society, London, 427 p.

Guilbaud, G. and Iggo, A. (1985) The effect of lysine acetylsalicylate on joint capsule mechanoreceptors in rats with polyarthritis. Exp. Brain Res. 61, 164 – 168.

Guilbaud, G., Iggo, A. and Tegner, R. (1985) Sensory receptors in ankle joint capsules of normal and arthritic rats. Exp. Br. Res. 58, 29 – 40.

Handwerker, H. O., Iggo, A. and Zimmermann, M. (1975) Segmental and supraspinal actions on dorsal horn neurons responding to noxious and non-noxious skin stimuli. Pain 1, 147 – 165.

Handwerker, H. O., Adriaensen, H., Gybels, J. and Van Hees, J. (1984) Nociceptor discharges and pain sensations: results and open questions. In: B. Bromm (Ed.), New Approaches to Pain Measurement in Man. Elsevier, Amsterdam.

Höfkelt, T., Skirboll, L., Lundberg, J. M., Dalsgaard, C-J., Johansson, O., Pernow, B. and Jansco, G. (1983) Neuropeptides and pain pathways. In: J. J. Bonica, U. Linblom and A. Iggo (Eds.), Advances in Pain Research and Therapy. Vol. 5, Raven Press, New York, pp. 227 – 246.

Iggo, A. (1985) Sensory receptors in the skin of mammals and their sensory functions. Rev. Neurol. (Paris) 141, 599–613.

Kosterlitz, H. W. (1983) Opioid peptides and pain – an update. In: J. J. Bonica, U. Linblom and A. Iggo (Eds.), Advances in Pain Research and Therapy, Vol. 5. Raven Press, New York, pp. 199–208.

Le Bars, D., Dickenson, A. H. and Besson, J. M. (1983) Opiate analgesia and descending control system. In: J. J. Bonica, U. Linblom and A. Iggo (Eds.), Advances in Pain Research and Therapy, Vol. 1. Raven Press, New York, p. 341.

Mendell, L. M. (1966) Physiological properties of unmyelinated fiber projections to the spinal cord. Exp. Neurol. 16, 316–322.

Meyerson, B. A. (1983) Electrostimulation procedures: effects, presumed rationale, and possible mechanisms. In: J. J. Bonica U. Linblom and A. Iggo (Eds.), Advances in Pain Research and Therapy, Vol. 5. Raven Press, New York, pp. 495–534.

Torebjörk, H. E., Schady, W. and Ochoa, J. (1984) Sensory correlates of somatic afferent fibre activation. Hum. Neurobiol. 3, 15–20.

Vallbo, Å. B., Olsson, K. Å, Westberg, K-G. and Clark, F. J. (1984) Microstimulation of single tactile afferents from the human hand. Sensory attributes related to unit type and properties of receptive fields. Brain 107, 727–749.

Wall, P. D. and Sweet, W. H. (1967) Temporary abolition of pain in man. Science 155, 108–109.

Wall, P. D., Scadding, J. W. and Tomkiewicz, M. M. (1979) The production and prevention of experimental anesthesia dolorosa. Pain 6, 175–182.

Yaksh, T. L. and Reddy, S. V. R. (1981) Studies in the primate on the analgesic effects associated with intrathecal actions of opiates, α-adrenergic agonists and baclofen. Anesthesiology 54, 451–467.

Burrows/Elton/Stanley (eds.) Handbook of Chronic Pain Management
© *1987 Elsevier Science Publishers B.V. (Biomedical Division)*

3

Non-opioid neurotransmitters in pain perception and analgesia

RITA B. MESSING and GEORGE L. WILCOX

Department of Pharmacology, Medical School, University of Minnesota, Minneapolis, MN 55455, U.S.A.

Introduction

Studies of stress-induced analgesia, or endogenous pain control mechanisms provide unequivocal evidence for non-opioid mediated mechanisms of pain perception and control (see Bodnar et al. 1980; Chance 1980; Terman et al. 1984). Further, opiates exert effects on functioning of virtually all neurotransmitter systems (see Loh and Ross 1979). Consistently, two brain and spinal cord monoamines have been implicated, either as modulators of pain perception in their own right, or as mediators of opiate effects on pain perception. These are serotonin (Messing and Lytle 1977) and norepinephrine (see below). Thus, we will briefly review recent evidence that these monoamines are involved in nociception and analgesia, before turning to other recent evidence that non-opioid peptides, primarily substance P, may also be of critical importance.

Serotonin (5-hydroxytryptamine)

Pharmacology

Current conceptions of 5-hydroxytryptamine (5-HT) neuronal functioning provide many sites and mechanisms for drug effects on these neurons (Messing and Lytle 1977; Fuller 1980). These include manipulating biosynthesis by changing levels of precursor amino acids tryptophan and 5-hydroxytryptophan (5-HTP), or by affecting the synthetic enzyme tryptophan hydroxylase with the inhibitor para-chlorophenylalanine (pCPA). Other drugs are available to cause release of serotonin (parachloroamphetamine [PCA], fenfluramine), or to inhibit its uptake (fluoxetine, zimelidine). Still other drugs selectively destroy serotonin-containing neurons (halogenated amphetamines, 5,6- or 5,7-dihydroxytryptamine [5,6-DHT, 5,7-DHT]). Finally, there are drugs that stimulate (quipazine) or antagonize (mianserin, cinanserin, ketanserin, methysergide, cyproheptadine, pirenperone, metergoline) receptors. However, two receptor subtypes have been distinguished, and the above-named antagonists work most potently at the 5-HT_2 receptor. Serotonin itself has high affinity only for the 5-HT_1 site, thought to mediate postsynaptic inhibitory effects of 5-HT in the CNS (Peroutka et al. 1981), a role the monoamine plays at most identified sites postsynaptic to serotonin-containing neurons. The 5-HT_2 receptor is the type most often found in the periphery. In the CNS, 5-HT_2 sites mediate the excitatory effects of 5-HT (Peroutka et al. 1981). Thus, more complete understanding of serotonin actions awaits the development of drugs which act selectively at the 5-HT_1 receptor.

EFFECTS IN ASSAYS OF NOCICEPTION

In general (Messing and Lytle 1977), manipulations that enhance brain and/or spinal cord serotonergic neurotransmission produce analgesia and increase morphine-induced antinociception. However, these effects are not seen in all assays, and inconsistencies appear between groups of investigators, and even within a laboratory (for some recent work see Dennis and Melzack 1980; Ogren and Holm 1980; Berge 1982; Ogren and Berge 1984). Some differences are doubtless due to the different drugs used by these investigators, and possible different effects at the two receptor types mentioned above. Related to this is the possibility that systemic injections have multiple, sometimes inconsistent effects. In general, far more consistent data have been obtained using local (e.g. intrathecal) drug administration (see below).

MEDIATION OF ENDOGENOUS PAIN CONTROL SYSTEMS

A similar situation exists for serotonin mediation of endogenous pain control systems (studied either as stress-induced or stimulation-produced analgesia). Intact serotonin neurons and serotonergic neurotransmission are necessary for analgesia to occur in many, but not all of these assays. Analgesias produced by stimulation of different brain areas (e.g. dorsal raphe versus periaqueductal gray) appear to be neurochemically as well as neuroanatomically different. Naloxone blocks only the former (Terman et al. 1984), while 5-HT depletion with pCPA blocks analgesia induced by either stimulation of the periaqueductal gray, an effect that can be reversed by treatment with the precursor 5-HTP (Akil and Liebeskind 1975), or of the dorsal raphe (Akil and Mayer 1972). Spear et al. (1985) have shown that opioid and 5-HT systems mediate different forms of stress-induced analgesia in neonatal rats. Again, positive and negative effects on 5-HT neurotransmission generally increase or decrease stress-induced analgesia, respectively (Snow et al. 1982; Spear et al. 1985). Consistent with this is the finding of Hayes et al. (1977) that depression of 5-HT neuronal activity by injection of the agonist lysergic acid diethylamide (LSD) decreased analgesia produced by stimulation of the dorsal raphe. Nevertheless, it is difficult to specify the effects of many of these agents a priori, and it is sometimes the case that an agonist (5-methoxy-N,N-dimethyltryptamine; 5-MeODMT), which generally has analgesia enhancing effects (see below), may attenuate stress-induced analgesia, while cyproheptadine and methiothepin may enhance it (Hutson et al. 1983).

MEDIATION OF OPIATE ANALGESIA

An extensive literature indicates that serotonin is involved in morphine analgesia (Messing and Lytle 1977). Increased 5-HT neurotransmission induced by systemic (Messing et al. 1975; Larson and Takemori 1977; Sugrue, 1979) or intrathecal (see below) administration of serotonin reuptake inhibitors, causes a potentiation of morphine analgesia in a variety of assays, as does administration of 5-HTP (Tulunay et al. 1976). Conversely, serotonin depletion induced by a low tryptophan diet (Phebus and Lytle 1978), by pCPA (Tulunay et al. 1976; Taber and Latranyi 1981), by neurotoxic destruction (using PCA or 5,7-DHT) of 5-HT neurons (Tulunay et al. 1976; Mohrland and Gebhart 1980) or by surgical destruction of raphe nuclei (Chance et al. 1978; York and Maynert, 1978) all reduce morphine analgesia. In fact, there is a near unanimity that 5-HT is involved in mediating morphine effects, even among investigators who do not find that manipulations of 5-HT alone result in nociceptive alterations. This situation also extends to some other opiate drugs, but not to all of them. Thus, 5-HT seems to be a mediator of analgesic effects of D-ala^2-leu^5-enkephalin (BW 180C) (Lee et al. 1978) and pentazocine (Taber and Latranyi 1981) but not of methadone, pethidine, meperidine or codeine (Chance et al. 1978; Lytle et al. 1978; Sugrue 1979). These data, of course, complement the growing body of evidence for multiple opioid analgesic systems. More important, the robustness of the apparent serotonin mediation of morphine analgesia provides hope (see below) that appropriate enhancement of 5-HT neurotransmission may prove a useful clinical adjunct to morphine and similar opiates in treatment of chronic pain.

OPIATE AND STRESS EFFECTS ON SEROTONIN METABOLISM

It has been known for a relatively long time that acute morphine administration induces increases in the metabolism of brain catechol- and indoleamines (cf. Messing et al. 1978a). This apparent increase in turnover is not associated with any changes in the activities of synthetic enzymes, and precursor availability has been shown to be of importance for monoamine metabolism (cf. Fernstrom et al. 1974; Gibson and Wurtman 1977). Further, it has been known for some time that decreases in brain tryptophan availability, which are associated with lower levels of serotonin metabolism, are also associated with lower pain thresholds (Lytle et al. 1975; Messing et al. 1976a; see Table 1). In recent years, it has also been shown that several different types of stress, which are most likely capable of inducing analgesia, are also associated with higher levels of brain tryptophan and brain serotonin metabolism (Weil-Fugazza et al. 1980; Kennett and Joseph 1981), although stress-induced analgesia was not measured in these studies. Conversely, it has been shown that neonatal food deprivation (which presumably results in an increase in brain tryptophan; Knott et al. 1973) causes analgesia and increased serotonin metabolism (Spear and Scalzo 1985; Spear et al. 1985), although levels of brain tryptophan were not measured in these studies (see Table 1). Similarly, numerous studies have measured central nervous system tryptophan and 5-hydroxyindoles after (presumably) analgesic doses of morphine or opioid peptides (Table 1), and have found that increases in serotonin metabolism after morphine or opioids can be partially (but not entirely) accounted for by a morphine or opioid-induced rise in tryptophan (Garcia-Sevilla et al. 1978, 1980; Messing et al. 1978a, b; Crossley and Slater 1979; Weil-Fugazza et al. 1979; Godefroy et al. 1980). These effects have generally, but not always been found to be naloxone-reversible. Also, Messing et al. (1978b) have found that morphine induces an increase in brain tryptophan and 5-HT metabolism in cerebellum, an area of the rat brain which is devoid of morphine receptors. Thus, it is likely that the effect of morphine on brain tryptophan and 5-hydroxyindoles is indirect, and that 5-HT and opioid pain inhibitory systems are distinct, even if interdependent (see also sections on Mediation of endogenous pain control systems and Localization). Finally, it is of some interest, in view of the lack of effect of serotonin depletion on analgesic effectiveness of some opiates (see above), that not all opiates influence levels of brain tryptophan (Crossley and Slater 1979).

TABLE 1
Brain tryptophan and nociception.

Manipulation	Brain tryptophan	Pain response	Reference
1) Consumption of a tryptophan			
deficient diet	↓	↑	Lytle et al. (1975)
+ nutritional rehabilitation	n	n	
+ tryptophan	n	n	Messing et al. (1976a)
+ valine	ne	ne	
2) Valine administration	↓	↑	Messing et al. (1976a)
3) Stress			
a) Restraint	↑	(↓)	Kennett and Joseph (1981)
+ valine	n	(n)	
b) Freund's Adjuvant	↑	(↓)	Weil-Fugazza et al. (1980)
c) Neonatal Food or	(↑)	↓	Spear et al. (1985)
maternal deprivation			Spear and Scalzo (1985)
4) Opiate administration			Crossley and Slater (1979)
a) Morphine	↑	(↓)	Messing et al. (1978a,b)
+ Freund's Adjuvant	↑↑	(↓↓)	Godefroy et al. (1980)
+ Naloxone	n	(n)	Weil-Fugazza et al. (1979)
b) β-endorphin	↑	(↓)	Garcia-Sevilla et al. (1978, 1980)
c) Enkephalins	↑	(↓)	
+ naloxone	n	(n)	
d) Naloxone	↓	(↑)	

↑ = increase; ↓ = decrease; n = reversal of main treatment effect towards normal control levels; ( ) = inferred change, based on data available in other papers, but not actually measured in accompanying reference; ne = no effect.

A paper by Weil-Fugazza et al. (1984) has shown that extremely high levels of tail shock administered to anesthetized rats result in only small increases in CNS 5-HT metabolism with no change in tryptophan levels, and that these effects are actually reversed by a low, probably nonanalgesic dose of morphine. These data, apparently contradicting earlier work of these investigators (see above) may be the result of an overloading and exhaustion of the system by the ultra-high and prolonged stress of anesthesia and electroshock.

LOCALIZATION

Systemic administration of substances affecting serotonin metabolism and release invariably has multiple central and peripheral effects which may not all be synergistic (see Messing and Lytle 1977). In general, far more consistent and reproducible data have been obtained when substances have been given locally in the CNS. Numerous studies have shown that 5-HT containing neurons with cell bodies in the nucleus raphe magnus, projecting to the spinal cord, play an important modulatory role in regulation of pain perception, and opiate analgesia. First, direct (intrathecal) administration of 5-HT into spinal cord produces antinociception (Hylden and Wilcox 1983a; Wang 1977; Yaksh and Wilson 1979) and depression of spinothalamic tract neurons (Jordan et al. 1978). Second, intrathecal administration of 5-HT reuptake inhibitors (Larsen and Christensen 1982; Botney and Fields 1983) or of 5-HTP or of quipazine (Yaksh and Wilson 1979) also elevates pain thresholds, while intrathecal methysergide administration antagonizes these effects (Yaksh and Wilson 1979). As mentioned above, destruction of 5-HT cell bodies in the nucleus raphe magnus with 5,7-DHT reduces spinal cord serotonin content and also abolishes or attenuates morphine antinociception if morphine is administered systemically or into the brain (Chance et al. 1978; Mohrland and Gebhart 1980; Vasko, et al. 1984). However, if morphine is administered directly into the cord, serotonin does not appear to mediate analgesic effects (Larsen and Christensen 1982; Vasko et al. 1984). Further, microinjection of morphine into the periaqueductal gray and/or systemic injections of morphine increases spinal cord serotonin metabolism and release (Shiomi et al. 1978; Yaksh and Tyce 1979). Carstens et al. (1981) have found that pCPA or methysergide reduce or abolish inhibition of spinal dorsal horn neurons produced by stimulation of the midbrain periaqueductal gray, again implicating serotonin as a mediator of analgesia caused by stimulation of this area. Conflicting data do occur when drugs affecting 5-HT neurotransmission are given to spinally transected rats. Zemlan et al. (1980) found that the agonists quipazine or 5-MeODMT were analgesic only during the first few postoperative days, whereas Berge (1982) observed longer term analgesic effects with 5-MeODMT in spinally transected rats, and some evidence of receptor supersensitivity.

Studies of supraspinal 5-HT mechanisms are not as numerous, nor are the important pathways as well worked out, but it is also clear that ascending 5-HT systems, originating from cell bodies in the dorsal and medial raphe, also are involved in nociception and analgesia (Dubuisson and Melzack 1977; Rodgers, 1977; Chance et al. 1978; Shyu et al. 1984; see also Messing and Lytle 1977).

HUMAN STUDIES

Overall, a strong case can be made that drugs which enhance serotonergic neurotransmission may have potential therapeutic use either by themselves or in conjunction with opiates. The two classes of drugs which have the greatest potential usefulness are precursor amino acids and 5-HT reuptake inhibitors. This is further supported by clinical data indicating possible therapeutic usefulness of tricyclic antidepressants (Sternbach et al. 1976; Butler 1984). However, these drugs have many non-specific effects, and with the exception of zimelidine*, which had a therapeutic effect in a double-blind study in chronic pain patients (Johansson and von Knorring 1979), clinical trials have not yet been done with specific 5-HT reuptake inhibitors. Tryptophan and 5-HTP administration produce increases in brain serotonin, although 5-HTP is also decarboxylated in catecholamine containing neurons where the resulting 5-HT can be released as a 'false transmitter'. Further, while precursor administration causes higher levels of 5-HT, it does not follow that releasable serotonin is always increased (Lytle et al. 1975; Messing et al. 1975; Messing et al. 1976a). Nevertheless, there is ample evidence that tryptophan availability may be of importance for mediating analgesic effects of opiates, or during chronic pain or stress (see Table 1). Hosobuchi et al. (1980) have found that addition of tryptophan to the diet provided a useful supplementation to opiate treatment in chronic pain patients, although by itself, when acutely administered, the amino acid appears to have little effect (Sternbach et al. 1976). In contrast to treatments which work through noradrenergic mechanisms (see below), there is no evidence that any analgesia-enhancing treatment which is dependent upon serotonergic mechanisms (e.g. tryptophan or fluoxetine administration) results in behavioral suppression (animals) or sedation

---

* Zimelidine is no longer available for clinical use

(humans) at reasonable doses (Messing et al. 1975, 1976b, 1978c). Clearly, more human studies along these lines are of the utmost importance.

Norepinephrine

While investigations of the role of catecholamines in nociception and analgesia have a long history, it is only in recent years, as knowledge of adrenergic receptor pharmacology has increased, that a consistent story has begun to emerge. Space does not permit much detailed consideration of the evidence; but the overwhelming weight of it supports the notion that stimulation of α_2-adrenergic receptors in the spinal cord may be importantly involved in the production of analgesia at the spinal level induced by a supraspinal action of opiates. Analgesic brainstem stimulation increases release of spinal cord norepinephrine (NE) (Yaksh et al. 1984). NE, applied in the spinal cord, produces behavioral analgesia in rodents (Reddy et al. 1980; Hylden and Wilcox 1983b) and inhibition of spinothalamic tract cells in the primate (Willcockson et al. 1984). Yeung and Rudy (1983) found that supraspinally administered morphine interacts multiplicatively with spinally administered morphine. NE (Hylden and Wilcox 1983b) but not 5-HT (Hylden and Wilcox 1983a) interacts synergistically with morphine when administered together intrathecally. It is conceivable therefore, that the supraspinal-spinal opiate interaction is mediated by the spinal interaction between opiate and adrenergic agonists. This contention is supported by results showing that depletion of NE by 6-hydroxydopamine injection into the lateral reticular formation attenuates stress-induced analgesia (Bragin and Durinyan 1983), while reserpine-induced depletion of biogenic amines reduces the effect of morphine administered systemically or i.c.v. (Hu et al. 1984).

If morphine produces spinal analgesia by *release* of NE, one would presume that such an action would involve *activation* of neurons in a catecholamine-containing, bulbospinal system. However, since the opposite has been consistently demonstrated (cf. review by Duggan and North 1983), a mechanistic explanation of observed interactions is not yet possible. The presence of α_2-adrenergic autoreceptors on catecholamine-containing cells may underlie some of the controversy surrounding adrenergic analgesia. For example, Sagen et al. (1983) showed that analgesia, depending upon intact descending monoaminergic systems, was produced by supraspinally administered α-receptor antagonists. By contrast, stimulation of α_2-adrenergic receptors in the spinal cord produces analgesia, and their blockade with the specific α_2-antagonist yohimbine blocks effects of agonists (Reddy et al. 1980; Howe et al. 1983; Hylden and Wilcox 1983b; Sagen and Proudfit 1984). In general, systemically administered clonidine and yohimbine have effects similar to those seen after intrathecal administration (Paalzow 1978; Spaulding et al. 1979; Coderre and Rollman 1984; Marwaha 1984; Ossipov et al. 1984). However, anomalous results sometimes occur, such as an attenuation of stress-induced analgesia seen after clonidine administration (Snow et al. 1982), as might be expected from the fact that the drug has simultaneous access to spinal and supraspinal compartments.

The α_2-adrenergic receptor may be an autoreceptor, but in any case, stimulation of it seems to be involved with inhibition of noradrenergic activity (cf. Dwoskin and Sparber 1983). The idea that inhibition of noradrenergic activity mediates analgesia is consistent with findings that opiate administration to noradrenergic cell bodies in the locus coeruleus inhibits their activity, both in vivo (Bird and Kuhar 1977) and in vitro (Yoshimura and North 1983). Further, morphine and opioids inhibit release of NE in cerebral cortex (Taube et al. 1976; Arbilla and Langer 1978). Finally, it has been shown that clonidine administration increases plasma concentrations of β-

endorphin (Pettibone and Mueller 1981). Clonidine is known to attenuate signs of opiate withdrawal (Gold et al. 1978; Sparber and Meyer 1978).

It must be noted that studies of analgesic effects of systemically administered clonidine were done at doses which also result in general behavioral suppression in animals or sedation in humans (Meyer et al. 1977; Dwoskin and Sparber 1983), and that chronic administration of clonidine itself leads to tolerance and dependence (Meyer et al. 1976). However, recent preliminary data (Coombs et al. 1984) indicate that intrathecally administered clonidine may be useful, combined with morphine, for the control of cancer pain.

Peptides: tachykinins and other non-opioid peptides

Although substance P (SP) was isolated in the 1930's (von Euler and Gaddum 1931), demonstration of its involvement in the transmission of noxious information awaited its complete purification and synthesis (Chang and Leeman 1970). Otsuka et al. (1972) showed its presence in dorsal horn and dorsal roots and its ability to depolarize spinal cord neurons and Henry (1976) subsequently showed that SP selectively excited nociceptive neurons in the spinal cord. Immunohistochemical studies (Hökfelt et al. 1975) had showed that small somata, which presumably give rise to small diameter nociceptive afferent fibers, in dorsal root ganglia contain SP as well as other peptides. Electrical stimulation of nociceptive, but not non-nociceptive, afferent fibers promoted the release of SP in the perfused spinal cord of rats (Yaksh et al. 1980). Using microperfusion and natural stimulation, Takagi's group (Kuraishi et al. 1985) has found that immunoreactive SP is released from rabbit dorsal horn after noxious mechanical stimulation, but not after noxious thermal stimulation. This group suggested that SP may be selectively involved in the transmission of nociceptive information subserved by mechanical nociceptive afferent fibers, but not by thermal or polymodal nociceptors. However, SP was found in both nociceptive and non-nociceptive DRG cells in the cat (Leah et al. 1984), suggesting that SP is involved in non-nociceptive transmission as well. The overwhelming majority of studies of localization and release support some role of SP in the transmission of nociceptive information from primary afferent fibers to neurons in the dorsal horn, but its exact role and importance relative to other transmitter candidates awaits further study.

The local administration of exogenous SP to the spinal cord and to spinal neurons has proved to be valuable for the assessment of its role in nociceptive neurotransmission. Intrathecal injection of SP in mice (Hylden and Wilcox 1981) and rats (Seybold et al. 1982) produced counterirritative behavior similar to that elicited by the dermal injection of irritants. This behavior was blocked by simultaneous administration of opioid agonists and other spinally active analgesic agents, supporting the nociceptive nature of this manipulation (Hylden and Wilcox 1983b). Interestingly, δ-type opioid agonists were found to be particularly effective and more potent than μ or $\varkappa$ agonists in this SP test, making SP useful in the screening for centrally active δ opioid agonists (Hylden and Wilcox 1983b). Whereas NE monotonically inhibits this action of SP (Hylden and Wilcox 1983b), 5-HT inhibits at low doses but adds to and produces scratching behavior by itself at higher doses (Hylden and Wilcox 1983a). The susceptibility of SP's spinal action to these several classes of agents closely parallels the spinal analgesic activity of these agents in other antinociceptive tests. Furthermore, intrathecal administration of SP in rats decreases the latency to tail-flick in response to noxious heat (Yasphal et al. 1982). Both of these hyperalgesic events (decrease in tail-flick latency and elicitation of scratching behavior) occur within two minutes of SP administration. Some studies suggest that SP or some of its fragments are antinociceptive (Stewart et al., 1976; Doi and Jurna, 1982), but the time courses of these anti-nociceptive effects are slower and longer than the nociceptive effects. The longer time course suggests that the nociceptive event precipitates the anti-nociceptive effects as has been observed by LeBars and collaborators (1979). In support of this contention, Doi and Jurna (1982) found that naloxone blocked SP's antinociceptive action, suggesting the involvement of an endogenous opioid system in SP-induced antinociception.

Depletion of SP (along with depletion of other peptides) by capsaicin produces analgesia in some (Yaksh et al. 1979; Gamse 1982) but not all (Hayes et al. 1981; Buck et al. 1982) tests. Likewise, SP antagonists are active anti-nociceptive agents in some (Piercey et al. 1981; Akerman et al. 1982; Vaught et al. 1983) but not all (Post and Vaught 1983) tests. Failure of depletion and of antagonists to be active in all tests indicates that SP is not the only nociceptive neurotransmitter. Furthermore, SP appears to be involved in function other than nociception, as evidenced by induction of paralysis in the rat after intrathecal injection of SP antagonists (Akerman et al. 1982).

Other peptides have also been implicated in nociceptive neurotransmission. Somatostatin is localized in small dorsal root ganglion cell bodies similar to but individually distinct from those containing SP (Hökfelt et al. 1976; Tuchscherer and Seybold 1985). Somatostatin elicits scratching behavior in rats (Seybold et al. 1982) and mice (Wilcox 1983) when injected intrathecally; this activity of somatostatin is not blocked by SP antagonists (Vaught, personal communication). Furthermore, somatostatin-like immunoreactivity is released from the rabbit dorsal horn by noxious thermal stimulation but not by noxious mechanical stimulation (Kuraishi et al. 1985); furthermore, Leah et al. (1984) found somatostatin only in nociceptive cells in the cat. Thus, somatostatin may be involved selectively in the transmission of noxious thermal information from the primary afferent thermal or polymodal nociceptors.

Several other substances may be involved in the spinal transmission and modulation of noxious input. Bombesin elicits scratching behavior in rodents after intrathecal administration (Gmerek et al. 1983), which is not blocked by SP antagonists (Post and Vaught 1983). Cholecystokinin is co-contained in many dorsal root ganglion cells which contain SP (Tuchscherer and Seybold 1985), but it has been shown to produce only anti-nociception (Jurna and Zetler 1981). Neurotensin is contained in interneurons in the superficial dorsal horn (Seybold and Elde 1982) and produces anti-nociception after intrathecal administration in some tests (Hylden and Wilcox 1983c). A large group of SP-related peptides called the tachykinins (Erspamer 1981) have actions not unlike SP. This latter group includes SP, the amphibian peptide physalaemine, the molluskan peptide eledoisin, neuromedin K or neurokinin β which acts like the amphibian peptide kassinin, and substance K or neurokinin α (Buck et al. 1984). These peptides have been differentially characterized in peripheral tissues, but the selectivity, if any, of mammalian CNS tachykinin receptors is unknown. Neuromedin K, however, shares behavioral activities with SP when injected intrathecally in rodents (Vaught et al. 1983).

Neither capsaicin nor SP antagonists have proved to be useful analgesics in the treatment of chronic pain. Depletion or antagonism of peptide transmitters thought to be involved in the transmission of nociceptive information from primary afferent neurons apparently has consequences for systems other than the pain transmission system. Design of successful therapies awaits the identification of transmitters specifically associated with various modalities of pain and the production of pharmaceutical manipulators of these transmitters.

Conclusions

The perception of pain clearly depends upon the functioning of many neurohumoral systems. Studies of monoaminergic systems, because of a longer history and a greater variety of pharmacological tools, are already advanced enough to suggest that appropriate manipulations of these systems may be of clinical value for the control of pain. More recent data suggest that peptides other than opioids are involved in nociception, and still newer research indicates that amino acid neurotransmitters, e.g. glutamate, aspartate and γ-amino butyric acid, are also of importance (e.g. Cahusac et al. 1984; Willcockson et al. 1984). As more sophisticated drugs become available for manipulating peptidergic and amino acid neurotransmitter systems, their functions will become better understood, and hopefully, yet other, and more useful strategies for pain control will become available.

Acknowledgments

This work was partially supported by USPHS grants K07 ES00123 to RBM and R01 DA01933 to GLW.

References

Akerman, B., Rosell, S. and Folkers, K. (1982) Intrathecal [D-Pro^2,D-Trp^{7,9}] SP elicits hypoalgesia and motor blockade in the rat and antagonizes noxious responses induced by substance P. Acta Physiol. Scand. 114, 631 – 633.

Akil, H. and Liebeskind, J. C. (1975) Monoaminergic mechanisms of stimulation-produced analgesia. Brain Res. 94, 279 – 296.

Akil, H. and Mayer, D. J. (1972) Antagonism of stimulation-produced analgesia by p-CPA, a serotonin synthesis inhibitor. Brain Res. 44, 692 – 697.

Arbilla, S. and Langer, S. Z. (1978) Morphine and β-endorphin inhibit release of noradrenaline from cerebral cortex but not of dopamine from rat striatum. Nature 271, 559 – 561.

Berge, O-G. (1982) Effects of 5-HT receptor agonists and antagonists on a reflex response to radiant heat in normal and spinally transected rats. Pain 13, 253 – 266.

Bird, S. J. and Kuhar, M. J. (1977) Iontophoretic application of opiates to the locus coeruleus. Brain Res. 122, 523 – 533.

Bodnar, R. J., Kelly, D. D., Brutus, M. and Glusman, M. (1980) Stress-induced analgesia: Neural and hormonal determinants. Neurosci. Biobehav. Rev. 4, 87 – 100.

Botney, M. and Fields, H. L. (1983) Amitriptyline potentiates morphine analgesia by a direct action on the central nervous system. Ann. Neurol. 13, 160 – 164.

Bragin, E. O. and Durinyan, R. A. (1983) A study of the catecholaminergic systems of the lateral reticular nuclei and the serotoninergic systems of the raphe magnus in various types of analgesia. Pain 17, 225 – 234.

Buck, S. H., Miller, M. S. and Burks, T. F. (1982) Depletion of primary afferent substance P by capsaicin and dihydrocapsaicin without altered temperature sensitivity in rats. Brain Res. 233, 216 – 220.

Buck, S. H., Burcher, E., Shults, C. W., Lovenberg, W. and O'Donohue, T. L. (1984) Novel pharmacology of Substance K-binding sites: a third type of tachykinin receptor. Science 226, 987 – 989.

Butler, S. (1984) Present status of tricyclic antidepressants in chronic pain therapy. Adv. Pain Res. Ther. 7, 173 – 197.

Cahusac, P. M. B., Evans, R. H., Hill, R. G., Rodriquez, R. E. and Smith, D. A. S. (1984) The behavioral effects of an N-methylaspartate receptor antagonist following application to the lumbar spinal cord of conscious rats. Neuropharmacology 23, 719 – 724.

Carstens, E., Fraunhoffer, M. and Zimmermann, M. (1981) Serotonergic mediation of descending inhibition from midbrain periaqueductal gray, but not reticular formation, of spinal nociceptive transmission in the cat. Pain 10, 149 – 167.

Chance, W. T. (1980) Autoanalgesia: opiate and non-opiate mechanisms. Neurosci. Biobehav. Rev. 4, 55 – 67.

Chance, W. T., Krynock, G. M. and Rosecrans, J. A. (1978) Effects of medial raphe and raphe magnus lesions on the analgesic activity of morphine and methadone. Psychopharmacology 56, 133 – 137.

Chang, M. M. and Leeman, S. E. (1970) Isolation of a sialogic peptide from bovine hypothalamic tissue and its characterization as substance P. J. Biol. Chem. 245, 4784 – 4790.

Coderre, T. J. and Rollman, G. B. (1984) Stress analgesia: effects of pCPA, yohimbine, and naloxone. Pharmacol. Biochem. Behav. 21, 681 – 686.

Coombs, D.W., Savage, S., LaChance, D., Saunders, R., Jensen, L. and Gaylor, M. (1984) Intrathecal clonidine control of cancer pain when spinal morphine tolerance develops. Pain (Suppl. 2), S21.

Crossley, A. W. A. and Slater, P. (1979) The effect of morphine and some other narcotic analgesics on brain tryptophan concentrations. J. Neurosci. Res. 4, 423 – 429.

Dennis, S. G. and Melzack, R. (1980) Pain modulation by 5-hydroxytryptaminergic agents and morphine as measured by three pain tests. Exp. Neurol. 69, 260 – 270.

Doi, T. and Jurna, I. (1982) Intrathecal substance P depresses spinal motor and sensory responses to stimulation of nociceptive afferents – antagonism by naloxone. N.-S. Arch. Pharmacol. 319, 154 – 160.

Dubuisson, D. and Melzack, R. (1977) Analgesic brain stimulation in the cat: effect of intraventricular serotonin, norepinephrine, and dopamine. Exp. Neurol. 57, 1059 – 1066.

Duggan, A. W. and North, R. A. (1983) Electrophysiology of opioids. Pharmacol. Rev. 9, 219 – 281.

Dwoskin, L. P. and Sparber, S. B. (1983) Comparison of yohimbine, mianserin, chlorpromazine and prazosin as antagonists of the suppressant effect of clonidine on operant behavior. J. Pharmacol. Exp. Ther. 226, 57 – 64.

Erspamer, V. (1981) The tachykinin peptide family. Trends Neurosci. 4, 267 – 269.

Fernstrom, J. D., Madras, B. K., Munro, H. N. and Wurtman, R. J. (1974) Nutritional control of the synthesis of 5-hydroxytryptamine in the brain. In: CIBA Foundation Symposium, Aromatic Amino Acids in the Brain. Elsevier, Amsterdam, pp. 153 – 174.

Fuller, R. W. (1980) Pharmacology of central serotonin neurons. Ann. Rev. Pharmacol. Toxicol. 20, 111 – 127.

Gamse, R. (1982) Capsaicin and nociception in the rat and mouse: possible role of substance. Naunyn-Schmiedeberg's Arch. Pharmacol. 320, 205 – 216.

Garcia-Sevilla, J. A., Ahtee, L., Magnusson, T. and Carlsson, A. (1978) Opiate-receptor mediated changes in monoamine synthesis in rat brain. J. Pharm. Pharmacol. 30, 613 – 621.

Garcia-Sevilla, J. A., Magnusson, T. and Carlsson, A. (1980) Effects of enkephalins and two enzyme resistant analogues on monoamine synthesis and metabolism in rat brain. Naunyn-Schmiedeberg's Arch. Pharmacol. 310, 211 – 218.

Gibson, C. J. and Wurtman, R. J. (1977) Physiological control of brain catechol synthesis by brain tyrosine concentration. Biochem. Pharmacol. 26, 1137 – 1142.

Gmerek, D. E., Cowan, A. and Vaught, J. L. (1983) Intrathecal bombesin in rats: effects on behavior and GI transit. Eur. J. Pharmacol. 94, 141 – 143.

Godefroy, F., Weil-Fugazza, J., Coudert, D. and Besson, J.-M. (1980) Effect of acute administration of morphine on newly synthesized 5-hydroxytryptamine in spinal cord of the rat. Brain Res. 199, 415 – 424.

Gold, M. S., Redmond, D. E. and Kleber, H. D. (1978) Clonidine blocks acute opiate-withdrawal symptoms. Lancet 1, 599 – 602.

Hayes, A. G., Scadding, J. W., Kingle, M. S. and Tyers, M. B. (1981) Effect of neonatal administration of capsaicin on nociceptive thresholds in the mouse and rat. J. Pharm. Pharmacol. 33, 183 – 185.

Hayes, R. L., Newlon, P. G., Rosecrans, J. A. and Mayer, D. J. (1977) Reduction of stimulation-produced analgesia by lysergic acid diethylamide, a depressor of serotonergic neural activity. Brain Res. 122, 367 – 372.

Henry, J. L. (1976) Effects of substance P on functionally identified units in cat spinal cord. Brain Res. 114, 439 – 451.

Hökfelt, T., Kellerth, J. O., Nilsson, G. and Pernow, B. (1975) Experimental immunohistochemical studies on the localization and distribution of substance P in cat primary sensory neurons. Brain Res. 100, 235 – 252.

Hökfelt, T., Elde, R., Johansson, O., Luft, R., Nilsson, G. and Arimura, A. (1976) Immunohisto-chemical evidence for separate populations of somatostatin-containing and substance P-containing primary afferent neurons in the rat. Neuroscience 1, 131 – 136.

Hosobuchi, Y., Lamb, S. and Bascom, D. (1980) Tryptophan loading may reverse tolerance to opiate analgesics in humans: a preliminary report. Pain 9, 161 – 169.

Howe, J. R., Wang, J. Y. and Yaksh, T. L. (1983) Selective antagonism of the antinoceptive effect of intrathecally applied alpha adrenergic agonists by intrathecal prazosin and intrathecal yohimbine. J. Pharmacol. Exp. Ther. 224, 552–555.

Hu, G., Zhong, R. and Tsou, K. (1984) Dissociation of supraspinal and spinal morphine analgesia by reserpine. Eur. J. Pharmacol. 97, 129–131.

Hutson, P. H., Tricklebank, M. D. and Curzon (1983) Analgesia induced by brief footshock: blockade by fenfluramine and 5-methoxy-N,N-dimethyltryptamine and prevention of blockade by 5-HT antagonists. Brain Res. 279, 105–110.

Hwang, S., Kehl, L. J. and Wilcox, G. L. (1984) Analgesic properties of antidepressants given intrathecally. Pain (Suppl. 2), 158.

Hylden, J. L. K. and Wilcox, G. L. (1981) Intrathecal substance P elicits a caudally-directed biting and scratching behavior in mice. Brain Res. 217, 212–215.

Hylden, J. L. K. and Wilcox, G. L. (1983a) Intrathecal serotonin in mice: analgesia and inhibition of a spinal action of substance P. Life Sci. 33, 789–795.

Hylden, J. L. K. and Wilcox, G. L. (1983b) Pharmacological characterization of substance P-induced nociception in mice: modulation by opioid and noradrenergic agonists at the spinal level. J. Pharmacol. Exp. Ther. 226, 398–404.

Hylden J. L. K. and Wilcox, G. L. (1983c) Antinociceptive action of intrathecal neurotensin in mice. Peptides 4, 517–520.

Johansson, F. and von Knorring, L. (1979) A double-blind controlled study of a serotonin uptake inhibitor (Zimeldine) versus placebo in chronic pain patients. Pain 7, 69–78.

Jordan, L. M., Kenshalo, D. R. Jr., Martin, R. F., Haber, L. H. and Willis, W. D. (1978) Depression of primate spinothalamic tract neurons by iontophoretic application of 5-hydroxytryptamine. Pain 5, 135–142.

Jurna, I. and Zetler, G. (1981) Antinociceptive effect of centrally administered caerulein and cholecystokinin octapeptide (CCK-8). Eur. J. Pharmacol. 73, 323–331.

Kennett, G. A. and Joseph, M. H. (1981) The functional importance of increased brain tryptophan in the serotonergic response to restraint stress. Neuropharmacology 20, 39–43.

Knott, P. J., Joseph, M. H. and Curzon, G. (1973) Effects of food deprivation and immobilization on tryptophan and other amino acids in rat brain. J. Neurochem. 20, 249–251.

Kuraishi, Y., Hirota, N., Sato, Y., Hino, Y., Satoh, M. and Takagi, H. (1985) Evidence that substance P and somatostatin transmit separate information related to pain in the spinal dorsal horn. Brain Res. 325, 294–298.

Larsen, J.-J. and Christensen, A. V. (1982) Subarachnoidal administration of the 5-HT uptake inhibitor citalopram points to the spinal role of 5-HT in morphine antinociception. Pain 14, 339–345.

Larson, A. A. and Takemori, A. E. (1977) Effect of fluoxetine hydrochloride (Lilly 110140), a specific inhibitor of serotonin uptake, on morphine analgesia and the development of tolerance. Life Sci. 21, 1807–1812.

Leah, J., Cameron, A. and Snow, P. (1984) Peptides in C and Aδ fibres of identified modality. Pain S2, 145.

LeBars, D., Dickenson, A. H. and Besson, J.-M. (1979) Diffuse noxious inhibitory controls (DNIC). I. Effects on dorsal horn convergent neurones in the rat. Pain 6, 283–304.

Lee, R. L., Sewell, R. D. E. and Spencer, P. S. J. (1978) Importance of 5-hydroxytryptamine in the antinociceptive activity of the leucine-enkephalin derivative, D-Ala^2-Leu^5-enkephalin (BW 180C), in the rat. Eur. J. Pharmacol. 47, 251–253.

Liu, S.-J. and Wang, R. I. H. (1981) Increased sensitivity of the central nervous system to morphine analgesia by amitriptyline in naive and morphine-tolerant rats. Biochem. Pharmacol. 30, 2103–2109.

Loh, H. H. and Ross, D. H. (Eds.) (1979) Neurochemical mechanisms of opiates and endorphins. Adv. Biochem. Psychopharmacol. 20.

Lytle, L. D., Messing, R. B., Fisher, L. and Phebus, L. (1975) Effects of long-term corn consumption on brain serotonin and the response to electric shock. Science 190, 692–694.

Lytle, L. D., Phebus, L., Fisher, L. A. and Messing, R. B. (1978) Dietary effects on analgesic drug potency. In: M. L. Adler, L. Manara and R. Samanin (Eds.), Factors Affecting the Action of Narcotics. Raven, Press, New York, pp. 543–564.

Marwaha, J. (1984) Supersensitivity of analgesic responses to α_2-adrenergic agonists in genetically hypertensive rats. Brain Res. 304, 363–366.

Messing, R. B. and Lytle, L. D. (1977) Serotonin-containing neurons: their possible role in pain and analgesia. Pain 4, 1–21.

Messing, R. B., Phebus, L., Fisher, L. A. and Lytle, L. D. (1975) Analgesic effects of fluoxetine hydrochloride (Lilly 110140), a specific inhibitor of serotonin uptake. Psychopharmacol. Commun. 1, 511 – 521.

Messing, R. B., Fisher, L. A., Phebus, L. and Lytle, L. D. (1976a) Interaction of diet and drugs in the regulation of brain 5-hydroxyindoles and the response to painful electric shock. Life Sci. 18, 707 – 714.

Messing, R. B., Phebus, L., Fisher, L. A. and Lytle, L. D. (1976b) Effects of p-chloroamphetamine on locomotor activity and brain 5-hydroxyindoles. Neuropharmacology 15, 157 – 163.

Messing, R. B., Flinchbaugh, C. and Waymire, J. C. (1978a) Changes in brain tryptophan and tyrosine following acute and chronic morphine administration. Neuropharmacology 17, 391 – 396.

Messing, R. B., Flinchbaugh, C. and Waymire, J. C. (1978b) Tryptophan and 5-hydroxyindoles in different CNS regions following acute morphine. Eur. J. Pharmacol. 48, 137 – 140.

Messing, R. B., Pettibone, D. J., Kaufman, N. and Lytle, L. D. (1978c) Behavioral effects of serotonin neurotoxins: an overview. In: J. H. Jacoby and L. D. Lytle (Eds.), Serotonin Neurotoxins. Ann. N.Y. Acad. Sci. 305, 480 – 496.

Meyer, D. R., El-Azhary, R., Bierer, D. Ws., Hanson, S. K., Robbins, M. S. and Sparber, S. B. (1977) Tolerance and dependence after chronic administration of clonidine to the rat. Pharmacol. Biochem. Behav. 7, 227 – 231.

Miranda, F., Candelaresi, G. and Samanin, R. (1978) Analgesic effect of etorphine in rats with selective depletions of brain monoamines. Psychopharmacology 58, 105 – 109.

Mohrland, J. S. and Gebhart, G. F. (1980) Effect of selective destruction of serotonergic neurons in nucleus raphe magnus on morphine-induced antinociception. Life Sci. 27, 2627 – 2632.

Ogren, S.-O. and Berge, O.-G. (1984) Test-dependent variations in the antinociceptive effect of p-chloroamphetamine-induced release of 5-hydroxytryptamine. Neuropharmacology 23, 915 – 924.

Ogren, S.-O. and Holm, A.-C. (1980) Test-specific effects of the 5-HT reuptake inhibitors alaproclate and zimelidine on pain sensitivity and morphine analgesia. J. Neural Trans. 47, 253 – 271.

Ossipov, M. H., Malseed, R. T., Eisenman, L. M. and Goldstein, F. J. (1984) Effect of α_2 adrenergic agents upon central etorphine antinociception in the cat. Brain Res. 309, 135 – 142.

Otsuka, M., Konishi, S. and Takahashi, T. (1972) The presence of a motoneuron-depolarizing peptide in bovine dorsal roots of spinal nerves. Proc. Jpn. Acad. 48, 342 – 346.

Paalzow, G. (1978) Development of tolerance to the analgesic effect of clonidine in rats: cross-tolerance to morphine. Naunyn-Schmiedeberg's Arch. Pharmacol. 304, 1 – 4.

Peroutka, S. J., Lebovitz, R. M. and Snyder, S. H. (1981) Two distinct serotonin receptors with different physiological functions. Science 212, 827 – 829.

Pettibone, D. J. and Mueller, G. P. (1981) α-Adrenergic stimulation by clonidine increases plasma concentrations of immunoreactive β-endorphin in rats. Endocrinology 109, 798 – 802.

Phebus, L. and Lytle, L. D. (1978) Diet induced alterations in opiate analgesic drug potency. Proc. West. Pharmacol. Soc. 21, 361 – 364.

Piercey, M. F. Schroeder, L. A., Folkers, K., Xu, J.-C. and Horig, J. (1981) Sensory and motor functions of spinal cord substance P. Science 214, 1361 – 1363.

Post. L. J. and Vaught, J. L. (1983) Substance P antagonists: analgesia and inhibition of SP-induced scratching. Pharmacologist 23, 612.

Reddy, S. V. R., Maderdrut, J. L. and Yaksh, T. L. (1980) Spinal cord pharmacology of adrenergic agonist-mediated antinociception. J. Pharmacol. Exp. Ther. 213, 525 – 533.

Rodgers, R. J. (1977) The medial amygdala: serotonergic inhibition of shock-induced aggression and pain sensitivity in rats. Aggress. Behav. 3, 277 – 288.

Sagen, J. and Proudfit, H. K. (1984) Effect of intrathecally administered noradrenergic antagonists on nociception in the rat. Brain Res. 310, 295 – 301.

Sagen, J., Winker, M. A. and Proudfit, H. K. (1983) Hypoalgesia induced by the local injection of phentolamine in the nucleus raphe magnus: blockade by depletion of spinal cord monoamines. Pain 16, 253 – 263.

Seybold, V. S. and Elde, R. P. (1982) Neurotensin immunoreactivity in the superficial laminae of the dorsal horn of the rat: I. Light microscopic studies of cell bodies and proximal dendrites. J. Comp. Neurol. 205, 89 – 100.

Seybold, V. S., Hylden, J. L. K. and Wilcox, G. L. (1982) Intrathecal substance P and somatostatin in rats: behaviors indicative of sensation. Peptides 3, 49 – 54.

Shiomi, H., Murakami, H. and Takagi, H. (1978) Morphine analgesia and the bulbospinal serotonergic system: increase in concentration of 5-hydroxyindoleacetic acid in the rat spinal cord with analgesics. Eur. J. Pharmacol. 52, 335 – 344.

Shyu, K. W., Lin, M. T. and Wu, T. C. (1984) Possible role of central serotoninergic neurons in the development of dental pain and aspirin-induced analgesia in the monkey. Exp. Neurol. 84, 179 – 187.

Snow, A. E., Tucker, S. M. and Dewey, W. L. (1982) The role of neurotransmitters in stress-induced antinociception (SIA). Pharmacol. Biochem. Behav. 16, 47 – 50.

Sparber, S. B. and Meyer, D. R. (1978) Clonidine antagonizes naloxone-induced suppression of conditioned behavior and body weight loss in morphine-dependent rats. Pharmacol. Biochem. Behav. 9, 319 – 325.

Spaulding, T. C., Fielding, S., Venafro, J. J. and Lal, H. (1979a) Antinociceptive activity of clonidine and its potentiation of morphine analgesia. Eur. J. Pharmacol. 58, 19 – 25.

Spaulding, T. C., Venafro, J. J., Ma, M. G. and Fielding, S. (1979b) The dissociation of the antinociceptive effect of clonidine from supraspinal structures. Neuropharmacology 18, 103 – 105.

Spear, L. P. and Scalzo, F. M. (1985) Ontogenetic alterations in the effects of food and/or maternal deprivation on 5HT, 5HIAA and 5HIAA/5HT ratios. Dev. Brain Res. 18, 143 – 157.

Spear, L. P., Enters, E. K., Aswad, M. A. and Louzan, M. (1985) Drug and environmentally-induced manipulations of the opiate and serotonergic system alter nociception in neonatal rats. Behav. Neural Biol. 44, 1 – 22.

Sternbach, R. A., Janowsky, D. S., Huey, L. Y. and Segal, D. S. (1976) Effects of altering brain serotonin activity on human chronic pain. Adv. Pain. Res. Ther. 1, 601 – 606.

Stewart, J. M., Getto, C. J., Neldner, K., Reeve, E. B., Krivoy, W. A. and Zimmermann, E. (1976) Substance P and analgesia. Nature 262, 784 – 785.

Sugrue, M. F. (1979) On the role of 5-hydroxytryptamine in drug-induced antinociception. Br. J. Pharmacol. 65, 677 – 681.

Taber, R. I. and Latranyi, M. B. (1981) Antagonism of the analgesic effect of opioid and non-opioid agents by p-chlorophenylalanine (PCPA). Eur. J. Pharmacol. 75, 215 – 222.

Taube, H. D., Borowski, E., Endo, T. and Starke, K. (1976) Enkephalin: a potential modulator of noradrenaline release in rat brain. Eur. J. Pharmacol. 38, 377 – 380.

Terman, G. W., Shavit, Y., Lewis, J. W., Cannon, J. T. and Liebeskind, J. C. (1984) Intrinsic mechanisms of pain inhibition: activation by stress. Science 226, 1270 – 1277.

Tuchscherer, M. M. and Seybold, V. S. (1985) Immunohistochemical studies of substance P, cholecystokinin-octapeptide and somatostatin in dorsal root ganglia of the rat. Neuroscience 14, 593 – 605.

Tulunay, F. C., Yano, I. and Takemori, A. E. (1976) The effect of biogenic amine modifiers on morphine analgesia and its antagonism by naloxone. Eur. J. Pharmacol. 35, 1976.

Van Loon, G. R. and De Souza, E. B. (1978) Effects of β-endorphin on brain serotonin metabolism. Life Sci. 23, 971 – 978.

Vasko, M. R., Pang, I.-H. and Vogt, M. (1984) Involvement of 5-hydroxytryptamine-containing neurons in antinociception produced by injection of morphine into nucleus raphe magnus or onto spinal cord. Brain Res. 306, 341 – 348.

Vaught, J. L., Post, L. J., Jacoby, H. I. and Wright, D. (1983) Tachykinin-like central activity of Neuromedin K in mice. Eur. J. Pharmacol. 103, 355 – 357.

Von Euler, U. S. and Gaddum, J. H. (1931) An unidentified depressor substance in certain tissue extracts. J. Physiol. (London) 72, 74 – 87.

Wang, J. K. (1977) Antinociceptive effect of intrathecally administered serotonin. Anesthesiology 47, 269 – 271.

Weil-Fugazza, J., Godefroy, F. and Besson, J.-M. (1979) Changes in brain and spinal tryptophan and 5-hydroxyindoleacetic acid levels following acute morphine administration in normal and arthritic rats. Brain Res. 175, 291 – 301.

Weil-Fugazza, J., Godefroy, F., Coudert, D. and Besson, J.-M. (1980) Total and free serum tryptophan levels and brain 5-hydroxytryptamine metabolism in arthritic rats. Pain 9, 319 – 325.

Weil-Fugazza, J., Godefroy, F. and Le Bars, D. (1984) Increase in 5-HT synthesis in the dorsal part of the spinal cord, induced by a nociceptive stimulus: Blockade by morphine. Brain Res. 297, 247 – 264.

Wilcox, G. L. (1983) Antagonism between two behaviorally active peptides in rodent spinal cord. Proc. Int. Union Physiol. Sci. 15, 108.

Willcockson, W. S., Chung, J. M., Hori, Y., Lee, K. H. and Willis, W. D. (1984) Effects of iontophoretically released amino acids and amines on primate spinothalamic tract cells. J. Neurosci. 4, 732 – 740.

Yaksh, T. L. and Tyce, G. M. (1979) Microinjection of morphine into the periaqueductal gray evokes release of serotonin from the spinal cord. Brain Res. 171, 176 – 181.

Yaksh, T. L. and Wilson, P. R. (1979) Spinal serotonin terminal system mediates antinociception. J. Pharmacol. Exp. Ther. 208, 446 – 453.

Yaksh, T. L., Farb, D. H., Leeman, S. E. and Jessell, T. M. (1979) Intrathecal capsaicin depletes substance P in the rat spinal cord and produces prolonged thermal analgesia. Science 206, 481 – 483.

Yaksh, T. L., Jessell, T. M., Gamse, R., Mudge, A. W. and Leeman, S. E. (1980) Intrathecal morphine inhibits substance P release, in vivo, from mammalian spinal cord. Nature (London) 286, 155 – 156.

Yaksh, T. L., Howe, J. R. and Harty, G. J. (1984) Pharmacology of spinal pain modulatory systems. Adv. Pain Res. ther. 7, 57 – 70.

Yasphal, K., Wright, D. M. and Henry, J. L. (1982) Substance P reduces tail-flick latency: Implications for chronic pain syndromes. Pain 14, 155 – 167.

Yeung, J. C. and Rudy, T. A. (1980) Multiplicative interaction between narcotic antagonisms expressed at spinal and supraspinal sites of antinociceptive action as revealed by concurrent intrathecal and intracerebroventricular injections of morphine. J. Pharmacol. Exp. Ther. 215, 633 – 642.

York, J. L. and Maynert, E. W. (1978) Alterations in morphine analgesia produced by chronic deficits of brain catecholamines or serotonin: Role of analgesimetric procedure. Psychopharmacology 56, 119 – 125.

Yoshimura, M. and North, R. A. (1983) Substantia gelatinosa neurons hyperpolarized in vitro by enkephalin. Nature (London) 305, 529 – 530.

Zemlan, F. P., Corrigan, S. A. and Pfaff, D. W. (1980) Noradrenergic and serotonergic mediation of spinal analgesia mechanisms. Eur. J. Pharmacol. 61, 111 – 124.

Burrows/Elton/Stanley (eds.) Handbook of Chronic Pain Management
© *1987 Elsevier Science Publishers B.V. (Biomedical Division)*

4

Endorphins and cortisol in chronic pain

LARS TERENIUS

Department of Pharmacology, University of Uppsala, Uppsala, Sweden

Introduction

The history of the treatment of pain is a history of miracle cures and their failures. Despite medical progress, substantial numbers of patients have chronic, invalidizing pain. Such cases are treatment failures and research is needed to define the reasons for the failures and to suggest new therapies.

The discovery of the endogenous opioid peptides, the endorphins, a decade ago created new hope for chronic pain patients. At the basic science level there has also been a very dramatic increase in knowledge. The chemical structure of the opioid peptides, their distribution, their biosynthesis and its genetic regulation are known and the physiology of these peptides is rather well understood. Opioid peptides have also been synthesized and several hundred analogues have been tested as potential analgesics. This work has emphasized the existence of multiple opioid receptor types. Not only the classic morphine-(mu)-type receptor but also other receptor types some of which are more selective for the peptides can mediate pain relief. This may lead to a new generation of drugs which are more effective and/or have less side effects than morphine-type analgesics.

An important goal is to consider whether this new knowledge can be utilized to prevent the development of, or to reduce the number of patients with chronic pain. In view of previous failures of pharmacologic therapies, attention has been given to the possibility of stimulating the endogenous systems. Early work in this field focussed on endorphins as putative neurotransmitters gating the pain signal by neuron to neuron interaction. More recently, endorphins have been considered in a broader context, as links in pain modulatory neuronal systems and also as modulators at an endocrine level. Mechanistically, the endorphins are then considered in relation to the stress response. Pain is known to generate stress and stress also aggravates pain. This

---

Address for correspondence: Lars Terenius, Box 591, 751 24 Uppsala, Sweden.

chapter will discuss chronic pain and its relation to the endorphin systems, as well as the stress response, particularly with regard to endorphins and cortisol.

The endorphin families

The simplest endorphin is enkephalin with the sequence Tyr-Gly-Gly-Phe-X, where X is Met (Methionine) or Leu (Leucine). This pentapeptide sequence is the minimum for opioid activity and occurs in all endorphins. Like other bioactive peptides, endorphins derive from prohormones. Three such prohormones are known, each coded for by a separate gene. Each prohormone is pluripotent and by progressive proteolytic cleavage a large number of peptides may be formed. Table 1 lists some of the best known, altogether about 30 opioid peptides have been described (Bloom 1983). Proopiomelanocortin is unique in the sense that it also is the prohor-

TABLE 1
Amino acid sequences of opioid peptides (the common N-terminus is Tyr-Gly-Gly-Phe-X, where X = Leu or Met).

Prohormone	Peptide		
	Name	Amino acid X	Amino acid no.
Proopiomelanocortin	β-Endorphin	Met	31
Proenkephalin	Leu-enkephalin	Leu	5
	Met-enkephalin	Met	5
	Methorphamid	Met	8
Prodynorphin	Dynorphin A	Leu	17
	Dynorphin B	Leu	13
	α-Neoendorphin	Leu	10

PROOPIOMELANOCORTIN

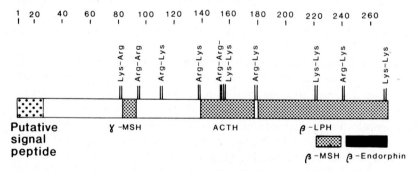

Fig. 1. Schematic structure of the prohormone for ACTH and β-endorphin, proopiomelanocortin. The protein is shown as a column with amino acid numbers on top. By proteolysis the protein is cleaved to smaller fragments; the signal peptide is cleaved off already at the ribosomal level. Note that the active hormone sequences are flanked by pairs of basic amino acids which are recognized by specific proteolytic enzymes. Proenkephalin and prodynorphin have a similar construction.

mone for the nonopioid hormones adrenocorticotropic hormone (ACTH) and melanocyte-stimulating hormone (MSH) (Fig. 1). Theoretically, this prohormone would generate one molecule of β-endorphin for each molecule of ACTH; in practice, tissue-specific enzymatic activity may alter the proportions. In general, proteolytic enzymes have an important regulatory role in the biosynthesis of neuropeptides (Loh et al. 1984).

Endorphins and pain

Immunohistochemical studies have indicated that enkephalin fibres are associated with pain pathways at several levels. In the dorsal spinal cord, enkephalin terminals are found to overlap with termination areas of nociceptive neurons (e.g. Hökfelt et al. 1977). Most enkephalin is in interneurons which apparently directly control the projection neurons. Biochemical and pharmacologic studies indicate that opiate receptors may also presynaptically control the release of transmitter from primary afferents. Dynorphin occurs in other interneurons with slightly different localizations; dynorphin peptides interact preferably with so-called $\varkappa$-receptors which mediate analgesia at the spinal level. Enkephalin fibres are also present in the medullary and midbrain (periaqueductal gray, PAG) circuitry, areas in which morphine microinjection can induce powerful analgesia. The PAG also receives innervation by β-endorphin fibres. A descending pathway from the midbrain and medullary areas projects to the spinal cord, providing a basis for a multilevel synergistic system for pain modulation (Basbaum and Fields 1984). Summarizing the distribution of opioid peptides and opiate receptors, we have defined the 'primary' level of interaction between pain pathways and the endorphin systems (Table 2). Enkephalin, dynorphin and β-endorphin fibres are also spread over many other CNS areas including basal ganglia and the hypothalamus. Opioid peptides may therefore influence mood and behaviour, as expected considering the psychotropic effects of morphine-like substances.

Pain, stress and the neuroendocrine system

As already indicated, the opioid peptides differ with regard to receptor type selectivity. They also differ with regard to metabolic stability. The enkephalins are the most unstable, easily degraded by various CNS enzymes whereas β-endorphin is the most stable, with several hours duration after intrathecal or intracerebral administration. There are β-endorphin fibres terminating in the wall of the third ventricle, suggesting that this peptide may be released in a neuroendocrine fashion. Endorphins are also formed in and released from endocrine tissues pro-

TABLE 2
Endorphins and pain: primary level of interaction – an overview.

Spinal cord	Enkephalin
	Dynorphin
Medulla	Enkephalin
Midbrain	Enkephalin
	β-Endorphin
Higher centres	Enkephalin
	β-Endorphin

viding a possible 'secondary level' interaction with pain and stress (Table 3). The hypophyseal secretion has been relatively well studied. Apparently β-endorphin secretion goes in parallel with that of ACTH, although some studies suggest absence of negative glucocorticoid feedback regulation of β-endorphin release. Enkephalins of the adrenal medulla are stored in the same cells as the catecholamines. The importance of this system is less well documented. The enkephalins are very unstable in plasma but it is conceivable that the proteolytic processing of proenkephalin is not complete in the adrenal and that longer, more metabolically resistant peptides are released. The hypothalamus-pituitary-adrenal axis can indirectly affect endocrine and probably neuronal endorphin biosynthesis; cortisol suppresses the expression of pro-opiomelanocortin but increases expression of proenkephalin (Civelli et al. 1983). Stress may also induce analgesia via opioid or nonopioid mechanisms. The former mechanism is inhibited by adrenalectomy (Terman et al. 1984).

Very little is known about the physiologic mechanisms which activate the different endorphin systems. Mild stimulation, e.g. by sensory activation, may contribute to a sense of well-being. Physical exhaustion or psychological stress could be triggering events for intense activation leading to inactivity and analgesia. In shock, endorphin release may have pathogenetic consequences (Holaday 1983). This escalation of activity may represent the physiologic domain. Pathologic states of prolonged hypo- or hyper-activation may lead to psychosomatic or psychiatric disorders. A state of hypo-activation may for instance be sensed as deprival and create a demand for substitution (therapy).

Endorphins and cortisol activity in chronic pain

Chronic pain is an operational definition. There is no reason to anticipate that there should be a common aetiology. Clinical criteria have been used to define subcategories such as 'organic' or 'psychogenic' chronic pain. Generally, there is a tendency to favour somatic approaches and describe the lesion rather than consider the pain patient. Certainly, any chronic pain syndrome will have both somatic and psychic components. Here, we will discuss the use of biochemical measurements in the chronic pain syndrome.

An early study by Lascelles et al. (1974) showed that patients in chronic pain tended to have higher than normal cortisol plasma levels. Although there was no significant difference between mainly 'organic' or 'psychogenic' cases, there was less diurnal variation in the former group. Unfortunately, this study does not indicate the duration or severity of pain in the individual patient, factors which clearly could have affected the results.

In a series of studies, our group has analyzed the possible involvement of endorphins in chronic pain. Endorphins were measured in the CSF on the assumption that they would provide an indicator of the global activity in the CNS. Since all endorphin systems could be of impor-

TABLE 3
Endorphins and pain (and stress): secondary level of interaction.

Neuroendocrine	
Pituitary, posterior lobe	Dynorphin
Endocrine	
Pituitary, anterior lobe	β-Endorphin
	(Dynorphin)
Adrenal	Enkephalin

tance and there is presently no basis for selecting any one of them, we chose to use a receptor assay which recognizes all the endorphins present, regardless of structure. However, a chromatographic fractionation step prior to the assay was found to be useful and so-called Fraction I endorphins appeared as possible indicators of endorphin activity (Terenius 1981). In a series of unselected patients attending a University Neurology Clinic, most presented with 'neurogenic' pain problems. They were subjected to extensive neurologic and psychiatric evaluation. In relation to control subjects, patients with pain of neurogenic origin had very low CSF endorphin levels; patients with a syndrome better explained in psychologic terms tended to show the opposite trend (Table 4). There was also a correlation with levels of the serotonin metabolite, 5-hydroxyindoleacetic acid. On the other hand, there was a negative correlation between the duration of the pain syndrome and endorphin levels. Other studies (Terenius 1981) have indicated relationships between CSF endorphin levels and tolerance to postoperative pain emphasizing the importance of constitutional factors.

A series of experimental and clinical studies have underscored the effectiveness of acupuncture and related techniques in relieving chronic pain. It is interesting, that these techniques are particularly effective in neurogenic pain, the condition with low endorphins. Acupuncture is known to stimulate endorphin and other pain modulatory systems in the CNS (Han and Terenius 1982) (see also Chapter 6).

Plasma endorphins have endocrine origin and their levels cannot be used to infer levels of activity in CNS. Beta-endorphin related peptides in plasma have been found to be higher in patients with chronic pain and major depressive disorder than in healthy volunteers indicating hyperactivity in the hypothalamus-pituitary-adrenal axis. Resistance to cortisol suppression in the dexamethasone suppression test (DST) examines the hypothalamic response to exogenously given steroid and has been advocated as a neuroendocrine marker for depression (Carroll et al. 1981). Atkinson et al. (1983) reported abnormal DST in 4/7 patients. France and Krishnan (1985) studied 80 chronic back pain patients with the DST. Thirty-five of these patients satisfied the DSM-III criteria of major depression; 40% of these patients had an abnormal DST. No patient with absence of major depression had abnormal DST. Other investigators have reported similar proportions of chronic pain patients with abnormal DST: 40% (Blumer et al. 1982), 26% (Salminen 1984) and 41% (von Knorring and Almay, personal communication). In the last study, 8/9 patients with abnormal DST were classified as psychogenic supporting the findings of France and Krishnan (1985) that an abnormal DST is related to depression.

TABLE 4

Endorphin activity (so-called Fraction I endorphins) in the CSF of patients with chronic pain, as compared with healthy volunteers and patients with major depressive disorder.

	< 0.6	0.6 – 1.2	> 1.2 pmol/ml*
Healthy volunteers	3	12	4
Neurogenic pain	29	2	2
Nociceptive pain	2	3	3
Psychogenic pain	3	9	10
Depressive disorders	–	3	12

* Measured as Met-enkephalin equivalents.

Neuroendocrinology of chronic pain syndromes – attempts at a synthesis

Pain is a *subjective* feeling. The reductionist approach is to describe pain at a 'cognitive' level (sensory characteristics and motor behaviour) at a 'physiologic' level (neuronal circuits and endocrine systems) or at an effector (neurotransmitter, modulator)/receptor level. It is a mistake to separate these levels like the concentric circles of electron orbitals around the atomic nucleus. What is advocated here is that evaluation of pain, and particularly chronic pain needs an integrated approach.

It is also accepted that many CNS functions are sensitive to stress and psychological discomfort. The endocrine status and its variation as for instance during the menstrual cycle can affect the mental well-being. It may still be less commonplace to consider pain under psychoneuroendocrine influence. However, even in a healthy individual there is a diurnal variation in nociceptive thresholds which are higher in the morning than in the evening (see further Terenius 1981). Biochemical studies of Scandinavian patients have indicated a circannual rhythm in CSF endorphins (von Knorring et al. 1982). Since differences occur already at the sensory/discriminative stage, reactive components of clinical pain may show even greater dependence on environmental and endocrine factors.

The biochemical markers of pain, stress and their modulation offer certain possibilities to categorize clinical pain. Chronic pain is a debilitating condition which may be a triggering event for depression. However, data reviewed here suggest neuroendocrine differences between chronic pain with depression and major depression with pain. Patients with neurogenic pain seem to be quite distinct both with regard to endorphin activity and the hypothalamus-pituitary-adrenal axis. They seem to be in a state of hypo-endorphin activity, which progresses with increasing disease duration. At a mechanistic level, pain is probably nonnociceptive. Nociceptive, chronic pain as secondary to ischaemia or malignancy is mechanistically easier to define. The chronic character and its association with severe, maybe terminal, illness is a strong psychic burden, which has neuroendocrine significance. Chronic pain where the psychic components dominate and there is no apparent somatic pathology is also a clinical reality. It is often termed psychogenic (as opposed to organic), a misnomer since every chronic pain syndrome has psychic components. Studies reviewed here suggest high endorphin activity and abnormal DST in these patients, which is paralleled with resistance to various sensory stimuli (cf. Terenius 1981).

In conclusion, neuroendocrinological investigations may be useful in categorizing chronic pain. The DST is already a versatile procedure. However, measurements of endorphin activity require the resources of a specialized laboratory, limiting their general applicability.

References

Almay, B. G. L., Johansson, F., von Knorring, L., Terenius, L. and Wahlström, A. (1978) Endorphins in chronic pain. I. Differences in CSF endorphin levels between organic and psychogenic pain syndromes. Pain 5, 153 – 162.

Atkinson, J. H., Kremer, E. F., Risch, S. C., Morgan, C. D., Azad, R. F., Ehlers, C. L. and Bloom, F. E. (1983) Plasma measures of beta-endorphin/beta-lipotropin-like immunoreactivity in chronic pain syndrome and psychiatric subjects. Psychiatr. Res. 9, 319 – 327.

Basbaum, A. I. and Fields, H. L. (1984) Endogenous pain control systems: brainstem spinal pathways and endorphin circuitry. Ann. Rev. Neurosci. 7, 309 – 338.

Bloom, F. E. (1983) The endorphins: a growing family of pharmacologically pertinent peptides. Ann. Rev. Pharmacol. Toxicol. 23, 151 – 170.

Blumer, D. Zorick. F. and Heilbronn, M. (1982) Biological markers for depression in chronic pain. J.

Nerv. Ment. Dis. 170, 425 – 428.

Carroll, B. J., Feinberg, M, Greden, T. F. et al. (1981) A specific laboratory test for the diagnosis of melancholia. Arch. Gen. Psychiatry 38, 15 – 22.

Civelli, O., Birnberg, N., Comb, M., Douglass, J., Lissitzky, J. C., Uhler, M. and Herbert, E. (1983) Regulation of opioid gene expression. Peptides 4, 651 – 656.

France, R. D. and Krishnan, K. R. R. (1985) The dexamethasone suppression test as a biologic marker of depression in chronic pain. Pain 21, 49 – 55.

Han, J. S. and Terenius, L. (1982) Neurochemical basis of acupuncture analgesia. Ann. Rev. Pharmacol. Toxicol. 22, 193 – 220.

Holaday, J. W. (1983) Cardiovascular effects of endogenous opiate systems. Ann. Rev. Pharmacol. Toxicol. 23, 541 – 594.

Hökfelt, T., Ljungdahl, Å., Terenius, L., Elde, R. and Nilsson, G. (1977) Immunohistochemical analysis of peptide pathways possibly related to pain and analgesia: enkephalin and substance P. Proc. Natl. Acad. Sci. USA. 74, 3081 – 3085.

Lascelles, P. T., Evans, P. R., Merskey, H. and Sabur, M. A. (1974) Plasma cortisol in psychiatric and neurologic patients with pain. Brain 97, 533 – 538.

Loh, Y. P., Brownstein, M. J. and Gainer, H. (1984) Proteolysis in neuropeptide processing and other neural functions. Ann. Rev. Neurosci. 7, 189 – 222.

Salminen, A. (1984) Regional Symp. World Psychiatr. Assoc., Helsinki 1984, Book of Abstracts (Eds. Hemmi, A. & Tukkanen, K.).

Terenius, L. (1981) Endorphins and pain. Front. Horm. Res. 8, 162 – 177.

Terman, G. W., Shavit, Y., Lewis, J. W., Cannon, J. T. and Liebeskind, J. C. (1984) Intrinsic mechanisms of pain inhibition: activation by stress. Science 226, 1270 – 1277.

Von Knorring, L., Almay, B. G. L., Johansson, F., Terenius, L. and Wahlström, A. (1982) Circannual variation in concentrations of endorphins in cerebrospinal fluid. Pain 12, 265 – 272.

Burrows/Elton/Stanley (eds.) Handbook of Chronic Pain Management
© *1987 Elsevier Science Publishers B.V. (Biomedical Division)*

5

Intrinsic pain inhibitory mechanisms: Central and environmental activation

ANTOINE DEPAULIS, ROBERT N. PECHNICK and JOHN C. LIEBESKIND*

Department of Psychology, University of California, Los Angeles, CA 90024, U.S.A.

Introduction

Encountering tissue damaging or tissue threatening (i.e. 'noxious') stimuli is virtually inevitable in the day-to-day lives of most organisms. It is not surprising, therefore, that a complex neural apparatus has evolved to protect the body's integrity against such harm. First to note is the existence of a sensory system specialized to carry impulses initiated by noxious stimuli. We call activity within this system 'nociception'. Actions provoked by nociception may be reflexive or much more complicated and involve even the highest centers of the brain. One complex reaction of the nervous system to a noxious stimulus is the conscious awareness of the stimulus, which we call 'pain'. In addition, it now appears that the brain has a neural substrate whose function is to suppress activity in the nociceptive system, and experiments are revealing this substrate's anatomy and its mechanisms of actions. It seems that, under some circumstances, it might be more adaptive to inhibit pain than to perceive it, for example, during certain strong drive states such as sexual arousal, aggression and fear, and especially during the performance of goal-directed behaviors associated with these drives. Under these circumstances, feeling pain could disrupt effective performance and pain suppression would have greater survival value to the organism and species than pain itself.

The demonstration that electrical stimulation of a portion of the medial brain stem can produce profound analgesia (Reynolds 1969; Mayer et al. 1971) gave the first solid evidence for an intrinsic pain-inhibitory system and began the systematic search for specific structures and pathways involved in this function. Early studies in this series also stimulated the search for neurohumoral factors that modulate pain, leading to the discovery of the endogenous opioid peptides, including the enkephalins and β-endorphin. The purpose of this chapter is to describe

---

* To whom correspondence should be addressed.

some elements of the anatomy, physiology and pharmacology of the intrinsic pain inhibitory system and to discuss various environmental stimuli that seem able to turn it on.

Stimulation-produced analgesia

Reynolds (1969) first observed that electrical stimulation of the mesencephalic periaqueductal gray matter resulted in sufficient analgesia to perform laparotomies in rats. Mayer et al. (1971) repeated and extended these observations, providing evidence that this stimulation-produced analgesia (SPA), had a specific antinociceptive effect not attributable to generalized sensory, attentional, emotional or motoric deficits. They showed also that SPA occurred in a restricted peripheral field such that noxious stimuli applied outside that field elicited normal defensive reactions. The analgesia produced by electrical stimulation of the midbrain periaqueductal gray can be equipotent to that induced by high doses of morphine. It has been found to eliminate behavioral responses to such varied noxious somatic and visceral stimuli as electric shocks applied to the tooth pulp and limbs, heating of the skin, and injection of irritants into the skin and abdominal cavity (for references see Cannon and Liebeskind 1979). Finally, it can be observed only seconds after stimulation is begun and may last for minutes or even hours after the stimulation is terminated.

These findings suggested the existence of a natural and powerful pain-inhibitory substrate in the periaqueductal gray matter. Subsequent demonstrations by Adams (1976), Richardson and Akil (1977), Hosobuchi et al. (1977) and others (see Young et al. 1984) that stimulation of homologous brain regions in man could relieve chronic pain symptoms greatly enhanced interest in this phenomenon. In human beings relief from chronic pain has been seen to outlast the period of stimulation by up to 24 hours (see Young et al. 1984).

Electrical stimulation of various structures has been shown to produce analgesia; however, stimulation of the periaqueductal gray matter has given the most consistent results and has been the area most extensively studied. This structure is in an excellent position to relay messages from the forebrain to the lower brain stem. It receives inputs from, among other places, the frontal and insular cortex, the amygdala and hypothalamus, nucleus cuneiformis, the pontine reticular formation, locus coeruleus, and the spinal cord. On the other hand, it has descending connections to the medullary reticular nuclei and the nucleus raphe magnus. These sites in the medulla are a major source of axons projecting principally via the dorsolateral funiculus to the dorsal horn of the spinal cord. The periaqueductal gray also has ascending projections to the intralaminar nuclei of the thalamus in a pattern similar to that known for the spinothalamic tract (see Basbaum and Fields 1984).

SPA appears to result from an active, rather than a passive process of inhibition. Neither lesions of the periaqueductal gray matter nor injections of local anesthetic into it produce an obvious deficit in pain responsiveness, indicating that electrical stimulation does not cause analgesia by producing a temporary lesion. The concept of a descending pain-inhibitory system was suggested by Melzack and Wall (1965), and evidence for it was provided by Mayer et al. (1971) who demonstrated that spinally-mediated nociceptive reflexes could be blocked by SPA. It was later found that responses of spinal cord dorsal horn cells to nociceptive stimuli were inhibited by SPA (Oliveras et al. 1974). Furthermore, lesions of the nucleus raphe magnus or the dorsolateral funiculus were found to inhibit SPA and to block its inhibitory effect on dorsal horn cells (Basbaum and Fields 1984). These results suggested that SPA acts by activating a descending or centrifugal control system. This pathway includes the raphe and other nearby reticular nuclei and descends via the spinal dorsolateral funiculus. These nuclei are not only sites at which SPA can be obtained but are important relays conveying centrifugal pain inhibitory messages deriving from more rostral brain structures to the final site of pain inhibition at the level of those spinal cord interneurons responsive to noxious stimuli.

With respect to the neurochemical mechanisms underlying SPA, the greatest amount of research has centered on the role of the endogenous opioid peptides. Analgesia induced by brain stimulation and that induced by opiate drugs appear to share some common sites and mechanisms of action. Areas of the brain from which SPA can be elicited are found to be rich in opioid peptides and opiate receptors (Snyder 1980). Furthermore, SPA in man can cause increases in opioid material in the cerebrospinal fluid (Akil et al. 1978; Hosobuchi et al. 1979). Microinjection of minute quantities of morphine into these same brain areas results in the development of analgesia (Yaksh and Rudy 1978). Also, both systemically and centrally administered morphine increases neural activity in the periaqueductal gray region (Urca et al. 1977), suggesting that opiate analgesia, like SPA, involves an active rather than a passive process of pain inhibition. Finally, lesions of the spinal cord dorsolateral funiculus, as well as lesions of the nucleus raphe magnus, disrupt morphine analgesia as well as SPA (Basbaum and Fields 1984).

In order to establish that SPA is mediated by endogenous opioid peptides three additional criteria must be met: SPA must show the development of tolerance with repeated stimulation; SPA and opiate analgesia must demonstrate cross-tolerance with each other; and SPA must be reduced by opiate antagonists. Tolerance has been found to develop to the analgesic effects of brain stimulation, and cross-tolerance has been observed between opiate analgesia and SPA (Mayer and Hayes 1975). Opiate antagonists such as naloxone also antagonize SPA, at least partially (Akil et al. 1976a). However, this latter finding has proven controversial: it appears that not all forms of SPA involve the stimulation-induced release of opioid peptides. 'Opioid' and 'nonopioid' forms of SPA seem to occur and appear to have different anatomical localizations in the brain (Cannon et al. 1982).

Physiological triggers of intrinsic analgesia systems

The analgesic effects of brain stimulation and opiate administration suggested that these manipulations in some way mimic the natural evocation of activity within an intrinsic pain modulatory system. A question of major importance, therefore, is what are the stimuli that normally activate this system. Painful stimuli are one obvious candidate, but some environmental stimuli not producing obvious pain can elicit analgesia. For example, in the heat of battle or athletic competition, insensitivity to pain following an injury has been reported. Because many such situations are stressful, it has been suggested that stress is a natural or physiological trigger of the intrinsic pain-inhibitory system. This phenomenon has been termed stress-induced analgesia (SIA).

The first demonstrations of SIA were made in rats by Akil et al. (1976b) and Hayes et al. (1978). Their results differed in one major respect: the sensitivity of SIA to reversal by narcotic antagonists. The analgesia observed by Akil et al. (1976) was blocked by pretreatment with the opiate antagonist naloxone, suggesting that opioid peptides are involved in SIA. However, the analgesia seen by Hayes et al. (1978) was not blocked by naloxone pretreatment, indicating a different, nonopioid mechanism. Subsequently, SIA was studied in response to many varied stressors, but the question of the involvement of endogenous opioid peptides remained unclear with some investigators reporting naloxone blockade and others failing to see this effect. In addition, Hayes et al. (1978) noted that not all stressors elicit analgesia. It is still not clear what are the specific characteristics that cause one type of stressor to elicit analgesia and others not.

A major problem in comparing the early studies of SIA was the variety of types of stressors used. Lewis et al. (1980) at least partly resolved the question of SIA sensitivity to naloxone by studying a single stressor, inescapable footshock of constant intensity. They found that they could elicit either naloxone-sensitive or naloxone-insensitive analgesia by varying the temporal pattern of the shock. This finding indicates that, like SPA, SIA has both an opioid form utilizing endogenous opioid peptides and a nonopioid form whose neurochemical mediators are currently unknown. The naloxone-sensitive analgesic response met two other important criteria for inferring the involvement of opioid peptides: it showed tolerance development with repeated administration of footshock, and it was reduced in morphine-tolerant rats, indicating the presence of cross-tolerance with morphine (Lewis et al. 1984). The nonopioid form of SIA, in addition to revealing no inhibition by naloxone, failed to show either tolerance or cross-tolerance with morphine. Further supporting the independence of these two forms of SIA is the lack of cross-tolerance between the opioid and nonopioid forms (Terman et al. 1984). As is the case for SPA (e.g. Akil and Liebeskind 1975), little is known about which neurotransmitters are involved in the opioid form of SIA. The neurochemistry of nonopioid SIA is even less well understood. Attempts have been made to determine what neurotransmitters are involved in this form of SIA and one candidate appears to be histamine (Terman et al. 1984).

The body responds to increased physical or psychological demands by activating the pituitary-adrenal cortical and sympathetic-adrenal medullary axes. The hormone products of these activations contribute to the adaptive response of the organism to stress by affecting energy production and the cardiovascular and immune systems (Axelrod and Reisine 1984). Because pain suppression can be viewed as an adaptive response to stress, it seems logical that these hormonal systems also play a role in SIA; and several lines of evidence support this hypothesis. β-Endorphin is highly concentrated in the pituitary, and stress has been shown to cause the co-release of pituitary opioids and adrenocorticotropic hormone (ACTH) (Guillemin et al. 1977). In addition, the adrenal medulla contains opioid peptides that are released under the same circumstances of sympathetic activation that elicit the release of catecholamines (Viveros et al. 1979). Therefore, stimuli that activate the pituitary-adrenal axis and the adrenal medulla also cause the release of endogenous opioids from the pituitary and adrenal medulla. In this regard, one opioid form of SIA was found to be attenuated in hypophysectomized animals (Lewis et al. 1984). Furthermore, it was found that complete adrenalectomy, adrenal demedullation and adrenal medullary denervation via celiac ganglionectomy also blocked this opioid form of SIA. Because demedullation and ganglionectomy had as great an effect as total adrenalectomy, it was concluded that this form of SIA is dependent on adrenal medullary opioids (Lewis et al. 1982). The behavioral data were supported by biochemical evidence showing that adrenal enkephalin-like material was decreased after footshock that elicited opioid SIA but not after footshock that elicited nonopioid SIA.

SIA and SPA appear to share many of the same mechanisms, suggesting that SPA is not just an experimental curiosity. Both opioid and nonopioid SIA as well as SPA are antagonized by lesions of the dorsolateral funiculus indicating that SIA, like SPA, relies at least in part on centrifugal pathways (Lewis et al. 1984). In addition, cross-tolerance develops between opioid forms of SPA and SIA (Terman et al. 1984). An interesting finding is that under surgical levels of anesthesia rats show a normal, spinally mediated tail-flick reflex and normal inhibition of that reflex by SPA and by certain forms of SIA (Terman et al. 1984). These findings indicate that the conscious perception of pain is not necessary for some forms of SIA to be activated, nor is consciousness required for at least some portions of the intrinsic pain inhibitory system to work.

Conclusion

It is clear that the central nervous systems of human beings and laboratory animals possess a highly organized mechanism for controlling nociception. Elucidating the neural and neurochemical bases of this mechanism might well lead to the development of new approaches to pain management. Perhaps the greatest promise for such development lies in investigating nonopioid analgesia. Activating this system should cause pain inhibition without the unwanted opiate sequelae of tolerance and dependence. Determining its neurochemistry is an essential first step in devising nonnarcotic analgesic drugs. The fact that opioid and nonopioid SIA have comparable magnitude suggests that such centrally acting nonnarcotics will be as potent as opiates.

Direct application of SPA techniques devised in laboratory animals has been made in pain patients (see references in Young et al. 1984). Although deep brain stimulation remains a costly and highly specialized treatment that will probably never have widespread application, still it has found a respected place in the arsenal of pain therapies. The apparent existence of a natural pain suppressive system, reinforced greatly by the effectiveness of the human SPA trials, gives hope that reliable, noninvasive means will be found for activating this function powerfully in man.

References

Adams, J. E. (1976) Naloxone reversal of analgesia produced by brain stimulation in the human. Pain 2, 161 – 166.

Akil, H. and Liebeskind, J. C. (1975) Monoaminergic mechanisms of stimulation-produced analgesia. Brain Res. 94, 279 – 296.

Akil, H., Mayer, D. J. and Liebeskind, J. C. (1976a) Antagonism of stimulation-produced analgesia by naloxone, a narcotic antagonist. Science 191, 961 – 962.

Akil, H., Madden, J., Patrick, R. L. and Barchas, J. D. (1976b) Stress-induced increases in endogenous opioid peptides; concurrent analgesia and its partial reversal by naloxone. In: H. W. Kosterlitz (Ed.), Opiates and Endogenous Opioid Peptides. Elsevier, Amsterdam, pp. 63 – 70.

Akil, H., Richardson, D. E., Barchas, J. D. and Li, C. H. (1978) Appearance of beta-endorphin-like immunoreactivity in human ventricular cerebrospinal fluid upon analgesic electrical stimulation. Proc. Natl. Acad. Sci. U.S.A. 75, 5170 – 5172.

Axelrod, J. and Reisine, T. D. (1984) Stress hormones: their interaction and regulation. Science 224, 452 – 459.

Basbaum, A. I. and Fields, H. L. (1984) Endogenous pain control systems: brainstem spinal pathways and endorphin circuitry. Ann. Rev. Neurosci. 7, 309 – 338.

Cannon, J. T. and Liebeskind, J. C. (1979) Descending control systems. In: R. F. Beers, Jr. and E. G. Basset (Eds.), Mechanisms of Pain and Analgesic Compounds. Raven Press, New York, pp. 171 – 184.

Cannon, J. T., Prieto, G. J., Lee, A. and Liebeskind, J. C. (1982) Evidence for opioid and nonopioid forms of stimulation-produced analgesia in the rat. Brain Res. 243, 315 – 321.

Guillemin, R., Vargo, T., Rossier, J., Minick, S., Ling, N., Rivier, C., Vale, W. and Bloom, F. (1977) Beta-endorphin and adrenocorticotropin are secreted concomitantly by the pituitary gland. Science 197, 1367 – 1369.

Hayes, R. L., Bennet, G. J., Newlon, P. G. and Mayer D. J. (1978) Behavioral and physiological studies of non-narcotic analgesia in the rat elicited by certain environmental stimuli. Brain Res. 155, 69 – 90.

Hosobuchi, Y., Adams, J. E. and Linchitz, R. (1977) Pain relief by electrical stimulation of the central gray matter in humans and its reversal by naloxone. Science 197, 183 – 186.

Hosobuchi, Y., Rossier, J., Bloom, F. E. and Guillemin, R. (1979) Stimulation of human periaqueductal gray for pain relief increases immunoreactive beta-endorphin in ventricular fluid. Science 203, 279 – 281.

Lewis, J. W., Cannon, J. T. and Liebeskind, J. C. (1980) Opioid and nonopioid mechanisms of stress analgesia. Science 208, 623 – 625.

Lewis, J. W., Tordoff, M. J., Sherman, J. E. and Liebeskind, J. C. (1982) Adrenal medullary enkephalin-like peptides may mediate opioid stress analgesia. Science 217, 557 – 559.

Lewis, J. W., Terman, G. W., Shavit, Y., Nelson, L. R. and Liebeskind, J. C. (1984) Neural, neurochemical and hormonal bases of stress-induced analgesia. In: L. Kruger and J. C. Liebeskind (Eds.), Advances in Pain Research and Therapy, Vol. 6. Raven Press, New York, pp. 277 – 288.

Mayer, D. J. and Hayes, R. L. (1975) Stimulation-produced analgesia: development of tolerance and cross-tolerance to morphine. Science 188, 941 – 943.

Mayer, D. J., Wolfle, T. L., Akil, H., Carder, B. and Liebeskind, J. C. (1971) Analgesia from electrical stimulation in the brain stem of the rat. Science 174, 1351 – 1354.

Melzack, R. and Wall, P. D. (1965) Pain mechanisms: a new theory. Science 150, 971 – 979.

Oliveras, J. L., Besson, J. M., Guilbaud, G. and Liebeskind, J. C. (1974) Behavioral and electrophysiological evidence of pain inhibition from midbrain stimulation in the cat. Exp. Brain Res. 20, 32 – 44.

Reynolds, D. V. (1969) Surgery in the rat during electrical analgesia induced by focal brain stimulation. Science 164, 444 – 445.

Richardson, D. E. and Akil, H. (1977) Pain reduction by electrical brain stimulation in man. I. Acute administration in periaqueductal and periventricular sites. J. Neurosurg. 47, 178 – 183.

Snyder, S. H. (1980) Brain peptides as neurotransmitters. Science 209, 976 – 983.

Terman, G. W., Shavit, Y., Lewis, J. W., Cannon, J. T. and Liebeskind, J. C. (1984) Intrinsic mechanisms of pain inhibition: activation by stress. Science 226, 1270 – 1277.

Urca, G., Nahin, R. L. and Liebeskind, J. C. (1977) Effects of morphine on spontaneous multiple unit activity: possible relation to mechanisms of analgesia and reward. Exp. Neurol. 66, 248 – 262.

Viveros, O., Dilberto, E.J., Jr., Hazum, E. and Chang, K-J. (1979) Opiate-like materials in the adrenal medulla: evidence for storage and secretion with catecholamines. Molec. Pharmacol. 16, 1101 – 1108.

Yaksh, T. L. and Rudy, T. A. (1978) Narcotic analgesics: CNS sites and mechanisms of action as revealed by intracerebral injection techniques. Pain 4, 299 – 359.

Young, R. F., Feldman, R. A., Kroening, R., Fulton, W. and Morris, J. (1984) Electrical stimulation of the brain in the treatment of chronic pain in man. In: L. Kruger and J. C. Liebeskind (Eds.), Advances in Pain Research and Therapy, Vol. 6. Raven Press, New York, pp. 289 – 293.

Burrows/Elton/Stanley (eds.) Handbook of Chronic Pain Management
© *1987 Elsevier Science Publishers B.V. (Biomedical Division)*

6

Endogenous opioid peptides and acupuncture analgesia

LIANFANG HE and XIAODING CAO

Laboratory of Neurophysiology, Research Department of Acupuncture, Shanghai Medical University, Shanghai 200032, People's Republic of China

Introduction

Acupuncture, an important branch of Chinese traditional medicine, was first systematically described in the Chinese medical classic, *Canon of Medicine of the Yellow Emperor*, which was published some 2000 years ago. Acupuncture therapy refers to the techniques of inserting fine needles into particular points of the body and stimulating the points either by hand manipulation or by applying electrical current through the needles. The practice of acupuncture for the relief of pain opened a new field with its application to surgical analgesia in the late 1950's. Systematic studies carried out in the past 20 years have revealed that the essence of acupuncture analgesia (AA) is mainly the activation of the endogenous antinociceptive system to modulate pain transmission and pain response. The most important advance of the study of AA within the last decade is the establishment of the participation of the endogenous opioid peptidergic system (EOPS). This chapter intends to review the information accumulated in this respect and to discuss the possible central circuits through which the endogenous opioid peptides (EOP) mediate AA.

Evidence for the involvement of EOP in AA

Substantial evidence has been given by three main series of experiments, the use of narcotic antagonists as probes, the measurement of EOP levels and the blocking of EOP degradation.

ANTAGONISM OF AA BY NALOXONE

Reversal by narcotic antagonists is a necessary condition for characterizing an analgesic manipulation as narcotic. Mayer et al. (1975, 1977) first reported that AA in humans was reversible by naloxone, a specific opiate antagonist. Pain threshold estimated by electrical stimulation of the tooth was increased significantly by acupuncture of Hegu points. This increase was completely reversed by naloxone 5 minutes after injection.

Huang et al. (1979) established a monkey model on which acupuncture significantly prolonged the latent period of the operant lever-pressing response to noxious stimulus, with naloxone effective in blocking analgesia. Naloxone antagonism was demonstrated also in other animal models such as the rabbit, mouse and rat.

He (1981) recorded noxious response from nucleus lateralis anterior of the rabbit thalamus. The response could be inhibited by iontophoretic etorphine and electroacupuncture (EA), and the inhibition was readily reversed by iontophoresis of naloxone. Results obtained from both humans and animals indicate that acupuncture may activate certain processes to release EOP onto their binding sites and a consequent interaction between them results in analgesia.

RELEASE OF EOP BY ACUPUNCTURE

Measurement of the EOP levels in the cerebrospinal fluid (CSF) is a potential approach to evaluate their release from the central nervous system (CNS). Sjölund et al. (1977) investigated changes of EOP content in the CSF during the period of analgesia induced by 'electroacupuncture' via surface electrodes in patients with chronic pain. Clement-Jones et al. (1980) found that low-frequency EA effectively alleviated recurrent pain and significantly increased CSF β-endorphin levels, but enkephalin levels were unaltered. Chen and Pan (1984) reported that EA increased the content of β-endorphin-like immuno-reactive substances in ventricular CSF in patients with brain tumour. There was a linear correlation between the percentage increase of β-endorphin-like immuno-reactive substances and the pain threshold or pain tolerance.

Since the isolation of opioid peptides from the blood, some laboratories began to study the plasma concentrations of EOP during EA. Malizia et al. (1979) reported that β-endorphin and adrenocorticotropic hormone (ACTH) were secreted into the peripheral blood during EA in healthy subjects. Xu et al. (1980) found that manual acupuncture resulted in a significant increase in opioid peptides in plasma, with correlation between the efficacy of AA and the plasma content of opioid peptides. Xi and Li (1983) found that serum levels of morphine-like substances in patients with chronic pain were lower than those in healthy pain-free subjects. EA raised the serum morphine-like substances towards normal in patients expressing good acupuncture effects but not in those with poor effects.

The role of plasma β-endorphin in AA is still obscure. Pomeranz et al. (1977) postulated that acupuncture might exert its analgesic actions by releasing endorphins from the pituitary into the blood. The circulatory endorphins were then thought to pass into the brain to produce analgesia. However, Fu et al. (1980) found that hypophysectomy did not alter the EA inhibition of phenylquinone-induced writhing in mice. Therefore, the functional significance of plasma opioid peptides in AA is still to be clarified.

POTENTIATION OF AA BY BLOCKING EOP DEGRADATION

Tsou et al. (1979a,b) reported that intraventricular injection of bacitracin, which retards destruction of enkephalin, greatly prolonged the analgesic effect of manual acupuncture in rabbits. Acupuncture plus bacitracin also resulted in increased enkephalin contents in the striatum and hypothalamus compared with controls. On the other hand, Wu et al. (1980) used the protein synthesis inhibitor cycloheximide, which is reported to interfere with the incorporation of [3H]tyrosine into enkephalin in vitro. Intraventricular injection of cycloheximide was found to have no significant effect on pain threshold, but greatly attenuated EA analgesia in rats. Cycloheximide decreased met-enkephalin content by 47% in the hypothalamus and by 20% in the striatum. EA increased met-enkephalin by 113 and by 222% respectively in these two brain regions. Following cycloheximide, EA increased met-enkephalin only by 28 and 123% respectively. These results indicate that EA activates the biosynthesis of enkephalins and the latter may play an active part in the process of analgesia.

Cheng and Pomeranz (1980) observed that an additive analgesic effects was produced by EA and D-amino acids (D-phenylalanine and D-leucine), which are peptidase inhibitors. The combined effect was blocked by naloxone. Takeshige et al. (1983) investigated the similarities among AA, morphine analgesia and periaqueductal gray (PAG) stimulation produced analgesia in rats. Individual variations in the effectiveness of these three kinds of analgesia were parallel and could be reduced by the administration of D-phenylalanine, suggesting a common basic mechanism underlying them.

Hyodo et al. (1983) demonstrated the enhancement of AA by phenylalanine in man. They found that D-phenylalanine markedly prolonged the pain threshold raising effect in healthy subjects, improved the therapeutic effect on low back pain and increased the success rate of AA in dental surgery.

Mediation of the endogenous opioid peptidergic system in the central mechanism of AA

Studies over the past few years indicate that there are a number of CNS sites rich in opiate receptors and opioid peptides participating in AA. The data from physiological, biochemical and pharmacological evidence will be briefly reviewed here to give a comprehensive description.

SPINAL CORD

The enkephalin system of the spinal cord is considered as part of the endogenous antinociceptive system relevant to opiate analgesia and brain stimulation-produced analgesia (Basbaum and Fields 1978), thus raising the possibility of its participation in AA. Han et al. (1982) injected intrathecally the IgG fraction from antisera against enkephalins prior to EA in rabbits and found that the EA effect was apparently seen on the head while that on the caudal section was markedly attenuated. Han and Xie (1984) observed that intrathecal injection of the endogenous opioid dynorphin produced a very potent analgesia which was naloxone reversible. Intrathecal administration of antidynorphin antibody markedly attenuated EA analgesia at the tail, leaving the analgesic effect intact in the head region. Rabbits made tolerant to EA by long-term EA stimulation no longer exhibited analgesia following dynorphin administration. A possible role of spinal enkephalin and dynorphin in AA is thus suggested.

LOWER BRAIN STEM

Ventromedial medulla. It has been established that the ventromedial medulla and its descending inhibitory pathway constitute a fundamental component in the central circuit responsible for the expression of AA. Transection of the spinal cord has been proved to abolish almost completely the inhibitory effect of acupuncture on nociceptive response (Du and Chao 1976; Pomeranz et al. 1977).

The dorsolateral funiculi (DLF) are derived from the nucleus raphe magnus (NRM) and its adjacent reticular formation (Basbaum and Fields 1979). It was found that a median lesion in the medulla including the NRM resulted in a significant diminution of AA (Du and Chao 1976), whereas stimulation of the raphe nuclei potentiated acupuncture inhibition (Du et al. 1978a). The NRM region though not rich in opiate receptors (Atweh and Kuhar 1977), contains numerous enkephalin perikarya (Conrath-Verrier et al. 1983). It is suggested that the enkephalin system of the NRM is part of the central antinociceptive system (Basbaum and Fields 1978). Its relevance for AA is suggested by several findings, e.g. effects of acupuncture on NRM neurons were blocked by intravenous naloxone (Zhang and Ku 1982), and iontophoresis of naloxone into the NRM could partially block the modulatory effects of acupuncture (Shi and Zhu 1983).

There is evidence that the serotonergic descending pathways in the DLF transmit inhibitory influence from the ventromedial medulla to the spinal cord and mediate AA. Du et al. (1978b) injected 5,6-hydroxytryptamine thus causing degeneration of 5-hydroxytryptamine (5-HT) nerve terminals in the spinal cord originating from the raphe nuclei. The inhibitory effect of acupuncture was reduced. The 5-HT axons project heavily onto the dorsal horn where the distributions of enkephalins and opiate receptors overlap and the nociceptive projecting neurons are localized (Fields 1981). This extensive anatomical correspondence provides a substrate for functional interaction between the EOPS and 5-HT system in pain transmission.

The above and many other results indicate that the ascending sensory impulses are blocked at the spinal cord level by acupuncture-induced descending impulses from the ventromedial medulla, the EOPS being a component link in the spinal cord-medulla-spinal cord circuit.

PERIAQUEDUCTAL GRAY

The landmark microinjection studies by Tsou and Jang (1964) stimulated a series of work leading to the finding of PAG as a region sensitive to local application of the opiates (see Yaksh and Rudy 1978). Available data have indicated that the PAG is a critical site for morphine analgesia and brain stimulation-produced analgesia, and at least part of its pain-modulating function is mediated by the ventromedial medulla (Fields 1981). It has also been established that acupuncture may utilize these same substrates.

Electrical stimulation of the PAG induces analgesia with a gradual development (Melzack and Melinkoff 1974) and a prolonged after-effect (Mayer et al. 1971) similar to AA. Stimulation of the PAG greatly potentiated AA (Huang et al. 1982) and lesion of the PAG greatly attenuated acupuncture inhibition (Takeshige et al. 1979).

Han et al. (1982), taking advantage of the high specificity of antibody-antigen reaction, injected anti-β-endorphin IgG or antienkephalin IgG into rabbits' PAG and found that either treatment could partially block the inhibitory effect of acupuncture on nociceptive response. However, antidynorphin antibody injection produced no significant effect (Han and Xie 1984). The data imply that acupuncture activates the brain to release enkephalins and β-endorphin onto their binding sites. The actual release of EOP by acupuncture was demonstrated by Zhang et al. (1981) and Chen et al. (1982). Increase of EOP levels of PAG perfusates during acupuncture was found to be related to the efficacy of analgesia.

There is general agreement that the PAG exerts its analgesic action through the ventromedial medulla, of which the major afferent connections originate in the PAG (Mantyh 1983). Acupuncture may modulate the inhibitory and excitatory influences of the PAG on the NRM, resulting in activation of the NRM. The work of Liu and Zhang (1984) on microinjection showed that local application of naloxone into the PAG could block the modulating effect of EA on the NRM neurons, suggesting the important role of the PAG-EOP system.

In general, the actions of exogenous opiates and enkephalins applied on their target neurons are inhibitory (Bradley et al. 1978). It is interesting to note that acupuncture inhibits most of the opiate-sensitive neurons in the PAG, and that iontophoresis of naloxone can readily block the inhibition (Dong and He 1983a; He and Dong 1983; Cao et al. 1984a). It is relevant to postulate that acupuncture activates certain brain areas such as the PAG to release EOP onto their binding sites resulting in an inhibition of the inhibitory interneurons and an activation of the output neurons. The descending inhibition of pain transmission through ventromedial medulla is thus accomplished.

DIENCEPHALON

Hypothalamic arcuate nucleus. According to Bloom et al. (1978) the cell bodies of the β-endorphin containing neurons are clustered in the arcuate and tuberal region. The fibres originating from the neurons distribute in a number of structures related to AA such as the lateral septal nucleus, nucleus accumbens, PAG and locus coeruleus. Quo et al. (1982) reported that electrolytic lesions of the arcuate weakened AA. There is evidence to suggest that the antinociceptive action of the arcuate is mainly mediated via its functional connection with the PAG-NRM system (Gao and Ku 1983 a,b).

Preoptic area. The preoptic area has been proved to have an antinociceptive function. Microinjection of morphine (Pert and Yaksh 1974) or β-endorphin (Tseng et al. 1978) into this area produced significant analgesic effect. Available data show that the preoptic area may play an active part in AA. Cao et al. (1982) demonstrated that the inhibitory effect of acupuncture was enhanced by simultaneous stimulation of the lateral preoptic area and was nearly abolished by destroying it. Wu et al. (1984) reported that most neurons recorded from the preoptic area were responsive to EA and most neurons which were inhibited by iontophoresis of etorphine were inhibited by EA as well. The results suggest that the effect of acupuncture is also related to the effect of EOPS in the preoptic area.

Stimulation of the preoptic area could modulate the activity of the PAG. This suggests that a connection between the preoptic area and the PAG may be implicated in AA (Cao et al. 1984b).

FOREBRAIN

Caudate nucleus (CN). Recent studies have provided substantial evidence indicating the involvement of the CN in pain modulation. Stimulation of the CN is able to raise pain threshold (Schmidek et al. 1971) and suppress pain responses (Lineberry and Vierck 1975) in chronic monkeys. Stimulation of the CN also produces satisfactory pain relief in patients suffering from intractable pain (Ervin et al. 1966; Chen et al. 1983). Recent research has revealed that the CN participates in AA. It was found in chronic rabbits that caudate lesion attenuated AA while caudate stimulation enhanced AA (see He and Xu 1981). The caudate contains abundant opiate peptides and opiate receptors (Simantov et al. 1976).

He et al. (1985) reported that acupuncture increased the release of EOP from the caudate, and microinjection of naloxone into the caudate blocked AA. They also noticed that there were caudate neurons responsive to both microiontophoresis and EA. The inhibition induced by EA could be reversed by microiontophoresis of naloxone, a phenomenon similar to that seen in the PAG and the preoptic area. These results indicate that the intracaudate opioid peptidergic system participates in AA.

In addition, several findings have suggested that the cholinergic (Ho et al. 1979; Lu et al. 1983) and dopaminergic (Zhou et al. 1981) systems also participate in AA. The interrelationship among opioid peptides, acetylcholine and dopamine needs to be clarified.

Available data have shown that the functional connection between the CN and the PAG-NRM system is related to the antinociceptive function of the CN (He et al. 1981; Dong and He 1983b). The work of Zhu and Liu (1984) suggests that PAG is an important link between the CN and the NRM.

Limbic nuclei. *Septal area:* Clinical observation has shown that stimulation of the septal area produced an analgesic effect on cancer pain (Gol 1967). Animal experiments have implicated this area in acupuncture inhibition of nociceptive responses (Mo and Ling 1979). The septal area is rich in opioid peptides and opiate receptors (Simantov et al. 1976; Finley et al. 1981). Naloxone microinjected into this area can partially block AA. The antinociceptive effect of the septal area is possibly brought forth by the activation of the opioid peptidergic system in the PAG, since naloxone microinjected into the latter blocks septal stimulation-produced analgesia (Huang et al. 1983).

Nucleus accumbens: Recent studies have revealed that the nucleus accumbens has an antinociceptive function and participates in AA. It is rich in opioid peptides and opiate receptors (Simantov et al. 1976). The accumbens projects to the lateral habenular nucleus (Powell and Leman 1976) and exerts an inhibitory effect on the latter (Kao and Wang 1985). This is probably part of the mechanism through which the accumbens mediates AA.

Nucleus amygdala: The amygdala is one of the forebrain structures containing the highest density of opiate receptors (Atweh and Kuhar 1977) and the highest concentration of opioid peptides (Simantov et al. 1976). Its possible involvement in AA is suggested by the findings that lesion of this nucleus (Zhai et al. 1981) or microinjection of naloxone into it results in the attenuation of acupuncture inhibition of nociceptive defence reaction.

Concluding remarks

There is now convincing evidence indicating that AA is produced via the activation of the central antinociceptive system. In this antinociceptive system, the ventromedial medulla and the spinal cord constitute a fundamental circuit, while the PAG occupies a strategic position to funnel all the influences from the high structures and to collect all the information from the spinal cord. In the whole process, the EOPS plays an important role at different levels of the CNS. The main activity of EOPS might be the inhibition of the inhibitory interneurons, thus bringing the output neurons into action.

Clinical observations (Chen 1981) and animal experiments (Chiang et al. 1975) have indicated that acupuncture signals are conveyed to the brain via the spinal ventrolateral funiculus, which is an important pathway transmitting pain sensation. This is understandable since acupuncture sensation also bears characteristics of pain sensation, such as the unpleasant feeling of soreness.

Axons of the extralemniscal system of the ventrolateral funiculus, on their way upward, project to various brain areas related to both algesia and analgesia (Melzack 1973). These areas are particularly rich in opioid peptides, the PAG being a good example. There is evidence suggesting that pain is a physiological factor which activates the EOPS (see Mayer 1979). It is probable that acupuncture elicits a kind of sensory input which is a physiological factor similar to pain. Its physiological significance is to enforce the antinociceptive function of the organism to combat against pain.

Acknowledgement

The authors wish to express their appreciation to Dr. Yao Tai for his critical review of the manuscript.

References

Atweh, S. F. and Kuhar, M. J. (1977) Autoradiographic localization of opiate receptors in rat brain. The brain stem. Brain Res. 12, 1 – 12.

Basbaum, A. I. and Fields, H. L. (1978) Endogenous pain control mechanisms: review and hypothesis. Ann. Neurol. 4, 451 – 462.

Basbaum, A. I. and Fields, H. L. (1979) The origin of descending pathways in the dorsolateral funiculus of the cord of the cat and rat: further studies on the anatomy of pain modulation. J. Comp. Neurol. 187, 513 – 532.

Basbaum, A. I. and Fields, H.L. (1984) Endogenous pain control systems: brainstem spinal pathways and endorphin circuitry. Ann. Rev. Neurosci. 7, 309 – 338.

Bloom, F. E., Rossier, J., Battenberg, E. L. F., Bayon, A., French, E., Henriksen, S. J., Sigging, G. K., Segal, D., Browne, R., Ling, N. and Guillemin, R. (1978) β-Endorphin: cellular localization, electrophysiological and behavioral effects. In: E. Costa and M. Trabucchi (Eds.), Advances in Biochemical Psychopharmacology, Vol. 18. Raven Press, New York, pp. 89 – 109.

Bradley, P. B., Gaton, R. J. and Lambert, Lynn A. (1978) Electrophysiological effects of opiates and opioid peptides. In: J. Hughes (Ed.), Centrally Acting Peptides. Macmillan, London, pp. 215 – 229.

Cao Xiaoding, Du Lina and Jiang Jianwei (1982) Role of different regions of preoptic area in electroacupuncture inhibition upon cortical potential evoked by tooth pulp stimulation. Acupunc. Res. (Suppl. 1) 37.

Cao Xiaoding, Wang Miaozhen and Jiang Jianwei (1984a) Effects of electroacupuncture and iontophoresis of etorphine and noradrenaline on neuronal activity in rabbits' periaqueductal gray matter (PAG). In: The Second National Symposium on Acupuncture and Moxibustion and Acupuncture Anesthesia, Abstracts (August 7 – 10, 1984) Beijing, China, p. 308.

Cao Xiaoding, Jiang Jianwei and Wang Miaozhen (1984b) Inhibition of neurons in periaqueductal gray matter (PAG) by lateral preoptic area stimulation. In: The Second National Symposium on Acupuncture and Moxibustion and Acupuncture Anesthesia, Abstracts (August 7 – 10, 1984) Beijing, China, p. 360.

Chen Baiying, Wang Deling and Pan Xiao-ping (1982) Changes of opiate-like substances (OLS) level in the perfusate of periaqueductal gray (PAG) after electroacupuncture and brain stimulation in rabbit. Acta Physiol. Sin. 34, 385 – 391.

Chen Bo-Ying and Pan Xiao-Ping (1984) Correlation of pain threshold and level of β-endorphin-like immunoreactive substance in human CSF during electroacupuncture analgesia. Acta Physiol. Sin. 36, 183 – 187.

Chen Gongbai (1981) Acupuncture anesthesia in neurosurgery. Chinese Med. J. 94, 423 – 430.

Chen Gongbai, Jiang Chengchuan, Li Shengchang, Yang Boyi, Jang Deming, Yan Jie, and He Lianfang (1983) The role of the human caudate nucleus in acupuncture analgesia. Acupunc. Electro-Ther. Res. 7, 255 – 265.

Cheng Richard S. S. and Pomeranz B. (1980) A combined treatment with D-amino acids and electroacupuncture produces a greater analgesia than either treatment alone: naloxone reverses these effects. Pain 8, 231 – 236.

Chiang Chen-yü, Liu Jen-yi, Chu Teh-hsing, Pai Yao-hui and Chang Shu-chich (1975) Studies on spinal ascending pathway for effect of acupuncture analgesia in rabbits. Sci. Sin. 18, 651 – 658.

Clement-Jones, V., MacLoughlin, L., Tomlin, S., Besser, G. M., Rees, L. H. and Wen, H. L. (1980) Increased β-endorphin but not met-enkephalin levels in human cerebrospinal fluid after acupuncture for recurrent pain. Lancet 2, 946 – 948.

Conrath-Verrier, M., Dietl, M., Arluison, M., Cesselin, F., Bourgoin, S. and Hamon, M. (1983) Localization of met-enkephalin-like immunoreactivity within pain-related nuclei of cervical spinal cord, brainstem and midbrain in the cat. Brain Res. Bull. 11, 587 – 604.

Dong Weichang and He Lianfang (1983a) Effects of microiontophoretic opiates and caudate stimulation on neurons in periaqueductal gray (PAG). Acta Physiol. Sin. 34, 63 – 70.

Dong Weiqiang and He Lianfang (1983b) The effects of acupuncture points and caudate stimulation on the activity of etorphine-sensitive neurons in periaqueductal gray matter. Acta Acad. Med. Pri. Shanghai 10, 119 – 124.

Du Huan-ji and Chao Yan-fang (1976) Localization of central structures involved in descending inhibitory effect of acupuncture on viscero-somatic reflex discharge Sci. Sin. 19, 137 – 148.

Du Huan-ji, Chao Yang-fang and Zheng Rui-kang (1978a) Inhibitory effect of raphe stimulation on viscerosomatic reflexes in cat and its relationship with acupuncture analgesia. Acta Physiol. Sin. 30, 1 – 9.

Du Huan-ji, Shen En, Dong Xinwen, Jiang Zhihua, Ma Weixiang, Fu Yifan, Jin Guozhang, Zhang Zhende and Han Yifan (1978b) Effect of acupuncture analgesia by injection of 5,6-dihydroxytryptamine in cat: a neurophysiological, neurochemical and fluorescence histochemical study. Acta Zool. Sin. 24, 11 – 20.

Ervin, F. R., Brown, C. E. and Mark, V. H. (1966) Striatal influence on facial pain, 2nd Int. Symp. Stereoencephalotomy (Vienna, 1965) Confin. Neurol. (Basel) 27, 75 – 86.

Fields, H. F. (1981) An endorphin-mediated analgesia system: experimental and clinical observations. In: J. B. Martin et al. (Eds.), Neurosecretion and Peptides. Raven Press, New York pp. 199 – 212.

Finley, J. C. W. Maderdrut, J. L. and Petrusz, P. (1981) The immunocytochemical localization of enkephalin in the central nervous system of the rat. J. Comp. Neurol. 198, 541 – 565.

Fu Tsu-ching, Halenda S. P. and Dewey, W. L. (1980) The effect of hypophysectomy on acupuncture analgesia in the mouse. Brain Res. 202, 33 – 39.

Gao Yuan-sheng and Ku Yun-hui (1983a) Mechanism underlying the excitatory effect of nucleus arcuatus hypothalami on PAG-NRM system and its significance in electroacupuncture in rats. Acta Physiol. Sin. 35, 409 – 415.

Gao Yuan-sheng and Ku Yun-hui (1983b) Mechanism underlying the inhibitory effect of rat nucleus arcuate hypothalami on unit discharge of locus coeruleus with reference to electroacupuncture. Acta Physiol. Sin. 35, 163 – 171.

Gol, A. (1967) Relief of pain by electrical stimulation of the septal area. J. Neurol. Sci. 5, 115 – 120.

Han Ji-sheng, Xie Guo-xi, Zhou Zhong-fu, Folkesson, R. and Terenius, L. (1982) Enkephalin and β-endorphin as mediators of electro-acupuncture analgesia in rabbits: an antiserum microinjection study. In: E. Costa and M. Trabucchi (Eds.), Regulatory Peptides from Molecular Biology to Function. Raven Press, New York, pp. 369 – 377.

Han Si-sheng and Xie Guo-xi (1984) Dynorphin: important mediator for electroacupuncture analgesia in spinal cord of the rabbit. Pain 18, 367 – 376.

He Lianfang (1981) Effect of iontophoretic etorphine and electroacupuncture on nociceptive response from nucleus lateralis anterialis of thalamus in rabbits. Acupunc. Electro-Ther. Res. 6, 151 – 157.

He Lianfang and Dong Weiqiang (1983) Activity of opioid peptidergic system in acupuncture analgesia. Acupunc. Electro-Ther. Res. 8, 257 – 266.

He Lianfang and Xu Shaofen (1981) Caudate nucleus and acupuncture analgesia. Acupunc. Electro-Ther. Res. 6, 169 – 181.

He Lianfang, Du Lina, Zhang Xuegui, Shi Zhenzhong, Jiang Jianwei and Wang Miaozhen (1981) Effect of naloxone microinjected into central grey on caudate stimulation produced analgesia. Acta Acad. Med. Pri. Shanghai 8, 81 – 84.

He Lianfang, Lu Ruiliang, Zhuang Shouyuan, Zhang Xuegui and Pan Xiaoping (1985) Possible involvement of opioid peptides of caudate nucleus in acupuncture analgesia. Pain, 23, 83 – 93.

Ho Lien-fang, Ho Xiao-ping and Shi Cheng-zhong (1979) Effect of intracaudate microinjection of scopolamine on electroacupuncture analgesia in the rabbit. Acta Physiol. Sin. 31, 47 – 51.

Huang Chenge, Li Xicheng, Zhang Changcheng, Liu Shengtian, Pan Xijuan and Zhou Zhonghui (1982) Effect of electrical stimulation of midbrain periaqueductal gray on acupuncture analgesia in rats. Acta Physiol. Sin. 34, 343 – 357.

Huang Xianfen, Wang Gennian, Yu Guihua and Mo Wanying (1983) Analgesic effect of septal stimulation in rabbits and the influence of naloxone microinjected into the periaqueductal gray. Acta Acad. Med. Pri. Shanghai 10, 199 – 203.

Huang Ye, Wang Qingwei, Zheng Jinze, Li Derong and Xie Guoyang (1979) Analgesia effect of acupuncture and its reversal by naloxone as shown by the method of operant conditioning responses in monkeys. In: National Symposia of Acupuncture and Moxibustion and Acupuncture Anaesthesia (June 1 – 5, 1979), Beijing, China, p. 485.

Hyodo Massayoshi, Kitade Toshikatsu and Hosoka Eikichi (1983) Study on the enhanced analgesic effect induced by phenylalanine during acupuncture analgesia in humans. In: J. J. Bonica et al. (Eds.), Advances in Pain Research and Therapy, Vol. 5. Raven Press, New York, pp. 577 – 582.

Kao Chang-qing and Wang Shao (1985) Effect of stimulation of nucleus accumbens and naloxone microinjection on nociceptive unit discharge in the lateral habenular nucleus. Acta Physiol. Sin. 37, 24 – 30.

Lineberry, C. G. and Vierck, C. J. (1975) Attenuation of pain reactivity by caudate stimulation in monkey. Brain Res. 98, 119 – 134.

Liu Xiang and Zhang Shouxin (1984) The influence of injection or microinjection of naloxone into PAG upon the effect of electroacupuncture on NRM neurons. In: The Second National Symposium on Acupuncture and Moxibustion and Acupuncture Anesthesia, Abstracts (August 7 – 10, 1984) Beijing, China. p. 372.

Lu Wenxiao, Zeng Dayun and Xu Shaofen (1983) Effect of cholinergic activity in caudate nucleus on acupuncture analgesia. Acupunc. Res. 8, 109 – 112.

Malizia, E., Andreucci, G., Paolucci, D., Crescenzi, F. Fabbri, A. and Fraioli, F. (1979) Electroacupuncture and peripheral β-endorphin and ACTH levels. Lancet 2, 535 – 536.

Mantyh, P. W. (1983) Connections of midbrain periaqueductal grey in monkey. II. Decending efferent projections. J. Neurophysiol. 49, 582 – 594.

Mayer, D. J. (1979) Endogenous analgesic systems: neural and behavioral mechanisms. In J. J. Bonica, J. C. Liebeskind and D. G. Albe-Fessard (Eds.), Advances in Pain Research and Therapy, Vol. 3. Raven Press, New York, pp. 385 – 410.

Mayer, D. J., Wolfle, T. L., Akil, H., Carder, B. and Liebeskind, J. C. (1971) Analgesia from electrical stimulation in the brainstem of the rat. Science 174, 1351 – 1354.

Mayer, D. J., Price, D. D. and Rafii, A. (1975) Acupuncture hypalgesia: evidence for activation of a central control system as a mechanism of action. In: 1st World Congr. Pain, Florence, Abstr. 276.

Mayer, D. J., Price, D. D. and Rafii, A. (1977) Antagonism of acupuncture analgesia in man by the narcotic antagonist naloxone. Brain Res. 121, 368 – 372.

Melzack, R. (1973) The physiology of pain. In: R. Melzack (Ed.), The Puzzle of Pain. Penguin Education, Great Britain, pp. 74 – 124.

Melzack, R. and Melinkoff, D. F. (1974) Analgesia produced by brain stimulation: evidence for prolonged onset period. Exp. Neurol. 43, 369 – 374.

Mo Wanying and Ling Ruijing (1979) Preliminary observation on the role of the septal area in altering the galvanic skin reflex during acupuncture in cat. In: National Symposia of Acupuncture and Moxibustion and Acupuncture Anesthesia (June 1 – 5, 1979), Beijing, p. 343.

Pert, A. and Yaksh, T. L. (1974) Sites of morphine induced analgesia in the primate brain: relation to pain pathways. Brain Res. 80, 135 – 140.

Pomeranz, B., Cheng, R. and Law, P. (1977) Acupuncture reduces electrophysiological and behavioral responses to noxious stimuli: pituitary is implicated. Exp. Neurol. 54, 172 – 178.

Powell, E. W. and Leman, R. B. (1976) Connections of the nucleus accumbens. Brain Res. 105, 389 – 403.

Quo Shiyu, Yin Weipin, Zhang Huiqin and Yin Qizhang (1982) Role of hypothalamic arcuate region in lip-acupuncture analgesia. Acta Physiol. Sin. 34, 71 – 77.

Schmidek, H. H., Fohanno, D., Ervin, H. R. and Sweet, W. H. (1971) Pain threshold alterations by brain stimulation in the monkey. J. Neurosurg. 35, 715 – 722.

Shi Qingyao and Zhu Lixia (1983) The influence of iontophorotic naloxone upon acupuncture effect on the nucleus raphe magnus. Acupunc. Res. 8, 89 – 95.

Simantov, R., Kuhar, M. J., Pasternak, G. W. and Snyder, S. H. (1976) The regional distribution of a morphine-like factor enkephalin in monkey brain. Brain Res. 106, 189 – 197.

Sjölund, B., Terenius, L. and Eriksson, M. (1977) Increased cerebrospinal fluid levels of endorphins after electroacupuncture. Acta Physiol. Scand. 100, 382 – 384.

Takeshige, C., Luo, C. P., Kamada, Y., Oka, K., Murai, M. and Hisamitsu, T. (1979) Relationship between midbrain neurons (periaqueductal central gray and midbrain reticular formation) and acupuncture analgesia, animal hypnosis. In: J. J. Bonica et al. (Eds.), Advances in Pain Research and Therapy, Vol. 3. Raven Press, New York, pp. 615 – 621.

Takeshige, C., Murai, M., Tanaka, M. and Hachisu, M. (1983) Parallel individual variations in effectiveness of acupuncture, morphine analgesia and dorsal PAG-SPA and their abolition by d-phenylalanine. In: J. J. Bonica et al. (Eds.), Advances in Pain Research and Therapy, Vol. 5. Raven Press, New York, pp. 563 – 569.

Tseng, L. F., Wei, E., Loh, H. and Li, C. H. (1978) β-Endorphin: central sites of analgesia and catalepsy. Fed. Proc. 37, 237.

Tsou Kang and Jang, C. S. (1964) Studies on the site of analgesic action of morphine by intracerebral microinjection. Sci. Sin. 13, 1099 – 1109.

Tsou Kang, Wu Shih-hsiang, Wan Fan-sheng, Ji Xin-quan, Chang Tsu-shuan, Lo Ee-sing and Yi Ching-cheng (1979a) Increased levels of endorphins in the cisternal cerebrospinal fluid of rabbits in acupuncture analgesia. Acta Physiol. Sin. 31, 371 – 376.

Tsou Kang, Zhao Dan-dan, Wu Shih-hsiang, Chang Tsu-shuan, Lo Ee-sing and Wan Fan-sheng (1979b) Enhancement of acupuncture analgesia with concomittant increase of enkephalins in striatum and hypothalamus by intraventricular bacitracin. Acta Physiol. Sin. 31, 377 – 381.

Wu Gencheng, Jiang Jianwei and Cao Xiaoding (1984) Effect of microiontophoretic etorphine, noradrenaline and electroacupuncture on spontaneous discharges of neurons in rabbit's preoptic area. Acta Physiol. Sin. 36, 552 – 558.

Wu Shih-hsing, Chang Tsu-shuan, Wan Fan-sheng and Tsou Kang (1980) Effect of intraventricular cycloheximide on acupuncture analgesia and brain methionenkephalin. Acta Physiol. Sin. 32, 79 – 81.

Xi Quefang and Li Qisong (1983) Changes in serum levels of morphine-like substances during acupuncture therapy on patients with pain and its relationship to curative effects. Shanghai J. Acupunc. Moxibus. 1, 12 – 15.

Xu Shulian, Xiang Manjun, Lu Zusun, Han Jisheng, Tang Jian and Zhao Silan (1980) The effect of manual acupuncture analgesia and its relation to blood histamine and suggestibility. Acupunc. Res. 5, 273 – 281.

Yaksh, T. L. and Rudy, T. A. (1978) Narcotic analgesics: CNS sites and mechanisms of action as revealed by intracerebral injection techniques. Pain 4, 299 – 359.

Zhai Xiaozhung, Chen Gongbai, Mo Wanying, Jiang Cheng-chuan, Li Shengchang and Xu Meifen (1981) Role of amygdala in acupuncture analgesia – experiment report on animals. Acupunc. Res. 6, 215 – 219.

Zhang Anzhong, Huang Dengkai, Zeng Dayun, Zhang Lingmai, Wang Deling, Zhu Gengen, Jiang Zheng-ying, Zhong Gaozen and Li Yanlu (1981) The changes of endorphins in perfusate of certain brain nuclei in rabbits during acupuncture analgesia. Acta Physiol. Sin. 33, 8 – 16.

Zhang Siaobing and Ku Yunhui (1982) Effects of electroacupuncture and stimulation of nucleus periventricularis and nucleus arcuatus hypothalami on unit discharge of nucleus raphe magnus. Acta Physiol. Sin. 34, 476 – 482.

Zhou Guangzhao, Wang Deling and Xu Shaofen (1981) Effect of dopaminergic system in caudate nucleus on acupuncture analgesia. Kexue Tongbao 26, 1143 – 1147.

Zhu Bing and Liu Xiang (1984) Influence of stimulation of the head of caudatum on the unit activities of neurons of nucleus raphe magnus in the rat and its probable pathway. Acta Physiol. Sin. 36, 157 – 164.

Burrows/Elton/Stanley (eds.) Handbook of Chronic Pain Management
© *1987 Elsevier Science Publishers B.V. (Biomedical Division)*

7

Quantitative models for the assessment of clinical pain: Individual differences scaling and sensory decision theory

W. CRAWFORD CLARK

New York State Psychiatric Institute and Department of Psychiatry, Columbia University, New York, NY 10032, U.S.A.

'But I've gotta use words when I talk to you'

Sweeney Agonistes

T.S. Eliot

Introduction

Correct interpretation of a patient's report of pain is one of the most important, and at the same time, one of the most difficult problems facing a practitioner. This chapter suggests conceptual approaches to the understanding of the patient's description of pain based on two quantitative models of the pain experience: Individual Differences Scaling (INDSCAL), which identifies the dimensions of global pain, and Sensory Decision Theory (SDT), which measures the patient's attitude towards reporting pain. The ways in which these models have guided our own thinking and clinical strategies will be described in two types of patients: those patients who experience constant pain and are usually depressed about it (e.g. patients with chronic back pain) and those patients who experience episodic pain and are anxious about its significance (e.g. patients with atypical headache and other pains).

Qualitative and quantitative evaluation of a patient's pain is extremely difficult. The practitioner cannot share the patient's urgent experience of pain; this must be inferred. The initial assessment of pain is most frequently based upon the patient's description, in combination with objective findings, and an evaluation of the patient's psychological status. We ask ourselves,

How valid is the patient's report of pain? Is he expressing mental anguish rather than physical pain? Is he by nature stoical or not? The primary problem here is not the patient's veracity, but the manifold meanings which people attach to the word pain. A person's complaint of pain is influenced by many variables in addition to the painful sensation itself. It is modified by learning processes established by the culture, by the family, and by the individual's personality. In addition to being an objective description, the report of pain is an interpersonal message: a cry for help, or a bid for attention, or an attempt to dominate another person. The patient has difficulty enough interpreting and conveying his own experience, but the clinician is faced with an even more arduous task; he must attempt to unravel the sensory, psychological and other components of the patient's message. This is particularly true where the patient's physical condition and his symptomatic complaints are at variance. Thus, physicians are required to make psychiatric as well as somatic diagnoses in patients who complain of persistent pain.

There are two basic problems in interpreting the patient's description of pain. The first is the vagueness and ambiguity inherent in the various words used to describe pain. Is pain to be conceptualized as a sensation, an emotion, or a mixture of these and other qualities? How many dimensions are there? The second problem is that of report bias; even within a specified meaning of pain, patients vary in their attitudes about reporting pain. Depending upon a variety of personal and social factors, some individuals will be stoical and others much less so. Increased understanding of these twin problems of meaning and report bias has recently been obtained by applying new analytical techniques to patients in pain. In the context of meaning, INDSCAL analysis suggests that clinical or global pain has at least three attributes: pure sensory pain, emotional distress and somatosensory qualities. With respect to response bias, SDT makes it possible to distinguish 'pain deniers' from 'pain amplifiers'. The conceptual approaches and empirical findings based on these models should prove helpful in the diagnosis and treatment of persistent pain of unknown or ambiguous etiology.

Individual differences scaling

The first step towards quantification of the chronic pain experience requires a better understanding of its dimensions. At present, even the number and the characteristics of the dimensions are in dispute. Some hold that pain has two dimensions: a sensory dimension and an emotional dimension, while others have suggested three dimensions: sensory-discriminative, motivational-affective, and cognitive-evaluative. For the clinician, interpretation of the patient's description of pain presents a semantic problem, because 'pain' is commonly used with at least two (but probably more) quite different meanings. As used with respect to the acute pain of a recent injury or in the laboratory, 'pain' often refers almost solely to *sensory pain*, that is, to the intensity of the noxious sensation itself without any of its other, adjunctive qualities. On the other hand, especially with reference to chronic pain, 'pain' may refer to *global pain*, the total pain experience which includes pure pain sensations, other somatosensory qualities, as well as emotional, cognitive, and motivational components. The dimensions of global pain have recently been examined by means of a new method, INDSCAL, which represents the components of global pain by a set of coordinates in multidimensional space. This approach makes irrelevant such questions as, Is this patient in pain or is he depressed? The question should be, What is the location (coordinates) of the patient in the multidimensional global pain space? Which dimensions of pain are most relevant for him? INDSCAL can identify the relative contributions made by the dimensions of global pain in various pain syndromes.

INDSCAL, a multidimensional scaling model and procedure developed by Carroll and Chang (1970), takes the subjects' similarity ratings made between all possible pairings of a set of *stimulus objects*, which may be either physical stimuli or verbal descriptors. The procedure yields the *group stimulus* space: a geometric configuration of points, as on a map, where each point corresponds to one of the stimulus objects. The distances between these points and their configuration in *r*-dimensional space reflect the relative similarities among these stimuli along the various dimensions. The group stimulus space allows inferences to be made about the structure or dimensions of the group's perceptual world. In addition to the group stimulus space, INDSCAL generates a *subject space* which represents a set of dimension weights for each subject, one point per subject. These individual subject weights represent the relative importance or salience of each dimension for a particular subject; they may be said to provide an address for each individual in the multidimensional group stimulus space.

Clark (1984) and Clark and Ferrer-Brechner (1985) used INDSCAL to compare the global pain dimensions of a group of patients suffering cancer-related pain and a matched group of healthy volunteers. The subjects made similarity judgments on a scale from 0 to 10 to all possible pairings (36) of the following descriptors: Burning, Cramping, Shooting, Sickening, Miserable, Annoying, Mild Pain, Intense Pain, and Unbearable Pain. As portrayed in Fig. 1, the cancer-pain patients yielded a 2-dimensional solution: a 'sensory pain magnitude' dimension, running from Mild Pain to Intense Pain and a 'qualities of pain' dimension with a somatosensory attribute at one pole (e.g. Burning) and an emotional distress attribute (e.g. Miserable) at the other. The healthy volunteers yielded a similar solution. However, there were interesting differences. For the cancer patients, Mild Pain lay closer to the emotional distress pole or attribute; for them, Mild Pain probably described their cancer pain when it was at its least, but nevertheless still

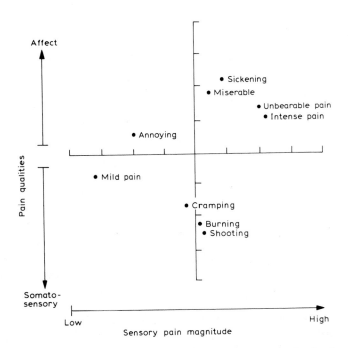

Fig. 1. Group stimulus space of patients suffering cancer-related pain.

distressing. In contrast, for the volunteers, Mild Pain was at the opposite, somatosensory qualities pole; for them Mild Pain was simply a sensation (e.g. a pin-prick) without any emotional quality. These findings are very encouraging and suggest that within the general global pain spaces, groups of patients with different syndromes will exhibit maps with different characteristics. These maps should prove valuable in diagnosis and treatment.

An important characteristic of INDSCAL is its ability to quantify individual differences by means of the subject weight space. The subject weights on each dimension give a quantitative estimate of the relative importance or salience of each dimension to the individual. The weights are the coordinate values specifying a subject's location with respect to the dimensions of the group stimulus space. As portrayed in Fig. 2, the subject weights of the cancer-pain patients F,J,G, were high on the sensory pain dimension and low on the qualities of pain dimension. In contrast, for patients I and H the qualities of pain dimension with its somatosensory and emotional attributes was more salient. Other patients, E and O, weighted the two dimensions equally; however, both of the two dimensions were more salient for patient E who was further from the origin, than for patient O, who was closer to the origin. (If a subject were to locate at the origin of the subject space, this would mean that none of the group dimensions were relevant to his pain.) Information pertaining to the subject space obtained during a patient's initial work-up could greatly improve the precision of the diagnosis and the tailoring of treatment. For example, a patient who weighted heavily on the sensory pain magnitude dimension could be expected to profit more from analgesics, while a patient who weighted heavily on the emotional distress attribute might prove to be a suitable candidate for psychotropic drugs or for psychotherapy.

Further research is needed; the use of a larger number of descriptors will undoubtedly add to the number of dimensions; for example, the emotional attribute discussed here may actually contain separate depression and anxiety attributes or dimensions. Types of patients who might be

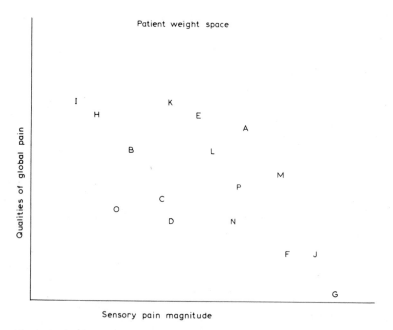

Fig. 2. Subject weight space of patients suffering cancer-related pain.

expected to weight on the anxiety or on the depression attributes are described later in this chapter. Although this study is just a beginning, this description of INDSCAL suggests a cognitive framework within which various types of patients with different loadings on the dimensions of global pain may be pictured.

Sensory decision theory model

In addition to the semantic difficulties associated with the definition of persistent pain, the decision process which influences a patient's report of pain must be considered. Here, the report of pain may be viewed as possessing separately identifiable sensory and attitudinal components. These two components are most clearly seen when SDT is used to analyze a subject's response to brief, calibrated noxious stimuli (e.g. thermal, electrical or pressure). As a working hypothesis, it is assumed that the responses of patients to such stimuli will reveal something about their reporting of pain in general, including their clinical pain. The SDT model is useful here because it yields two parameters of perceptual behavior. The *sensory-discriminative* index measures the accuracy with which an individual distinguishes amongst different stimulus intensities. The second parameter, the *pain criterion*, measures the willingness or reluctance of an individual to report pain. SDT is the only psychophysical method which yields separate quantitative measures that can be so readily identified with the neurosensory and the emotional components of pain. Later it will be demonstrated that patients who suffer from different types of chronic pain and who differ psychologically, differ on these two SDT measures.

The procedures for computing the parametric measures of discriminability, d', and criterion, L_x have been described by Clark (1974), and those for the non-parametric (distribution-free) measures of discriminability, $P(A)$, and criterion, B, by McNicol (1972). The basic concepts can be grasped very easily. An example of the stimulus-response, binary-decision matrix appears in

Stimulus-response matrix for the binary decision task

		RESPONSE	
		'Positive' e.g. 'pain', or 'high', or 'event A occurred'.	'Negative', 'no pain', or 'low', or 'B occurred'
S T I M U L I	*Signal,* e.g. Higher Intensity Stimulus, or any Event A	Hit (correct)	Miss (incorrect)
	Blank, e.g. Lower Intensity Stimulus, or any Event B	False alarm (incorrect)	Correct rejection (correct)

Fig. 3. Discriminability is related to the total proportion of correct responses (hits + correct rejections). Report bias is related to the total proportion of positive responses (hits + false alarms).

Fig. 3. In the simplest instance, either a signal or a blank is presented, and the observer responds 'yes, signal present' or 'no, signal absent', or equivalently 'pain' or 'no pain'. The items which comprise the signals and blanks may be physical stimuli of various calibrated intensities, or words (Yang et al. 1983) describing painful situations of various intensities, and so on. The responses may be 'high'/'low', or 'painful'/'not painful', etc. The subject judges anywhere from 12 to 100 signals and blanks presented randomly. Interference, or 'noise', is assumed to be present in amounts which vary randomly over time, thus creating two overlapping distributions of information. The subject's task is to decide whether the information sampled during an observation interval was produced by the signal or by the blank. To make this statistical decision, the subject sets a criterion, above which he responds 'yes' and below which he responds 'no'. The four possible decision outcomes appear in Fig. 3. The index of discriminability, d' or $P(A)$, measures the accuracy with which an individual distinguishes between signals and blanks. In the binary decision case the responses are scored correct or incorrect, and discriminability is determined by the proportion of the responses which are correct (the sum of hits plus correct rejections). Report bias, the subject's disposition to favor one of the response categories over the other, is related to the proportion of 'yes' responses (the sum of hits plus false alarms), to 'no' responses (the sum of misses plus correct rejections).

The discriminability index, d' or $P(A)$, is related to the functioning of the neurosensory system. High values suggest that neurosensory functioning is normal, low values suggest either that the signal-related neurosensory activity has been attenuated, as it might be by an analgesic, or that neural noise has increased, as might occur following an extended period of chronic pain. In a number of studies, analgesics such as morphine and codeine (Clark and Yang 1983) have been shown to decrease discriminability to thermal stimuli. Unlike the pain threshold, which is typically determined by the Method of Limits or Serial Exploration, d' or $P(A)$ have been shown to be essentially uninfluenced by changes in the subjects' expectation, mood, and motivation. Thus the discriminability parameter measures neurophysiological functioning independently of psychological variables.

The other measure of perceptual performance is the report criterion, L_x or B; it measures response bias, the willingness or reluctance of a subject to use a particular response. It is related to the subject's attitude toward painful experiences. A high criterion reflects stoicism, while a low criterion indicates that the subject readily reports pain even to a low stimulus intensity. Many studies (reviewed by Clark and Yang 1983) have demonstrated the effect of attitudinal variables on the criterion. A placebo described and accepted by the subjects as a powerful analgesic, raised the pain report criterion (stoicism) without altering d', suggesting that the placebo-induced reduction in pain report was not due to the effect of the placebo on neurosensory function, but was due to a criterion shift made in response to the social demand characteristics of the experimental situation. Other studies have shown that suggestion by the experimenter, depending upon its direction, can either raise or lower the pain report criterion, that various ethnocultural groups differ in where they set their criteria, and that anxious subjects set a low pain report criterion. In each of these studies the various experimental manipulations or psychological and cultural differences were without effect on the discrimination parameter. Thus, it may be concluded that the differences found in the pain reports did not reflect differences in underlying neurosensory activity related to the sensation of pain, but reflected only differences in the subjects' criterion for reporting the stimuli as painful.

The effect of chronic pain and stress on SDT parameters

The problem with understanding a patient's description of clinical pain is that the intensity of the 'stimulus' responsible for the pain report (e.g. nerve compression, muscle ischemia, etc.) cannot be independently quantified; often, indeed, the stimulus is completely unknown. Thus, we cannot tell whether the patient is exaggerating or minimizing his pain. However, some insight into the patient's attitude towards pain in general can be gained by using SDT to measure the patient's response to calibrated noxious stimulation. The hypothesis is that the patient's bias (high or low criterion) for experimental pain will reflect the bias (denier or amplifier) for reporting clinical pain. For reasons which will be discussed, patients experiencing severe pain will set a high criterion while patients whose primary problem is anxiety will set a low criterion. It is also expected that, as a result of stress, perhaps related to increased brain opioids and/or activity in the limbic-hypothalamic-pituitary-adrenal (LHPA) axis, patients experiencing severe sensory pain will demonstrate decreased discriminability of the physical stimuli.

Hospitalized psychiatric patients are obviously under considerable emotional stress, but are not suffering severe physical pain. Clark and Mehl (1976) used SDT to compare a group of psychiatric patients with matched healthy volunteers. The patients were less able to discriminate between the noxious thermal stimuli, lower d', and set a higher pain report criterion, L_x. SDT parameters were similar for various psychiatric diagnoses, and with respect to various medication groups. It was concluded that chronic emotional stress was responsible for poorer discriminability and a higher, more stoical, criterion. Janal et al. (1984) found that acute exercise stress produced hypoalgesia to tourniquet ischemic pain and to thermal stimulation, diminished discriminability, $P(A)$. A group of chronic back pain patients suffering pain in addition to emotional stress were studied by Yang et al. (1985). These outpatients had suffered chronic low back pain for a period of at least 6 months, caused by herniated lumbar discs, myofascial syndrome or osteoarthritis. They were compared with age and sex-matched healthy volunteer subjects. The patients stopped medication on the evening before testing. The subjects responded to brief calibrated radiant heat stimuli, along a scale from 'nothing' through various degrees of heat and pain to withdrawal. The patients set a much more stoical pain report criterion, higher B. That is, a given stimulus temperature which was described as 'Very Faintly Painful' by the patients, was considered to be 'Painful' by the normal controls. A reasonable explanation of the patients' high criterion is that, compared to their own clinical pain, the calibrated noxious stimuli were perceived as relatively innocuous. This interpretation would also help to explain why patients who demonstrated high criteria at admission showed the least improvement at follow-up; they were in greater physical pain and hence more difficult to treat successfully. The high criterion indicates that these chronic pain patients were experiencing considerable sensory pain. The patients were also found to have a much lower $P(A)$, showing that they were far less able than the controls to discriminate amongst the stimulus intensities. The sensory losses were extreme, being much greater than that produced in healthy volunteers by 10 mg of intravenous morphine (Yang et al. 1979).

It is also worth noting that the pattern of low discriminability, $P(A)$, and high criterion, B, found in these chronic pain patients is similar to that produced by analgesics, and suggests the presence of high levels of some endogenous analgesic(s) and/or high levels of neural noise. The hypoalgesic response which was found to the thermal stimuli is paradoxical: one would expect the failure of endogenous mechanisms to control clinical pain to be coupled with a failure to control experimental pain, resulting in a high $P(A)$ and a low B. The opposite finding of a low $P(A)$ and high B to noxious stimulation suggests that the endogenous analgesic mechanisms were triggered, but were insufficient to ameliorate the far more intense endogenous stimulus responsible for the back pain.

The appearance of hyperalgesia at the affected site in the presence of hypoalgesia elsewhere in the chronic pain patients suggests the possibility that the LHPA axis is involved. Stress without chronic pain has been shown in a number of studies (Clark et al. 1986) to produce hypoalgesia to experimental pain in man. In particular, Janal et al. (1984) studied a group of marathon runners before and after a 10 km run and found decreased discriminability, $P(A)$, to thermal stimulation. They also found that the runners were hypoalgesic to tourniquet ischemic pain and in a euphoric mood following the run. These latter two effects were not found following the administration of naloxone, indicating that the stress had increased levels of endogenous opioids. They also found that the run had elevated the plasma levels of β-endorphin, adrenocorticotropic hormone (ACTH) prolactin and growth hormone, demonstrating the effect of stress on LHPA axis activity. That emotional distress can cause LHPA axis dysfunction is well established. Risch et al. (1983) reported that depressed patients showed adrenal cortisol hypersecretion, flattened cortisol circadian periodicity, failure of dexamethasone to suppress plasma cortisol concentrations, as well as increased plasma ACTH and β-endorphin levels. Thus, altered LHPA axis function might also explain the diminished thermal discriminability found by Clark and Mehl (1976) in psychiatric patients. It is also of interest that Atkinson et al. (1983) found chronic pain patients to have the highest plasma levels of β-endorphin, followed by a group of psychiatric patients, who in turn had higher levels than healthy controls. Thus, the plasma β-endorphin levels found in these groups paralleled the amount of thermal hypoalgesia found with SDT in our chronic pain, psychiatric illness and healthy volunteer groups. It may be concluded that hypoalgesia to calibrated noxious thermal stimulation reflects levels of brain and LHPA axis activity in response to stress and clinical pain, and, furthermore, that low $P(A)$ and high B serve as markers for the presence of stress and clinical pain.

In relation to the attributes of pain found with INDSCAL, the thermal pain data suggest that the back pain patients are high on the sensory pain magnitude dimension. In addition, the measures of high psychological distress found on the Brief Symptom Index (BSI) (Derogatis and Melisaratos 1983) suggest that these patients are also high on the emotional attribute of the pain qualities dimension. Thus, in the patient weight space of Fig. 2 the chronic back patients would probably fall further from the origin along the line formed by patient E and the origin.

The effect of atypical pain and anxiety on SDT parameters

We have recently studied a small group of patients suffering persistent pain who are in many ways at the opposite end of the spectrum from the chronic back pain patients (Wharton et al. 1985). These anxiety-prone patients suffer from a variety of atypical pains of unknown etiology, such as muscle pain, headaches, facial or abdominal pain. The pains are often diffuse, migratory and episodic rather than continuous. Most of the patients appeared to have an overly responsive sympathetic nervous system: for example, restoration of normal skin temperature and circulation following immersion of the hand in ice-water was abnormally prolonged. These initial findings suggest abnormal sympathetic nervous system functioning, although, in general, not to the extent that a diagnosis of sympathetic dystrophy could be made. The patients often appeared to be far more concerned with the possible medical significance of the pain than with the pain itself. All had been referred for psychiatric evaluation after two to three subspecialty work-ups had proved inconclusive, and various treatment attempts had produced mixed results. They tended to have family histories of sudden traumatic deaths, of severe medical illnesses with pain as a prominent feature (e.g. cancer), and a personal history of disturbed interpersonal relationships, including divorce. All had avoided surgery for their pain, and none were in litigation. Most were highly successful professionals in stressful, competitive occupations (e.g. stock broker, manager, TV producer). On the BSI they usually scored high on the anxiety scale. They also revealed a specific anxiety towards the noxious stimulus testing session, which they anticipated with obvious and often freely expressed anxiety. On these tests they over-reacted, labeling mild stimuli as painful; in brief, they may be described as pain amplifiers. These patients were diagnosed as suffering from a well-defined, chronic, generalized anxiety disorder, DSM-III category 300.02.

As has been described, some insight into the patient's attitude towards reporting clinical pain can be gained by measuring the response to calibrated noxious stimulation. The atypical pain patients were remarkably over-responsive to noxious stimuli. SDT analysis of their responses to thermal stimulation revealed that their discriminability, $P(A)$, was close to normal, but that they set an extremely low pain report criterion, B. Thermal intensities which the healthy volunteers called moderately painful, and which the chronic back patients called slightly painful, were labeled by the atypical pain patients as severely painful. In addition, these patients were overly sensitive to cold-pressor pain; immersion of the hand in ice-water was tolerated only 18 seconds, compared to 58 seconds for normals. For tourniquet pain these patients gave their first pain report after 3 minutes of ischemia compared to 11 minutes for controls. Obviously, compared to healthy volunteers and chronic back patients, atypical pain patients reported much more pain to these calibrated noxious stimuli. Anxiety has different effects in clinical and laboratory pain. In clinical pain, anxiety can induce headaches, muscle spasm and other pains, a sensory not a psychological effect. However, the effect of the brief situational anxiety which is encountered in experimental pain studies is to lower the pain report criterion; it does not influence the discriminability index. The reason for the low criterion probably is that anxious subjects, fearful of injury, respond 'pain' to low intensity stimuli hoping to induce the experimenter to avoid higher intensity stimuli. It seems likely that patients who describe relatively innocuous physical stimuli as painful may also be misinterpreting their clinical pain. The sensory experience which they label pain would be described by others as not painful. These patients are not necessarily deliberately misleading the physician and may well be unaware of their motivation.

That anxiety and not pain is the main problem of these patients is also supported by their response to treatment. Many of these patients, including some who had not responded to analgesics or antidepressants, responded to tranquilizers in the benzodiazepine family, including the triazolo analog, alprazolam. Treatment also included a more cognitive rather than psychoanalytic style of psychotherapy and a discussion of the meaning of pain as defined by the calibrated noxious thermal, cold pressor and tourniquet stimulation. Reassessment 6 months later revealed improved tolerance for the noxious cold pressor and tourniquet stimuli, as well as a raised (more stoical) criterion for the thermal stimuli. The patients themselves stated that they were now much less anxious about the pain tests, and about their clinical pain. The changes might be labeled as learned stoicism. The learning experience also may have promoted a cognitive restructuring of the meaning of pain. Perhaps they were now able to make a more valid distinction between the sensory pain and the emotional distress dimensions. In the context of the INDSCAL analysis of global pain the treatment may have caused the patients to find the emotional pain axis less salient.

The anxious, pain amplifying patients have yet to be studied by the INDSCAL method. However, it seems quite clear that these patients would fall high on the emotional attribute of the dimension, and low on the sensory pain magnitude dimension. Thus, members of this atypical pain group would be expected to fall in the region of patients I and H in Fig. 2.

Summary

In summary, the chronic back and atypical pain patients differed in a number of ways, which become comprehensible in the light of the SDT and INDSCAL models. The chronic back patients set a stoical pain report criterion, were poor discriminators of thermal stimuli, were depressed rather than anxious, and were in considerable pain when tested. In contrast, the atypical pain patients set a low thermal pain report criterion, were normal discriminators of thermal stimuli, were anxious rather than depressed, and were experiencing relatively little pain when tested. The diminished thermal discriminability of the chronic pain patients suggests the possibility that they have high (but still ineffective) levels of endogenous analgesics, which have been induced by the pain. The chronic pain patients were much less amenable to psychiatric or behavioral intervention, while the atypical pain patients were much more open. The latter learned to raise their pain report criterion and to understand the meaning of pain as a sensory as well as an emotional experience. The response of pain patients to experimental pain provides some indication for treatment. If they set a stoical criterion and are poor discriminators, then analgesics and antidepressant medication merit consideration. Conversely, if the patient sets a low pain report criterion to noxious stimuli, and discriminates well, then an anxiolytic may be indicated.

On the basis of the dimensions of global pain found with INDSCAL, we may speculate on the differences which may exist between the chronic back and atypical pain groups. The meaning of global pain for the anxious atypical pain patients was closely related to the emotional attribute of the pain qualities dimension and not to the sensory pain magnitude dimension. In contrast, for the chronic back pain patients, global pain was on both the sensory magnitude and pain qualities dimensions. The different responses of the chronic pain and atypical pain patients to thermal stimulation and to treatment suggest that they occupy different regions in the global pain space. Further work with more verbal descriptors might yield two emotional dimensions, depression and anxiety. In this case, for the chronic pain patients, the pure sensory pain dimension and an emotional depression dimension might be equally salient, while in the global pain space of the pain amplifiers, only an emotional anxiety dimension would appear as salient. The fact that chronic back pain patients tended to fare better with non-narcotic analgesics and mild antidepressants, while the atypical pain patients tended to do best with axiolytics, supports the saliency of these respective dimensions to these two groups of patients.

The INDSCAL model using responses to verbal descriptors and the SDT model using responses to physical stimuli point to new means of understanding the complaint of pain. INDSCAL forces us to examine what a patient means by pain (which dimension the patient is on) and SDT allows us to view the response bias of the patient in reporting pain.

Acknowledgement

Much of the research described here was supported by USPHS Grants NIGM-26461, MH-30906 and NINC DS-20248.

References

Atkinson, J. H., Kramer, E. F., Risch, S. C., Morgan, C. D., Azad, R. F., Ehlers, C. L. and Bloom, F. E. (1983) Plasma measures of beta-endorphin/beta-lipotropin-like immunoreactivity in chronic pain syndrome and psychiatric subjects. Psychiatr. Res. 9, 319–327.

Carroll, J. D. and Chang, J. J. (1970) Analysis of individual differences in multidimensional scaling via an N-way generalization of 'Eckart-Young' decomposition. Psychometrika 35, 283–319.

Clark, W. C. (1974) Pain sensitivity and the report of pain: an introduction to sensory decision theory. Anesthesiology 40, 272–287.

Clark, W. C. (1984) Applications of multidimensional scaling to problems in experimental and clinical pain: an introduction. In: B. Bromm (Ed.), New Approaches to Pain Measurement in Man. Elsevier Science Publ., Amsterdam, pp. 349–369.

Clark, W. C. and Ferrer-Brechner, T. (1985) A multidimensional scaling (INDSCAL) approach to pain in cancer patients and controls. Am. Psychol. Assoc. Los Angeles, CA, August.

Clark, W. C. and Mehl, L. (1976) Thermal pain: sensory (d') and criterion (L_x) differences between psychiatric patients and normals. 21st Internat. Congress of Psychol., Paris, France, July.

Clark, W. C. and Yang, J. C. (1983) Applications of sensory decision theory to problems in laboratory and clinical pain. In: R. Melzack (Ed.), Pain Measurement and Assessment. Raven Press, New York, pp. 15–25.

Clark, W. C., Yang, J. C. and Janal, M. N. (1986) Altered pain and visual sensitivity in humans: the effects of acute and chronic stress. In: D. Kelly (Ed.), Stress-Induced Analgesia. Ann. NY Acad. Sci.

Derogatis, L. R. and Melisaratos N. (1983) The brief symptom inventory: an introductory report. Psychol. Med. 13, 595–605.

Janal, M. N., Colt, E. W. D., Clark, W. C. and Glusman, M. (1984) Pain sensitivity, mood and plasma endocrine levels in man following long-distance running: effects of naloxone. Pain 19, 13–25.

McNicol, D. (1972) A Primer of Signal Detection Theory. George Allen & Unwin, London, England.

Risch, S. C., Janowsky, D. S., Judd, L. L., Gillin, J. C. and McClure, S. F. (1983) The role of endogenous opioid systems in neuroendocrine regulation. Psychiatr. Clin. North Am. 6, 429–441.

Wharton, R. N., Clark, W. C. and Yang, J. C. (1985) Pain amplification as a response to certain types of persistent pain. Am. Pain Soc., Dallas, TX, October.

Yang, J. C., Clark, W. C., Ngai, S. H., Berkowitz, B. A. and Spector, S (1979) Analgesic action and pharmacokinetics of morphine and diazepam in man: an evaluation by sensory decision theory. Anesthesiology 51, 495–502.

Yang, J. C., Wagner, J. M. and Clark, W. C. (1983) Psychological distress and mood in chronic pain and surgical patients: a decision theory analysis. In: J. J. Bonica et al. (Eds.), Advances in Pain Research and Therapy, Vol. 5. Raven Press, New York, pp. 901–906.

Yang, J. C., Richlin, D., Brand, L., Wagner, J. and Clark, W. C. (1985) Thermal sensory decision theory indices and pain threshold in chronic pain patients and healthy volunteers. Psychosom. Med. 47, 461–468.

Burrows/Elton/Stanley (eds.) Handbook of Chronic Pain Management
© *1987 Elsevier Science Publishers BV (Biomedical Division)*

8

A new method of research in the cross-cultural psychology of pain: An Italian case study

FAUSTO MASSIMINI[1], PAOLO INGHILLERI[2] and
MINALY CSIKSZENTMIHALYI[3]

[1] *Department of Psychology, University of Turin, Turin,* [2] *Institute of Psychology, Faculty of Medicine, University of Milan, Milan, Italy and* [3] *Department of Behavioral Sciences, University of Chicago, Chicago, Illinois, U.S.A.*

Researchers dealing with the area of pain in cross-cultural psychology are faced with a series of problems. First of all they need to gather data sufficiently homogeneous and comparable to those of other cultures or sub-cultures. Next they need terms and methods appropriate and understandable to the cultural and behavioral situation of the country or social group researched. Thirdly, particularly in laboratory studies, some of the techniques and interpretations of data may refer to the cognitive and emotional definition of pain of the researcher and his culture, rather than to those of the individuals tested.

Let us look at some of the problems more closely. We need to consider a) whether the meaning of pain is the same for both the researcher and the individual tested; b) whether it is given a physical or a psychological interpretation, or, as in the case of the Navajos (Reichard 1974), it is accepted as a total, inseparable, psychophysical experience; c) in a given country or culture, what are the cognitive, emotional and social characteristics of pain; d) interpretation of the threshold of pain, i.e. at which point is a noxious stimulus interpreted as pain in various cultures? We encountered these problems in our field research among various cultures; the Asmat tribe in western New Guinea, the Navajos in North America and the north-eastern cultures in Thailand. The relevant bibliography confirms it (Rajadhon 1968; Reichard 1974; Parratt 1976; Trenkenschuh 1978).

Correspondence should be addressed to: F. Massimini or P. Inghilleri, Istituto di Psicologia, Facolta Medica, Universita di Milano, Via F. Sforza 23, 20122 Milano, Italy.

These problems of methodology concern all areas of cross-cultural psychology (Triandis and Draguns 1980) and are also relevant to the cross-cultural study of pain. It seems necessary to find a method of research measuring states of consciousness and subjective experience in the course of daily living (Reis 1983). The collection of data must correspond to the cultural parameters of the sample group and at the same time be comparable to analogous data coming from different cultures.

Behavioral sciences have three broad research techniques at their disposal: a) measurement and research involving only observable behavior. In this case it is assumed that the researchers cannot investigate the individual's private life without altering the observed phenomena. These techniques are typical of the behaviorist school and of K. Lewin's followers. They are rigorously scientific but cannot study the intra-psychic aspects of the experience. b) Self-reports of behavior. This is an effective method for studying the individual's private and public life. In this case too, however, the focus of the study is behavior; the cognitive, emotional and affective aspects are ignored. c) Procedures to measure intra-psychic variables by self-assessment questionnaires. Research on personality has yielded psychometric methods to investigate, measure and analyze thoughts and emotions. Even in this case, however, there are methodological problems and possible criticisms. Various authors (Yarmey 1979; Fiske 1981) stress the dubious validity of data referring to subjective past experience recalled after a lapse of time.

Moreover, psychometric research has generally dealt with the study of stable personality traits rather than current daily experience, sometimes neglecting the study of how real situations and contexts influence subjective reality. So the three broad research techniques present a series of problems which are accentuated in the case of cross-cultural pain research.

The Experience Sampling Method

In recent years, M. Csikszentmihalyi and colleagues of the University of Chicago's Committee on Human Development have developed a procedure called Experience Sampling Method (ESM) (Csikszentmihalyi et al. 1977; Csikszentmihalyi and Graef 1980; Csikszentmihalyi 1982; Larson and Csikszentmihalyi 1983; Csikszentmihalyi and Larson 1984). This measurement and research procedure tends to partially overcome the abovementioned methodological problems. It seems to fulfill some of the basic requirements of research in cross-cultural psychology. ESM is a research instrument for the study of what people do, think and feel in their daily lives. It consists of asking the individuals to supply systematic self-reports at random times during the waking hours of their daily lives. The individuals are given questionnaire sheets and an electronic pager, often used to page doctors for urgent calls. With the pager it is possible to beep the individuals at random times according to a standard schedule, with a beep sent within every 2 hours from 8 a.m. to 10 p.m. (for research purposes it is possible to vary the time periods). When the individuals hear the beep, they fill out a sheet regarding their objective situation and subjective state at that particular moment. The questions concerning the objective situation include items relative to what they are doing, where they are and with whom. The answers are open-ended. Later, the researcher codes the answers according to specifically prepared categories and codes.

The questions regarding subjective states include items relative to thought content, cognitive, emotional and motivational states, and the perception of the present situation in interacting with others. Some of the answers are open-ended; for others differential semantic scales are used. The filling out of the questionnaire after each beep takes about 2–3 minutes.

The ESM has the following unique features when compared with other methods: a) it provides self-reports about on-going, real-life situations. b) It provides random observations representative of every aspect of waking life. It minimizes response sets typical of testing situations, laboratories, clinical settings or even daily reporting periods. c) In addition to what people do, and where, it measures a number of theoretically-based psychological dimensions: cognitive efficiency, quality of emotions and volitional states. At the same time, the ESM can accommodate any number of additional measures depending on specific research goals.

As far as the ESM's reliability and validity are concerned, see the work of Larson and Csikszentmihalyi (1983) and Csikszentmihalyi and Larson (1984). The Italian version of the ESM was developed by the authors of this chapter in direct collaboration with the University of Chicago. It seems evident that the ESM may be used to study individuals suffering from chronic or acute pain, either by using the basic version of the procedure or by adding specific items as required. The items are mainly open-ended and easily read, even with respect to the differential semantic scales; the test is given and completed in the course of daily living. For these two reasons, the ESM largely overcomes the bias possible in applying the test in different cultural contexts. It is, nonetheless, necessary first to do a correct translation in the language of the country where the method is being used and then proceed to an accurate standardization.

The use of the beeper creates a sense of urgency, and provides the impetus to fill in the questionnaires at the time rather than putting them off for a more opportune moment. One of the problems of self-reports, even if they are required to be filled in hourly by the subject, is that the subjects sometimes forget to fill them in at the time, and then resort to retrospective recollection.

Since the beep occurs at random intervals, i.e. sometimes at 45 minutes, and sometimes at 5 minutes, while sometimes after 2 hours' interval, no habitual adjustment to the procedure is possible and the account of the activities, thoughts and feelings reflects more closely the daily existence of the individual. Having concurrent recording of activities, thoughts and emotions provides ongoing multiple correlations between these variables.

The radio signal schedules are pre-arranged and sent to many subjects at once by an answering service, usually up to 30 subjects may be beeped at once. The random distribution of beeps is programmed by a computer. On receipt of responses, and after subsequent coding, SPSS program is used to attain statistical results.

The importance of this method from a cross-cultural viewpoint is that it demonstrates not only the differences but also the similarities between individuals and groups.

Case study – Sante

This study presents data on behavior, thoughts and emotions of an individual before and after a traffic accident, resulting in pain and probably some initial shock. Sante had been studied by the authors using the ESM prior to his accident as part of an Italian research into the possible usefulness of this method. He was therefore familiar with the use of the procedure, recording, etc. We present reports of his daily life for a period prior to the accident and a period post-accident (Figs. 1 and 2). As indicated by the graphs we recorded his activities, emotions, cognition and motivation. The accident resulted in physical consequences, pain, a cast, relative immobility. There were non-significant mood changes (Fig. 1) as he did not become more irritable or sad or depressed. The cognitive efficiency (Fig. 2) was decreased initially after the accident, presumably due to shock, but increased considerably in the following days as he needed to adjust to his altered condition. The thought content varied accordingly and focussed less on school and more on his present physical situation. (Tables 1 and 2).

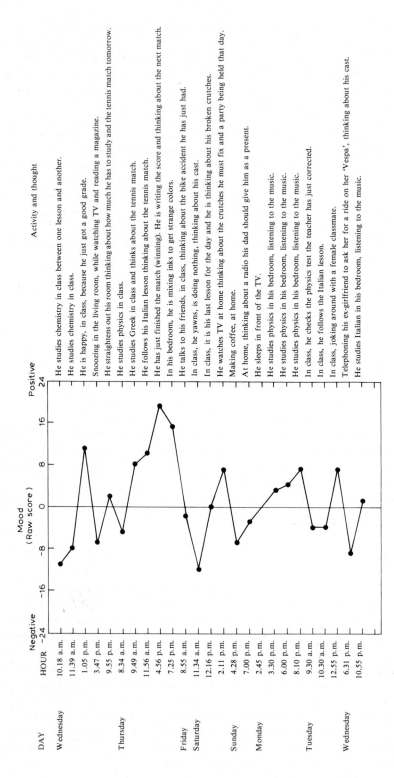

DAY	HOUR		Activity and thought
Wednesday	10.18 a.m.		He studies chemistry in class between one lesson and another.
	11.39 a.m.		He studies chemistry in class.
	1.05 p.m.		He is happy, in class, because he just got a good grade.
	3.47 p.m.		Snoozing in the living room, while watching TV and reading a magazine.
	9.55 p.m.		He straightens out his room thinking about how much he has to study and the tennis match tomorrow.
Thursday	8.34 a.m.		He studies physics in class.
	9.49 a.m.		He studies Greek in class and thinks about the tennis match.
	11.56 a.m.		He follows his Italian lesson thinking about the tennis match.
	4.56 p.m.		He has just finished the match (winning). He is writing the score and thinking about the next match.
	7.25 p.m.		In his bedroom, he is mixing inks to get strange colors.
Friday	8.55 a.m.		He talks to his friends, in class, thinking about the bike accident he has just had.
Saturday	11.34 a.m.		In class, he yawns, is doing nothing, thinking about his cast.
	12.16 p.m.		In class, it is last lesson for the day and he is thinking about his broken crutches.
	2.11 p.m.		He watches TV at home thinking about the crutches he must fix and a party being held that day.
	4.28 p.m.		Making coffee, at home.
Sunday	7.00 p.m.		At home, thinking about a radio his dad should give him as a present.
Monday	2.45 p.m.		He sleeps in front of the TV.
	3.30 p.m.		He studies physics in his bedroom, listening to the music.
	6.00 p.m.		He studies physics in his bedroom, listening to the music.
	8.10 p.m.		He studies physics in his bedroom, listening to the music.
Tuesday	9.30 a.m.		In class, he checks the physics test the teacher has just corrected.
	10.30 a.m.		In class, he follows the Italian lesson.
	12.55 p.m.		In class, joking around with a female classmate.
Wednesday	6.31 p.m.		Telephoning his ex-girlfriend to ask her for a ride on her 'Vespa', thinking about his cast.
	10.55 p.m.		He studies Italian in his bedroom, listening to the music.

Fig. 1.

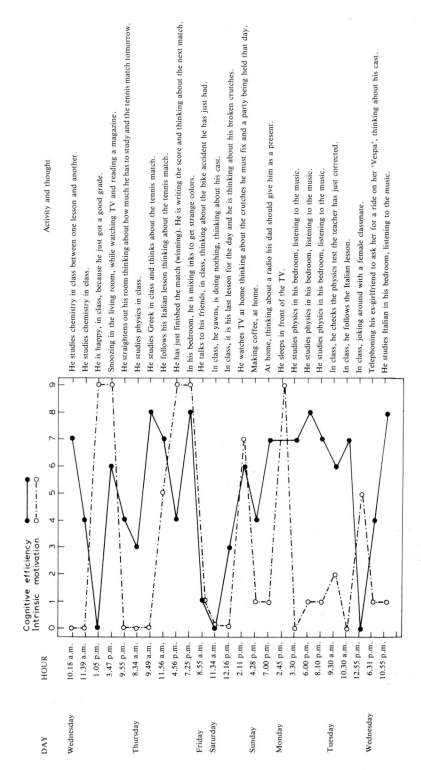

Fig. 2.

This example is of interest because it provides detailed information of mood swings in a pain-free adolescent, and an indication that some individuals do not respond as negatively to pain and immobility as might have been assumed without the use of this tool. Possibly, a study of another individual, who focusses on pain and is overwhelmed by the experience, would have yielded opposite data. We suggest therefore that this method provides information which is not available by other means.

TABLE 1

Activity before the accident	
School activities at school	50%
Loafing around	20%
Small leisure activities at home	10%
Marking the score of the tennis match	10%
Sleeping	10%

Activities after the accident	
Studying at home alone	26.66%
Studying at home with peers	6.66%
School activities at school	13.33%
Talking to friends	6.66%
Talking to friends on the phone	6.66%
Watching TV	6.66%
Loafing around	6.66%
Thinking	6.66%
Making himself a cup of coffee	6.66%
Sleeping	6.66%
Doing nothing	6.66%

TABLE 2

Thoughts before the accident	
Thoughts inherent to study and school	60%
Active sports	20%
Planning leisure time	10%
Sleeping	10%

Thoughts after the accident	
Thoughts inherent to study and school	33.33%
His own physical condition	13.33%
Thinking about his crutches	13.33%
Receiving a car radio as a gift	6.66%
Friends of the opposite sex	6.66%
Himself, personal psychological situation	6.66%
Eating	6.66%
The news	6.66%
Sleeping	6.66%

References

Csikszentmihalyi, M. (1982) Toward a psychology of optimal experience. In: L. Wheeler (Ed.), Review of Personality and Social Psychology, Vol. 2. Sage, Beverly Hills, California.

Csikszentmihalyi, M. and Graef, R. (1980) The experience of freedom in daily life. Am. J. Commun. Psychol. 8, 401 – 414.

Csikszentmihalyi, M. and Larson, R. (1984) Being Adolescent. Basic Books, New York.

Csikszentmihalyi, M., Larson, R. and Prescott, S. (1977) The ecology of adolescent activity and experience. J. Youth Adoles. 6, 281 – 294.

Fiske, D. (1981) Measuring the Concept of Personality. Aldine, Chicago.

Larson, R. and Csikszentmihalyi, M. (1983) The experience sampling method. In: H. Reis (Ed.), New Directions for Naturalistic Methods in the Behavioral Sciences. Jossey-Bass, San Francisco, pp. 41 – 56.

Lewin, K. (1951) Field theory in social science; selected theoretical papers. D. Cartwright (Ed.). Harper & Row, New York.

Parratt, J. (1976) Papuan Belief and Ritual. Vantage Press, New York.

Rajadhon, P. A. (1968) Essay on Thai Folklore. Editions Duang Kamol, Bangkok.

Reichard, G. A. (1974) Navaho Religion, 2nd edn. Princeton University Press, Princeton, Bollingen Series.

Reis, H. (Ed.) (1983) New Directions in the Behavioral Sciences Jossey-Bass, San Francisco.

Trenkenshuh, F. A. (Ed.) (1978) An Asmat Sketch Book, 2nd edn., No. 1 – 6. Hastings, Crossier Mission.

Triandis, H. C. and Draguns, J. G. (1980) Handbook of Cross-Cultural Psychology, No. 1 – 6. Allyn and Bacon, Boston.

Yarmey, D. (1979) The Psychology of Eyewitness Testimony. Free Press, New York.

Burrows/Elton/Stanley (eds.) Handbook of Chronic Pain Management
© *1987 Elsevier Science Publishers B.V. (Biomedical Division)*

9

Cognition and pain

MATISYOHU WEISENBERG

Department of Psychology, Bar-Ilan University, Ramat-Gan, Israel

Introduction

During the past 10 years, a greatly increased emphasis has been placed upon cognitive theory and techniques for dealing with psychological problems. Most notable has been the application of cognitive theory to the problems of coping with stress (cf. Roskies and Lazarus 1980), depression (cf. Beck 1976; Beck et al. 1979) as well as its broad clinical application to a variety of psychological problems (cf. Meichenbaum 1977).

The field of pain control also has been strongly influenced by cognitive and cognitive-behavioral approaches. Cognitions have been defined as 'A generic term embracing the quality of knowing which includes perceiving, recognizing, conceiving, judging, sensing, reasoning and imagining' (Stedman's Medical Dictionary 1976, p. 295). Many of the procedures used are concerned with the way the patient perceives, interprets, and relates to his pain rather than with the elimination of the pain stimulus per se. That is, the cognitions the person possesses in regard to his pain are what is of importance. For more lengthy, recent reviews of the cognitive-behavioral approaches to pain control the reader is referred to Turk et al. (1983) or Weisenberg (1984).

Theoretically, other established pain-control procedures recently have been reinterpreted on the basis of cognitive factors that might underlie them. For example, successful treatment of tension headache by means of biofeedback has been associated with patient beliefs of self-efficacy and changes in locus of control rather than with changes in physiology (Holroyd et al. 1984). Andrasik and Holroyd (1983) had taught tension-headache patients to either increase, decrease or achieve a stable level of forehead tension. Direction of forehead change did not effect successful outcomes that were maintained even at a 3-year follow-up. Success was viewed as due to the mediating psychological changes achieved rather than to changes in physiology as originally proposed by Budzynski et al. (1973).

In the area of hypnosis and pain control the cognitive rather than the dissociation approach (Hilgard 1973) has been favored as a means of explaining response differences between high and low hypnotically susceptible subjects (Spanos et al. 1984a, b). High or low hypnotic susceptibility subjects were assigned either to 1) a suggestion group where they were asked to imagine their hand as numb and insensitive, 2) a distraction task group (shadowing words read quickly), or 3) a control group without special instructions. Cold-pressor pain ratings between high and low hypnotic susceptible subjects differed for the suggestion group whereby the high susceptibles showed greater pain reduction. However, the distraction task was equally effective for both high and low hypnotic susceptibles compared with the control subjects. Both suggestion and distraction were viewed as changes in cognition. Low susceptible subjects were seen, however, as being poorer in their use of imaginal abilities. However, high and low susceptible subjects equally were capable of using attention diversion. Thus, different cognitive strategies might apply to different types of subjects. This latter point was taken further by D'Eon and Perry (1984) who found that hypnotic susceptibility level or cognitive strategy per se was not important in reducing reactions to pressure pain stimulation. What was most important was whether or not the subject had a choice of which strategy he would use.

Cognitions and pain theory

Conceptually, the gate-control theory (Melzack and Wall 1965, 1982) is still the most relevant for an understanding of the cognitive aspects of pain. Although the theory has been criticized on the basis of the specific neurophysiological mechanisms involved, conceptually it is widely accepted. Pain phenomena are viewed as consisting of several components. Pain has a sensory component similar to other sensory processes. It is discriminable in time, space, and intensity. However, pain also has an essential aversive-cognitive-motivational and emotional component that leads to behavior designed to escape or avoid the stimulus. Different neurophysiological mechanisms have been described for each system.

Great importance is attached to central nervous system processes, including learning, memory, and a host of perceptual functions. Higher cortical areas are involved in both discriminative and motivational systems influencing reactions on the basis of cognitive evaluation and past experience. More than any other theoretical approach, gate-control emphasizes the tremendous role of psychological variables and how they affect the reaction to pain. Especially with chronic pain, successful pain control often involves changing the cognitive-motivational components while the sensory component remains intact. Hypnosis, anxiety reduction, desensitization, attention distraction, as well as other cognitive-behavioral approaches can be effective alternatives and supplements to pharmacology and surgery in the control of pain. Their effect is felt mostly on the cognitive-motivational components of pain.

Cognitions, psychological theories, and pain control

Some of the earlier work on pain control primarily was designed to test derivations from psychological theory. For example, Zimbardo et al. (1966, 1969) tested derivations from the theory of cognitive dissonance to show how commitment, choice, and justification can affect pain reactions.

Attribution theory states that people seek causes or explanations for the observed events that take place around them. Thus, Davison and Valins (1969) showed how pain tolerance can be increased when subjects are taught to attribute pain tolerance changes to their own efforts as opposed to the effects of a pill.

Attribution of control as due to internal rather than external factors has been used as a key factor in the clinical treatment of low back patients (Gottleib et al. 1977). Patients with low back pain exhibit a learned helplessness as a result of their disability which tends to become reinforced by masses of medication and dependency on others. Patients are taught self-regulation rather than drug regulation for dealing with their problems as part of a comprehensive treatment program.

Control as a variable has been shown to be important in both laboratory and clinical settings. Perceived control has been associated with anxiety reduction and predictability (Bowers 1968; Staub et al. 1971). Clinically, it has been applied successfully even with post-surgical patients who were permitted to administer their own analgesic (Keeri-Szanto 1979).

In a recent review, Thompson (1981) defines control as a belief that a person has at his disposal a response that can influence the aversiveness of an event. Thompson concludes that behavioral control, in which the person knows he has a behavioral response to reduce aversiveness, does not reduce painfulness or stressfulness, but does increase tolerance of a noxious stimulus and post-event effects. Cognitive control does have uniform positive effects on an aversive event. Some cognitive strategies are more effective than others. Information about an aversive event will not necessarily reduce the pain, but could have some beneficial effect when paired with a means of coping.

For treatment of chronic pain the main ingredient may indeed be the feeling of control that is provided to subjects such as in the low back pain program of Gottleib et al. (1977). Melzack and Perry (1975), for example, conducted a clinical study of alpha training, hypnosis, and suggested benefits with three groups of chronic pain patients. Neither hypnosis per se nor alpha alone produced significant pain reduction. What was important was the creation of a sense of control.

Recently, Weisenberg et al. (1985) were able to demonstrate that control to be effective in pain reduction required some optimal level of control. The optimal level of control was found to be partially dependent upon such variables as a person's existing anxiety level and perceived self-efficacy of pain control.

Theoretically, the work of Roskies and Lazarus (1980) and Bandura (1977) relates to the issue of the cognitive control of pain. According to Roskies and Lazarus (1980), how a person psychologically copes with stress depends upon his cognitive view of the situation. This cognitive evaluative view, referred to as appraisal, is a dynamic process that changes according to the person's perceived anticipated consequence of an event, its importance to his well-being, and the perceived resources he has available to cope with the threat. The appraisal process changes as events change.

Coping has been classified according to the mode of action used (direct action, action inhibition, information search, intrapsychic processes) and according to the function it serves (problem-oriented or palliative regulation of the emotional response). Changing how a person thinks and feels in a given situation is viewed as an effective means of problem-solving.

Along with other cognitive theorists (cf. Beck 1976; Ellis 1962), belief systems are seen as exerting influence upon the cognitive appraisal. Emotion is a consequence of the cognitive appraisal (cf. Beck 1976). To handle stress, the person must learn to modify his appraisal of the environment and to manage his stress more effectively. Eliminating stress per se is not as important as learning to cope with it and to master it. Coping involves both what a person does and what he thinks and says to himself rather than simply what he does. This is in contrast to the behavioral view of Fordyce (1976) who says that if there is no pain behavior there is no problem of pain.

Effective coping depends upon a person's assessment of his competence. It is not enough to possess the relevant skills. The person must *believe* that he has them and believe he is capable of applying them as needed. This latter notion Bandura (1977) has referred to as self-efficacy. A person's belief in his own effectiveness will determine whether he will try to cope or avoid a situation that he views as beyond his coping ability. Efficacy expectations also can determine how much effort a person will invest and how long he will persist in the face of aversive experiences.

Laboratory studies of pain have drawn greatly from Roskies and Lazarus, and Bandura. Much of the emphasis has been on changing how subjects view the pain stimulus. In assessing the effectiveness of the cognitive strategies as used in pain perception in laboratory studies, Tan (1982) has related outcomes to the six major categories of cognitive strategies referred to by Turk (1978).

1) Imaginative inattention asks the subject to ignore the pain by using imagery that is incompatible with the pain, e.g. enjoying a pleasant day at the beach. Six studies were reported by Tan as showing this procedure to be more effective than a control for increasing pain tolerance or decreasing subjective reports of pain. In three studies imagery and control groups did not differ.

2) Imaginative transformation of pain asks the subject to interpret what he is feeling as something other than pain. Based upon pain tolerance, self-report and/or physiological measures, three studies showed this approach as superior to the control groups, while in three studies they were equal.

3) Imaginative transformation of context asks the subject to change the setting of the aversive stimulation, e.g. being chased by enemy agents. One study showed this procedure to be equal to the control group for increasing pain tolerance.

4) Attention-diversion (external) asks the subject to focus upon physical characteristics of the environment, e.g. counting ceiling tiles. One study showed this procedure to be more effective than the control, while two showed it to be equal for increasing pain threshold or tolerance or reducing self-report of pain.

5) Attention-diversion (internal) asks the subject to use self-generated thoughts, e.g. doing mental arithmetic. One study showed this strategy to be more effective, while three studies showed this approach to be equal to the control group for increasing pain tolerance, reducing self-reports of pain and/or changing physiological measures.

6) Somatization asks the person to focus upon the part of the body being stimulated in a detached manner. Four studies showed this approach to be superior to a control with none showing it to be equal based upon pain tolerance and/or self-report measures.

Based upon Turk's (1978) analysis there are 15 studies showing more effective pain tolerance for cognitive strategies, while 12 studies showed that these strategies were not superior to control groups.

Reviews by Tan (1982) and Turk et al. (1983) essentially support Turk's conclusion. One of the problems in assessing cognitive approaches is that control subjects are not passive, but tend to use their own cognitive strategies spontaneously (cf. Scott and Barber 1977; Scott 1978). Other factors that can influence outcome include perceived efficacy (Girodo and Wood 1979) and perceived involvement (Jaremko 1978). As Tan (1982) points out, studies also differ in terms of type of pain stimulus, different measures, different instructions and experimental demands and different experimental designs.

Meichenbaum and Turk (1976), Meichenbaum (1977), and Turk (1978) developed what they call stress-inoculation training. Stress-inoculation attempts to deal with individual differences by offering subjects a variety of different strategies. Subjects choose those strategies which they feel most capable of using. There is a period of training prior to exposure to the pain situation. During the education phase, subjects are told of the different components of pain as used in gate-control theory, and subjects are provided with different coping strategies to use for each component. Subjects are taught relaxation and slow breathing. They can choose from such strategies as attention-diversion or somatic focusing. Imagery manipulations are taught to change the pain stimulation by reinterpreting what is being experienced. Subjects are taught how to generate self-statements to deal with the different phases, such as preparing for pain, confronting pain, and self-reinforcement for having coped. Examples of such statements are: 'What is it you have to do?' (preparation statement). 'Just relax, breathe deeply, and use one of the strategies' (confrontation statement). 'You handled it pretty well' (reinforcing self-statement).

Prior to actual confrontation with the pain stimuli, subjects are given the opportunity to practice using different strategies while imagining they were being stimulated. Subjects are also asked to role-play giving advice to a new subject. The entire training procedure took one hour. Subjects were then exposed to ischemic pain. Compared to a pretest of 17 minutes, post-training tolerance increased to 32 minutes. Meichenbaum and Turk refer to earlier evidence that 10 mg of morphine were only capable of increasing ischemic pain tolerance by 10 minutes compared to the 15 minutes obtained here. Control subjects did not shown any significant increase. Greater detail in the use of stress-inoculation approaches can be found in Turk et al. (1983).

Horan et al. (1977) performed a component analysis of stress-inoculation. Separate groups were provided the educational component, coping skills training, the full stress-inoculation procedure, no treatment control or a repeated exposure condition, in which the cold-pressor was presented six times. Results indicated that the education component was not effective by itself, while the coping skills group resulted in an increased threshold and tolerance. Education as part of stress-inoculation, however, was more effective than coping skills alone. Repeated exposure appeared to reduce the effectiveness of the preparation. Generalization to pressure algometer was not obtained.

In a follow-up study, Hackett et al. (1979) found that multiple exposure in stress-inoculation is less effective than one-time exposure. When instructions were included to enhance generalization, pain tolerance generalization for pressure algometer was obtained.

Hackett and Horan (1980) questioned the contribution of the self-instructional component. This component was largely ignored by subjects during the stressor itself. Perhaps the perceived efficacy of the treatment procedure was not conveyed to subjects.

Clinically, Wernick et al. (1981) assessed the effectiveness of a stress-inoculation procedure for eight severely burned patients compared to eight patients not provided special training. Burns represent a severe challenge to coping ability. Not only is the original wound painful, but the treatment itself is very painful. The stress-inoculation treatment group showed significant differences on nine dependent measures, while the no-treatment group did on two – physical self-rating and emotional self-rating. Although this study has a number of methodological problems, it is a demonstration of stress-inoculation effectiveness under difficult conditions.

Other clinical studies and applications

Cognitive-behavioral approaches now have been used for a variety of clinical problems either as the main treatment approach or as part of a combined treatment. Problems include, among others, headache (Brown 1984), prepared childbirth (Melzack 1984), preparation for surgery (Faust and Melamed 1984), low-back pain (Turk and Flor 1984), burns (Wernick et al. 1981), cancer (Turk et al. 1983), combined programs (Khatami and Rush 1982). Detailed instructions for the application of pain-control strategies have appeared in a variety of books and manuals (cf. McCaffery 1979; McCaffery et al. undated; Sternbach 1983; Turk et al. 1983).

Concluding comment

This brief review of studies, as well as others not mentioned, does support the effectiveness of cognitive strategies in clinical settings. What remains unclear, however, is what the critical ingredients should be, as many of the studies used combined procedures or did not have control groups. Dependent measures also are not consistently used across studies, leaving doubt as to what outcomes can be expected. What is also unclear are just which cognitive approaches or techniques work under which conditions. Serious questions still remain concerning just which cognitive ingredients are critical. What is missing is a clear theoretical statement that would tie the different cognitive aspects together. Bandura's (1977) self-efficacy approach is one possibility. Perhaps the specific cognitive strategy per se is of lesser importance. What is important is that the person believe it helps. Another alternative would be that some cognitive strategies do possess active ingredients that go beyond belief. The belief factor is necessary, however, to insure the use of the strategy. Whichever view is correct, cognitive-behavioral techniques are still of great value in pain control.

References

Andrasik, F. and Holroyd, K. A. (1983) Specific and nonspecific effects in the biofeedback treatment of tension headache: 3-year follow-up. J. Consult. Clin. Psychol. 51, 634–636.
Bandura, A. (1977) Self-efficacy: toward a unifying theory of behavioral change. Psychol. Rev. 84, 191–215.
Beck, A. T. (1976) Cognitive Therapy and the Emotional Disorders. International Universities Press, New York.
Beck, A. T., Rush, A. J., Shaw, B. F. and Emery, G. (1979) Cognitive Therapy of Depression. Guilford Press, New York.
Bowers, K. S. (1968) Pain, anxiety, and perceived control. J. Consult Clin. Psychol. 32, 596–602.
Brown, J. M. (1984) Imagery coping strategies in the treatment of migraine. Pain 18, 157–167.
Budzynski, T. H., Stoyva, J. M., Adler, C. S. and Mullaney, D. J. (1973) EMG biofeedback and tension headache: a controlled outcome study. Psychosom. Med. 35, 484–496.
Davison, G. S. and Valins, S. (1969) Maintenance of self-attributed and drug-attributed behavior change. J. Personal. Soc. Psychol. 11, 25–33.
D'Eon, J. L. and Perry, C. W. (1984) The role of imagery and coping cognitions in response to pressure pain as moderated by choice of pain control strategy. Paper presented at the meeting of the American Psychological Association, Toronto.
Ellis, A. (1962) Reason and Emotion in Psychotherapy. Lyle Stuart, New York.
Faust, J. and Melamed, B. G. (1984) Influence of arousal, previous experience and age on surgery preparation of same day of surgery and in-hospital pediatric patients. J. Consult. Clin. Psychol. 52, 359–365.
Fordyce, W. E. (1976) Behavioral Methods for Chronic Pain and Illness. C. V. Mosby, St. Louis.
Girodo, M. and Wood, D. (1979) Talking yourself out of pain: the importance of believing that you can. Cog. Ther. Res. 3, 23–33.
Gottleib, H., Strite, L. C., Koller, R., Madorsky, A., Hockersmith, V., Kleeman, M. and Wagner, J. (1977) Comprehensive rehabilitation of patients having chronic low back pain. Arch. Phys. Med.

Rehab. 58, 101 – 108.

Hackett, G. and Horan, J. J. (1980) Stress inoculation for pain: what's really going on? J. Consult. Psychol. 27, 107 – 116.

Hackett, G., Horan, J. J., Buchanan, J. and Zumoff, P. (1979) Improving exposure generalization potential of stress inoculation for pain. Percep. Motor Skills 48, 1132 – 1134.

Hilgard, E. R. (1973) A neodissociation interpretation of pain reduction in hypnosis. Psychol. Rev. 80, 396 – 411.

Holroyd, K. A., Penzien, D. B., Hursey, K. G., Tobin, D. L., Rogers, L., Holm, J. E., Marcille, P. J., Hall, J. R. and Chila, A. G. (1984) Change mechanisms in EMG biofeedback training: cognitive changes underlying improvements in tension headache. J. Consult. Clin. Psychol. 52, 1037 – 1053.

Horan, J. J., Hackett, G., Buchanan, J. D., Stone, I. and Demchik-Stone, D. (1977) Coping with pain: a component analysis of stress inoculation. Cog. Ther. Res. 1, 211 – 221.

Jaremko, M. E. (1978) Cognitive strategies in the control of pain tolerance. J. Behav. Ther. Exp. Psychiatr. 9, 239 – 244.

Keeri-Szanto, M. (1979) Drugs or drums: what relieves postoperative pain? Pain 6, 217 – 230.

Khatami, M. and Rush, A. J. (1982) A one-year follow-up of the multimodal treatment for chronic pain. Pain 14, 45 – 52.

McCaffery, M. (1979) Nursing Management of the Patient with Pain. J. B. Lippincott, Philadelphia, PA.

McCaffery, M., Morra, M. E., Gross, J. and Moritz, D. A. (undated) Dealing with Pain: A Handbook for Persons with Cancer and Their Families, American Cancer Society Connecticut Division. Yale Comprehensive Cancer Center, New Haven, CT.

Meichenbaum, D. (1977) Cognitive Behavior Modification. Plenum Press, New York.

Meichenbaum, D. and Turk, D. (1976) The cognitive-behavioral management of anxiety, anger, and pain. In: P. O. Davidson (Ed.), The Behavioral Management of Anxiety, Depression, and Pain. Brunner/Mazel, New York, p. 1.

Melzack, R. (1984) The myth of painless childbirth. Pain 19, 321 – 337.

Melzack, R. and Perry, C. (1975) Self-regulation of pain. The use of alpha-feedback and hypnotic training for the control of chronic pain. Exper. Neurol. 46, 452 – 469.

Melzack, R. and Wall, P. D. (1965) Pain mechanisms: a new theory. Science 150, 971 – 979.

Melzack, R. and Wall, P. D. (1982) The Challenge of Pain. Penguin Books, Middlesex, England.

Roskies, E. and Lazarus, R. S. (1980) Coping theory and the teaching of coping skills. In: P. O. Davidson and S. M. Davidson (Eds.), Behavioral Medicine: Changing Health Lifestyles. Brunner/Mazel, New York, p. 38.

Scott, D. S. (1978) Experimenter-suggested cognitions and pain control: problem of spontaneous strategies. Psychol. Rep. 43, 156 – 158.

Scott, D. S. and Barber, T. X. (1977) Cognitive control of pain: four serendipitous results. Percep. Motor Skills 44, 569 – 570.

Spanos, N. P., Kennedy, S. K. and Gwynn, M. I. (1984a) Moderating effects of contextual variables on the relationship between hypnotic susceptibility and suggested analgesia. J. Abnorm. Psychol. 93, 285 – 294.

Spanos, N. P., McNeil, C., Gwynn, M. I. and Stam, H. J. (1984b) Effects of suggestion and distraction on reported pain in subjects high and low on hypnotic susceptibility. J. Abnorm. Psychol. 93, 277 – 284.

Staub, E., Tursky, B. and Schwartz, G. E. (1971) Self-control and predictability: their effects on reactions to aversive stimulation. J. Pers. Soc. Psychol. 18, 157 – 162.

Stedman's Medical Dictionary, 3rd edn. (1976) Williams & Wilkins, Baltimore.

Sternbach, R. A. (1983) How Can I Learn to Live with Pain When it Hurts so Much? Scripps Clinic and Research Foundation, La Jolla, CA.

Tan, S. Y. (1982) Cognitive and cognitive-behavioral methods for pain control: a selective review. Pain 12, 201 – 228.

Thompson, S. C. (1981) Will it hurt less if I can control it? A complex answer to a simple question. Psychol. Bull. 90, 89 – 101.

Turk, D.C. (1978) Cognitive-behavioral techniques in the management of pain. In: J. P. Foreyt and D. P. Rathjen (Eds.), Cognitive Behavior Therapy: Research and Application. Plenum Press, New York, p. 199.

Turk, D. C. and Flor, H. (1984) Etiological theories and treatment for chronic back pain. II. Psychological models and interventions. Pain 19, 209 – 233.

Turk, D. C., Meichenbaum, D. and Genest, M. (1983) Pain and Behavioral Medicine: A Cognitive-Behavioral Perspective. Guilford Press, New York.

Weisenberg, M. (1984) Cognitive aspects of pain. In: P. D. Wall and R. Melzack (Eds.), Textbook of Pain. Churchill Livingstone, Edinburgh.

Weisenberg, M., Wolf, Y., Mittwoch, T., Mikulincer, M. and Aviram, O. (1985) Subject versus experimenter control in the reaction to pain. Pain 23, 187 – 200.

Wernick, R. L., Jaremko, M. E. and Taylor, P. W. (1981) Pain management in severely burned adults: a test of stress inoculation. J. Behav. Med. 4, 103 – 109.

Zimbardo, P. G., Cohen, A. R., Weisenberg, M., Dworkin, L. and Firestone, I. (1966) Control of pain motivation by cognitive dissonance. Science 151, 217 – 219.

Zimbardo, P. G., Cohen, A. R., Weisenberg, M., Dworkin, L. and Firestone, I. (1969) The control of experimental pain. In: P. G. Zimbardo (Ed.), The Cognitive Control of Motivation. Scott, Foresman, Glenview, IL, p. 100.

Burrows/Elton/Stanley (eds.) Handbook of Chronic Pain Management
© *1987 Elsevier Science Publishers B.V. (Biomedical Division)*

10

Behavioural approaches in pain management

DENNIS C. TURK[1] and DONALD MEICHENBAUM[2]

[1] Center for Pain Evaluation and Treatment, University of Pittsburgh School of Medicine, Pittsburgh, Pennsylvania, U.S.A., and [2] Department of Psychology, Faculty of Arts, University of Waterloo, Waterloo, Ontario, Canada

Prior to the later half of the 19th century, the importance of psychological factors in the experience of pain had received substantial attention. Aristotle classified pain as an emotion and the Stoic philosophers suggested that pain could be 'overcome' through logic and 'rational repudiation'. The philosopher Immanuel Kant, described the utility of attention diversion to cope with pain in the 18th century. In fact, prior to the late 1800's, all treatments for pain might be associated largely with psychological factors because the treatments prescribed often had no active ingredient and may even have been detrimental. For example, the physician's pharmacopeia included oil derived from ants, human perspiration, crocodile dung, and just about every organic and inorganic substance known; and surgeons employed leeching, blister raising, and cupping to ameliorate pain. Perhaps the most striking point to note when examining the range of treatments utilized is that for at least some individuals the therapeutic regimen had some beneficial effects. This latter point underscores the important contribution of psychological factors that have sometimes been disparagingly referred to as only 'placebo effects'. Recent evidence has begun to reveal that so-called placebo effects do have a physical basis perhaps by increasing production of endogenous opioids (e.g. Levine et al. 1978; Chen 1980).

The lack of interest in the contribution of psychological factors appears to be related to advances in sensory psychophysics and physiology. With increased sophistication in these areas, psychological factors were relegated as reactions to sensory stimulation and consequently considered as being of secondary importance. Even with accumulating knowledge about sensory physiology and the development of a plethora of medical, surgical, and pharmacological interventions, permanent and consistent amelioration of chronic pain has remained elusive. Patients with ostensibly the same syndrome respond quite differently to their condition and to the treatments prescribed or performed. Thus, although we have achieved tremendous sophistication in our understanding of sensory processes and in the development of somatic treatments, there continues to be a substantial number of patients who do report pain despite the best efforts of physicians and surgeons. Moreover, there continue to be pain syndromes for which the physical bases are obscure (e.g. Malow et al. 1981; Flor and Turk 1984). This frustrating state of affairs has led to the development of a dichotomy of somatic (true) pain and functional or psychogenic (imaginary) pain. Psychogenic pain is often viewed as being within the domain of psychiatry and psychology and not that of somatic medical specialties.

In the mid-1960's, three trends resulted in renewed interest in the contribution of psychological factors to the pain experience. Melzack and his collaborators (Melzack and Wall 1965; Melzack and Casey 1968) proposed a model of pain, the Gate Control Theory, that emphasized the important contribution of psychological factors as well as sensory phenomena in the experience of pain. They suggested that cognitive-evaluative factors (e.g. the patient's appraisal of sensory stimulation, the context in which the stimulation was induced, along with prior learning) and motivational-affective factors (e.g. anxiety, distress, desire to avoid noxious sensory input) modulate the experience of pain. That is, pain was both centrally and peripherally mediated. The Gate Control Theory has received a great deal of attention and it has not been without its critics (e.g. Nathan 1976). Yet, this theory has served to renew interest in the potential contribution of psychological variables.

The second impetus to interest in psychological factors came from a quite different source, namely, Fordyce's (1968) formulation of an operant conditioning model of chronic pain. Fordyce suggested that since pain is a subjective experience it can never be observed, rather what is observable are 'pain behaviours'. Pain behaviours consist of specific communications that a patients emits that indicate the presence of pain. These behaviours include both verbal statements and non-verbal indicants (e.g. limping, rubbing a painful body part, grimacing). According to Fordyce, these behaviours are learned, perhaps initially as a protective mechanism or as a way to receive attention for the subjective experience. However, over time, these pain behaviours become positively reinforced whereas other behaviours, 'well-behaviours' (e.g. activity, work) are negatively reinforced and eventually are extinguished. Chronic pain patients continue to complain and express distress, often with increasing urgency required to obtain attention, and they become more sedentary with their lives becoming more and more restricted. As was the case with the Gate Control theory, Fordyce's Operant Model has received much attention but it has also attracted critics who suggest that it is superficial (Pinsky 1980) or inadequate (Linton et al., in press).

Finally, the development of sophisticated computers, sensitive psychophysiological monitoring equipment, and the demonstration that autonomic processes, once believed to be involuntary, could be controlled by the individual led to increased interest in biofeedback training as in the case of patients suffering from migraine headaches, low back pain, and temporomandibular pain dysfunction syndrome. These developments reflected increased interest in the ability of pain patients to learns to 'self-control' physiological processes and thereby their pain.

Each of these three trends has fostered a set of treatments for chronic pain. Melzack and Wall's Gate Control Theory (1965) emphasized the need to consider cognitive and affective as well as sensory factors when treating pain. Fordyce's (1968) operant conditioning model emphasized reinforcement of well-behaviours and the extinction of pain behaviours, and biofeedback emphasized the importance of teaching patients control of their physiological processes putatively related to the cause of the pain. Since the development of these approaches, a multitude of studies has appeared supporting the efficacy of each and a number of reviews have been published that summarize the relative efficacy of the approaches (e.g. Turk et al. 1979, 1983; Hall 1982; Turner and Chapman 1982a, b; Keefe and Hoelscher, in press).

Many variations of psychologically-oriented treatments have evolved ranging from family psychotherapy to assertiveness training to cognitive restructuring to relaxation training. These have been used alone or in conjunction with innovative surgical procedures, acupuncture, nerve blocks, transcutaneous nerve stimulators, dorsal column stimulators, ultrasound, and so forth. It is interesting to contemplate how such a diversity of interventions can all produce similar beneficial effects. In a sense, we can learn from the treatments prescribed prior to the 19th century, for they too were diverse and had some therapeutic effects. What we are suggesting is that there may be a common set of factors that underlies the positive effects reported for the diversity of treatment modalities.

Turk and his colleagues (Genest and Turk 1979; Turk et al. 1983, 1986) have suggested that several factors appear to be common across treatment approaches. First, they suggest that all psychologically-based treatments and even somatic treatments either directly or indirectly affect patients' conceptualizations of their pain problem. Practitioners attempt to present a conceptualization of pain, either formally or informally, that establishes the rationale for the treatment offered. Thus, the operant-conditioning therapist provides a conditioning model to conceptualize the patient's current pain. Practitioners who rely on biofeedback present a conceptualization of pain based on maladaptive psychophysiological hyperactivity. And the cognitive-behavioural therapist working within the Gate Control Theory, suggests that the experience of pain is an interaction among thoughts, feelings, behaviour, and sensory phenomena. The important point underlying each approach is that a workable conceptualization of pain emerges between the therapist and patient (and in some instances family members). The type of questions and assessment procedures the therapist uses, the treatment rationale offered, and the various treatment procedures employed all contribute to the implicit (re)conceptualization process.

Each of the behavioural approaches, operant conditioning, biofeedback, and cognitive behaviour modification have at least four characteristics in common.

1) They offer a conceptualization to the patient that is likely to differ from the one the patient brings with him or her. Implicitly or explicitly, the therapist attempts to shape the patient's conceptualization to one that is consistent with that of the therapist and the treatment offered. For example, many pain patients have a conception of illness that is based on an acute disease model. Pain is viewed as a primary symptom being caused by something discrete and out of the patient's direct control (e.g. a pathogen, tissue damage). Pain is expected to be susceptible to specific medical treatments that will exert their beneficial effects in a relatively brief period of time (viz. 'there is a pill for every ill'). According to this model, things are done to the patient, and the patient has little or no role in potentiating or eliminating pain. This acute model places minimal responsibility on the patient and encourages and rewards passivity. The acute model conveys the message that the patient's pain is largely beyond his or her ability to change and out of his or her control. The reconceptualization process is designed to help patients develop a self-management perspective by helping them collect and then evaluate data that implicate the role of psychological factors in the experience of pain. Patients are not mere victims of pain, but how they appraise sensations and their ability to cope will influence the level and intensity of their pain experience. The various behavioural treatments, each in their own way, convey that patients are not helpless in dealing with their pain. Although the specific procedures used by various behaviour therapists differ, a common objective is to nurture a reconceptualization process.

2) They each provide an optimistic view that encourages hope and that combats demoralization. They foster a sense of learned resourcefulness as compared to learned helplessness.

3) They encourage the patient's active participation in the treatment process, placing some responsibility for the success of the treatment on the patient.

4) They assist the patient in the acquisition of new skills or behaviours or attempt to increase

or strengthen existing ones. For example, in cognitive behavioural treatment pain patients are taught such diverse skills as relaxation, attention diversion by means of imagery and non-imagery techniques, intra- and interpersonal coping skills. A central feature of these training procedures is the inclusion of relapse prevention or the need to anticipate and subsume possible future setbacks and failures into the training regimen. As reviewed by Turk et al. (1983), the initial results of such multifaceted training programmes have been quite encouraging.

Illustrative of this cognitive behavioural approach are studies by Herman and Baptiste (1981), Rybstein-Blinchik and Grzesiak (1979), and Turner (1982) who successfully treated patients who suffered from chronic pain complaints. The combined use of cognitive restructuring, relaxation, guided imagery and stress management were successful in reducing reports of pain severity, the intake of analgesic medication, anxiety levels, while increasing self-reports of ability to tolerate pain and participation in normal activities. These improvements were evident in the brief follow-up periods (several months). As Turk et al. (1983) note, such studies require more extensive clinical trials and much work along these lines is now underway.

Behavioural treatment programmes are likely to prove effective insofar as a number of general conditions are met: a) there is a fit between the patient's conceptualization of their problem and the rationale of the treatment being offered; b) the expected value of more adaptive behaviour for the patient is emphasized rather than the worth of these behaviours for the practitioner; c) the patient has or can be provided with the necessary skills to carry out more adaptive responding; d) the patient believes that the treatment components will be effective in alleviating problems; e) the patient believes that he is competent to perform the skilled acts that make up the treatment regimen; and f) there is sufficient intrinsic and extrinsic reinforcement for the maintenance and generalization of the skills incorporated within the treatment regimen. The patient's beliefs may be even more important than the specific behavioural modalities employed. Insufficient attention has been given to these 'non-specific factors' in the enthusiasm for the intricacies of the treatment modalities per se (e.g. the size of the electrodes, the nature of the distracting image, characteristics of the homework assignments).

In summary, a variety of diverse lines of evidence has implicated the role of psychosocial factors in the exacerbation and maintenance of pain. In recent years, many behaviour therapy procedures have been developed to treat pain patients. These procedures can be viewed as supplements to somatic forms of treatment. In fact, in combination they may have important synergistic effects. As Turk and Holzman (1986) note, there is a tendency for a merging of views, where multicomponent treatments that employ a host of techniques are the norm. Treatment programmes that attend to both the sensory and behavioural components of pain are more likely to be successful.

As research continues, the arbitrary distinction between so-called psychogenic and somatic perspectives is breaking down. Simplistic dichotomies between structural versus functional; peripheral mediation versus central mediation, mind versus body are being put aside. The work of behaviour therapists has underscored the need for such an integrative interdisciplinary treatment perspective.

References

Chen, A. C. N. (1980) Behavioral and brain evoked potential (BEP) evaluation of placebo effects: contrasts of cognitive mechanisms and endorphin mechanisms. Paper presented at the second general meeting of the American Pain Society, New York.

Flor, H. and Turk, D. C. (1984) Etiological theories and treatments for chronic back pain. I. Somatic factors. Pain 19, 105 – 121.

Fordyce, W. E., Fowler, R. S., Lehmann, J. and DeLateur, B. (1968) Some implications of learning in problems of chronic pain. J. Chron. Dis. 21, 179 – 190.

Genest, M. and Turk, D. C. (1979) A proposed model for group therapy with pain patients. In: D. Upper and S. M. Ross (Eds.), Behavioral Group Therapy: An Annual Review. Research Press, New York, pp. 237 – 276.

Hall, W. (1982) Psychological approaches to the evaluation of chronic pain patients. Aust. N.Z. J. Psychaitry 16, 3 – 9.

Herman, E. and Baptiste, S. (1981) Pain control: mastery through group experience. Pain 10, 79 – 86.

Keefe, F. J. and Hoelscher, T. (1987) Biofeedback in the management of chronic pain syndromes. Biofeedback Society of America (in press).

Levine, J. D., Gordon, N. C. and Fields, H. L. (1978) The mechanism of placebo analgesia. Lancet 1, 654 – 657.

Linton, S. J., Melin, L. and Gotestam, K. G. (1987) Behavioral analysis of chronic pain and its management. In: M. Hersen, R. Eisler, and P. Miller (Eds.), Progress in Behavior Modification, Vol 18. Academic Press, Orlando (in press).

Lipton, J. A. and Marbach, J. J. (1984) Ethnicity and the pain experience. Soc. Sci. Med. 19, 1279 – 1298.

Malow, R. M., Olson, R. E. and Greene, C. S. (1984) Myofascial pain dysfunction syndrome: a psychophysiological disorder. In: C. Golden, S. Alcaparras, F. Strider and B. Graefer, (Eds.), Applied Techniques in Behavioral Medicine. Grune & Stratton, New York, pp. 101 – 133.

Melzach, R. and Casey, K. L. (1968) Sensory, motivational, and central control determinants of pain: a new conceptual model. In: D. Kenshalo (Ed.), The Skin Senses. Charles C. Thomas, Springfield, Illinois, pp. 121 – 139.

Melzack, R. and Wall, P. D. (1965) Pain mechanisms: a new theory. Science 50, 971 – 979.

Nathan, P. W. (1976) The gate-control theory of pain: a critical review. Brain 99, 123 – 158.

Pinsky, J. (1980) The behavioral consequences of chronic intractable benign pain. Behav. Med. 7, 12 – 20.

Rybstein-Blinchik, E. and Grzesiak, R. C. (1979) Reinterpretive cognitive strategies in chronic pain management. Arch. Phys. Med. Rehab. 60, 609 – 612.

Turk, D. C. and Holzman, A. D. (1986) Commonalities among psychological approaches in the treatment of chronic pain: specifying the metaconstructs. In: A. D. Holzman and D. C. Turk (Eds.), Pain Management: A Handbook of Psychological Treatment Approaches. Pergamon Press, Elmsford, New York, pp. 257 – 268.

Turk, D. C., Meichenbaum, D. and Berman, W. H. (1979) The application of biofeedback for the regulation of pain: a critical review. Psychol. Bull. 86, 1322 – 1338.

Turk, D. C., Holzman, A. D. and Kerns, R. D. (1986) Treatment of chronic pain: emphasis on self-management. In: K. A. Holroyd and T. L. Creer (Eds.), Self-Management of Chronic Disease: A Handbook of Clinical Interventions and Research. Academic Press, Orlando, pp. 441 – 472.

Turk, D. C., Meichenbaum, D. and Genest, M. (1983) Pain and Behavioral Medicine: A Cognitive-Behavioral Perspective. Guilford Press, New York.

Turner, J. A. (1982) Comparison of group progressive-relaxation training and cognitive-behavior therapy for chronic low back pain. J. Consult. Clin. Psychol. 50, 757 – 765.

Turner, J. A. and Chapman, C. R. (1982a, b) Psychological interventions for chronic pain: a critical review I. and II. Pain 12, 1 – 46.

Burrows/Elton/Stanley (eds.) Handbook of Chronic Pain Management
© *1987 Elsevier Science Publishers B.V. (Biomedical Division)*

11

Emotional variables and chronic pain

DIANA ELTON

Department of Psychology, University of Melbourne, Victoria 3052, Australia

Introduction

Psychological factors play an important role in pain experience, and there is considerable evidence, that anxiety, depression, low self-esteem, hysteria and anger, can cause an increase in pain (Elton et al. 1983). Distinction between the perceptual, cognitive and emotional variables in pain experience is convenient for expository purposes, but is purely artificial, as they are all interconnected (Schachter and Singer 1962; Arnold 1970). As shown by Ellis and Harper (1975), there can be no sustained emotion without thought, which maintains the emotional state. Equally, there can be no thought without a prior perception of the event by the individual. Even if such perception seems objectively irrational, it may have subjective reality for the patient, and may influence thoughts, feelings and behaviour. Excessive emotional reactions have a profound effect on the function of the autonomic nervous system, particularly the sympathetic nervous system, and its endocrine interconnections. It has been recognized by workers in the area of stress (Selye 1976) that many pathological conditions are associated with stress reactions. The fight or flight response of the body results in increased neural stimulation, and a production of complex biochemical substances, which disturb the homeostasis of the body. Negative emotional states can stimulate the production of adrenaline and noradrenaline, corticoids, and other biochemicals. They can speed up the activity of the heart, increase blood pressure, change functional activity of the stomach, and other organs. Therefore, they can also increase muscular tension and the experience of pain.

This chapter will address itself to the discussion of the role of anxiety, depression and low self-esteem in the experience of pain. Both experimental and clinical evidence will be presented.

Pain and anxiety

Experimentally induced pain may be helpful in identifying emotions associated with pain, although such studies cannot be used as an analogue for the study of clinical pain. Sternbach

(1975) discussed the strong association between emotional variables and pain, and suggested that almost any procedure that reduces the pain report in experimental studies may be interpreted as reducing anxiety, tension or fear.

Experimental studies indicated, that when the subjects were given a feeling of control over the experimental procedure, the pain threshold increased (Hill et al. 1952; Mandler and Watson 1966). When the instructions given prior to the experiment reduced anxiety, the subjects' pain thresholds were higher (Wolff and Horland 1967). A single session of relaxation prior to the second application of a painful stimulus, substantially reduced both pain threshold and pain tolerance of subjects (Elton and Stanley 1976). Similar findings were reported in studies of the effect of hypnosis on experimental pain (Hilgard and Hilgard 1975). These findings can explain the usefulness of clinical treatment of pain by relaxation, biofeedback, cognitive reinterpretation, and hypnosis.

In clinical studies, there was significant correlation found between the severity of anxiety and pain (Leventhal and Everhardt 1980). In studies of labour, it was found that anxious women suffer from more pain during labour, than those who do not feel anxiety (Klusman 1975; Wilson-Evered and Stanley 1986). Stam et al. (1984) showed the predominance of anxiety in patients with temporomandibular joint pain, and found that treatment by relaxation alleviated the symptoms. Similar findings were noted by Trifiletti and Calgary (1984), Parker et al. (1984) and Weisenberg et al. (1984). Studies of postoperative pain also revealed that when the patients' anxiety abated, recovery was quicker, and pain reports decreased (Martinez-Urrutia 1975; Pickett and Clum 1982). Peoples and Burnside (1982) showed that involvement of spouses in relaxation and imagery after surgical intervention had beneficial results, presumably because there was greater motivation to practice relaxation, when another person participated as well, and encouragement may have been provided. Abatement of anxiety, by treatment with muscular relaxation resulted in relief from phantom limb pain in 14 patients in a study by Sherman et al. (1979).

This small sample of the relevant literature indicates that anxiety plays a powerful role in maintenance and augmentation of pain. Both experimental and clinical evidence indicate that individuals in pain show considerable anxiety. Psychometric studies point to pre-existing anxiety traits in cases of prolonged and severe pain (Elton et al. 1983).

While both anxiety and depression may be present in some pain patients, it is argued that anxiety predominates in acute pain patients, as they are concerned with the implications of their pain, and worry about possible disability and social problems. On the other hand, in chronic pain patients, depression predominates, and some researchers (Sternbach 1978) argued that there is a correlation between the biochemical reactions of the body in pain and in depression. In both conditions, there was evidence of withdrawal of interests, weakening of relationships, increased somatic preoccupation, appetite disturbance, irritability, sleep disturbance, hopelessness and despair.

Pain and depression

Timmermans and Sternbach (1974) showed that there is a close relationship between depression and pain, and that relief of depression is associated with relief from pain. While they could not specify the exact mechanism of this association, they argued that depression may operate to reduce pain threshold.

In line with this report, Joffe and Sandler (1967) discussed depression as one of the important correlates in children suffering from psychosomatic symptoms. A Melbourne study, investigating atypical dental pain, which resisted normal dental procedures revealed that many of the patients were suffering from depression, and treatment by antidepressants relieved the symptoms (Gerschman and Reade 1987). This finding has support in the work of Lesse (1983).

Some researchers dispute the centrality of depression in chronic pain experience. As suggested by Merskey (1987), a tendency to develop psychosomatic symptoms without antecedent physical causes can be attributed to diverse psychological processes, such as tension, conversion symptoms and various other personality traits.

There are studies which suggest that depressive personalities do not appear to be more prone to pain than non-depresssed individuals. In a study of two clinical cases, Ben-Tovim and Schwartz (1981) indicated that these depressed patients reported feeling unable to experience either emotion or pain. The authors stated that the state of emotional indifference may have led to an increase in the level of endorphin in the cerebrospinal fluid (CSF). This study was supported by Philips and Jahanshahi (1985) who argued that despite the common somatic components between pain and depression, depression was not found to be higher in a group of 360 migraine and headache sufferers. The authors proposed that the patterns which had higher association with pain were avoidance and complaining behaviour. They suggested that depression levels were highest with the onset of the complaint, and abated when the pain continued for some years, then showed greater intensity in those who suffered for 20 – 30 years.

Further doubts on the role of emotions in headaches was cast by Arena et al. (1984), who studied 75 chronic headache sufferers (21 migraineurs, 32 headache sufferers and 22 combined). Each subject kept a diary of mood states, including depression, anxiety and anger. The headache activity was measured daily on a 6-point scale, from 0 to 5. Data were collected for 28 – 35 days. The results showed that anger had no effect on pain activity in migraine sufferers, and anxiety and depression did not significantly alter the tension headache activity. The authors suggested that situational factors (which they did not specify clearly) may be associated with increase of pain activity. They admitted the obvious limitations of the study, such as examination of only a small number of variables and demand characteristics of the situation. Their alternative explanation, that worry, unconscious repressed anger and rage are possible precursors of pain is unconvincing, as the distinction between worry and conscious anxiety is tenuous.

In a promising study by Harrigan et al. (1984), 17 migraine sufferers were studied at the Headache Center at the University of Cincinnati. The variables were mood states and migraine activity. Patients recorded mood and headache scores three times daily over a period of 21 – 75 days (mean number of days = 52). The pain was measured on a 5-point scale, from 0 to 4. Mood states included fullness vs. emptiness of life, receptivity towards and stimulation by the world, personal freedom vs. external constraint, harmony vs. anger, sociability vs. withdrawal, present work, tranquility vs. anxiety, energy vs. fatigue, elation vs. depression and control vs. lack of control. The results indicated that some mood states were correlated with pain, and could be used as consistent predictors. A feeling of fatigue is often associated with pain. Constraint, feeling trapped, hemmed in and frustrated offered further predictions. The authors suggested that the need to maintain control over difficult situations may result in fatigue, which in turn may lead to increased pain activity.

Further problems in investigation of the relationship between depression and pain could arise because some pain patients may not be aware of being depressed. There is convincing evidence that pain may be a manifestation of masked depression. Blumer and Heilbronn (1982) attempted to categorize chronic pain as a variant of depressive disease. Unlike acute pain, which is 'a disease in itself, rather than a symptom of something else', chronic pain has been attributed to central mechanisms. While the pain patient may consider the condition a purely physical problem, the condition often resists standard medical care procedures. Blumer and Heilbronn argued, that predominant symptoms of depression, anguish, suffering and hopelessness, are also to be found in chronic pain. Psychological testing may show chronic pain patients to be depressed, althought they do not experience a depressed mood, as it has been masked by somatic symptoms (Sternbach 1978). These studies are supported by the finding, that many pain patients lose their symptoms if given antidepressant medication (Ward et al. 1979). Often when patients attribute their depression to pain, a study of premorbid personality indicates that the depression preceded pain. Chronic pain may be viewed as neither primary nor secondary to depression, but rather as a synchronous expression of a mood state. Blumer and Heilbronn described a Swedish study, where high endorphin levels in CSF were found both in depression and in pain.

Weighty evidence for the presence of masked depression in pain patients was presented by Lesse (1983), who argued that often this condition is misdiagnosed, as there is insufficient knowledge of its antecedents and manifestations. He described masked depression in terms of sadness, melancholy, dejection, despair, despondency or gloominess, and argued that it presents primarily in Western society in middle-class menopausal, intelligent women.

In a review of the relationship between depression and pain, Roy et al. (1984) cited lack of conformity in findings. They pointed out that there are three kinds of evidence for such a relationship: a) presence of pain in depressed subjects; b) presence of depression in pain subjects; and c) efficacy of antidepressant medication in the treatment of chronic pain. Depression was defined as a clinically demonstrable condition. The authors' review showed that on each of these criteria there was a divergence of findings between different workers. While some reported presence of depression in 100% of subjects, others showed much lower percentages, and one study reported only a 13% correlation. Many studies were, according to the reviewers, poorly designed, insufficiently controlled and lacking proper operational definitions. They stated that the only pain condition which showed consistent relationship between pain and depression is head pain, where 85% of sufferers were found to be depressed. The authors accepted the efficacy of antidepressants in the treatment of chronic pain, but considered a possibility of analgesic effects of antidepressants. They contended that some of the confusion in the field may be due to methodological issues, as most depression scales do not contain measurements of pain.

While differing points of view were presented, the author supports the view, that there is a relationship between depression and chronic pain, as she has found that most of her patients showed some evidence of overt or masked depression.

Self-esteem and chronic pain

Elton et al. (1978) investigated the relationship between self-esteem and chronic pain. In line with Engel (1958), they argued that pain may be learned as a form of coping in early childhood, and may predispose the patient towards a development of pain-prone personality. If children learn that pain is rewarded by a caring attitude, or greater attention by the parents, they are more likely to use pain to gain attention and caring when other means of attaining them have failed. The authors accepted the finding of Joffe and Sandler (1967) that it is easier to endure tangible, physical pain than a state of inner unrest, guilt and low self-esteem. Pain, in these patients, may provide a way out of facing difficult situations and decisions. Elton et al.'s study compared four groups: chronic pain patients, acute pain patients (aged approximately 40 years), a pain-free group matched for age and socio-economic status, and a group of first year university students. Each group comprised 20 individuals. It was found that the 'pain-prone' group had a significantly lower self-esteem than the other three groups. There was little difference in self-esteem between the acute pain group and the pain-free individuals, showing that while illness may foster negative feeling states, self-esteem is not affected significantly by illness and pain. When, on the other hand, the patients doubt their ability to cope with life's problems, they may be prone to escape into pain, as means of avoiding difficulties. Pain may be used as means of explaining their perceived failures to achieve desired goals. The self-esteem of university students did not differ significantly from self-esteem of the other control groups, showing that age and socio-economic status did not result in differences on this dimension. Treatment aimed solely at improvement of self-esteem showed significant reduction in pain activity, and on post-test there was no significant difference between the groups. This study indicated that self-esteem may be an important variable in pain experience. It implied the need to consider the inner state of pain patients, if they fail to improve under standard medical care.

It is of interest, that while Lesse (1983) described in detail the correlates of masked depression, and an overwhelming evidence of its presence in a 17-year study of 1465 patients, some of the antecedents of masked depression he offered were: feelings of inadequacy, worthlessness, guilt, negative self-image and excessive criticism of self and others. These parameters have been quoted in Elton et al.'s study of self-esteem, and it is possible that if more attention had been directed to self-esteem of the patients presenting with pain, the masked depression may not have developed.

Other emotional states which affect the pain experience are hysteria (Merskey 1965) which may predispose to undue attention to pain. While there was a relationship between neuroses and pain, this was less evident in the case of psychoses. The relationship between emotional states and pain led Merskey and Spear (1967) to differentiate between organic and 'psychogenic' pain. The authors considered psychogenic pain to be associated with emotional factors, and an absence of clearly evident peripheral or central stimulation. While this distinction may be useful, it is doubtful whether there is any organic pain which is devoid of psychological processing. This was highlighted by Merskey (1984).

Aggression, and passive-aggressive dependency are also important factors in pain experience, and may predispose the patients to abnormal illness behaviour (Sternbach 1974). As long as the patients retain a blaming attitude towards others, they are less likely to take over responsibility for their own inprovement.

Summary

There is convincing evidence that emotional variables play an important role in pain experience. Unless they are considered by the helping professions, some patients may be unable to benefit from whatever help is offered in a form of medication, surgery or other interventions. While researchers differ on which is the most crucial emotional variable associated with chronic pain, the author suggests that anxiety, depression and low self-esteem may predispose towards a pain-prone personality.

References

Arena, J. G. Blanchard, E. B. and Andrasik, F. (1984) The role of affect in the etiology of chronic headache. J. Psychosom. Res. 28, 79 – 86.

Arnold, M. B. (1970) Feelings and Emotions. Academic Press, New York.

Ben-Tovim, D. I. and Schwartz, M. S. (1981) Hypoalgesia in depressive illness. Br. J. Psychiatry 138, 37 – 39.

Blumer, D. and Heilbronn, M., (1982) Chronic pain as a variant of depressive disease. The pain prone disorder. J. Nerv. Ment. Dis. 170, 381 – 394.

Ellis, A. and Harper, R. A. (1975) A New Guide to Rational Living. Wiltshire, Hollywood, Ca.

Elton, D. and Stanley, G. V. (1976) Relaxation as a method of pain control. Aust. J. Physiother. 22, 121 – 123.

Elton, D., Stanley, G. V. and Burrows, G. D. (1978) Self-esteem and chronic pain. J. Psychosom. Res. 22, 25 – 30.

Elton, D., Stanley, G. V. and Burrows, G. D. (1983) Psychological Control of Pain. Grune and Stratton, Sydney.

Engel, G. L. (1958) Psychogenic pain. Med. Clin. North Am. 26, 1481 – 1496.

Gerschman J. A. and Reade, P. C. (1987) Management of chronic oro-facial pain syndromes. In: G. D. Burrows, D. Elton and G. V. Stanley (Eds.), Handbook of Chronic Pain Management. Elsevier Science Publ., Amsterdam, pp. 321 – 330.

Harrigan, J. A., Kues, J. R., Ricks, D. F. and Smith, R. (1984) Moods that predict coming migraine headaches. Pain 20, 385 – 396.

Hilgard, E. R. and Hilgard, J. R. (1975) Hypnosis in the Relief of Pain. William Kaufmann, Los Altos, Ca.

Hill, H. E., Kornetsky, C. H., Flanary, H. G. and Winkler, A. (1952) Studies of anxiety associated with anticipation of pain. 1. Effects of morphine. Arch. Neurol. Psychiatry 67, 612 – 619.

Hughes, M. (1984) Recurrent abdominal pain and childhood depression: clinical observations of 23 children and their families. Am. J. Orthopsychiatry 54, 146 – 155.

Joffe, W. G. and Sandler, G. (1967) On concepts of pain, with special reference to depression and psychogenic pain. J. Psychosom. Res. 11, 69 – 75.

Klusman, L. E. (1975) Reduction of pain in child birth by alleviation of anxiety during pregnancy. J. Consult. Clin. Psychol. 213, 162 – 165.

Lesse, S. (1983) The masked depression syndrome – results of a seventeen-year study. Am. J. Psychother. 37, 457 – 475.

Leventhal, H. and Everhardt, D. (1980) Emotion, pain and physical illness. In: C. E. Izard (Ed.), Emotion and Psychopathology. Penguin, New York, pp. 263 – 299.

Mandler, G. and Watson, D. L. (1966) Anxiety and the interruption of behavior. In: C. D. Spielberger (Ed.), Anxiety and Behavior. Academic Press, New York, pp. 166 – 173.

Martinez-Urrutia, A. (1975) Anxiety and pain in surgical patients. J. Consult. Clin. Psychol. 213, 437 – 442.

Merskey, H. (1965) The characteristics of persistent pain in psychological illness. J. Psychosom. Res. 9, 291 – 298.

Merskey, H. (1984) Psychological approaches to the treatment of chronic pain. Postgrad. J. Med. 60, 886 – 899.

Merskey, H. (1987) Pain, personality and psychosomatic complaints. In: G. D. Burrows, D. Elton and G. V. Stanley (Eds.), Handbook of Chronic Pain Management. Elsevier Science Publ., Amsterdam, pp. 137 – 146.

Merskey, H. and Spear, E. G. (1967) Pain: Psychological and Psychiatric Aspects. Tindal and Cassell, London.

Parker, J. C., Karol, R. L., Doerfler, L. A. and Truman, H. S. (1983) Pain unit director: role issues for health psychologists. Profess. Psychol. Res. Prac. 14, 232 – 239.

Philips, H. C. and Jahanshahi, M. (1985) The effects of persistent pain: the chronic headache sufferer. Pain 21, 163 – 176.

Peoples, J. and Burnside, J. P. (1982) The effect of therapist and spouse assisted emotive imagery on post-surgical pain and adjustment. Monograph, Virginia Polytechnic Institute and State University.

Pickett, C. and Clum, G. A. (1982) Comparative treatment strategies and their interaction with locus of control in the reduction of postsurgical pain and anxiety. J. Consult. Clin. Psychol. 50, 439 – 441.

Roy, R., Thomas, M. and Matas, M. (1984) Chronic pain and depression: a review. Compr. Psychiatry 25, 96 – 105.

Schachter, S. and Singer, J. E. (1962) Cognitive, social and physiological determinants of emotional state. Psychol. Rev. 69, 379 – 399.

Selye, H. (1976) The Stress of Life. McGraw-Hill, New York.

Sherman, R. A., Gall, N. and Gormly, J.   (1979)   Treatment of phantom limb pain with muscular relaxation training to disrupt the pain-anxiety-tension cycle. Pain 6, 47 – 55.

Stam, H. J., McGrath, P. A. and Brooke, R. I.   (1984)   The treatment of temporomandibular joint syndrome through control of anxiety. J. Behav. Ther. Exp. Psychiatry 15, 41 – 45.

Sternbach, R. A.   (1974)   Pain and depression, In: A. Kiev (Ed.), Somatic Manifestations of Depressive Disorders. Excerpta Medica, Amsterdam, pp. 107 – 119.

Sternbach, R. A.   (1975)   Psychological aspects of pain and the selection of patients. Clin. Neurosurgery 21, 323 – 333.

Sternbach, R. A.   (1978)   The Psychology of Pain. Raven Press, New York.

Sternbach, R. A.   (1981)   Fundamental of psychological methods in chronic pain. Pain S.162 (Abstr.) 197.

Timmermans, G. and Sternbach, R. A.   (1974)   Factors in human chronic pain: an analysis of personality and pain reaction variables. Science 184, 806 – 807.

Trifiletti, R. J. and Calgary, U.   (1984)   The psychological effectiveness of pain management procedures in the context of behavioral medicine and medical psychology. Genet. Psychol. Monogr. 109, 251 – 278.

Ward, N. G., Bloom, V. L. and Friedel, R. O.   (1979)   The effectiveness of tricyclic antidepressants in the treatment of coexisting pain and depression. Pain 7, 331 – 341.

Weisenberg, M., Aviram, O., Wolf, Y. and Raphaeli, N.   (1984)   Relevant and irrelevant anxiety in the reaction to pain. Pain 20, 371 – 383.

Wilson-Evered, E. and Stanley, G. V.   (1986)   Stress and arousal during pregnancy and childbirth. Br. J. Med. Psychol. 59, 57 – 60.

Wolff, B. B. and Horland, A. A.   (1967)   Effects of suggestion upon experimental pain: a validational study. J. Abnorm. Psychol. 72, 402 – 407.

Burrows/Elton/Stanley (eds.) Handbook of Chronic Pain Management
© *1987 Elsevier Science Publishers B.V. (Biomedical Division)*

12

Cultural factors in chronic pain management

KENNETH D. CRAIG[1, *] and MARGO G. WYCKOFF[2, **]

[1]*Department of Psychology, University of British Columbia, Vancouver, Canada, and*
[2]*Swedish Hospital Medical Center, and Providence Hospital Medical Center, Seattle, Washington, U.S.A.*

Pain and suffering are central features of human existence independent of the person's culture, but their form and expression are strongly dependent upon cultural variations. Pain as a result of accidents, diseases, and other peoples' actions is an altogether too common experience for many, if not most, people throughout their lives. Human culture has evolved in part as a means of reducing this form of human misery. Through collective action people are best able to minimize the sources and consequences of deprivation, disease and debility. Regrettably, neither the technologically sophisticated approaches to pain management that have evolved in Western cultures nor the intervention strategies used in societies that have not focused on biophysical solutions (Foster 1978) have proven wholly successful.

The major challenges of pain and suffering make it inevitable that new solutions will be explored and tried by different cultures and subcultures within them. Given striking differences in the natural environments where humans have chosen to live, and the ongoing transmission of historical precedents within cultures over time, it is not surprising that a substantial range of culture-specific approximations to solutions to the challenges of pain have evolved. While all people may share the same *disease* states, in the sense that this refers to pathophysiological pro-

Address for correspondence: * Kenneth D. Craig, Professor of Psychology, No. 2509 – 2136 West Mall, University of British Columbia, Vancouver, B.C. Canada V6T 1Y7
** Margo G. Wyckoff, Springbrook Professional Building, 4540 Sand Point Way N.E., Seattle, Washington, D.C. 98105, U.S.A.

cesses, patterns of *illness* behavior differ substantially, in the sense that this term should be reserved to describe the personal, interpersonal, and cultural reactions to disease (Kleinman 1980). The concept of illness behavior was first introduced by David Mechanic in 1962 in a classic study which postulated that individuals perceive, evaluate and act upon physical symptomatology in different ways. These responses depend upon cultural and social conditioning, the availability of coping skills and, possibly, immediate and long-term gains from the illness experience.

The term 'culture' refers to the beliefs, customs, interpersonal relationships and behavior patterns that distinguish groups of people that share common patterns from one and other. The concept identifies both a common characteristic that all humans share − a capacity to learn complex cognitive and behavioral practices − and the potential for unique patterns that distinguish groups from each other. The expression has been used broadly in research on pain. Studies tend to cut across linguistic, geographic, religious, and racial groupings when comparisons have been made, as in the case of Zborowski's comparisons of 'Old Americans', Jews, Italians and Irish immigrants and descendants resident in New York City (1969). There is considerable scope for more precise definition of cultural groups and substantial need for investigation of other groups, as in Kotarba's (1983) intriguing studies of the subcultures of professional athletes and manual laborers experiencing chronic pain.

Ethnic and cultural variables join many other psychological and social variables that must be considered by the clinician when investigating the psycho-social-biological etiologies of chronic pain (Engel 1977; Chapman and Wyckoff 1981). Anxiety, depression, coping skills, marital and family factors, and vocational and economic realities all play an important role in the total presentation of suffering (Wyckoff 1978a). They represent other important determinants of pain experience and expression embedded within cultural processes. The predicament of a woman who was referred to a Pain Clinic for extreme pain in her legs consequent to a fall 3 years previously illustrates these complexities. She had been to eight different physicians, was addicted to her pain medications, and could not walk a distance more than one block, necessitating her son and daughter-in-law to do her shopping and housework. Upon examination it was determined that she had taken her fall when climbing the church steps to her son's wedding. She admitted to despising her daughter-in-law and she regretted the reality of her son leaving the family home to marry. She stated 'I was afraid that he would never come home to me again' (Wyckoff 1978b). Thus, in the search for the sources of individual differences in pain experience and expression, psychosocial variables other than cultural factors assume an important role. Nevertheless, the concept of culture is powerful because it serves to integrate psychosocial variables, attracts attention to their importance, and identifies a basis for important differences to be observed among patients during the delivery of care.

As pain persists for any given patient, the impact of the social environment on patterns of pain behavior increases. Acute pain provokes a readily identifiable pattern of vocalization, grimace, gesticulation and reflex withdrawal in most people (Craig and Prkachin 1983; Patrick et al. 1985). These actions commonly lead to relief from pain, identify for others the hurt person's dilemma, and permit observers to deliver care or to escape similar distress. If the pain persists, these actions rapidly habituate (Craig and Patrick 1985). In the case of chronic pain, whether it is persistent, recurrent, or progressive (Turk et al. 1983), its dramatic behavioral manifestations may only be observable when there are acute exacerbations or the chronic pain sufferer is engaged in the act of seeking additional care. Here, the individual becomes engaged in the process of convincing others about the urgency of the problems and the necessity of delivering relief. Pain-afflicted people may choose to communicate their private states of distress, if they judge such actions would be in their best interests, or conceal pain if, in their experience, the consequences would be damaging to their interests. Thus, activity designed to be instrumental in eliciting care or release from stressful situations would be expected to conform to culture specific social display rules rather than reflexively expressing acute distress.

People afflicted with chronic pain express their distress by pursuing those means of pain relief developed through personal experience within the context of their culture. In Western cultures, patients commonly exhaust the sanctioned resources − the health professional's repertoire of medical knowledge and skills − then turn to nonsanctioned, but readily available, sources of relief (Kotarba 1983). These may include the hazards of excessive reliance on analgesic drugs or polydrug abuse, alternate nonmedical health care activities (naturopathy, acupuncture, etc.), or folk practices (meditation, faith healing, yoga, spiritual healers, etc.). In many ways, contemporary, comprehensive pain clinics have combined conventional and various forms of alternate health care through the delivery of multidisciplinary care. Demand for alternate sources of health care can be expected to continue until the major challenges of chronic pain are resolved.

Inter- and intra-cultural variation in pain behavior

Professionals, scientists and lay people frequently believe individual differences in pain expression are attributable to the sufferer's ethnocultural heritage. Given the inadequacies of the relatively few studies that are available (Wolff and Langley 1968), there seems to be a good possibility that many of these beliefs are founded on unsubstantiated social anecdotes, clinical impressions, and cultural stereotypes, rather than an empirical knowledge-base. In consequence, statements about the experience and expression of pain in different cultural groups need to be made with great care, and treatment predicated upon these beliefs should be undertaken with considerable caution. Assuming, for instance, that in any cultural group, women exaggerate pain introduces the risk of not providing pain relief for an ordinarily conservative woman who presents with strong complaints. Rather, it is more helpful to recognize that people may use different descriptors with which to convey their experience of suffering and that these descriptors are often just as reflective of personal, behavioral styles and language ability as intensity of pain. A patient who has a rich ability to utilize verbal language could be viewed by the caregiver as different from the more eidetic sufferer, when, in fact, the more verbal patient might well be suffering less than the other.

Zborowski (1969) provided the seminal descriptions of ethnocultural variations in pain and illness behavior in his contrasts of Italian, Jewish, Irish and 'Old American' patients. It is important to note that the subjects of this classic investigation were all male, World-War II veterans in a large New York City hospital. While the findings were complex and the descriptions of the ethnic groups intricate, it was generally the case that the Jewish and Italian patients expressed their pain in a strong, emotive manner and some had tendencies to exaggerate their pain experiences. In contrast, Irish patients had an accepting, matter-of-fact attitude and tended to engage in pain denial, and the 'Old Americans' tended to be quiet and stoical. The evidence indicated that cultural identification led to the adoption of relatively discrete patterns of pain and illness behavior. However, the studies did not clarify whether these behavioral patterns would be descriptive of other populations of people with these ethnic backgrounds in other settings. Without recognizing this there would be a substantial risk of generating and contributing to inaccurate stereotypes and prejudicing patient treatment.

Fortunately, other investigators (Tursky and Sternbach 1967; Sternbach and Tursky 1965;

Zola 1966) using the same ethnic groups, but with subjects differing in important characteristics (e.g. 'housewives' in the case of Sternbach and Tursky), have reported complementary findings. The combined evidence suggests that people of Mediterranean cultural extraction are more likely to be aware of and to communicate symptoms of physical discomfort than Northern European peoples. Other investigators have provided detailed descriptions of other cultural groups (Weisenberg 1982; Meinhardt and McCaffery 1983).

It is also important to recognize that general descriptions pose major risks to patients by stereotyping their reactions solely as a function of cultural history. In considering individuals one must examine the unique personal backgrounds and cultural contexts in which patients live. Pilowsky and Spence (1977) observed that Greek patients consulting a general practitioner in Australia displayed more hypochondriacal attitudes, disease conviction, and a preference for somatic rather than psychological explanations of their symptoms than patients of Anglo-Saxon background. However, Greek patients who had become acculturated to Australian customs provided evidence of changing towards the values and beliefs of the dominant Anglo-Saxon culture. They stood intermediate to the above-named groups on the various measures and discrimination between them and the Anglo-Saxon patients became difficult. Zborowski (1969) similarly observed that successive generations of a family subsequent to immigration increasingly resembled the host culture in their pain behavior. Pilowsky and Spence (1977) noted that the differences between ethnic groups represented appropriate and adaptive reactions to economic and social demands imposed upon them, as well as socialization within a particular society. Recent immigrants were more likely to assume the lower socioeconomic status jobs of manual laborers who require good health for employment. Hence, preoccupation with physical health and emotional distress when it is threatened would represent an adaptive response.

Lambert et al. (1960) demonstrated that ethnic groups can display an even more immediate change in pain expression contingent upon situational demand. Using induced pain, Jewish and Protestant groups were found not to differ during a baseline pain tolerance assessment. However, when the experimenters implied that the subjects' religious group could not tolerate pain as well as other religious groups, both Jews and Protestants displayed a dramatic increase in pain tolerance. Clearly, the global descriptions of ethnocultural variations in pain expression need to be considered with reference to the social, economic and political contexts of peoples' lives.

The evidence that pain expression and experience are highly reactive to situational demand has further implications. Those differences between cultural groups that have been reported do not necessarily represent enduring qualities of individuals. They can be characterized as the collective, optimal adjustment to the immediate demands of the situation for the group studied. For example, minority groups may choose for reasons of ethnic rivalry to present themselves as relatively stoical when assessed by a member of the dominant culture (Poser 1963). Thus, individuals in pain may present themselves as capable of substantially different levels of discomfort if the situational and social context changes.

It also is not unusual for patients from minority cultures to be fearful of describing the psychological impact of their pain for fear of being labeled 'crazy'. Typically, these patients are nervous about psychometric testing and unwilling to be open about their reading abilities. It is not only necessary for clinicians to feel comfortable with and respectful of other cultures, but also to make efforts to include minority care-givers on their treatment staffs.

An often overlooked, but productive exchange with patients can be generated by asking them how they were taught to deal with pain by their families. If this investigation is made with respect, a wealth of helpful information may be shared. Often, healers, religious practitioners, or other important figures in the patient's life can assist in the treatment – thus providing care with cultural sanctions.

GROUP CHARACTERIZATIONS AS DESCRIPTIVE OF INDIVIDUALS

A clinician responsible for the care of any single patient must recognize that additional personal factors interact with ethnocultural heritage. Assuming that the findings on cultural variations in pain described here apply to particular patients bears the risk of misrepresentation and overgeneralization. All patients' belief systems and behavioral patterns will have been influenced during socialization, but global characterizations of cultural groups do not satisfactorily describe the range of variation within them. Indeed, at times the differences between ethnic groups are so small as to be meaningless when contrasted with the broad ranges of individual variations within the groups. Knowledge of the group differences would not allow prediction of the behavior of any particular person in the group. In most studies, many patients or subjects within groups that were characterized as displaying lesser pain tolerance would have exceeded the pain tolerance of participants in the groups that were characterized as more tolerant. Clinicians and investigators must recognize this by paying careful attention to *intra*group variability, even when searching for *inter*group differences, and by attending to overlapping distributions. The stereotypes may be more illusory than real and may propagate misconceptions that lead to prejudicial discrimination since our perception of people dictates the treatment they receive.

ORIGINS OF THE VARIATIONS

Virtually all humans experience pain and communicate distress to others, but the form varies with the unique physical and social environments in which they are raised. The impact of the physical environment becomes salient when one recognizes that *homo sapiens* has been a remarkably adaptive species capable of surviving in extraordinary ecological niches. The Inuit of Northern Canada encounter extremes of prolonged cold weather, whereas the Aborigines of the Australian outback must endure the searing heat of the desert. No less demanding than the environmental rigours are different belief systems and sociocultural restraints imposed upon those who experience pain or are ill. These would seem to be most conspicuous during childhood when parents and others charged with child-rearing responsibilities make demands upon children to conform to those patterns of pain and illness behavior that approximate the behavioral solutions that have proven most effective for adults.

Expressive behavior would appear to have evolved phylogenetically as adaptive, prepotent reactions to pain that marshall aid for the individual in distress and enable conspecifics to recognize imminent danger (Melzack and Dennis 1980; Craig 1984a). From birth, human infants are responsive to noxious stimuli and display vocal and nonvocal behavior that adults interpret as signs of pain (Craig 1980; Owens 1984). Initially, infant pain behavior appears to be reflexive, more spontaneous and diffuse, whereas later pain behavior becomes goal-directed and coordinated. Thus, in a contrast of reactions of infants in the first and second years of life to immunization needle injections, Craig et al. (1984) found the latter to cry and scream for a shorter span of time, orient towards the locus on their bodies where the needle stick occurred, visually track their mothers and the nurse responsible for the injection to a greater extent, and protect and touch the wounded area more often. As perceptual, cognitive, and behavioral capacities for interaction with the invironment emerge in the first year of life, and pain expression begins to display instrumental qualities, one would expect parents and other caretakers to systematically shape the patterns of expression.

Parents and other caretakers provide social models for those forms of pain complaint that represent their personal resolution to the challenges of painful injury and disease. In support of these role models they would act promptly and with conviction to ensure children conformed to their exemplars and demands (Craig 1978, 1983). Children are vulnerable to morbid accidents and have ample opportunity to learn about the dangers of their worlds, the consequences of injuries, and self-care activities. Cuts, scrapes, bruises, burns, twisted joints, stomach aches, and other crises are far too common for most children as a result of poor sensori-motor coordination, risk taking, limited capacity to anticipate danger, and the willingness of some peers and adults to inflict pain upon them.

Societies differ in the extent to which they have evolved patterns of work, recreation and health care practices that call for exposure to physical risk and pain and different styles of response. Contact sports such as rugby or football self-select for staunch, forbearing participants. Prophylactic health care practices may require exposure to pain, as during heel lancing to provide blood samples or needle injections for immunization purposes. Firewalking is found in communities around the world (e.g. Southeastern Asia, China, the Balkans, and, today, in California), Chinese children practice acupuncture upon themselves, and self-mutilative religious, decorative, and sexual rituals are practiced in many communities. For example, flagellants may assault themselves for religious or erotic purposes, and tattooing or scarification may symbolize manliness or beauty. Practices that appear esoteric to members of other cultures but are routine cultural activities to members of the communities in which they are accepted events, would have their own justification, perhaps only comprehensible within the culture where they are practiced.

At these times, children would observe their parents and others' reactions to them when they were at risk or experiencing painful distress. Witnessing children in pain can be an emotionally alarming experience for most adults, and they can be expected to exert considerable effort to reduce pain, minimize the threat to children's well-being and to inculcate their own concepts of the meaning of pain and how one can cope with it. Variability in adults' reactions to children in pain would lead to the promotion of variable sensitivity in children's reactions. Thus, the social contexts in which children experience pain would be expected to have a potent impact on the experience and expression of pain and patterns of pain complaint unique to the child's family and culture would be perpetuated.

Even as adults people continue to be exposed to environmental contingencies and social modeling that exert an influence on pain expression. For example, Zborowski (1969) noted in his studies of hospital patients that physicians and nurses favored the 'Old American' model of illness behavior and expected their patients to conform to this role model at home and in the hospital. Bond (1980) described the pressures in British hospitals towards enduring pain with little or no complaint as follows, 'Stoicism in a pain sufferer is rewarded with admiration, sympathy, and more material expressions of approval, notably administration of pain relieving medications. In contrast, complaints of pain, especially if regarded as excessive or unnecessary are punished by expressions of disapproval, both verbal and practical, in the form of withholding analgesics or administration of placebo substances (p. 54)'. Health professionals are in a position to utilize programmed social structures to enhance well behavior. Failure to recognize the impact of the social environment on patients could lead to the unwitting imposition of ethnosyncratic biases on patients and unfortunate discriminatory effects.

The cultural variations challenge both the assessment and treatment skills of clinicians. On the one hand, the complexities of understanding the essentially private nature of painful experiences are compounded by communication problems and the likelihood of different concepts and world views structuring the nature of the experience. On the other hand, even if the clinician is successful in comprehending the qualities and severity of pain being experienced, cultural differences will complicate the delivery of care whether biologically oriented or psychosocial intervention is attempted.

Assessment. The measurement and assessment of pain has not proven to be an easy task (Melzack 1983). Pain is a highly personal and intimate experience whose phenomenology is communicated to others with difficulty. Affective qualities in particular are not described readily through descriptive language and observers of pain are obliged to understand and empathize through the use of verbal and nonverbal evidence that is inherently ambiguous (Craig and Prkachin 1983). In addition, people who are suffering are often sensitized to the need to enlist care and their communications become predicated upon situational demand as much as subjective experience. There is considerable scope for confused communication and misinterpretation, particularly when the differences in cultural conventions for language and nonverbal communication are considered.

To provide sympathetic care for members of other cultures the observer must learn the signals members of that group use to communicate pain. While some features of these signals, such as facial grimaces, might have an invariant biological basis (Craig and Patrick 1985) and would be the same across cultures, there would be display rules and conventions unique to cultures that would have been learned. When stoical forbearance is socially appropriate, clinicians may have to attach greater meaning to self-report.

From the perspective of the clinician, judgments about pain severity, appropriate treatment regimes, and patient compliance reflect the clinician's cultural background and history of experience with patients. If the clinicians' judgments are dominated by the values and standards of his or her own culture there is a risk of ethnocentric bias. Clinicians must be cautious about setting up their own culture as the normative standard. There would be potential for implicitly viewing other behavior patterns as deviant and discriminating against minority group practices. Zborowski (1969) reported that nurses and aides were intolerant of atypical patterns of pain expression and tended to shape conformity to dominant cultural patterns of expression. Inimical comparisons based on cultural stereotypes can lead to broad moral judgments when pain tolerance and fortitude become equated with strong personal character and superior endowment.

To compensate for the risks of judgmental error it is important that clinicians recognize that both the sufferer *and* the health care provider perceive illness behavior differently as a result of social learning in different sociocultural contexts. A great deal can be accomplished by making translation available. Given the risk of misperception based on stereotypes, local norms for pain communications should be collected and made available. When health professionals work repeatedly with members of particular ethnic groups, consultation with the community can disclose the conventions, normative standards, practices and resources in the community. By opening networks of reciprocal communication, health professionals may come to discover that conventional treatment to them is as esoteric to members of minority groups as would be the practices characteristic of minority groups to the health professionals.

Treatment. Similar precautions need to be exercised in the delivery of treatment services for pain. Minority group membership should alert the clinician to the risks of mistreatment. Sensitivity to unique qualities of the individual need to be emphasized. There may be a risk of imposing group stereotypes on the individual, even if local norms were available. The presence of variation within any group must be recognized. Groups commonly seen as dramatically portraying their distress will also have members who are reluctant to admit distress. Failure to recognize individuality could lead to denial of treatment.

Treatments offered must reflect a sensitivity toward and a celebration of differences among people. Most cultures value self-esteem and group esteem although behavioral manifestations of these values may differ. Being open to what patients and/or families regard as appropriate and functional coping, and helping structure methods to assist these as objectives is a primary task of the caregiver.

This is most necessary when dealing with vocational realities for chronic pain patients. Arriving at a mutually agreed upon definition of 'work' is a necessary starting point. This, by its very nature includes not only cultural attitudes, but self-role and familial expectations. Work is not merely a paycheck, it is an existential statement about one's identity.

Finally, the ultimate objective of treatment is to decrease the experience of suffering and to increase the patient's sense of wellness and participation in life. All cultural paths, though they may appear different in some ways, and similar in others, lead to the same expectation – that of personal coherence and social belongingness.

CONCLUDING OBSERVATIONS

This perspective on cultural factors in chronic pain management is based upon acceptance of cognitive and affective components as fundamental to the experience of pain, in addition to sensory qualities. Patterns of experience and behavioral expression are recognized as the consequences of personal social histories and the environments in which people live. Cultural learning would primarily affect cognitive and affective dimensions of pain with the influence on sensory qualities secondary. Traditional medical management of pain, in the form of pharmacological, surgical and additional conservative management strategies, and outdated sensory specificity models of pain (Melzack and Wall 1984), have focused upon interruption and modulation of sensory qualities. Almost incidentally, it has been observed (Craig 1984b) that many strategies for attenuating pain have a substantial impact on emotional qualities of the experience (e.g. analgesic and psychotropic drugs, psychosurgery, relaxation and biofeedback training, cognitive-behavioral interventions, hypnosis and psychotherapy). Sensitivity to cultural variation – in cognition, affect and behavior – has promoted an appreciation of alternative treatment modalities.

Acknowledgement

This work was supported by grants from the Social Sciences and Humanities Research Council of Canada.

References

Bond, M. R. (1980) The suffering of severe intractable pain. In: H. W. Kosterlitz and L. Y. Terenius (Eds.), Pain and Society. Verlag Chemie, Weinheim, pp. 53 – 62.

Chapman, C. R. and Wyckoff, M. (1981) The problem of pain: a psychobiological perspective. In: S. N. Haynes and L. Gannon (Eds.), Psychosomatic Disorders. Praeger, New York, pp. 32 – 78.

Craig, K. D. (1978) Social modeling influences on pain. In: R. A. Sternbach (Ed.), The Psychology of Pain. Raven Press, New York, pp. 72 – 109.

Craig, K. D. (1980) Ontogenetic and cultural determinants of the expression of pain in man. In: H. H. Kosterlitz and L. Y. Terenius (Ed.), Pain and Society. Verlag Chemie, Weinheim, pp. 39 – 52.

Craig, K. D. (1983) Modeling and social learning factors in chronic pain. In: J. J. Bonica, U. Lindblom, and A. Iggo (Eds.), Advances in Pain Research and Therapy, Vol. 5. Raven Press, New York, pp. 813 – 826.

Craig, K. D. (1984a) Ontogenetic and phylogenetic determinants of the expression of pain. In: W. Paton, J. Mitchell and P. Turner (Ed.), Proceedings of the IUPHAR 9th International Congress of Pharmacology, 1984. Macmillan, London, pp. 351 – 358.

Craig, K. D. (1984b) Emotional aspects of pain. In: P. D. Wall and R. Melzack (Eds.), Textbook of Pain. Churchill Livingstone, Edinburgh, pp. 153 – 161.

Craig, K. D. and Patrick, C. J. (1985) Facial expression during induced pain. J. Pers. Soc. Psychol. 48, 1080 – 1091.

Craig, K.D. and Prkachin, K. M. (1983) Nonverbal measures of pain. In: R. Melzack (Ed.), Pain Measurement and Assessment. Raven Press, New York, pp. 173 – 179.

Craig, K. D., McMahon, R. S., Morison, J. D. and Zaskow, C. (1984) Developmental changes in infant pain expression during immunization injections. Soc. Sci. Med. 19, 1331 – 1337.

Engel, G. L. (1977) The need for a new medical model: a challenge for biomedicine. Science 196, 129 – 136.

Foster, G. (1978) Disease etiologies in non-Western medical systems of belief. Am. Anthropol. 80, 660 – 693.

Kleinman, A. (1980) Patients and Healers in the Context of Culture. University of California Press, Berkeley.

Kotarba, J. A. (1983) Chronic Pain: its social dimensions. Sage, Beverly Hills.

Lambert, W. E., Libman, E. and Poser, E. G. (1960) The effect of increased salience of group membership on pain tolerance. J. Pers. 28, 350 – 357.

Mechanic, D. (1962) The concept of illness behavior. J. Chronic Dis. 15, 189 – 194.

Meinhardt, N. T. and McCaffery, M. (1983) Pain, a Nursing Approach to Assessment and Analysis. Appleton-Century-Crofts, New York.

Melzack, R. (Ed.) (1983) Pain Measurement and Assessment. Raven Press, New York.

Melzack, R. and Dennis, S. G. (1980) Phylogenetic evolution of pain expression in animals. In: H. W. Kosterlitz and L. Y. Terenius (Eds.), Pain and Society. Verlag Chemie, Weinheim, pp. 13 – 25.

Owens, M. E. (1984) Pain in infancy: conceptual and methodological issues. Pain 20, 213 – 230.

Patrick, C.J., Craig, K. D. and Prkachin, K. M. (1985) Observer judgments of acute pain: facial action determinants. J. Pers. Soc. Psychol. (in press).

Pilowsky, I. and Spence, N. D. (1977) Ethnicity and illness behavior. Psychol. Med. 7, 447 – 452.

Poser, E. G. (1963) Some psychosocial determinants of pain tolerance. Paper presented at the 16th International Congress of Psychology, Washington, D. C.

Sternbach, R. A. and Tursky, B. (1965) Ethnic differences among housewives in psychophysical and skin potential responses to electric shock. Psychophysiology 1, 241 – 246.

Turk, D. C., Meichenbaum, D. and Genest, M. (1983) Pain and Behavioral Medicine. Guilford Press, New York.

Tursky, B. and Sternbach, R. A. (1967) Further physiological correlates of ethnic differences in responses to shock. Psychophysiology 4, 67 – 74.

Weisenberg, M. (1982) Cultural and ethnic factors in reaction to pain. In: Il Al-Issa (Ed.), Culture and Psychopathology. University Park, Baltimore, pp. 187 – 198.

Wolff, B. B. and Langley, S. (1968) Cultural factors and the response to pain: a review. Am. Anthropol. 70, 494 – 501.

Wyckoff, M. G. (1978a) Chronic pain, toward an understanding of maladaptive illness behavior. Unpublished doctoral dissertation, Vaion Graduate School.

Wyckoff, M. G. (1978b) The chronic pain experience: case illustrations. In: N. Bracht (Ed.), Social Work in Health Care. Haworth Press, New York.

Zborowski, M. (1969) People in Pain. Jossey-Bass, San Francisco.

Zola, J. K. (1966) Culture and symptoms: an analysis of patients presenting complaints. Am. Sociol. Rev. 31, 615–630.

Burrows/Elton/Stanley (eds.) Handbook of Chronic Pain Management
© *1987 Elsevier Science Publishers B.V. (Biomedical Division)*

13

The social meanings of chronic pain

PAUL E. BRODWIN and ARTHUR KLEINMAN

Department of Anthropology, Harvard University, William James Hall, Cambridge,
Massachusetts, U.S.A.

Introduction

Chronic pain poses great difficulties in accurate diagnosis and effective treatment. Psychological suffering and social disruption in these patients' lives are 'non-medical' factors which can threaten the successful management of pain disorders and lead to an ambivalent and frustrating relationship between pain patients and their physicians (Kotarba and Seidel 1984, p. 1393). We believe that the application of medical social science based on anthropological research can help explain these persistent problems. In this chapter, we show how chronic pain affects key areas of a patient's life outside the clinic. *Chronic pain draws its meaning from four social settings: the patient's family, ethnic/cultural community, work site, and health care organization.* Knowing the importance of these can help the clinician plan more effective interventions, and make the management of chronic pain more productive and less frustrating for both clinician and patient.

Pain illness and pain disease

From the standpoint of medical anthropology, chronic pain takes two forms: pain *illness* and pain *disease* (Kleinman et al. 1978). Pain *disease* refers to the doctor's perspective on the patient's suffering. Examples of pain disease include identifiable pathologies (osteoporosis, rheumatoid arthritis, lumbrosacral disc disease) or symptom clusters (migraine headaches or myofascial syndrome). The disease is a scientific biomedical account – an organic lesion, dysfunction, or degeneration – which guides the treatment decisions of the health care team.

Pain illness, however, comprises the patient's account of his/her experience. Verbal complaints, specific disabilities, lifestyle changes, and accompanying fears and anxieties all constitute the pain illness. This popular, non-professional understanding of pain and its effects on daily life often guides patients' decision about who to consult and which treatments to follow.

Unlike pain disease, pain illness is not the simple reflection of underlying physiological events. It rather represents culturally-grounded perceptions of the types of pain, the meanings of pain as threat, loss, or gain (cf. Lipowski 1969) and the possible responses to pain, both in the family and among biomedical and alternative healers.

Pain illness and pain disease thus represent two separate domains of knowledge about and behavioral responses to chronic pain. Anthropological studies suggest that conflicts between chronic pain patients and their clinicians arise from the illness/disease discrepancy. Malpractice claims, poor compliance, polypharmacy, and poor clinical care may result if clinicians neither attempt to learn the patient's illness model nor successfully translate the biomedical disease model into lay terms (Blumhagen 1982; Kotarba 1983). While time constraints in the clinic and the exclusive disease orientation of medical training make this an elusive goal, we offer some clinical guidelines to negotiation between disease and illness models for chronic pain.

To begin with, both disease and illness perspectives offer answers (explanatory models) to the same basic questions of care: 1) etiology, 2) onset of symptoms, 3) pathophysiology, 4) course of illness, and 5) treatment (Kleinman 1980). Differences of opinion in any of the five areas can create radically different expectations about the clinical encounter. However, clinicians can systematically elicit the patient's model by asking some such questions as:

1) What do you think caused your pain?
2) Why do you think it started when it did? What else was happening in your life at that time?
3) What do you think your chronic pain does to you (your body, your emotional reactions)? How do you think your pain works?
4) How severe is your pain? Will it have a short or long course?
5) What kind of treatment do you think you should receive?
6) What results do you hope to receive from this treatment?
7) What are the chief problems (at work, at home, with friends) your continued pain has caused you?

After becoming familiar with the patient's 'illness' perspective, the clinician should identify major discrepancies between the illness and disease models. Will problems in communication or compliance occur because of divergent accounts of the origin of pain? Must the physician negotiate between lay and medical accounts of pathophysiology in order to ensure compliance and patient satisfaction? How might patient and physician address different expectations for treatment (e.g. desire for total cure vs. symptomatic relief with occasional relapses)? These are empirical questions, to be answered anew in each case. In general, however, such comparisons will indicate which aspects of the disease model need clearer exposition, and what types of patient education are most effective (Kleinman et al. 1978).

Illness meanings of chronic pain: a schematic view

Comparisons between the illness and disease of chronic pain should not imply, however, that the illness is a mistaken or irrational version of the medical disease model. Pain *illness* is rather the outcome of a complex interaction of biological, psychological, and socio-cultural causes. Figure 1 maps out these factors, and illustrates some general social science principles for the clinical management of chronic pain.

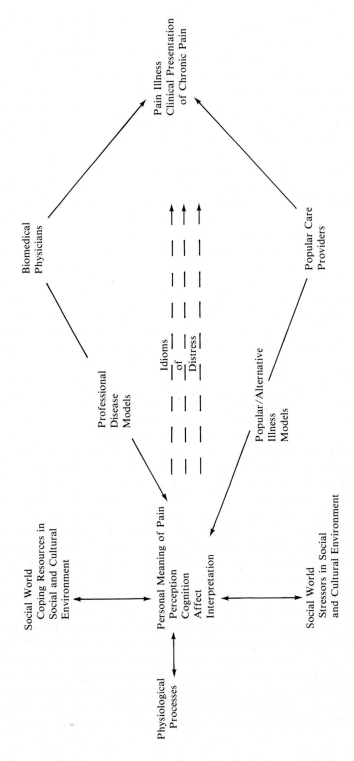

Fig. 1. The illness meanings of chronic pain (adapted from Good and Kleinman 1985).

1) While chronic pain symptoms usually have a physiological base, they become noticeable, emotionally salient, and personally meaningful only in the context of a patient's *social world*.

2) The patient's experience of pain depends on the *stressors* in his/her social and cultural environment. In the context of social isolation or a job with great physical demands, chronic pain produces specific emotional reactions: a renewed loneliness or anxiety about one's livelihood. Cultural beliefs can also act as stressors: a religious belief portraying pain as a punishment for sins can lead to guilt over and even denial of the severity of pain (Zola 1966). Stressful family dynamics contribute to these personal meanings. A patient's pain may be used as a scapegoat in a conflict-ridden or non-communicative family (cf. the concept of 'sick-role homeostasis' in Waring 1976).

3) Similarly, the *resources* in the socio-cultural environment affect the personal meanings of chronic pain. A supportive family can turn pain from a threat into an occasion for closeness or emotional growth. A religion extolling the nobility of suffering can cast pain as marker of piety. An adequate disability compensation system in the workplace may even make chronic pain an opportunity for time-off or financial gain.

4) The *health care system* shapes the patient's interpretation of chronic pain. Different medical models influence the patient to attend to certain patterns of pain, and hence actually experience the pain in different ways (cf. Mechanic 1972). A chiropractor, a neurosurgeon, and a behavioral psychologist each communicate to their patients distinct ways of viewing pain. While one patient hopes for a non-invasive cure, another fears the implications of a 'chronic' diagnosis and a third attempts to control pain by mood or lifestyle changes. These reactions depend largely on the illness meanings from professional and popular health care providers (Kotarba 1983).

5) The meanings and emotional reactions to chronic pain are highly idiosyncratic. They may not be easily understandable even by other family members, let alone a physician. A patient must therefore communicate the pain illness using shared *idioms of distress* (Nichter 1981). Common to many members of a culture, these idioms are conventional devices used to communicate personal discomfort. The Chinese idiom of somatization, for example, influences depressed and/or demoralized individuals to dampen overt emotional suffering and amplify instead bodily complaints (Kleinman 1980; Katon et al. 1982). Zborowski (1952) highlighted other idioms of distress found in America: e.g. the overt expression of fears and anxiety about pain, among Italian and Jewish patients, and the denial of emotional reactions among 'Old Americans'. Religiously-based idioms of persecution and suffering are sometimes used by Iranian and other Middle-Eastern peoples (Good 1977). While the idiom of distress should not be reduced to an ethnic stereotype (see Craig and Wyckoff, Chapter 12), patients necessarily exploit such idioms to communicate the private experience of pain in a conventional, socially-accepted fashion. In short, idioms of distress make possible the public expression of pain, constrain the private meanings of pain, and add meanings drawn from the popular culture to subjectively-felt pain.

These diverse social and cultural variables endow each patient's experience of chronic pain with specific personal meanings. These meanings arise in certain social contexts, and they connect the experience of the symptoms to the individual's entire life-world. Moreover, because the physiological bases of chronic pain are often difficult to treat, while it continually obtrudes in all areas of the patient's life, the 'illness meanings' of pain are crucially important to the clinician. Understanding the meaning patients give to the experience of their pain will aid the clinician in devising therapeutic goals and predicting where obstacles in treatment will occur.

The following case exemplifies some of the *illness meanings* of chronic pain:

Miss L., a single white 33-year old, has suffered migraine headaches for 4 years. They began during her former job, and she blames their onset to work stress and a difficult adjustment to urban life. An only child, she was raised in rural Vermont, and remembers her childhood as happy but isolated. Miss L.'s mother, who also suffered migraines, was her only confidante until Miss L. left home.

One year ago, Miss L. left her old job to pursue a career in children's illustration, her real interest. When her headaches persisted, despite less stressful work, she began to think they reflected an inability to deal with aggressive people and her own anger (an inability she traces to her childhood isolation). She has since entered psychotherapy. She takes pain medication every night, but would like to stop; she fears eventual side effects or addiction and does not want to handle social anxiety with a drug. During severe episodes, her boyfriend solicitously cares for her, while she recuperates in a quiet, darkened room. (From authors' research.)

Whereas an account of Miss L.'s *disease* would discuss vasodilatation and dysfunctional nociceptors (Sicuteri 1981), an account of her *illness* would focus on 1) the connection she draws between headaches and social anxiety; 2) the role of headaches in leaving a secure but stressful job to pursue a riskier but more rewarding career; 3) her memories of her mother and childhood isolation; and 4) the way headaches allow both legitimated isolation and loving attention from her boyfriend.

Most experienced clinicians will recognize these sources of illness meanings for chronic pain, and will acknowledge their importance for later treatment (e.g. adherence to suggested lifestyle changes and drug prescriptions). Yet, how can they systematically assess such issues? As Fig. 1 suggests, *the meanings of chronic pain arise and become stabilized in particular social contexts.* Asking patients how pain becomes important in these settings gives clinicians a window to the illness meanings of chronic pain. We describe below chiefly the effects of family variables on the meaning of chronic pain, and briefly mention the ethnic group, work site and health care system. While illness meanings also reflect the patient's personality and learning experience, we suggest that a strictly psychological approach gives an incomplete picture.

Family meanings of chronic pain

The patient's family and close friends provide a crucial context for chronic pain. For example, behavioral psychologists have shown that the responses of family members to pain patients can significantly affect the course and disability of chronic pain syndromes (Sternbach 1968; Fordyce 1976). Sympathy, increased attention, and nurturance from family members constitute the 'secondary gains' of chronic pain, which reinforce undesirable pain behaviors (e.g. medication intake, guarded movements, grimacing, time spent in bed). One study of chronic pain patients revealed some of the following secondary gains: controlling others, justifying dependency, earning rest, avoiding sex, gaining attention, punishing others, controlling anger, and avoiding close relationships (Hudgens 1979). Clinicians have therefore attempted operant-conditioning interventions in this context (Fordyce et al. 1973; Keefe 1982), and have even enlisted other family members as therapeutic agents to help 'extinguish' unwanted pain behaviors. In one program, the family was taught how to identify pain behaviors, to consistently ignore them, and to reinforce activity and other 'well' behaviors (Roberts and Reinhardt 1980).

However, the family also influences the meaning of pain at an earlier stage in a patient's illness, even before the appearance of the symptom. Chronic pain patients have often witnessed similar suffering among their kin. In one study, 68% of such patients had at least one other family member with chronic pain, compared with 44% of non-pain (but chronically ill) controls (Violon and Giurgea 1984). Identification and modeling can thus be important sources for the meaning of pain. Other research shows that a patient's family, spouse, and spouse's family have significantly more pain complaints than those of matched non-pain controls (Mohamed et al. 1978). Intriguingly, even the bodily location of pain was more similar between chronic pain patients and their kin than between non-pain controls and their families.

Do particular family traits correlate with or even predispose to chronic pain syndromes? Engel (1959) and Szasz (1957) offer psychodynamic speculations about early childhood experience and later problems with non-organic pain, but there are few empirical studies. Merskey reported that psychiatrically-ill patients with chronic pain, when compared to other non-pain psychiatric patients, disproportionately came from large families, married more often, and had a somewhat higher rate of maladjustment and sexual difficulty in marriage (Merskey and Spear 1967). Others have also noted the correlation between large family size and chronic pain (cf. Gonda 1962). In a study with a more causal hypothesis, Hughes and Zimin (1978) demonstrated the effect of families' 'idiom of distress' upon the pain complaints of children with abdominal pain. These families habitually dealt with conflict and emotional disturbances through bodily sensations, physical explanations, and medico-surgical procedures among all family members; their children's chronic pain thus fits an established pattern.

This research echoes the findings of Minuchin (e.g. Minuchin et al. 1978) about the family factors maintaining children's psychosomatic disorders (diabetes, asthma, and especially anorexia nervosa). 'Psychosomatic families' – characterized by enmeshment, overprotectiveness, and rigidity – encourage children to exemplify family conflicts by their physical symptoms. Moreover, Minuchin and his colleagues claim that such dysfunctional family organization applies across all types of psychosomatic illness. This view of the 'psychosomatic system' – the communicative difficulties and family conflicts which both create and are supported by the child's symptom – has much to teach us about the family meanings of chronic pain.

These studies yield one crucial clinical lesson: individuals learn how to name, interpret, and respond to particular pain disorders from the experience of family members. The following case illustrates this point:

Mr. B., a 28-year old white museum curator, has had worsening pain in the cervical spine for 3 years. Recently, he noticed muscular tenderness and 'painful flashes' in his shoulders and hips. Although his local physician dismissed these as transient symptoms, they recalled to Mr. B. the suffering of his brother, who has serious spondylitis. Mr. B. became quite alarmed about his new symptoms, and incensed at his doctor's inaction. After many telephone calls, his brother told Mr. B. of a specialist in a distant city. After visiting this doctor, Mr. B. learned that his pains in fact were not consistent with spondylitis, and was counselled to change his sleeping posture. The pains soon disappeared, but Mr. B. remains suspicious of his local physician, and has begun looking for a new doctor. (From authors' research.)

Although clinician and patient meet alone in the consulting room, the patient's trusted social circle has already given advice for treatment, and will soon jointly evaluate the effectiveness of intervention. These family negotiations help the patient decide 'what possible label should be applied, how severe the episode is, what help-seeking behavior is appropriate, and when action should be taken' (McKinlay 1981; see Katon and Kleinman 1982 for a fuller discussion). For a chronic pain sufferer, the family will evaluate the cost of care against family finances, the appropriateness of care against the family's health beliefs, and the potential disruption of specific treatments against the needs of other family members (Kotarba 1983 cf. Chrisman 1977). In this sense, the patient and his/her family jointly manage the chronic pain before and after medical treatment.

Families of chronic pain patients give meaning not only to the search for relief, but also to the assessment of the pain itself. Recent research shows that family members and pain patients largely agree about the duration of pain, effect of pain on activities, and daily fluctuations in pain (Swanson and Maruta 1980). Moreover, chronic pain patients and their spouses share certain types of psychological distress, which again suggests their conjoint assessment of the pain (Shanfield et al. 1979). Finally, the multiple losses of job and income resulting from incapacitating pain would affect the entire family, and this impact on other members will shape the meaning of the pain for the patient. Since agreement between patient and family about the meaning of pain can produce resistance to treatment and shared dissatisfaction with results (Swanson and Maruta 1980), clinicians must attend closely to the family setting of chronic pain.

The family meanings of chronic pain thus unfold along a number of stages. Within the family, an individual's pain is (at least partially) learned, named, evaluated, expressed in a particular idiom, and brought to a clinician. However, just as the family affects the pain, the pain reciprocally affects the family. Behaviorist psychology has stressed the pathological effect of chronic pain on family functioning: the manipulative 'pain games' of patients who use their symptoms to dominate other family members or escape responsibilities (Menges 1981). Most of this literature focuses on the secondary gains of chronic pain (cf. Fordyce 1976, and above).

However, this approach tells only half the story. Along with the patients' secondary gains, other family members also derive benefits (or, 'tertiary gains'). For example, a father's chronic back problem suddenly worsens the day before a planned visit to a disliked relative (Kotarba 1983, p. 87). A husband's protracted pain from a fractured acetabulum forces him to retire early, but places his wife in a caretaking role and legitimizes her desire to get a part-time job. The 'tertiary gain' for this woman — who had previously complained of emotional distance from her husband and social isolation — make her husband's return to health much more difficult (Bokan et al. 1981). These examples show that *pain behavior is never restricted to the identified patient, but always becomes embedded in family dynamics and the needs and desires of kin.* This may result in a dysfunctional family system, but in many cases opens up new role options for other family members or accomplishes certain goals of the family as a whole.

Chronic pain and ethnicity

Ethnic groups, as well as families, impart specific meanings to the chronic pain experience. Since Craig and Wyckoff's paper (Chapter 12) thoroughly reviews this issue, we offer only one comment and a clinical *vade mecum*. Ethnic groups do not exist as homogeneous wholes. In addition to the cross-cutting variables of social class, gender, age, etc. we introduce the distinction between ideological and behavioral ethnicity (Stein and Hill 1977; Harwood 1981). Within the same group, some individuals display their ethnic identity in most daily activities, while others have largely assimilated to the dominant national culture, and invoke their ethnic heritage only on specific occasions (e.g. religious holidays or political rallies). Moreover, the clinical situation will bring out different tendencies in the same group or even the same individual.

We strongly caution clinicians against relying on static descriptions of American ethnic groups in managing chronic pain. Lists of cultural/ethnic traits should rather serve as preliminary guidelines in establishing the relevant categories for a particular patient with a specific complaint (cf. Maranhao 1984). Ideally, clinicians should assess the importance of ethnicity for chronic pain patients according to some of the following variables (adapted from Lipton and Marbach 1984):

I: 'Non-ethnic' demographic variables
      Age; Education; Income; Gender; Social class.

II: 'Ideological' vs. 'Behavioral' ethnicity
      Generation American;
      Domestic arrangement (nuclear vs. extended family);
      Proportion of friends in same ethnic group;
      Importance of daily upholding ethnic customs/traditions.

III: 'Ethnic' health care practices
      Degree of exposure to/trust of biomedicine;
      Reliance on members of same ethnic group in making health care decisions.

Chronic pain, work, and the health care setting

Chronic pain is a private disorder. There usually exists neither gross trauma nor obvious physical reasons for disability. Therefore, chronic pain patients must constantly decide how much to reveal and to whom about the extent of their suffering. Certain work settings make this an especially crucial decision. Kotarba (1983) studied blue-collar workers and professional athletes with chronic pain. In order to keep their jobs, workers in these occupations must disguise the true extent of chronic pain. The surreptitious use of lay therapies (hot baths, massage) and self-medication (alcohol and illegally obtained potent analgesics) flourishes in these groups. Because these patients feel their economic survival threatened by chronic pain, they must usually hide their symptoms from employers and even co-workers. Pain thus becomes part of a concealed and potentially damaging self-identity. Such patients may have great reluctance in revealing to their physicians the true severity and impairment caused by pain. Clinicians treating such individuals must be aware of the obstacles to effective care posed by these work-related meanings of chronic pain.

Some occupations, however, exert just the opposite effect. In rigidly organized work settings, with little individual control over the conditions of work or opportunities for advancement, pain complaints may be the only legitimate idiom of protest against the system. Chronic pain may provide the only leverage to negotiate time off from work, change in work routines or location, and disability payments (Kleinman 1982). While most clinicians know of the familiar 'disability neurosis', they should inquire about this second work-related meaning of chronic pain whenever patients hold jobs that seem overly rigid or minimally rewarding.

A brief mention of the health care system as a source of illness meanings for chronic pain cannot do justice to the literature on the topic. When chronic pain sufferers seek medical treatment, they encounter clinicians who construct the meaning of chronic pain for their patients by espousing particular technologies and specific philosophies of sickness and health. Thus the trajectory of somatic amplification is frequently a transactional result of doctor-patient relationships. Kotarba (1983) places the clinical construction of chronic pain against the backdrop of the professionalization of various non-M.D. clinicians. He discusses the appeal of chiropractic and osteopathy for chronic pain patients, and shows how the divergent expectations of patient and clinician in modern 'Pain Centers' contribute to the labeling of 'good' and 'bad' patients (hence, the moral meaning of chronic pain). Fagerhaugh and Strauss (1977) analyze the social organization of hospital personnel and patients with chronic pain. They demonstrate the inappropriateness of an acute care model, as well as the political and persuasive activities that surround pain management.

Clinical social science recommendations

1) Clinicians should legitimate patients' experience of chronic pain. By simply spending more *time* listening to a patient's pain story, and by rooting out their own negative countertransference reactions (e.g. the stereotype of non-compliant, 'problem' patients), clinicians will more quickly see the potential obstacles in treatment.

2) Assessment of chronic pain patients must include a thorough, ethnographic-style, open-ended description of pain in the patient's own life-world. The clinician should learn the patient's *illness* as well as the *disease*. Eliciting patient and family explanatory models of the illness may be useful here (Kleinman 1980). An explanatory model for pain covers what the individual/family think causes the pain, how it works in the body, what its major effects are on their lives, what future problems they fear, and what treatment they want. Patients will readily offer these accounts to the empathetic physician, who can then compare them point by point to the disease model. Clinicians should actively negotiate between the models: presenting the disease model in lay terms, and incorporating the illness model into the treatment plan to guide management decisions.

3) Through the above and through careful evaluation of other sources of information (medical record, consultants' reports, illness diary, psychological tests), the clinician should systematically assess the local contexts of pain. She/he should examine how the patient's family, ethnic group, work-site, and health care setting contribute to the meaning of chronic pain, and how such meanings may amplify or dampen the actual pain complaint (Kleinman 1982).

4) Clinicians should negotiate with patient and family about interventions to alter these meanings and contexts. This will require supplementing biomedical and behavioral treatment with social interventions (e.g. psychotherapy, social work referrals, job counselling, marital and family therapy, and, with permission, even dealing directly with the patient's employers).

Conclusion

Chronic pain represents a heterogeneous group of pathologies and syndromes. Clinicians need to attend closely to the biology, psychology, and social context of a chronic pain patient in order to plan an effective treatment and rally the patient's cooperation. This chapter has claimed that the 'patient's point of view' – the illness meanings of chronic pain – reflects each of these disparate levels. Furthermore, the meanings of pain arise and become stabilized in particular social contexts. Of course, these four contexts (family, ethnic/cultural group, work site, and health care system) overlap and can completely encompass each other. We separate them here not only for clarity, but also to demonstrate that some major problems in chronic pain management can be resolved by taking each of them into account.

References

Adam, K. S. and Walshe, J. W. B. (1978) Psychogenic pain: an overview. In: C. Peck and M. Wallace (eds.), Problems in Pain. Pergamon Press, Sydney, pp. 141 – 150.
Blumhagen, D. (1982) The meaning of hyper-tension. In: N. J. Chrisman and T. W. Maretzki (Eds.), Clinically Applied Medical Anthropology. D. Reidel Publ. Co., Boston, pp. 297 – 323.
Bokan, J., Ries, R. and Katon, W. (1981) Tertiary gain and chronic pain. Pain 10, 331 – 335.

Chrisman, N. (1977) The health-seeking process: an approach to the natural history of illness. Culture Med. Psychiatry 1, 351 – 377.

Engel, G. L. (1959) 'Psychogenic' pain and the pain prone patient. Am. J. Med. 26, 899 – 918.

Fagerhaugh, S. Y. and Strauss, A. (1977) Politics of pain management: staff-patient interaction. Addison-Wesley Publ. Co., Menlo Park, California.

Fordyce, W. E. (1976) Behavioral Methods for Chronic Pain and Illness. Mosby Press, St. Louis, MO.

Fordyce, W. E., Fowler, R. S., Lehmann, J. F. et al. (1973) Operant conditioning in the treatment of chronic pain. Arch. Phys. Med. Rehab. 54, 399 – 408.

Gonda, T. A. (1962) The relation between complaints of persistent pain and family size. J. Neurol. Neurosurg. Psychiatry 25, 277 – 281.

Good, B. (1977) The heart of what's the matter: the semantics of illness in Iran. Culture Med. Psychiatry 1, 25 – 58.

Harwood, A. (1981) Ethnicity and Medical Care. Harvard University Press, Cambridge, Mass.

Hudgens, A. J. (1979) Family-oriented treatment of chronic pain. J. Marit. Fam. Ther. 5, 67 – 78.

Hughes, M. C. and Zimin, K. (1978) Children with psychogenic abdominal pain and their families. Clin. Pediatr. 17, 569 – 573.

Katon, W., Kleinman, A. and Rosen, G. (1982) Depression and somatization: a review. Parts I and II. Am. J. Med. 72, 127 – 135, 241 – 246.

Keefe, F. J. (1982) Behavioral assessment and treatment of chronic pain: current status and future direction. J. Consult. Clin. Psychol. 50, 896 – 911.

Kleinman, A. (1980) Patients and Healers in the Context of Culture. University of California Press, Berkeley.

Kleinman, A. (1982) Neurasthenia and depression: a study of somatization and culture in China. Culture Med. Psychiatry 6, 117 – 191.

Kleinman, A. and Kleinman, J. (1985) Somatization: the interconnections between culture, depressive experiences, and the meanings of pain. In: A. Kleinman and B. Good (Eds.), Culture and Depression. University of California Press, Berkeley, pp. 429 – 490.

Kleinman, A., Eisenberg, L. and Good, B. (1977) Culture, illness, and care. Ann. Intern. Med. 88, 251 – 258.

Kotarba, J. (1983) Chronic Pain: its Social Dimensions. Sage Press, Beverly Hills, CA.

Kotarba, J. and Seidel, J. (1984) Managing the problem pain patient: compliance or social control. Soc. Sci. Med. 19, 1393 – 1400.

Lipowski, Z. (1969) Psychosocial aspects of disease. Ann. Intern. Med. 71, 1197 – 1206.

Lipton, J. and Marbach, J. (1984) Ethnicity and the pain experience. Soc. Sci. Med. 19, 1279 – 1298.

Maranhao, T. (1984) Family therapy and anthropology. Culture Med. Psychiatry 8, 255 – 281.

McKinlay, J. B. (1981) Social network influences on morbid episodes and the career of help-seeking. In: L. Eisenberg and A. Kleinman (Eds.), The Relevance of Social Science for Medicine. D. Reidel Publ. Co., Boston, pp. 77 – 110.

Mechanic, D. (1972) Social psychologic factors affecting the presentation of bodily complaints. N. Engl. J. Med. 286, 1132 – 1139.

Menges, L. J. (1981) Psychological aspects of chronic pain. In: S. Lipton and J. Miles (Eds.), Persistent Pain: Modern Methods of Treatment (Volume 3). Grune and Stratton, New York, pp. 87 – 98.

Merskey, H. and Spear, F. A. (1967) Pain: Psychological and Psychiatric Aspects. Bailliere, Tindall, and Cassell, London.

Minuchin, S., Rosman, B. and Baker, L. (1978) Psychosomatic Families: Anorexia Nervosa in Context. Harvard University Press, Cambridge.

Mohamed, S., Weisz, G. and Waring, E. (1978) The relationship of chronic pain to depression, marital adjustment, and family dynamics. Pain 5, 285 – 292.

Nichter, M. (1981) Idioms of distress. Culture Med. Psychiatry 5, 379 – 408.

Roberts, A. and Reinhardt, L. (1980) The behavioral management of chronic pain: long-term follow-up with comparison group. Pain 8, 151 – 162.

Shanfield, S. B., Heiman, E. M., Cope, D. N. and Jones, J. R. (1979) Pain and the marital relationship: psychiatric distress. Pain 7, 343 – 351.

Sicuteri, F. (1981) Persistent non-organic central pain: headache and central panalgesic. In: S. Lipton and J. Miles (Eds.), Persistent Pain: Modern Methods of Treatment, Vol. 3. Academic Press, London, pp. 119 – 140.

Stein, H. F. and Hill, R.   (1977)   The Ethnic Imperative: Examining the New White Ethnic Movement. Pennsylvania State University Press, University Park, Pennsylvania.

Sternbach, R. A.   (1968)   Pain: A Psychophysiological Analysis. Academic Press, New York.

Swanson, D. and Maruta, T.   (1980)   The family's viewpoint of chronic pain. Pain 8, 163 – 166.

Szasz, T.   (1957)   Pain and Pleasure: A Study of Bodily Feelings. Basic Books, New York.

Violon, A. and Giurgea, E.   (1984)   Familial models for chronic pain. Pain 18, 199 – 203.

Waring, E.   (1976)   The role of family in symptom selection and perpetuation in psychosomatic illness. Presented at the 11th European Conference on Psychosomatic Medicine, September, 1976.

Zborowski, M.   (1952)   Cultural components in response to pain. J. Soc. Iss. 8, 16 – 30.

Zola, I.   (1966)   Culture and symptoms: an analysis of patients presenting complaints. Am. Sociol. Rev. 31, 615 – 636.

Burrows/Elton/Stanley (eds.) Handbook of Chronic Pain Management
© *1987 Elsevier Science Publishers B.V. (Biomedical Division)*

14

Religion, meditation and pain

GORDON STANLEY

Department of Psychology, University of Melbourne, Victoria, Australia

Introduction

Pain patients do not exist in isolation from their socio-cultural context (Elton and Stanley 1982). Religion is one widespread and important aspect of human culture and in this chapter we will consider the role that religious factors can play in modifying the reactive component of pain. In so doing we will adopt a functionalist perspective appropriate to a concern with the practical aspects of pain management. As a consequence, it is not our intention to engage in the evaluation of different religious beliefs or practices, but rather to draw attention to the part that they may play in the experience of pain.

Pain is a universal aspect of the human condition and it is not surprising that it has been given considerable attention in most religious systems (Lewis 1957; Yinger 1970). The history of religion is replete with examples of concern with pain and pain control (Yinger 1977; Lowie 1924). Religious rituals may enable pain to be either suppressed or expressed depending on the context and the particular belief system.

Levels of explanation

Modern Western medicine has centred on what was wrong with the patient in terms of symptoms. This symptomatic approach has involved a search for mechanism without consideration of subjective meaning. With pain, the search is for the disease process in terms of biological mechanism. Hence the patient often feels confronted by a technologist who is not interested in or capable of interpreting the significance of the condition in ultimate terms. Frank (1973) has pointed out that the traditional religious healer has addressed the anxiety patients have about the meaning of pain for their understanding of purpose and the nature of existence. In dealing directly with the existential aspects of illness, the religious professional has a function complementary to that of the physician and other health care workers (see Rappaport and Rappaport 1981).

As discussed in other chapters in this volume, the reactive component of pain is reduced effectively by various psychological procedures. Many religious practices appear to function in similar ways to these techniques. This is not to say that a psychological account of the effect of such religious practices is a sufficient explanation of the phenomena. Psychological accounts are at a different level of explanation than religious accounts (Stanley and Bartlett 1978) and represent an attempt to bring the important functional implications of religion into a scientific framework where they can be studied and understood.

Even in those situations where it can be assumed reasonably that the religious practice is functioning in essentially the same manner as a recognized and well-understood psychological procedure, there may be people for whom a religious framework is a necessary condition for their acceptance of the procedure. In our research with chronic pain patients (Elton et al. 1980) we occasionally found patients who spontaneously interpreted standard psychological procedures in terms of their own religious framework. While not positively encouraging such interpretation we were reluctant to reject it for to do so may have led to rejection of the treatment.

Some patients have an objection in principle to hypnotherapeutic techniques as they feel it will involve a handing over of self-control to another person. This is particularly true for some very conservative religious believers. Chaplains with appropriate understanding can be helpful in addressing the essentially theological concerns of such patients. Professionals who are not religious may not appreciate how significant such worries may be for the patient's acceptance of and progress in a proposed treatment. Equally, there are many patients for whom any association of a therapeutic practice with religion is unnecessary and for whom it would be counter-productive.

Altered states and meditation

Altered states of consciousness achieved through religious practices may be given their empirical verification by the participant's demonstration of an ability to suppress normal pain. Melzack (1973) described Indian ceremonies in which a person is suspended by hooks inserted into flesh without visible appearance of pain. Many non-Western cults have religious ceremonies in which people walk on burning coals or insert spikes into their flesh without the normal pain reactions (Elton et al. 1983, p. 48).

It is worth pointing out that such feats generally occur after a considerable preparatory phase in which the participant may engage in frenzied dancing or a meditative procedure which leads to a trance-like state in which acute pain reactions are blocked. In Christian traditions, speaking in tongues frequently occurs with faith healing of painful conditions (Hollenweger 1972). Again, a similar process may be occurring although tongue-speaking is not always associated with a trance-like state of dissociation (Stanley et al. 1978).

Noting a relationship in the literature between religion and pain reduction, Tiger (1985) speculated about the possibility of religious ritual influencing some 'obscure internal mechanism that releases endorphins' (p. 62). Such a mechanism was considered to produce its effects primarily through the social connectedness of religious participation, together with a 'chemically mediated cognitive bias' (p. 63). While having some plausibility, at this stage this speculation is not sufficiently explicit in detail to be evaluated. There appears to be no direct empirical evidence for the presumed role of endorphins in states of religious ecstacy.

In recent years, there has been a growth of interest in meditative procedures as practiced in Eastern religions. Such procedures have been promoted and studied extensively in the West.

Goleman (1977) provided a useful comparison of a dozen systems of meditation. There are many differences in procedure and in the interpretation of the significance of the state of consciousness achieved through the process of meditation. Despite these differences, Goleman (1977) asserts that 'all meditation systems are variations on a single process for transforming consciousness. The core elements of this process are found in every system and its specifics undercut ostensible differences among the various schools of meditation' (p. 106).

Greatest differences are found in the preparation for meditation. Religious groups differ in requirements for purification and withdrawal from the world of everyday events. More secularized systems such as Transcendental Meditation (TM) see meditation as a part of the person's normal daily round. The process of meditation itself is achieved through retraining attention so that the person is required to concentrate on a single percept, be it visual or auditory in origin. This concentration leads to a loss of usual sense awareness, attention to the one object to the exclusion of all other thoughts and an intensely rapturous feeling. Controlled breathing and fasting and the cognitive set induced by the religious instruction all combine with the attentional focus to produce the altered state of awareness. With practice the meditative state can occur more easily and it becomes possible for the person to 'maintain prolonged meditative awareness in the midst of his other activities. As the states produced by his meditation meld with his waking activity, the awakened state ripens. When it reaches full maturity, it lastingly changes his consciousness, transforming his experience of himself and of his universe' (Goleman 1977, p. 118).

In an important review Shapiro (1982) compared meditation to other clinical self-control techniques. He concluded that while meditation produced a state of relaxation with a reduction in physiological arousal, there was no evidence from EEG, autonomic or metabolic indication that it represented a unique state. For a range of conditions meditation appeared to be as effective as hypnosis, biofeedback and progressive relaxation.

There are major difficulties in assessing the comparative effectiveness of therapeutic techniques in general and these become more acute when the technique has a religious or quasi-religious commitment associated with it. Holmes (1984) reviewed the literature in terms of the adequacy of controls for drawing conclusions about the efficacy of treatment based on meditation. He concluded that 'the published experimental research on the influence of meditation on somatic arousal did not reveal any evidence that meditating subjects attained lower levels of somatic arousal than did resting subjects. Furthermore, the review did not reveal any evidence that subjects who had meditated had less somatic response to stressful situations than did subjects who had not meditated. These conclusions are in sharp contrast to the widely held beliefs about the effects of meditation' (Holmes 1984, p. 8).

The conclusions drawn by Holmes (1984) from the literature have been questioned by Benson and Friedman (1985), Shapiro (1985), Suler (1985) and West (1985). It would seem that at this stage the evidence for meditation producing distinct physiological effects is not substantial and that at best its effectiveness is parallel to other self-control techniques in common use. Shapiro (1985) points out that there may well be subjective factors, difficult to measure, which make meditation a preferred treatment for some patients. Meditation with its emphasis on focussed attention probably acts as a cognitive distractor from pain and is similar to other distraction approaches to pain control (McCaul and Malott 1984).

Religion and suffering

Religion can act to legitimize the suffering aspects of pain. Pain can be seen as being deserved and can be sustained by guilt and poor self-esteem (Engel 1958; Elton et al. 1983, pp. 42 – 44). Within Christianity the self-flagellations of the penitent or the stigmata were seen as ways of gaining forgiveness and identification with the suffering of Christ (Thomson 1980). While such practices are not common today, there is often concern with pain and suffering as avenues for spiritual development (Fichter 1981).

Much of the evidence for religion playing a part in the response to pain is descriptive and anecdotal. An exception is an interesting experiment by Lambert et al. (1960). They carried out an investigation of the effect of religious identification on ischaemic pain. By placing hard-rubber spikes in the pressure cuff of a sphygmomanometer pain induction occurred as the experimenter increased cuff pressure. The pressure was released when the subjects said they could no longer tolerate the pain. Half of them were Jewish and half Christian. After an initial measurement of pain tolerance the Jewish subjects were informed that it had been claimed that Jews could not tolerate as much pain as Christians and that the study was designed to see if it were true. The Christians were told the opposite. Members of both groups tolerated significantly more pain on the second occasion. Control group members for whom religious membership was not salient did not change their pain tolerance significantly on the second trial. Alternative groups of Christians and Jews were instructed that their groups could tolerate more pain than the other. With this instruction the Christians took significantly more pain on the second trial while the Jews did not change their tolerance on the second trial. This research is important in showing that even in a laboratory significant effects of religious identification on pain tolerance can be demonstrated.

Some theologians represent suffering as a refining process which builds character and acts as 'an avenue to joy' (Hageman 1966). If the patient construes the pain as the deserved fruits of sin or as morally cleansing, then effective pain modification treatment may be impossible without consideration of the moral and theological dimension. A goal of the chaplain may be to help the individual deal with guilt without resorting to the process of somatization.

Many contemporary religious writers consider suffering something to be overcome by means of faith (MacNutt 1977). This more positive emphasis can be of assistance in pain control. Sensitive use of the religious dimension in dealing with chronic pain patients requires considerable skill on the part of a chaplain and is best carried out in the context of a multidisciplinary and multimodal approach to the patient.

Summary

Religion allows the question of the meaning of pain and suffering to be addressed. As a universal aspect of human culture it has long been concerned with pain. This concern can enable pain to be reduced or augmented. While meditative practices facilitate the control of pain, the process does not appear to be distinctively different in its effects from other relatively well-studied psychological methods. For some patients meditation may be a preferred method of treatment. Some religious beliefs can produce an augmented pain response where the pain is seen as deserved or spiritually desirable. In such cases a chaplain may play a useful role in the approach to pain management by dealing with the theological dimension.

References

Benson, H. and Friedman, R. (1985) A rebuttal to the conclusions of David S. Holmes's article: 'Meditation and somatic arousal reduction'. Am. Psychol. 40, 725 – 728.

Elton, D. and Stanley, G. V. (1982) Cultural expectations and psychological factors in prolonged disability. In: J. Sheppard (Ed.), Advances in Behavioural Medicine, Vol. 2. Cumberland College of Health Sciences, Sydney.

Elton, D., Burrows, G. D. and Stanley, G. V. (1980) Chronic pain and hypnosis. In: G. D. Burrows and L. Dennerstein (Eds.), Handbook of Hypnosis and Psychosomatic Medicine. Elsevier/North-Holland Biomedical Press, Amsterdam, pp. 269 – 292.

Elton, D., Stanley, G. and Burrows, G. D. (1983) Psychological Control of Pain. Grune and Stratton, Australia.

Engel, G. L. (1958) Psychogenic pain. Med. Clin. North Am. 42, 1481 – 1496.

Fichter, J. H. (1981) Religion and Pain. Crossroad, New York.

Frank, J. D. (1973) Persuasion and Healing. Johns Hopkins University Press, Baltimore.

Goleman, D. (1977) The Varieties of the Meditative Experience. Irvington Press, New York.

Hageman, L. (1966) Suffering – an avenue to joy. Humanitas 9, 84 – 96.

Hollenweger, W. J. (1972) The Pentecostals. Augsburg Publishing, Minneapolis.

Holmes, D. S. (1984) Meditation and somatic arousal reduction. A review of the experimental evidence. Am. Psychol. 39, 1 – 10.

Lambert, W. E., Libman, E. and Poser, E. G. (1960) The effect of increased salience of a membership group on pain tolerance. J. Pers. 28, 350 – 357.

Lewis, C. S. (1957) The Problem of Pain. Fontana, Glasgow.

Lowie, R. (1924) Primitive Religion. Boni and Liveright, New York.

McCaul, K. D. and Malott, J. M. (1984) Distraction and coping with pain. Psychol. Bull. 95, 516 – 533.

MacNutt, F. (1977) The Power to Heal. Ave Maria Press, Notre Dame.

Melzack, R. (1973) The Puzzle of Pain. Penguin, Middlesex.

Rappaport, H. and Rappaport, M. (1981) The integration of scientific and traditional healing. Am. Psychol. 36, 774 – 781.

Shapiro, D. H. (1982) Comparison of meditation with other self-control strategies – biofeedback, hypnosis, progressive relaxation: a review of the clinical and psychological literature. Am. J. Psychiatr. 139, 267 – 284.

Shapiro, D. H. (1985) Clinical use of meditation as a self-regulation strategy; comments on Holmes's conclusions and implications. Am. Psychol. 40, 719 – 722.

Stanley, G. and Bartlett, W. K. (1978) Notes on the Psychology of Religion. Deakin University, Geelong, Australia.

Stanley, G., Bartlett, W. K. and Moyle, T. (1978) Some characteristics of charismatic experience: glossolalia in Australia. J. Sci. Stud. Relig. 17, 269 – 278.

Suler, J. R. (1985) Meditation and somatic arousal: a comment on Holmes's review. Am. Psychol. 40, 717.

Thomson, W. A. R. (1980) Faiths That Heal. Adam and Charles Black, London.

Tiger, L. (1985) Survival of the faithful. The Sciences 25, 61 – 63.

West, M. A. (1985) Meditation and somatic arousal. Am. Psychol. 40, 717 – 719.

Yinger, Y. M. (1970) The Scientific Study of Religion. Macmillan, New York.

Yinger, Y. M. (1977) A comparative study of the substructures of religion. J. Sci. Stud. Relig. 16, 67 – 86.

Burrows/Elton/Stanley (eds.) Handbook of Chronic Pain Management
© *1987 Elsevier Science Publishers B.V. (Biomedical Division)*

15

Dietary factors in chronic pain management

OLOV LINDAHL

Lambarö, Vallingby, Sweden

Introduction – theoretical background

This chapter differs in its approach from the usual treatment of pain theory and pain management. It is based on an explanation of the origin of pain which was introduced by Lindahl in his doctoral thesis in 1961, and which was further developed in subsequent work (Lindahl 1962, 1970, 1974, 1985). According to this work, all peripheral pain results from an acid change in the surroundings of the nerve endings. This change can be caused by a number of different tissue processes, all present in conditions of pain and all giving rise to an acid pH. In tissue damage or necrosis, for example, acid components are freed from the cell contents after destruction of the cell membrane. The content of all cells (inside the cell membrane) is more or less acid. In ischaemic conditions, such as claudication and infarction, the reaction becomes acid due to anaerobic metabolism in which acid metabolites accumulate. In certain malignant tumours the interstitial pH has been shown to be acid. With infection, the metabolism also occurs in an acid environment due to damage to the cell membranes and release of the acid cell content. An acid pH has been demonstrated by different authors and methods in all these conditions.

In Lindahl's thesis it was shown that in human experimental subjects a pH of 6.5 evoked significant pain, and a pH of 5.5 intensive pain, in the skin. In different pain conditions the pH can go down to 4.5 – as, for example, in fracture haematomas.

With this background, it would seem natural to treat pain conditions by trying to change the pH in an alkaline direction by, for example, giving the patient sodium bicarbonate by mouth. Unfortunately this does not work very well. The reason is that in every acid condition the metabolism already is trying to compensate for the change in pH. In the blood and interstitial fluid a series of buffer mechanisms are at work, and in the majority of pain conditions circulation is maximally increased, as, for example, in inflammatory states and in fractures.

Alkaline substances taken by mouth or intravenously do not change the local situation, as increased circulation to the painful areas and the buffer systems are already working at maximal levels. In cases of ischaemia, the lack of circulation is of course a hindrance in the compensation of the local acidosis. And in inflammation the most essential treatment must be stabilization of the cell membrane and prevention of cellular necrosis.

In one type of pain condition, however, the administration of alkaline substances by mouth has a definite effect on the pain. I have called this condition *varialgia*, and it is defined by the following parameters: the pain has no typical localization; it can exist in all parts of the body but normally not in inner organs; the location of the pain can change from one place to another; the pain varies in intensity; it often changes with the weather and may keep the patient awake at night; it is often worst in the morning. When sleeping, the patient wakes up very early in the morning. The patient feels stiff in the morning and has difficulty moving around. Unlike functional pain, it is often less pronounced after the patient has gotten up from bed in the morning and started his daily activities. There is no patho-anatomical basis for this pain condition, but is can be localized in the same region in which, for example, a normally pain-free osteo-arthritis exists. The pain can also be of this character in sciatica, and the condition can then be called varialgic sciatica (Lindahl 1966).

Most physicians have seen patients of this type, with uncharacteristic, moving, varying and diffuse pain syndromes which are very resistant to conventional treatment. It is a common concept that this type of pain is of nervous origin. Lack of understanding, lack of sleep, and no cure often *make* the patient nervous, which then seems to verify the first diagnosis. In patients with rheumatoid arthritis (RA) the same symptoms are common, but this disease is not included in the concept varialgia.

For 20 years, I have treated patients with these symptoms by giving them alkaline-ash food and alkaline medications by mouth. Over the years I have used different compositions, but all according to the same general principle that the patient is given proton acceptors in a dose of about 100 mEq per day. The preparation consists of a mixture of salts of potassium, calcium and magnesium with lactate, citrate or carbonate. At the same time it is important to eliminate acid-ash food and acid medications such as acetylsalicylic acid, hydrochloric acid (in achylia) and thiazide preparations (in hypertension and/or oedema).

The results are very good as about 70% of the patients become pain-free within $2-6$ months. The success of the treatment is significantly correlated to a change in the daily excretion of protons in the urine. This means that the effect cannot be explained as a placebo effect. Details of the results and the treatment are published elsewhere (Lindahl 1966, 1970, 1974).

When the excretion of protons in the urine is controlled over a longer period, it is usual in this condition for a huge store of protons to be excreted during a time period of up to 6 or even 12 months. Normally the daily urine contains $50-100$ mEq of protons. The same amount is also excreted week after week when the patient is given 100 or even 200 mEq of proton acceptors per day. This means that an excess of stored protons is being eliminated from the body and this can go on for a very long period. During this time the pain symptoms vary and are sometimes even worse. When the reaction in the urine finally changes from acid to alkaline, the symptoms often disappear at the same time as this change occurs. Normally the administration of $100-200$ mEq of proton acceptors changes the reaction of the urine from acid to alkaline in one or several days.

Calculation of the excess excretion of protons indicates that more than 20,000 mEq of protons can be stored in the body. The most probable place for this storage seems to be bone tissue and the collagen system (Langgård 1965). It is well known that bone tissue is lost (resulting in osteomalacia/porosis) by acidification. The bone tissue functions as an ion-changer, but at the expense of calcium. It has also been shown that alkalinization can prevent osteoporosis due to inactivity.

The administration of alkaline medicine is the essential part of the treatment, but it is also important to change the patient's dietary habits in the same direction. Acid-ash food such as cereals, including bread, should be excluded, and alkaline-ash food such as vegetables should be increased.

The treatment is complicated by the fact that pain relief can take a long time. It sometimes takes more than 6 months before alkalinization of the urine is obtained. The diagnosis – the criteria for the disease – is also not precise enough to guarantee that only patients with disturbance of the acid-base balance are included. This means that some patients do not respond to the treatment even when alkalinization is completed.

It is very easy to forget that different drugs, such as aspirin, give rise to substantial acidification. The patients often forget to report that they have taken this drug as it is considered a normal part of life and not a medicine. It is hardly possible to achieve an alkalinization at the same time as aspirin is being ingested!

Application and results of treatment

Within biological medicine we have the conception that some diseases which are not cured by conventional treatment can be helped with alternative, non-conventional methods, such as a radical change in diet.

There are two painful conditions in which the results of nutritional treatment are very good and are verified by means of scientific methods. These are premenstrual syndrome (PMS) and rheumatoid arthritis (RA).

Premenstrual syndrome. These patients have a reduction of gammalinolenic and dihomgammalinolenic acid in their blood (Horrobin 1983). This means that production of the 'good' prostaglandin E_1 is lower than normal. As it is difficult to give prostaglandin E_1 as a medicine (it works only when given intravenously), it has been natural to try to give gammalinolenic acid by mouth instead. This acid is easily converted to prostaglandin E_1 in the body. Gammalinolenic acid is very rare in nature and is normally found only in human milk. It has also been localized in evening primrose oil. This oil is commercially available as Efamol® in England. The substance has been tested in PMS in four double-blind tests, all with positive results (Horrobin 1982, 1984). The dose is 8 capsules per day. This dose can usually be lowered to $2-6$ capsules when the symptoms have disappeared. Sometimes taking the preparation for only a fortnight prior to menses is sufficient. Up to 85% of the patients experience relief from this treatment.

Rheumatoid arthritis. This disease is indeed a chronically painful condition, and many patients become successively worse in spite of conventional treatment. In these cases I have found that a very radical change of diet can help most of the patients (Lindberg 1979; Lindahl and Myrnerts 1979). The pain and joint swelling decreases and disappears, but of course any joint destruction present is not influenced. The results take quite a long time, and improvement is successively achieved over a period of at least $3-5$ years. This treatment is best administered by a nutritionist trained in this method, but I can outline the general guidelines here. The diet is a radical vegan diet. The following foodstuffs are not allowed: meat, fish and other animal products, including milk, cheese, cream and butter, pure sugar, table salt, coffee, tea, chocolate, all cereal products, beans, apples, citrus fruits, alcohol and tobacco. Drugs, especially aspirin and cortisone, must be excluded as soon as possible – which means when the symptoms decrease. Allowed are: all vegetables and fruits not mentioned above, berries and buckwheat. These products should primarily be raw or cooked for only a short time and, if necessary, chopped up in a mixer. The treatment is begun with a fasting period of $1-2$ weeks and this is repeated twice every year.

The theoretical background to this very radical regimen is that patients with RA have acquired a food allergy and a change in the intestine which allows large molecules to enter the blood stream and heavily load the immune system.

The results obtained with this regimen have been tested in a series of clinical trials, some of which have not yet been published. The cases chosen for these tests have all been RA, defined by the American Rheumatoid Association as definite or classical RA. In a prospective randomized series, the diet group was significantly better than the control group on conventional medication in respect to activity index, joint index and erythrocyte sedimentation rate (Hamberg et al. 1981). There are various criticisms of this study. While the results are interesting, for more controlled studies a doubleblind trial might be of use. Furthermore, patients were only observed for a short time – a period of one month. The improvement could then be explained as a result of the initial fasting for one week, which is known to produce a radical improvement in RA. We have now conducted two different investigations in which the patients were treated one and 2 years, respectively, with the same regimen. The same results have also been obtained in these two series. There is a significant improvement in comparison with the initial status in respect to joint index, activity index, erythrocyte sedimentation rate and a series of other laboratory variables. This is only a preliminary report of the results which are to be published later.

Of course, the lack of control in the two latter studies is a drawback. It would be impossible, however, to keep a control group intact over such a long period of time. All these patients had had their disease for more than 3 years and had become progressively worse. We believe, therefore, that the results demonstrate that a very radical change in diet may eradicate pain and other symptoms in RA.

References

Hamberg, J., Lindahl, O., Lindwall, L. and Öckerman, P. A. (1981) Fasta och hälsokost vid reumatoid arthrit – en kontrollerad undersökning, Swed. J. Biol. Med. 3, 6 – 17 (in Swedish with a short summary in English).

Horrobin, D. F. (1982) Prostaglandin E$_1$ and the nutritional regulation of its formation. Swed. J. Biol. Med. 1, 13 – 17.

Horrobin, D. F. (1983) The role of essential fatty acids and prostaglandins in the premenstrual syndrome. J. Reprod. Med. 28, 465 – 468.

Horrobin, D. F. (1984) Placebo-controlled tests of evening primrose oil. Swed. J. Biol. Med. 3, 13 – 17.

Langgård, H. (1965) Bindevaevets Elektrolytforhold (Danish dissertation). Borgens Forlag, Copenhagen.

Lindahl, O. (1961) Experimental skin pain. Acta Physiol. Scand. 51 (Suppl 179).

Lindahl, O. (1962) Pain – a chemical explanation. Acta Reum. Scand. 8, 161 – 169.

Lindahl, O. (1966) Metabolic treatment in diffuse pain (Varialgia). Acta Reum. Scand. 12, 153 – 160.

Lindahl, O. (1970a) Experimental muscle pain by chemical stimulus. Acta Orthop. Scand. 40, 741 – 750.

Lindahl, O. (1970b) Changes in the acid-base balance in metabolic treatment for pain. Acta Orthop. Scand. 41, 8 – 16.

Lindahl, O. (1974a) Pain – a general chemical explanation. Adv. Neurol. 4, 45 – 47.

Lindahl, O. (1974b) Treatment of pain by changing the acid-base balance. Adv. Neurol. 4, 559 – 561.

Lindahl, O. (1985) The pain concept in orthopaedics. Clin. Orthop. (in press).

Lindahl, O. and Myrnerts, R. (1979) Treatment of rheumatoid arthritis with a dietary regimen. Swed. J. Biol. Med. 2, 11 – 15.

Lindberg, E. (1979) Alimentary factors in rheumatoid arthritis. Swed. J. Biol. Med. 1, 13 – 18.

Burrows/Elton/Stanley (eds.) Handbook of Chronic Pain Management
© 1987 Elsevier Science Publishers B.V. (Biomedical Division)

16

Abnormal illness behaviour and chronic pain

ISSY PILOWSKY

*Department of Psychiatry, The University of Adelaide, Royal Adelaide Hospital, Adelaide,
South Australia 5000, Australia*

When a doctor evaluates a patient's health status, he is called upon not only to decide whether an illness is present, but also whether the patient's illness behaviour is appropriate to his health situation. This is, of course, a complex process, which includes negotiation with the patient so that an agreed understanding can be reached as to whether a sick role can be granted and, if so, of what type. Occasions sometimes arise when the doctor and patient cannot reach agreement, and indeed the patient is unable to agree with any doctor who does not accept the patient's own view of his health status even though it is wrong.

In order to comprehend the issues at stake in this difficult area, the following definitions are useful:

1) *Illness*:
   An illness is an organismic state which fulfills the requirements of a relevant reference group for admission to a sick role (Pilowsky 1978).
2) Illness behaviour refers to the ways in which individuals experience, perceive, evaluate and respond to aspects of themselves which they are predisposed to evaluate in terms of health and illness (Mechanic 1962; Pilowsky 1969).
3) Abnormal illness behaviour is the persistence of an inappropriate or maladaptive mode of perceiving, evaluating and acting in relation to one's own state of health, despite the fact that a doctor (or other appropriate social agent) has offered a reasonably lucid explanation of the nature of the illness and the appropriate course of management to be followed, based on a thorough examination and assessment of all parameters of functioning (including the use of special investigations where necessary), and taking into account the individual's age, educational and sociocultural background.

The sick role is a partially and conditionally legitimated social role, which is conferred on an individual provided he recognizes that it is 'undesirable' and cooperates with an appointed agent of society for the purpose of regaining optimal health (Parsons 1964).

We can see, therefore, that an important part of a doctor's role is to establish whether a person is entitled to a sick role and, furthermore, how many 'sick role units' he is eligible for.

The decision that a person's illness behaviour is abnormal is clearly a difficult one to make, and the clinical steps to be taken are described later in this chapter. If the illness behaviour is regarded to be abnormal, then the diagnostic process may proceed further, to decide whether the person has one of a number of conditions recognized as syndromes by a particular classificatory system, such as DSM-III or ICD-9.

Abnormal illness behaviours (AIB) can be grouped in terms of 1) whether the motivation is predominantly conscious or unconscious; 2) whether illness is affirmed or denied; or 3) whether the focus is somatic or psychological.

In this chapter, we will only consider forms of AIB in which illness is affirmed and the focus is somatic.

The possible diagnoses in this category are listed below using DSM-III terms:

A) Motivation predominantly conscious
   1) Malingering
   2) Chronic factitious syndrome with physical symptoms (Munchausen's syndrome)
   3) Factitious disorder with physical symptoms.
B) Motivation predominantly unconscious
   1) Neurotic (Somatoform disorders)
      Somatization disorder
      Conversion disorder
      Psychogenic pain disorder
      Hypochondriasis.
   2) Psychotic
      Hypochondriacal delusions associated with
      (a) Major depressive disorder with mood congruent psychotic features
      (b) Schizophrenic disorder
      (c) Monosymptomatic hypochondriacal psychoses.

It is well known that doctors will often be extremely reluctant to make a diagnosis of an illness such as hypochondriasis or psychogenic pain for fear that they have overlooked some somatic pathology. It should be borne in mind, however, that AIB refers to a discrepancy between the patient's view of his health status and the objective evidence for disease. It does not imply a complete absence of any pathology at all (Beaber and Rodney 1984).

Furthermore, it implies that the doctor has proceeded through the following steps:

1) An evaluation of the person's somatic functioning.
2) An appraisal of the person's psychological, emotional and social functioning.
3) An appraisal of the person's cultural background and belief system (particularly with regard to illness).
4) A presentation to the person of the doctor's appraisal and conclusions as to his health status and any measures to be undertaken, in a comprehensible form.
5) An evaluation of the patient's response to this presentation in terms of its appropriateness.
6) A phenomenological analysis of the basis for the patient's response.

It will be appreciated that the above presupposes that the doctor is able to match the patient's illness behaviour against the type of illness behaviour to be expected in the particular situation.

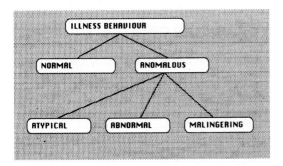

Fig. 1. Possible clinical significance of illness behaviour.

In practice, the doctor proceeds through a series of diagnostic steps (Fig. 1). He first decides whether the illness behaviour is 'normal' or 'anomalous', i.e. not what he would expect in the circumstances. However, further evaluation and negotiation may lead him to decide that the illness behaviour is appropriate and perhaps readily modifiable with proper explanation and counselling. If it remains anomalous, it may be classified into one of three main categories. Firstly, it may be decided that the patient is 'malingering', i.e. does not have an illness at all. This is an extremely difficult decision to make, but fortunately, clearcut consciously motivated malingering appears to be rare in ordinary civilian practice.

Secondly, the doctor may decide that the illness behaviour is 'atypical' but, nonetheless, adaptive and not a response which will interfere with management. This decision can only be made if the 'usual' illness behaviour is well known, and is thus easier in the context of conditions in which the pathophysiology is well delineated, such as diabetes or hypertension, and where the patient's response to the illness may be statistically unusual but not necessarily maladaptive.

Thirdly, the doctor may decide that the illness behaviour is 'abnormal'. The most satisfactory way to decide this, is on the basis of the phenomenology of the illness behaviour, i.e. the way the person experiences his health status and what he believes and thinks about it.

The most clearcut form of AIB is seen in the patient with hypochondriacal delusions, e.g. the patient who is absolutely convinced that he has cancer and cannot be reassured to the contrary. However, not all forms of AIB are of this classical type.

As mentioned earlier, AIB can involve not only the inappropriate affirmation of illness but, also, its denial. Furthermore, the focus may be on psychiatric rather than physical illness. For the purpose of this chapter, however, only somatically focussed, disease affirming AIB will be considered, beginning with the forms in which reality testing is clearly impaired and proceeding to the neurotic types.

Psychotic abnormal illness behaviour

Delusional ideas about disease may at times be a part of a schizophrenic disorder. Indeed, hypochondriacal ideas may be a prominent feature of the early stages of the illness and may be associated with highly abnormal ideas about bodily functions. Pain is often a salient feature of such presentations.

Perhaps the commonest association between hypochondriacal delusions and a psychotic illness, occurs in psychotic depression (major depressive disorder with mood congruent delusions).

The patient manifests highly abnormal and fixed beliefs about the presence of disease, such as cancer or pathology, such as blocked bowels or rotting internal organs. These ideas are associated with marked depression and biological features, such as insomnia, loss of appetite and psychomotor retardation. The delusions are often not presented spontaneously, and must be sought for.

Monosymptomatic hypochondriasis (atypical somatoform disorder, dysmorphophobia) does not appear to be common, but often takes the form of a preoccupation and dissatisfaction with some aspect of physical appearance. Pain is sometimes a feature.

Non-psychotic abnormal illness behaviour

In these conditions, pain is usually prominent and, at times, the only major symptom. There are two important diagnoses which are generally considered, viz. hypochondriasis and conversion disorder. More recently, (in DSM-III) two further diagnoses have been formulated: psychogenic pain disorder and somatization disorder.

HYPOCHONDRIASIS

Hypochondriasis is a condition in which the individual shows a concern with his health (somatic or emotional) which is excessive and inappropriate. The concern persists despite the provision of reassurance by a doctor, and may take the form of an obsessional idea, a phobia or a morbid preoccupation. In the case of an obsession (which is a relatively rare form of presentation), the patient regards the idea as alien and tries to resist it. In the case of a phobia, the patient fears illnesses which may befall him, such as a heart attack or a stroke. These ideas are usually regarded as irrational by the patient, in calmer moments. Where a morbid preoccupation is the only symptom, the condition may be regarded as 'primary hypochondriasis' (Pilowsky 1967, 1970).

CONVERSION DISORDERS

Conversion disorders are classically regarded as those in which there is a loss of a physical function in the absence of a somatic aetiology, following on emotional stress, in a predisposed individual. Frequently quoted examples are paralysis of a limb, blindness and aphonia. In clinical practice, however, it now appears that pain is the commonest form of conversion disorder. When this is the most prominent or only symptom, DSM-III suggests the condition be regarded as a psychogenic pain disorder.

As mentioned above, 'somatization disorder' is a more recently introduced term and is not yet generally accepted. It is described as a condition occurring mainly in women with an onset before the age of 30 years. The symptoms include those referable to the gastrointestinal system, female reproductive organs, cardiopulmonary system as well as pain, conversion symptoms and the belief in having been sickly for 'a good part of his or her life'.

Indeed, the description of this disorder suggests a mixture of hysterical personality, hypochondriasis, conversion disorder and anxiety disorder in a individual with a tendency to seek and accept health care as a method of coping.

Distinguishing between these conditions is not always easy. The main feature distinguishing between hypochondriasis and the other disorders (conversion, psychogenic pain and somatization) is that the hypochondriacal patient is preoccupied with ideas about health and disease,

ILLNESS BEHAVIOUR QUESTIONNAIRE REPORT FORM

NAME: __A.A._____ DATE: _____

AGE: ___49_____ POPULATION: __Pain Clinic____
                                                    (e.g. inpatient, outpatient)

DIAGNOSIS: __Psychogenic Pain Disorders_____

SCALES

	GH	DC	P/S	AI	AD	D	I	AS	DA	DF	WI
Raw Scores	1	5	0	1	1	5	1	3	10	93.7	10
Range	0–9	0–6	0–5	0–5	0–5	0–5	0–6	0–20	0–11	0–100	0–14
% Scores	11	83	0	20	20	100	17	15	91	94	71

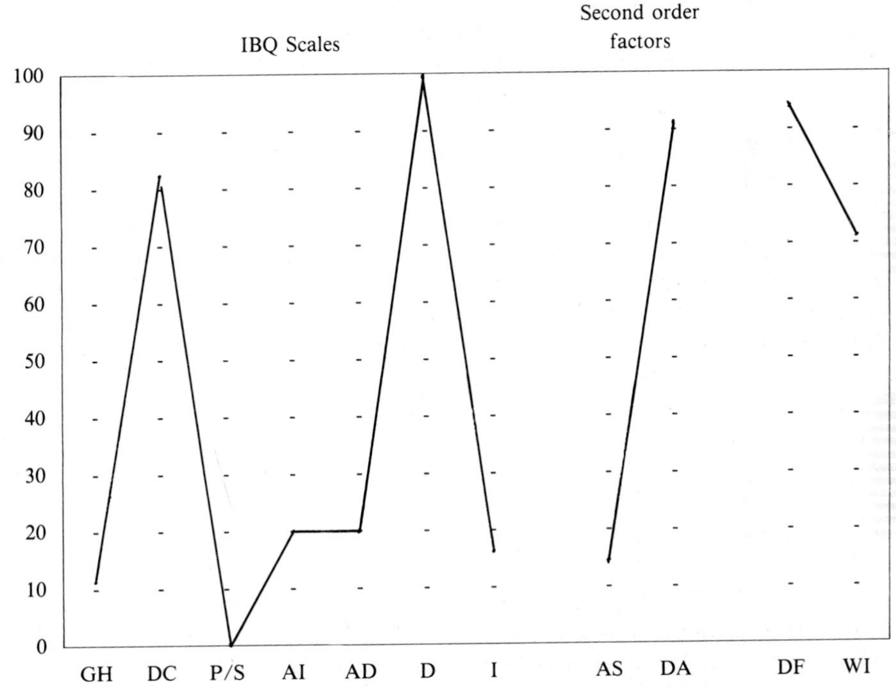

IBQ Scales / Second order factors

Key

GH – General Hypochondriasis
DC – Disease Conviction
P/S – Psychological (high score) vs. Somatic Focusing
AI – Affective Inhibition
AD – Affective Disturbance
D – Denial
I – Irritability

AS – Affective State (GH + AD + I)
DA – Disease Affirmation (DC + (5 – P/S))
DF – Discriminant Function 53.8 + 5.7 (DC) – 10.2 (P/S) – .6 (AI) + 2.4 (D). (Likelihood of a conversion reaction)
WI – Whiteley Index (Likelihood of a Hypochondriacal syndrome)

INTERPRETATION BY: _____

Enquiries: Professor I. Pilowsky, University of Adelaide, Department of Psychiatry, Royal Adelaide Hospital, Adelaide, South Australia, 5001.

Fig. 2. IBQ profile of patient referred to multidisciplinary pain clinic.

whereas the others usually deny such a concern, but rather emphasize their experience of symptoms and their disability.

Screening for AIB (the Illness Behaviour Questionnaire)

The Illness Behaviour Questionnaire (IBQ) can be used as an aid to screening for anomalous forms of illness behaviour and aiding more precise clinical decisions as to whether the illness behaviour is normal, atypical, abnormal or malingering.

The IBQ provides scores on 7 first order scales, two second order scales, a discriminant function and a hypochondriasis scale. The primary scales are: general (phobic) hypochondriasis, disease conviction, psychological vs. somatic focussing, affective inhibition, affective disturbance (dysphoria), denial (and displacement) and irritability. The second order scales are disease affirmation and affective state. The discriminant function scale indicates the probability of a conversion (or psychogenic pain) disorder and the hypochondriasis scale (Whiteley Index) is a measure of disease preoccupation and phobia (Pilowsky 1967; Pilowsky and Spence 1975, 1981).

The IBQ profile seen in patients referred to a multidisciplinary clinic for what is usually diagnosed as a 'psychogenic pain disorder' is fairly typical with a high disease conviction score, a low psychological vs somatic focussing score (indicating a prominent conversion element; (Fig. 2).

In conclusion, it should be emphasized that abnormal illness behaviours should not be diagnosed lightly, and it is most important not to confuse anomalous or atypical illness behaviour with the truly abnormal forms. Clearly, a great deal of research needs to be done to delineate the spectrum of illness behaviours which occurs in association with various dysfunctions in a variety of sociocultural situations, so that the diagnosis of abnormal illness behaviours may be more confidently operationalized.

References

Beaber, R. J. and Rodney, W. M. (1984) Underdiagnosis of hypochondriasis. Psychosomatics 25, 39–46.

Mechanic, D. (1962) The concept of illness behavior. J. Chron. Dis. 15, 189–194.

Parsons, T. S. (1964) Social Structure and Personality. Collier Macmillan, London.

Pilowsky, I. (1967) Dimensions of hypochondriasis. Br. J. Psychiatry 113, 89–93.

Pilowsky, I. (1969) Abnormal illness behaviour. Br. J. Med. Psychol. 42, 347–351.

Pilowsky, I. (1970) Primary and secondary hypochondriasis. Acta Psychiatr. Scand. 46, 273–285.

Pikowsky, I. (1978) A general classification of abnormal illness behaviours. Br. J. Med. Psychol. 51, 131–137.

Pilowsky, I. and Spence, N. D. (1975) Patterns of illness behaviour in patients with intractable pain. J. Psychosom. Res. 19, 279–287.

Pilowsky, I. and Spence, N. D. (1981) Manual for the Illness Behaviour Questionnaire (IBQ). University of Adelaide, Adelaide.

Burrows/Elton/Stanley (eds.) Handbook of Chronic Pain Management
© 1987 Elsevier Science Publishers B.V. (Biomedical Division)

17

Pain, personality and psychosomatic complaints

H. MERSKEY

Department of Psychiatry, University of Western Ontario, London Psychiatric Hospital, London, Ontario, Canada

Introduction

Pain has long been though to be produced or promoted by emotional factors (Merskey and Spear 1967; Sternbach 1968). Not surprisingly, there is an extensive literature on the personality of patients with chronic pain. Personality testing, particularly with the Minnesota Multiphasic Personality Inventory (MMPI) is widespread in chronic pain clinics. A tendency to develop psychosomatic complaints in the absence of a physical cause may be attributed to various types of psychological process such as hallucinations, conversion symptoms and tension states. Hence, it is relevant to ask to what extent stress or personality features produce symptoms through each of these routes. However, there are two very important complicating factors. First, pain from a lesion may itself be a cause of stress and perhaps emotional and personality change. Second, selection factors play a recognized part in determining who comes for treatment. This last point is relatively neglected and few writers in the field of pain have given it enough attention. I deal first here with selection factors.

Selection factors

Characteristics of temperament and personality influence the composition of almost all medical populations. In a few cases patients suffer an overwhelming disorder of sudden onset which ineluctably results in hospital admission. Subarachnoid haemorrhage is one example, but even coronary thrombosis does not invariably lead to admission. Some patients with the latter have no pain, others ignore warning signs or treat a full-blown coronary pain as 'indigestion'. Thus, even such a very acute and serious condition does not automatically produce a complete and fully representative sample in hospital in the hands of the treatment team. When we consider more chronic conditions selection is even more prominent. A man with migraine may say to himself, 'I have that terrible problem again I must see if the doctor can do anything more about it'. Or he may reflect, 'My Mother was always going to the doctor with her headaches and vomiting and got no benefit. I'll take the day off work and be alright to-morrow'. The effect of such differences in approach on the population of migraine clinics does not have to be imagined. It has been well recorded inasmuch as it is very clear that the patients in a migraine clinic tend to be more anxious, more hypochondriacal and more persistent in seeking relief than patients with migraine in the community.

The evidence for this difference between migraine patients and those in the community is now quite readily available. At first, authors working with highly selected populations of migraine patients, recognized abnormalities in their patients, e.g. Touraine and Draper (1934) who studied 50 patients with typical migraine, held that it occurs in subjects who are deliberate, hesitant over positive decisions, insecure, perfectionist, and unduly worrying. Amongst their patients, intelligence was high, the women had not had a successful heterosexual life, and the men had a low sexual drive. The migraine attack was seen as a conflict between the desire to escape from mother's influence and the compulsion not to leave her. Knopf (1935) described 'goody goody, ambitious, reserved, and repressed' patterns in the childhood of migraine patients combined with adult features of being 'dignified, domineering and resentful with very little sense of humour'. These sorts of descriptions were followed by the late H.G. Wolff (Wolff 1937, 1948). He particularly emphasized the presence of a rigid, ambitious, perfectionist personality with headache resulting from a variety of stresses. Klee (1968) in patients in a migraine clinic, found that emotion was a precipitant of severe attacks of migraine in at least 72% of his 50 patients examined in person. Thus a general pattern of belief that migraine was associated with a particular personality became very popular. However, when Henryk-Gutt and Rees (1973) studied their series of patients from a pain clinic and another series found by survey methods in a population of postal workers, it became evident that migraine clinic patients were much more anxious and neurotic than the random sample. The random sample was not completely random but was much nearer to normal emotionally than the migraine clinic group. Finally, a survey by Crisp et al. (1977) in an actual general practice population showed that migraine patients were scarcely any different from a general practice population. There was a statistically significant increase in anxiety in migraine patients but its quantitative significance was slight. These phenomena have been demonstrated in other fields. Pond and Bidwell (1959) examined patients with epilepsy in general practices. They found that the family practitioners had been far more ready to refer patients for a neurological opinion if they were psychologically ill. In other words, although the diagnosis was not in doubt, patients with emotional difficulties were referred to neurologists twice as often as those without emotional difficulties. In general practice, by the technique of having patients keep a symptom diary, it has been shown by Banks et al. (1975) that as few as 3% of all symptoms are reported to doctors. Patients exercise considerable discretion in selecting which symptoms they think need medical attention. Not all instances of headache and vomiting are a matter for consultation. Thus, the decision to seek treatment for pain of any type has to be understood against the background of the patient's ideas about whether or not he needs medical help.

Another field in which the relevance of psychological factors as a cause has been questioned in respect of pain is that of the temporomandibular pain and dysfunction syndrome (TMPDS). This syndrome is marked by pain in the face particularly in the maxillary region, clicking of the joints in some patients and tenderness or restriction of limitation in mouth opening. Agerberg and Carlsson (1972) showed that 39% of a normal population had clicking, 12% had pain in the face on wide opening of the jaw and 7% had limitation of movement. Heloe and Heloe (1979) showed that pain affected 5% of male 25-year old patients and 11% of females. Two percent of the men and 5% of the women sought treatment. This results in a 1:6 ratio of men to women in the clinic compared with a 1:2 ratio in the community. In clinical practice females typically present far more often with a complaint of TMPDS than do males, e.g. 86.5% in our own series (Salter et al. 1983). It has long been suggested that TMPDS is a condition in which psychophysiological dysfunction is important in producing the symptom. In other words, it has been held that it is produced by stress and anxiety. It is at least as likely that anxiety and stress produce a willingness, on the part of patients who have this symptom for other reasons, to present it to dentists and doctors. In confirmation of that view we found (Salter et al. 1983) that only 48% of a population of patients with TMPDS could be classified as psychiatric patients, using very liberal cut-off points on the General Health Questionnaire-28, a screening measure for psychological illness. Speculand et al. (1983) found likewise that the abnormal illness behaviour patterns of patients with this condition were more like those of general practice patients than that of a chronic pain population; and Feinmann (1984) using a clinical interview schedule (a systematic psychiatric interview) found that whilst 55% of her patients with facial pain had psychological illness, 45% did not have it according to that measure.

Perhaps the most definite evidence of these selection effects is to be found in the work of Crook et al. (1984). They have shown that chronic pain is extremely common, affecting as many as 11% of a survey population. The psychological characteristics of this population are different in a number of ways from the patients who present to a pain clinic. This subject still needs further work but it is evident that selection factors are of considerable importance in determining the psychological characteristics of patients undergoing treatment for pain.

THE PSYCHOGENESIS OF PAIN

It should not be thought, despite the foregoing, that the writer believes that pain is not caused by psychological illness. Pain may be generated by psychological factors and is commonly due to an emotional state. If it is not directly caused by an emotional state it may be made worse by one. For example, migraine is definitely worse in phases of depression (Selby and Lance 1960). There is also much historical and other evidence of the association of pain with psychiatric diagnoses. Pain may be produced by ideas alone. This has often been discussed before, e.g. Merskey and Spear (1967), Merskey (1981). This mechanism of production of pain by ideas may be hysterical although the alternative theoretical or conceptual bases for it could be considered. Freud (1893–1895) was one of the first to note its occurrence and to describe pain as the symbolic result of emotional conflict. Further, the anecdotal evidence that pain sometimes appears in individuals in moments of stress without a physical basis is quite common (Merskey 1981). Much more often it appears that pain is found in association with other personality features suggestive of hysteria. Very rarely pain results from a hallucination and quite often, although perhaps less often than is usually considered, it may be the result of a muscle tension mechanism or vascular mechanism induced by emotion. But the shadow of selection limits all conclusions of this type and the full extent of these mechanisms has never been thoroughly defined.

Despite the above, some of the evidence for the psychogenesis of pain can be listed. Recognition of the causation of pain by the emotions is of great antiquity. One rather striking quotation from Thomas Sydenham (1697) is as follows: 'When the mind is afflicted by some grievous accident, the animal spirits run into disorderly motions . . .' and the sick person develops a headache. Extensive collections of painful symptoms were characterized as hysteria, throughout the 19th century, e.g. by Dubois (1830), Landouzy (1846), Briquet (1859), and in the 20th century by Guze and his colleagues (1970). Some of these conditions are now recognized as organic but the pattern of hypochondriacal behaviour and numerous physical complaints, especially pain, without an adequate somatic basis, have traditionally been thought to be hysterical and associated with other classical neurological symptoms, such as astasia, ataxia, abasia, paralysis, anaesthesia, blindness and deafness which are clearly more related to hysterical mechanisms than to any organic disease. Such symptoms can be shown to occur when the bodily structure is intact and capable of function although the patient believes otherwise. Some of those symptoms recognized in previous centuries may also have been psychophysiological rather than hysterical but the pattern today still indicates that many of them have no recognizable or likely organic basis.

Innumerable MMPI reports suggest also that there is a characteristic pattern of abnormality in patients with pain. Typically, the hypochondriasis scale is elevated above the mean, depression is somewhat elevated and the hysteria scale is elevated more than depression but not as much as hypochondriasis. Provided the patient does not have organic illness this is acceptable evidence that the symptoms are of a hysterical type. It is not proof however. Unfortunately, many MMPI findings are mistakenly interpreted from pain clinics and other centres. The test is standardized on the basis that no physical illness is present when the hypochondriasis scale is read as evidence of hypochondriasis. If a patient with physical illness ticks off questions − as on the hypochondriasis scale − which confirm that he has back pain or pain in other joints, this will appear in the test result, if incorrectly interpreted, as suggesting that he is psychologically ill. Moreover, a segment of the questions on the hysteria scale in fact is used also for the hypochondriasis scale. Thus it follows, almost as the night the day, that if the hypochondriasis scale is elevated, the hysteria scale will follow upwards in its wake. Some authors recognize this phenomenon (Naliboff et al. 1982; Watson 1982) but it has been insufficiently considered.

Other psychological tests do not quite commit the same error but are also liable to be influenced by the physical state of the individual. Thus, organic disorder may wake people but wakefulness and insomnia tend to be seen as signs of depression in scales like the Wakefield Depression Inventory and the Beck Depression Inventory. The Maudsley Personality Inventory, the Eysenck Personality Inventory, the Middlesex Hospital Questionnaire (now known as the Crown-Crisp Experiential Index) and the Irritability/Depression and Anxiety Questionnaire (Snaith et al. 1978) are all subject somewhat to this problem, although not nearly to the same extent as the MMPI. The Eysenck Personality Questionnaire is designed to avoid it. The General Health Questionnaire has correction factors published for use in this setting, e.g. Finlay-Jones and Murphy (1979). If we make allowance for these problems it seems likely nevertheless that the many published studies using these alternative tests, as well as the MMPI, confirm the presence of some indications of hypochondriasis and depression in pain patients.

An alternative approach is based upon physical examination and psychiatric interview. In that case, the results may be influenced by observer bias but at least the observer is able to detect the symptoms in the patient in front of him which may be due to physical disorder. The early studies, e.g. Walters (1961); Merskey (1965a, b); Spear (1967), all relied on this technique as have some later ones, e.g. Large (1980). It is agreed that there is a positive and definite association between pain and psychological illness in which the psychological illness seems to generate the painful condition. In still other studies (e.g. Woodforde and Merskey 1972; Sternbach et al., 1973; Pelz and Merskey 1982) starting with patients who have physical illness it has been demonstrated that evidence exists conversely of the origin of psychological symptoms from the presence of pain.

The field of anthropology also contributes a little to our knowledge of the production of pain. The Couvade syndrome (Couvade is a Basque word meaning 'to sit on eggs') describes the behaviour of men who complain of abdominal and other symptoms during their wives' pregnancies. The occurrence of pain in such men has been well recorded (Bardhan 1965; Trethowan and Conlon 1965). Likewise, hysterical symptoms at one time in a group of individuals have been shown to be followed at another time by headache and pain complaints which seem to reflect a psychological function (Rawnsley and Loudon 1964).

An alternative formulation for the psychological aspects of pain is offered by Fordyce (1976) who describes many of the features of the behaviour of pain patients as 'operant'. One drawback to the operant approach (although it has some advantages) is that it neglects the subjective experience of the individual – at least in theory. Another drawback is that it loses the opportunity to distinguish in the terms which we are using between depression, anxiety, hysteria and so forth. The notion of operant mechanisms may in fact cover any or all of the above psychological terms at different times. However, the attempt to describe many phenomena as operant is yet another indication of the importance of behavioural or psychological matters in the production of pain. It clearly recognizes the importance of environmental factors, incentives, and family effects amongst others, in the production or maintenance of pain.

Pain also has a significant relationship with depression. The effort to measure this has resulted in varying figures. Surveys with rather stringent questionnaires such as the Levine-Pilowsky Depression Questionnaire produce findings like 10% of patients in a pain clinic having significant degrees of depression (Pilowsky et al. 1977). Chapman et al. (1979) with the same test found that patients seen in private practice had no more depression than a normal population. In a series of headache patients seen by a neurologist, only 7% of patients show recognizable depression on the Levine-Pilowsky Depression Questionnaire (Merskey et al. 1986, unpublished). At the other extreme, Blumer and Heilbronn (1982) suggest that 'pain-prone patients' all have a 'depression spectrum disorder'.

I consider that only a minority of patients with chronic pain have a depressive illness by the criteria of either ICD-9 or DSM-III. However, in patients who have painful lesions, some evidence of depression is often found even though it does not amount to full scale depressive illness in a psychiatric sense. Thus, Pelz and Merskey (1982) noted that in patients with lesions in a pain clinic, 54 out of 83 (65%) recognized that they were irritable. Twenty-six percent said that they were moderately or quite a bit 'distressed' or troubled by feeling 'blue'. On another questionnaire (SCL-90), 32% indicated 'feeling annoyed or irritated'. Thus, some subjective mood changes not amounting to full-scale depression are common in patients with pain where lesions are also to be found.

The above suffices to show both that psychological mechanisms of pain exist and that pain may cause emotional change. It is conceptually important to recognize that all pain is a psychological experience. The local change in the body is not pain but rather an alteration in nerve fibres or nerve conduction of impulses and so forth. It is for this reason that the International Association for the Study of Pain defined pain as, 'An unpleasant sensory and emotional experience associated with actual or potential tissue damage or described in terms of such damage' (IASP 1979).

Importance of pain as a symptom

Chronic pain affects 11% of a normal population (Crook et al., 1984). Everyone experiences acute pain and pain is the most common symptom in medicine. Repeated studies have shown that it has a significant association with psychological illness. This is reviewed elsewhere (Merskey 1980). Several mechanisms by which pain may develop have been outlined already. Thus, as indicated, it may follow from a schizophrenic hallucination or other type of hallucination although all those sorts of pain are very rare (Watson et al. 1981). Secondly, it may result from a muscle contraction process and is then often known as tension pain, and anxiety, similarly produced by autonomic dysfunction and anxiety. Thirdly, for reasons discussed at some length above, pain may follow from hysterical mechanisms. Any one of these mechanisms already mentioned may also serve to increase the pain from a physical disturbance which is already present (Walters 1961).

Although figures are lacking on this point, it is probably one of the most important in clinical work. Further, as described above, the selection process results in patients with emotional problems presenting with pain as a basis for their concern, although it may not be the whole source of their difficulty. The relative frequency of these different occurrences is not known. Although we now have the figure mentioned for the frequency of pain in the population and there are many figures for pain in hospital attenders, we have no estimate as to how often pain is due to one cause or another. Spear (1967) made the effort to distinguish the probable pain mechanisms in a series of psychiatric patients and his results were as follows: 80 patients had pain attributed to muscle tension; 58 to conversion; 31 to an organic lesion and 11 each to chemical or vascular causes. Thirty-one patients were not able to be assessed. To my knowledge this is the only study undertaken on this point. It is unpublished except in a thesis and it relates only to one series of psychiatric patients (132 patients with 222 pains). In my own series of patients seen in a similar setting, with an emphasis on chronic cases, more patients had a diagnosis relating to conversion symptoms (43 out of 100) and less to anxiety (27 out of 100) or other discrete causes. Evidence from pain clinics or headache clinics, e.g. Harper and Steger (1978) suggests that personality problems are more important in many cases than a muscle tension mechanism. In the latter study, MMPI scores were more closely associated with the occurrence of headache than was muscle contraction demonstrated through the EMG.

Personality and types of pain complaint

The relationship between pain and personality may be partly inferred from some of the foregoing discussion. Anxious individuals and obsessional ones tend to have illnesses marked by anxiety and depression and would accordingly be prone to tension pain. There do not appear to be any specific formal studies demonstrating the relationship between anxious personalities and tension pain but it is noted incidentally, in many of the investigations which have shown a link between anxiety and pain. Hysterical symptoms however, have only a limited relationship with the classical hysterical personality. The usual features of the latter in the literature are held to be frigidity and exhibitionism in females, attention seeking behaviour, suggestibility, labile and histrionic attitudes, mendacity with self-centredness, vanity (Chodoff and Lyons 1958; DeAlarcon 1973). The association of these traits with conversion symptoms (and inferentially with pain) was challenged by Chodoff and Lyons (1958) who found that only 3 out of 17 patients with conversion symptoms had hysterical personality as defined above. Ljungberg (1957) had found, before Chodoff and Lyons, that many patients with conversion symptoms or classical hysterical symptoms did not have evidence of hysterical personality. In his study, approximately 20% had such evidence and another 20% had an immature or 'asthenic' personality. About 43% of the men he followed and 47% of women exhibited abnormal personalities. Thus, no uniform personality type exists which is prone to hysterical reactions but certain abnormal personalities might be found more often in company with hysterical symptoms. This was demonstrated also by Merskey and Trimble (1979) who showed that in a group of 24 patients with classical conversion symptoms 5 out of 24 (21%) had hysterical personality and the same number showed passive immature dependent personalities. A control group of 24 psychiatric patients had no such personality types but seven obsessionals (29%) versus one obsessional in the hysterical group. Thus, a significant difference was discernible between patients with conversion symptoms in respect of their personalities and the personalities of patients who did not have conversion symptoms. We can suppose by extension of the argument that when pain is due to a conversion process it may well have an association with hysterical personality. This is certainly the traditional view based upon some of the evidence presented already and is incorporated, in a way, in the idea of the polysymptomatic hypochondriacal patient which has been developed to produce the stereotype of the Briquet syndrome or somatization disorder in the American Psychiatric Association Diagnostic and Statistical Manual (Third Edition: DSM-III).

Depressive personalities do not appear necessarily prone to pain symptoms. Indeed chronic depression may not be associated with anything like sustained headache. If depressive personality is associated with a pain symptom then any of the available mechanisms might be considered as an explanation. The depression could produce a hallucination in an extreme case and I have seen this and commented on it at other times. It is however rare. The context of a depression can lead to the production of conversion symptoms (Slater 1965; Merskey 1979). There is no reason to think that depressive patients get such sorts of pain particularly often but it is at least theoretically possible. Anxiety is common with depression however and a muscle tension mechanism might well be active in a fairly large proportion of those patients with depression and pain from the depression.

Hypochondriasis may best be distinguished from hysteria by the fact that the patient with hypochondriasis, in theory at least, tends to be more concerned with the presence of a symptom, despite reassurance that it is not dangerous or troublesome. Patients with hysteria on the other hand, are theoretically liable to be satisfied or even pleased with the fact that they have their complaint. Traditionally, this is recognized in the expression 'belle indifference', although the patients with belle indifference may represent a rather small proportion only of patients with hysterical complaints. Anyhow, hypochondriacal patients certainly persist in seeking attention and hypochondriacal aspects characterize many patients in pain clinics. Overprotection in childhood (Levy 1943) was postulated as a cause of hypochondriasis. In a controlled study using a standardized instrument, the Parental Bonding Instrument of Parker (1979), Baker and Merskey (1982) have shown that overprotection is much more marked in the childhood experience of patients with hypochondriasis, at least as the patients see it.

Alternative diagnostic categories for a number of these conditions have been provided by the DSM-III. For example, somatoform disorders represent a complete division. The present structure of this system has a number of disadvantages. Somatoform strictly would mean 'having the form of a body'. This is not really what is meant by those conditions which are marked by somatic complaints. Nor does the word 'psychosomatic' cover them adequately since psychosomatic tends to imply change in the bodily state produced by the psychological mechanism. Blushing is a good example of a psychosomatic symptom. Hysterical and hypochondriacal complaints without clearly defined psychophysiological causes also do not come into this group. One of the problems with the whole of DSM-III and also with other systems which are useful for research is that they tend to insist on cut-off points; the latter are is valuable for comparative investigations but patients who come above or below the cut-off point may be rather arbitrarily separated from each other.

The diagnosis of somatization disorder is another of those which have been introduced in the DSM-III. It is of course a development from the Briquet syndrome description by Guze and his colleages (Guze 1970). The category has usefulness for practical purposes and for research purposes with the limitations already specified. The category of hypochondriasis is generally similar in both the APA and the International system (ICD-9). One disadvantage of the APA hypochondriasis category is that one may not diagnose it in the presence of a psychotic illness which has to take precedence. However, hypochondriacal behaviour may often reflect an important part of the phenomena in patients with psychosis. Accordingly, it might be desirable if patients with a diagnosis of schizophrenia or other major psychosis but who are also hypochondriacal could have hypochondriasis used as a secondary diagnosis in their case.

The category of psychalgia which is also present in the DSM-III overlaps somewhat with hysteria and with anxiety. It does give a vivid and accurate description of a subset of pain clinic patients. The same phenomena are found in varying degrees in patients with other diagnoses, even depression, and sometimes patients who may have an organic illness that has been missed. Moreover, the psychalgia category is relatively easily diagnosed – probably too easily. These small points concerning the diagnoses of the DSM-III show how difficult it is to establish well-defined and useful categories relating to pain and personality and to diagnosis. Diagnosis is always a practical matter however and may result in some arbitrary decisions being taken which are nonetheless beneficial.

One final aspect of pain and personality remains to be considered. It has been shown, as mentioned earlier, that the persistence of chronic pain is liable to change the temperament of an individual (Woodforde and Merskey 1972). Pain of course changes the behaviour of animals. O'Kelly and Steckley (1939) have shown that when rats are kept together in a cage and the bars of the cage floor are electrified, the rats are liable to bite each other. The behavioural change in the direction of aggression, irritability and depression is common in patients who have chronic painful lesions. It is to be understood on common sense grounds as a reaction to the distressing experience. Sometimes these patients appear to score high on 'lie' scales in tests like the MMPI and are then said to be defensive and to be covering up about themselves. This is not necessarily the best interpretation. It could simply be the case that patients who develop physical illness which is debilitating and unpleasant may have had very good or effective premorbid personalities and may be quite accurate in saying how much they have changed for the worse. Although there is always a tendency to see the past with rose-tinged spectacles, we cannot assume that patients are wearing them. Most important we have to recognize that a complaint of pain accompanied by some difficulty of behaviour may well reflect the severity of the complaint rather than the abnormality of the personality.

References

Agerberg, G. and Carlsson, G. E. (1972) Functional disorder of the masticatory system. I. Distribution of symptoms according to age and sex judged from investigation by questionnaire. Acta Odont. Scand. 30, 597–613.

Baker, B. and Merskey, H. (1982) Parental representations of hypochondriacal patients from a psychiatric hospital. Br. J. Psychiatry 141, 233–238.

Banks, M. H., Beresford, S. H. A., Morrell, D. C., Waller, J. J. and Watkins, C. J. (1975) Factors influencing demand for primary medical care in women age 20–40 years; a preliminary report. Int. J. Epidemiol. 4, 189–255.

Bardhan, P. N. (1965) The couvade syndrome. Br. J. Psychiatry 111, 908–909.

Blumer, D. and Heilbronn, M. (1982) Chronic pain as a variant of depressive disease: the pain-prone disorder. J. Nerv. Ment. Dis. 170, 381 – 406.

Briquet, P. (1859) Traité de l'Hystérie. J. B. Baillière et Fils, Paris.

Chapman, C. R., Sola, A. E. and Bonica, J. J. (1979) Illness behavior and depression compared in pain center and private practice patients. Pain. 6, 1 – 7.

Chodoff, P. and Lyons, H. (1958) Hysteria, the hysterical personality and 'hysterical' conversion. Am. J. Psychiatry 114, 734 – 740.

Crisp, A. H., Kalucy, R. S., McGuinness, B., Ralph, P. C. and Harris, G. (1977) Some clinical, social and psychological characteristics of migraine subjects in the general population. Postgrad. Med. J. 53, 691 – 697.

Crook, J., Rideout, E. and Browne, G. (1984) The prevalence of pain complaints in a general population. Pain 18, 299 – 314.

DeAlarcon, R. (1973) Hysteria and hysterical personality: How come one without the other? Psychiat. Q. 47, 258 – 275.

Dubois d'Amiens, E. G. (1933) Histoire Philosophique de l'Hystérie. Deville Cavellin, Paris, pp. 141 – 292.

Feinmann, C., Harris, M. and Cawley, R. (1984) Psychogenic pain: presentation and treatment. Br. Med. J. 228, 436 – 438.

Finlay-Jones, R. A. and Murphy, E. (1979) Severity of psychiatric disorder and the 30-item General Health Questionnaire. Br. J. Psychiatry 134, 609 – 616.

Fordyce, W. E. (1976) Behavioral Methods in Chronic Pain and Illness. C.V. Mosby Co., St. Louis.

Freud, S. (1893 – 1895) (1955) Studies in Hysteria. Complete Psychological Works. Standard Edition, Vol. 2. Hogarth, London.

Guze, S. B. (1970) The role of follow-up studies: their contribution to diagnostic classification as applied to hysteria. Semin. Psychiatry 2, 392 – 402.

Harper, R. C. and Steger, J. C. (1978) Psychological correlates of frontalis EMG and pain in tension headache. Headache 18, 215 – 218.

Heloe, B. and Heloe, L. A. (1979) Frequency and distribution of myofascial pain dysfunction syndrome in a population of 25-year olds. Commun. Dent. Oral Epidemiol. 7, 357 – 360.

Henryk-Gutt, R. and Rees, W. L. (1973) Psychological aspects of migraine. J. Psychosom. Res. 17, 141 – 153.

International Association for the Study of Pain (Subcommittee on Taxonomy) (1979) Pain Terms: A list with definitions and notes on usage. Pain 6, 249 – 252.

Klee, A. (1965) A Clinical Study of Migraine with Particular Reference to the Most Severe Cases. Munksgaard, Copenhagen.

Knopf, O. (1935) Preliminary report on personality studies in thirty migraine patients. J. Nerv. Ment. Dis. 82, 270 – 285, 400 – 414.

Landouzy, H. (1846) Traité Complet de l'Hystérie. J. B. Baillière et Fils, Paris.

Large, R. G. (1980) The psychiatrist and the chronic pain patients: 172 anecdotes. Pain 9, 253 – 263.

Levy, D. M. (1943) Maternal Overprotection. Columbia University Press, New York.

Ljungberg, L. (1957) Hysteria. Acta Psychiatr. Scand. (Suppl.) 112.

Merskey, H. (1965a) The characteristics of persistent pain in psychological illness. J. Psychosom. Res. 9, 291 – 298.

Merskey, H. (1965b) Psychiatric patients with persistent pain. J. Psychosom. Res. 9, 299 – 309.

Merskey, H. (1979) The Analysis of Hysteria. Baillière, Tindall, London.

Merskey, H. (1980) The role of the psychiatrist in the investigation and treatment of pain. Research Publications. In: J. J. Bonica (Ed.), Pain. Raven Press, New York, pp. 249 – 260.

Merskey, H. (1981) Headache and hysteria. Cephalalgia 1, 109 – 119.

Merskey, H. and Spear, F. G. (1967) Pain: Psychological and Psychiatric Aspects. Baillière, Tindall & Cassell, London.

Merskey, H. and Trimble, M. (1979) Personality, sexual adjustment and brain lesions in patients with conversion symptoms. Am. J. Psychiatry 136, 179 – 192.

Naliboff, B. D., Cohen, M. J. and Yellen, A. N. (1982) Does the MMPI differentiate chronic illness from chronic pain? Pain 13, 333 – 341.

O'Kelly, L. E. and Steckley, L. C. (1939) A note on long enduring emotional responses in the rat. J. Psychol. 8, 125. Cited by Hutchinson, R. R., Ulrich, R. E. and Azrin, N. H. (1965) Effects on age and related factors or the pain-aggression reaction. J. Comp. Physiol. Psychol. 59, 365 – 369.

Parker, G. (1979) Parental characteristics in relation to depressive disorders. Br. J. Psychiatry 134, 138 – 147.

Pelz, M. and Merskey, H. (1982) A description of the psychological effects of chronic painful lesions. Pain 14, 293 – 301.

Pilowsky, I., Chapman, C. R. and Bonica, J. J. (1977) Pain, depression and illness behaviour in a pain clinic population. Pain 4, 183 – 192.

Pond, D. A. and Bidwell, B. H. (1959) A survey of epilepsy in 14 general practices. II. Social and psychological aspects. Epilepsia 1, 285 – 299.

Rawnsley, K. and Loudon, J. B. (1964) Epidemiology of mental disorder in a closed community. Br. J. Psychiatry 110, 830 – 839.

Salter, M., Brooke, R. I., Merskey, H., Fichter, G. F. and Kapusianyk, D. H. (1983) Is the temporo-mandibular pain and dysfunction syndrome a disorder of the mind? Pain 17, 151 – 166.

Selby, G. and Lance, J. W. (1960) Observations on 500 cases of migraine and allied vascular headache. J. Neurol. Neurosurg. Psychiatr. 23, 23 – 32.

Slater, E. (1965) Diagnosis of 'hysteria'. Br. Med. J. 1, 1395 – 1399.

Snaith, R. P., Constantopoulos, A. A., Jardine, M. Y. and McGuffin, P. (1978) A clinical scale for the self-assessment of irritability. Br. J. Psychiatry 132, 164 – 171.

Spear, F. G. (1967) Pain in psychiatric patients. J. Psychosom. Res. 11, 187 – 193.

Speculand, B., Goss, A. N., Hughes, A., Spence, N. D. and Pilowsky, I. (1983) Temporo-mandibular joint dysfunction: pain and illness behaviour. Pain 17, 139 – 150.

Sternbach, R. A. (1968) Pain: A Psychological Analysis. Academic Press, New York.

Sternbach, R. A., Wolf, S. R., Murphy, R. W. and Akeson, W. H. (1973) Traits of pain patients: the low-back 'loser'. Psychosomatics 14, 226 – 229.

Sydenham, T. (1697) Dr. Sydenham's Complete Method of Curing Almost All Diseases, and Description of Their Symptoms: To Which are Now Added Five Discourses of the Same Author Concerning the Pleurisy, Gout, Hysterical Passion, Dropsy, and Rheumatism, 3rd edn. Newman & Rich Parker, London, pp. 149 – 174.

Touraine, G. A. and Draper, G. (1934) The migrainous patient. J. Nerv. Ment. Dis. 81, 1 – 23, 182.

Trethowan, W. H. and Conlon, M. F. (1965) The couvade syndrome. Br. J. Psychiatry III, 57 – 66.

Walters, A. (1961) Psychogenic regional pain alias hysterical pain. Brain 84, 1 – 18.

Watson, G. D. (1982) Neurotic tendencies among chronic pain patients: an MMPI item analysis. Pain 14, 365 – 385.

Watson, G. D., Chandarana, P. C. and Merskey, H. (1981) Relationships between pain and schizophrenia. Br. J. Psychiatry 138, 33 – 36.

Wolff, H. G. (1937) Personality factors and reactions of subjects with migraine. Arch. Neurol. Psychiatry 37, 895.

Wolff, H. G. (1948) Headache and Other Head Pain. Oxford University Press, London.

Woodforde, J. M. and Merskey, H. (1972) Personality traits of patients with chronic pain. J. Psychosom. Res. 16, 167 – 172.

Burrows/Elton/Stanley (eds.) Handbook of Chronic Pain Management
© 1987 Elsevier Science Publishers B.V. (Biomedical Division)

18

Management of chronic pain: The anesthetist's role

MARK MEHTA[1] and MENNO E. SLUIJTER[2]

[1]United Norwich Hospitals, Norwich, U.K., and [2]Lutherse Diakonessen Ziekenhuis, Amsterdam, The Netherlands

Acute and chronic pain

Pain is a unique, emotional experience usually associated with tissue damage or disease and expressed in terms relating to these conditions (Merskey and Spear 1967). The cause is often evident and appropriate measures directed at the source usually lead to rapid and complete resolution of the symptoms. This is acute pain, but here we are concerned with an entirely different entity (Sternbach 1981) which is much more difficult to manage because the etiology is often obscure and appropriate corrective measures for the root of the problem are not readily available. Chronic pain has been recognized as a national disease of the greatest social and economic significance (Bonica 1985). It is responsible for considerable dislocation of industry, economic loss in subsidies and industrial benefits, together with escalating costs in medical health care.

TREATMENT

There has been a great surge of interest in the treatment of chronic pain in the last 20 – 25 years, fostered to a large extent by the founding of the International Association for the Study of Pain (I.A.S.P.). Journals like '*Pain*' and textbooks (Sternbach 1974; Cousins and Bridenbaugh 1980; Swerdlow 1983; Wall and Melzack 1984) on the subject are helping to spread the growth of knowledge and practical experience of treating pain.

PRINCIPLES

Certain principles must be observed before treatment of any kind is undertaken (Mehta 1986):

1) Investigations and diagnosis always take preference over treatment in the first instance.

2) Treat a patient and not his pain. The patient's social, economic and emotional needs are just as important as his physical ailments and must be carefully considered.
3) The ultimate choice of treatment must depend on the patient's own wishes as well as on available skills and equipment. Elderly patients in particular must not be submitted to an operation or long uncomfortable procedure they do not really want.
4) Treatment should not incapacitate and potential risk should be carefully weighed against prospects of lasting pain relief.
5) Patients should always give informed consent for treatment, which has been explained in simple and non-scientific terms.
6) Unlike in acute pain, complete pain relief is often not assured. In many cases the best that can be achieved is a modest remission of symptoms. Patients should be informed about their prognosis before treatment is undertaken.

The anesthetist's role in chronic pain management

Anesthetists are trained primarily in the care of patients undergoing surgery, but many of their skills acquired in the operating theatre are eminently suitable in the management of other clinical problems such as intensive care and pain relief (Swerdlow et al. 1978). For pain, these contributions consisted mainly of nerve blocks and analgesic drugs, but experience has shown that a wider range of expertise is required for the resolution of more difficult cases. In the first place it is important to understand the personality and emotional turmoils some of these individuals are experiencing without becoming too preoccupied with particular symptoms or the technical details of some elaborate procedure. The underlying pathology and mechanism of pain must also be appreciated together with the therapeutic options available for curing the disease or modifying its effects. Clinicians engaged in this work must therefore acquire a great deal of information, some of which is outside their normal training and experience.

It has been said that all those who treat pain patients may have to relate to them in many roles, such as psychotherapist, priest, confessor, counsellor and friend, but such versatility should not blind the anesthetist to need for expert help when this is required (Boulton 1978). Bonica (1977) recognized, about 40 years ago, that a wide base and a multidisciplinary approach were essential for chronic pain and this remains true at the present time. An essential nucleus consists of a surgeon, physician, neurologist, psychiatrist and an anesthetist, but individual units vary considerably and also there are considerable differences in opinion regarding the organization and running of a pain relief service (Murphy 1980; Lipton 1981; Mehta 1981a).

Methods available for pain treatment

Non-invasive methods

Melzack and Wall's gate theory in 1965 added great impetus to the recognition of non-invasive techniques, which do not rely on destruction of nerve tissue by surgery, neurolytic injections or thermocoagulation. Many of these are simple methods, easy to apply in any situation and relatively free from complications (Mehta 1978). Some, like acupuncture and ice massage are forms of hyperstimulation analgesia. This is a term used by Melzack (1975) to describe periods of brief, intense sensory stimulation, which cause temporary discomfort, but long-term relief of more severe chronic pain possibly by spinal inhibition or recruitment of central biassing mechanisms. Others, like transcutaneous electrical nerve stimulation (TENS) rely on afferent nerve stimulation modifying pain response partly by release of endogenous opiates and partly by recruitment of inhibitory mechanisms regulating sensory mechanisms in the dorsal horn of the spinal cord (Liebeskind et al. 1974). The concept is not new, having been used by Scribonius Longus in the Socratic era with torpedo fish for the relief of arthritic pain and headache (Kane and Taub 1975).

TENS is simple, relatively inexpensive and uncomplicated. However, this does not mean it should be applied indiscriminately without proper appreciation of the diagnosis or personality of the patient. Elderly people, unless carefully instructed and reassured, are often frightened of electrical devices and there are others, who expect instant and complete relief comparable, for instance, with nerve block and will not persevere with the method. Analgesia often builds up slowly over several weeks (Wynn-Parry 1980). Electrodes need to be sited carefully, after trial and error in the dermatomal distribution of the pain, and optimum effects are only achieved if the patient experiences paraesthesia in response to the initial stimulation.

TENS is effective in about 30 – 40% of patients with chronic pain, but a great deal depends on proper instruction and selection of patients. It is particularly suited to pain of neurogenic origin, particularly peripheral nerve injuries, causalgia and post-herpetic neuralgia (Loeser et al. 1975; Bates and Nathan 1980). Myofascial injuries, chronic back pain and radiculopathies are improved (Rutkowski et al. 1977) and there are some reports of success with difficult central pain states, such as spinal injuries, phantom limb pain (Miles and Lipton 1978) and brachial plexus avulsion injuries (Wynn-Parry 1980). In most cases, a modest remission of symptoms in analgesic drug requirements is the best that can be expected, but this is a considerable bonus for many patients who are unable to get relief in any other way. TENS is contraindicated for the emotionally unstable, psychoneurotics and those who are dependent on narcotics. Poor results are obtained in those with terminal cancer, widespread and poorly localized pain, particularly of visceral origin and post-irradiation pain.

Acupuncture has been practised in China for over 3000 years and it is an integrated part of their tradition and culture. It cannot be translated in isolated form into Western medicine. Acupuncture undoubtedly produces analgesia even though the practice is often associated with distraction by counter-irritation, suggestion and, occasionally, mass hypnosis. Investigations have shown that pain is mediated through nerves rather than meridians (Melzack et al. 1977; Nathan 1978), and that there are specific neurotransmitters (Han and Terenius 1982) which may be responsible for release of endogenous polypeptides, serotonin and other biochemical agents. Acupuncture is not a reliable alternative to conventional methods of anesthesia, even in China where it is used for less than 10% of surgical operations (Bonica 1977). Nevertheless, acupuncture has its uses in the treatment of chronic pain. Conditions which are likely to respond are musculoskeletal pain associated with spasm, tension states and migrainous headaches. It has also been recommended for phantom limb pain. Acupuncture may be more effective in altering attitudes to pain rather than modification of the underlying disease (Toomey et al. 1977). This may explain beneficial effects in anxiety and chronic depression. Details of the technique are described elsewhere (Chu et al. 1979; Wensel 1980).

Other non-invasive methods include vibration, massage, counter-irritation with ointments or pain-relieving sprays like ethylchloride, and application of heat or ice packs. A trial of these methods is recommended for every case of severe post-herpetic neuralgia (Nathan and Wall 1974). Into this category also come ultrasound, shortwave, microwave and other techniques performed by the modern physiotherapist.

Trigger points are localized areas of muscle irritation with patchy edema, platelet aggregation and focal necrosis (Simons 1976). They may give rise to troublesome pain both locally and at sites far removed from them (Travell 1976). Stimulation by finger-tip pressure, needle insertion or local anesthetic injection arouses brief, intense pain which gives way to prolonged relief in many cases. This is followed by a full range of active and passive movements (Wynant 1979). A number of apparently insoluble problems are solved with this simple approach, but precise localization of the site is necessary and this may require a long and diligent search.

Non-invasive methods also include central methods in the treatment of chronic pain. The intensity of human suffering is determined primarily by the mind and is not necessarily related to the quality or quantity of noxious afferent stimulation. Oriental cultures have recognized this by emphasizing the need for mental control and discipline in overcoming pain. This is facilitated by yoga, transcendental meditation, biofeedback, induced relaxation, hypnosis and guided imagery. Psychotherapy and allied procedures are described elsewhere in this book. Many anesthetists use hypnosis, relaxation and biofeedback as valuable adjuncts to other methods. Pain is made less distressing by these means.

Finally there is alternative or fringe medicine. It is fashionable to decry unconventional approaches to medicine, which do not appear to have a proper scientific basis. Nevertheless, complementary medicine, as it is better described has much to offer when the more usual lines of treatment are ineffective. Some exponents are sincere and well-trained, as in osteopathy and chiropractice, while others merely prey on the vulnerability of chronic invalids to any new form of treatment. Anesthetists should have some knowledge of these methods, which make interesting reading (Stanley 1979), so that they can usefully advise their patients.

ANALGESICS AND ALLIED DRUGS

Analgesic drugs remain the bedrock of pain therapy because they are easily available and there is a wide choice to select from in any particular case. Nevertheless, there are recognized limitations to long-term prescription of these agents. Problems of addiction, dependence and tolerance are prevalent and many patients are referred to a pain relief clinic because control with analgesic drugs is unsatisfactory. Drug dependence does not matter for terminal cancer pain and there are many excellent publications describing the use of opiates and other agents for this purpose (Twycross and Lack 1983) (see also Chapters 19 and 32). Vomiting or dysphagia may preclude oral medication and other routes of administration, such as sublingual or rectal, can be very useful in such circumstances. In general, the whole subject of analgesic drug therapy covers far too much ground to be covered adequately in a brief report such as this. Details are available elsewhere (Jaffe and Martin 1980) (see also Chapters 19 and 32).

Opiate receptors exist in many parts of the nervous system, particularly in the substantia gelatinosa (Yaksh 1981). This has led to a novel approach to pain relief by spinal or extradural injections of small doses of opiates (Behar et al. 1979), which last longer than conventional local anesthetics without significant respiratory or circulatory depression (Cousins et al. 1979a). Narcotics attach almost exclusively to these dorsal horn sites causing a predominantly nociceptive blockade with mild blunting of cutaneous sensation, just sufficient for a skilled observer to detect segmental spread of the spinal narcotic (Bromage et al. 1980). Motor and autonomic function are unaffected, but initial enthusiasm for these techniques has been clouded by reports of occasional hypotension or respiratory depression several hours after the injection (Davies et al. 1980). This may occur at a time when the patient is not under direct supervision, is entirely unpredictable and due to slow rostral spread after passive diffusion and redistribution in the CSF

(Bromage et al. 1981). Other side effects such as vomiting, pruritus and urinary retention, are less troublesome and not potentially dangerous. All these complications, which are more frequent after subarachnoid injection, can be treated promptly and efficiently if the patient is under close observation for at least 12 hours afterwards. Certainly there is no justification for undertaking this procedure unless these facilities are available. Opinions vary about the choice of agent and route of administration, even though most experience has been gained with extradural morphine in preservative-free solution. Unfortunately, this opiate is poorly lipid soluble and transference to receptors in the spinal cord is slow, with a tendency to accumulate in the CSF. Analgesia is more widespread and less intense than it is with more soluble drugs like diamorphin and fentanyl, but there is greater danger of rostral spread with delayed respiratory depression following involvement of receptors in the brain stem. Morphine, 2 – 4 mg in 5 – 10 ml of 10% dextrose or normal saline, will give approximately 12 – 16 hours analgesia in most cases, whereas 100 – 150 μg fentanyl provides more intense segmental analgesia for only 3 – 4 hours. Other opiates like methadone and pethidine are intermediate in their effects. Many anesthetists therefore now favor a highly soluble, short-acting drug like fentanyl administered in continuous epidural infusion at a rate of approximately 25 – 50 μg/hour (Bromage 1984).

Brief mention must be made of agents which are not normally classified as analgesics (Budd 1981). Steroids enhance pain relief by lessening inflammation, improving appetite and general well being. Psychotropic drugs, apart from their intrinsic value in countering anxiety and depression may have direct analgesic properties due to interference with 5-hydroxytryptamine (5-HT) uptake in the descending amine pathway. This may explain the beneficial effects of tricyclic antidepressants combined with phenothiazines in the treatment of post-herpetic and phantom limb pain (see also Chapter 1). Anticonvulsants are established in the treatment of trigeminal neuralgia, but drugs like carbamazepine and phenytoin are equally effective in other similar conditions with paroxysmal, lancinating pain triggered by minimal afferent stimuli such as neuromas (Swerdlow 1980). Recent advances in neuropharmacology have also shown that transmission of noxious impulses may be blocked by administration of enzyme inhibitors like D-phenylalanine, D-leucine and hydrocinnamic acid, which prevent the destruction of enkephalins in the spinal cord. This enhances the effects of techniques like TENS and acupuncture. Similarly, intravenous naloxone, an opiate antagonist, has been shown to ameliorate intractable central pain, as for example after a cerebrovascular accident. The drug needs to be given slowly and cautiously, with monitoring of blood pressure and pulse, because much larger doses than normal are required for this purpose (4 – 8 mg). A recent report also advocates the use of anticholinesterases for this notoriously difficult pain state (Schott and Loh 1984).

PROLONGED NEURAL BLOCKADE

Prolonged neural blockade can be achieved by injecting neurolytic agents like phenol or alcohol or by applying heat or cold. The injection of neurolytic agents is suitable for simple blocks as in abdominal wall pain due to cutaneous nerve entrapment in the rectus sheath (Mehta and Ranger 1971) but in more complicated blocks these agents should only be injected into preformed tissue spaces, such as the arachnoid space or the tissue compartments enveloping the sympathetic ganglia. If there is no preformed tissue space the spread of the injected fluid is unpredictable, and so is its effect. X-ray monitoring is recommended for neurolytic blocks to ensure the solution is deposited in the right place (Mehta 1981b).

Freezing a peripheral nerve interrupts the flow of pain impulses, but does not alter its gross anatomical structure (Lloyd et al. 1976). There is no permanent sensory loss or motor dysfunction and complete recovery always takes place, usually within 12 weeks (Barnard 1980). Analgesia is of variable duration, commonly for 3 – 4 weeks, but in a few patients has lasted several months. The Spembley-Oxford cryoprobe is 15 SWG in diameter, it is bevelled at the tip and contains an electric sensing device which facilitates accurate siting of the tip in selected nerve tissue. Using nitrous oxide as the refrigerant, the temperature is lowered to – 60°C usually for two 60 sec. cycles. In practice, more extensive cooling can be undertaken without deleterious effect.

Thermal lesions are obtained by applying high frequency electric current to an electrode. Fine electrodes (22 or more SWG), incorporating delicate thermocouples for accurate temperature measurement, are introduced percutaneously under the X-ray screen in close proximity to the nerve. Accuracy is checked by eliciting sensory and motor responses to preliminary electrostimulation. Since electrodes of this fine diameter can be introduced without preliminary infiltration with local anesthetics, full use can be made of this facility contributing significantly to the efficacy and safety of the method. The extent of the burn is determined by the central temperature of the lesion, and this is meticulously controlled by manipulations of the lesion generator. The resulting lesion consists of a small area of necrosis immediately around the tip and this is surrounded by a much larger zone in which heat selectively destroys the fine nerve larger zone in pain (Letcher and Goldring 1968; Smith et al. 1981).

Treatment of inoperable cancer pain

METHODS DIRECTED AT THE SOURCE

These include surgery, deep X-ray treatment, cytotoxic and hormonal drugs. Anesthetists are not directly involved, but are fully aware of their value in overall management.

ANALGESIC DRUGS

The use of analgesic drugs has been discussed on page 150 (see also Chapter 32). Since opiates can be freely used in this type of pain the result is satisfactory in the majority of cases. If it is not, prolonged neural blockade may be considered. In making this decision both the effect of drug therapy and the chances of success of neural blockade have to be taken into account.

PROLONGED NEURAL BLOCKADE

Pituitary ablation. Destruction of the pituitary gland is achieved by surgery and other methods, but anesthetists became interested when Moricca (1974) described alcohol injections for this purpose. This approach has now been superseded by techniques with a fine cryoprobe (Duthie et al. 1983) or with a 20 SWG radiofrequency electrode which has been specially constructed for this purpose. These methods are considerably safer avoiding visual complications resulting from uncontrolled spread of alcohol. Significant pain relief is often obtained without suppression of hormonal function and its mechanism is not fully understood. Transient elevations in ACTH and possibly also alpha endorphin in blood and CSF occur after the procedure, but are not maintained for many days afterwards. Whatever the mode of action, pituitary destruction provides excellent pain relief for over 70% of patients with advanced and disseminated cancer. Breast and prostatic cancer cases do best, sometimes with tumor regression, but there is also a small incidence of success in other patients with malignant secondaries, who should not be denied the benefits of this technique when pain control by other means is unsatisfactory.

PERCUTANEOUS CORDOTOMY

Surgical incision of the anterolateral tract has been replaced in many cases by radiofrequency denervation, mainly under local anesthesia with light intravenous sedation (Lipton and McLennon 1980). This important method of pain relief can therefore be offered to the elderly and those in poor general condition. A fine cordotomy electrode is introduced in the C1 – C2 interspace and advanced to pierce the spinal cord approximately 1 – 2 mm anterior to the dentate ligament, which has been outlined by prior injection of an emulsion containing iophendylate and water. Electrostimulation confirms the accuracy of needle placement and when X-ray appearances and both motor and sensory testing are satisfactory, small incremental burns are made at the tip of the electrode until analgesia to pin prick is achieved on contralateral side.

This is a difficult technique to master, but very worth while, with over 75% of patients experiencing pain relief for up to 2 years. It is better reserved for severe unilateral pain in those with inoperable cancer.

Intrathecal injections. Intrathecal injections of phenol or alcohol are useful because the technique is simple and widely available (Papo and Visca 1979; Swerdlow 1979). The method is more reliable than extradural block and it is particularly indicated for pain of limited segmental distribution. Neurological complications, especially rectal and urinary incontinence, are avoided by careful sensory testing or X-ray monitoring after preliminary injection of 0.1 – 0.2 ml of myodil and appropriate tilting of the table to ensure drift of the hyperbaric mixture away from the lower sacral nerves (Maher and Mehta 1977). In general, the short-term results are good, but these are not sustained for long periods of time (Wood 1984). The method is principally reserved for those with a near-to-terminal illness.

Coeliac plexus block. Afferent information from the abdominal organs is conducted via thin nerve fibers, travelling with the sympathetic system. Since all these fibers are crossing the coeliac plexus, this is an ideal location for blocking abdominal pain resulting from inoperable cancer. Originally the procedure was described as a blind technique, but X-rays and computerized tomography may be extremely useful (Moore et al. 1981). After accurate placement of the needles and checking of the position with the aid of a contrast medium either 6% phenol or 50% alcohol is injected. This is a successful procedure usually rendering the patient free of pain for a period of at least 3 – 6 months. If pain remains this usually means that the tumor has grown into the posterior abdominal wall and that other forms of treatment have to be considered.

PERCUTANEOUS PARTIAL RHIZOTOMY

This procedure is described on page 158. It should ideally be confined to one or two segmental levels and since malignant pain usually has a wider segmental distribution partial rhizotomy is only useful in a few specific situations:

1) Destruction of a vertebral body by a secondary, usually resulting in pressure on the corresponding exiting segmental nerve.
2) Unilateral pain at the C2 – C5 level. Pain in this region cannot be interrupted by performing

a percutaneous cordotomy, since the incoming fibers ascend two or three segments in the spinal cord before they cross over to join the anterolateral tract.

3) Pain in the lower sacral segments after an apparently successful rectosigmoid resection for carcinoma. As long as it is uncertain whether or not the pain is due to a recurrence of tumor, one would hesitate to do a lower end neurolytic block. A partial rhizotomy is a more elaborate alternative, but it carries less risk to the bladder function.

Pain of non-malignant origin

Once again diagnosis is all-important in the treatment of pain of non-malignant origin. Every effort should be made and the anesthetist can often be of help by performing prognostic blocks, injecting minimal quantities of a local anesthetic solution, preferably under X-ray control and using a contrast medium before injecting the local anesthetic to verify proper positioning of the needle.

Depending on the diagnosis, a strategy now has to be developed. The principles outlined on page 147, 148 must be kept in mind, and psychological factors must be considered. Next, the type of pain is important. This may be one of the following:

1) Central pain
2) Denervation pain
3) Pain in which the sympathetic system is involved
4) Pain due to high input of noxious stimuli

CENTRAL PAIN

Central pain is caused by pathology inside the central nervous system, for instance the thalamic syndrome, caused by a cerebrovascular accident. Drug treatment and non-invasive methods, as discussed above, are in order for the treatment of this type of pain. A recent report mentions the possibility of pituitary ablation (Levin et al. 1983) but otherwise there is no place for invasive treatment.

DENERVATION PAIN

Denervation pain is caused by a deficit in the normal afferent input, which maintains the equilibrium in the dorsal horn. Post-herpetic neuralgia, phantom limb pain, the various types of pain in paraplegic patients and pain resulting from traumatic or surgical section of a nerve come into this category. Once again, this is the field of drug treatment and non-invasive methods. Radiofrequency lesion in the dorsal root entry zone (Nashold 1979) is a new form of treatment, particularly indicated for post-herpetic neuralgia, pain due to traumatic avulsion of nerve roots and pain in paraplegic patients. Since this is a purely neurosurgical procedure, it is only briefly mentioned here.

Chemical neurectomy is used for the relief of pain and spasticity in multiple sclerosis, traumatic paraplegia and other neurological disorders (Maher 1964; Dimitrijevic and Nathan 1968). Reduction in the number of afferent stimuli impinging on the spinal cord causes reflex hypotonia, which eases the patient's discomfort and facilitates nursing hygiene to avoid troublesome bedsores. When the patient is bed-ridden and has no useful bladder function, a better result is achieved by injecting 1 ml of 10% phenol in glycerine and deliberately applying the solution to the anterior nerve roots.

THE SYMPATHETIC NERVOUS SYSTEM

Blocks of the autonomous nervous system are performed either at the level of the spinal ganglia or by intravenous regional perfusion of a limb. The perfusion technique is a modification of Bier's block for regional anesthesia (Hannington-Kiff 1974). Sympathectomy is effective in a wide variety of conditions, notably rest pain due to peripheral vascular ischemia or gangrene, where it also facilitates demarcation and separation of necrotic tissue (Reid et al. 1970). It is also indicated for causalgia and reflex sympathetic dystrophies, but its value in intermittent claudication is debatable (Fyfe and Quinn 1975). However, pain relief is usually achieved with this method in chronic pancreatitis due to infection or alcoholism and for dysesthesia in the long bones which is a feature of Paget's disease. Stellate ganglion blocks are disappointing, for cerebrovascular incidents, for which there is no apparent reason, are occasionally caused by a viral infection causing vasospasm of the inferior cerebellar artery. A dramatic response may be obtained with chemical sympathectomy. The results in tinnitus and Meniere's syndrome are more disappointing. Some painful scars and post-amputation pain may also improve with this treatment.

Sympathectomy by neurolytic or radiofrequency heat lesions is as effective as surgery (Reid et al. 1970), applicable to elderly or infirm patients and affords considerable economy in hospital beds. In the majority of cases, full activity can be resumed soon afterwards and patients can go home later in the day. The technique of lumbar sympathectomy is well described (Hughes-Davies and Redman 1976; Cousins et al. 1979b.) Injection with 6% phenol or alcohol gives more lasting relief than repeated blocks with local anesthetics, but the use of an X-ray image intensifier is mandatory to avoid untoward complications. Stellate ganglion block is a more complicated procedure. However, the modified low-dose, paratracheal approach at C6 (Caron and Litwiller 1975) is a considerable advance on previous techniques. Once again, X-ray screening is essential and only 1 – 1.5 ml of 6% phenol mixed with Conroy 280 should be used for the block. Great care is taken to ensure that the solution spreads in the correct plane and there is no lateral extension onto the brachial plexus. The accompanying Horner's syndrome is reported to disappear in a matter of months. One of the authors (M. E. Sluijter) has seen a permanent Horner's syndrome after this procedure in two patients despite taking all precautions and now prefers to make a 70°C radiofrequency lesion in the stellate ganglion in such cases.

Radiofrequency lesions in the sympathetic chain may also be useful in low back problems (see page 157) and in thoracic pain following mastectomy and irradiation.

PAIN DUE TO INCREASED INPUT OF NOXIOUS STIMULI

Many types of pain belong to this group, and a complete overview is not possible within the context of this chapter. Again, the first choice of treatment may be drug treatment or non-invasive methods. If these methods fail invasive methods come into consideration. Some examples will be briefly discussed.

Facial pain. The treatment of trigeminal neuralgia has changed dramatically over the last decades. Techniques such as electrocoagulation of the Gasserian ganglion following Kirschner's technique, section of the nerve or injections of alcohol into the ganglion or into one of the peripheral divisions are now obsolete. The method of choice nowadays is decompression of the nerve in the occipital fossa as described by Jannetta (1977), which is highly successful without causing any sensory loss. This however is not always possible, since many patients suffering from this affliction are of advanced age and since even younger patients sometimes worry about the prospect of an intracranial procedure. Also, the method is not entirely free from complications. If an operation is not wanted or contraindicated a selective radiofrequency heat lesion can be performed in the Gasserian ganglion (Sweet and Wepsic 1974). A 22 SWG electrode with a 2 mm active tip is introduced into the foramen ovale under X-ray guidance using a transverse projection and an oblique one parallel to the course of the needle. The electrode is manipulated until the tip is located in the area of the ganglion serving the trigger zone, as confirmed by electrostimulation. Heat lesions with increasing central temperature are then made until the trigger area becomes slightly hyperesthetic. No more is needed for a good result. Larger lesions result in dysesthesia or anesthesia dolorosa and should be avoided. The results are good in over 80% of cases. Recurrence after a year or so does occur, especially if one tends to be conservative during lesioning. By that time, sensory loss has usually disappeared and the procedure can be repeated.

Other facial pains, although usually less severe, are often much more difficult to treat. Cluster headache can be treated successfully by injecting alcohol into the sphenopalatine ganglion (Devoghel 1981). This causes severe pain for some days after the injection, and the results of making a radiofrequency lesion in this area are equally good. Again, a 22 SWG electrode is inserted under the zygomatic arch and advanced under X-ray control until the tip lies in the sphenopalatine foramen. On electrical stimulation the patient should feel tingling in or right under the nose. In this way a safe distance from the maxillary nerve and from the branches serving the palate can be assured.

Atypical facial pain is in fact probably a group of pain syndromes from various origins. Psychosomatic factors are notoriously important and one should always probe for emotional milestones at the time of onset before considering invasive therapy. Also many of these pains are in fact a manifestation of a cervical syndrome and disappear if this is properly treated. Diagnostic blocks can be of great help to clear up the conduction pattern. Radiofrequency lesions, either of the sphenopalatine ganglion or of one of the cervical segmental nerves have good results provided the results of the diagnostic blocks are unequivocal.

Back and neck pain. So complicated is the problem of back and neck pain that the subject can only be treated superficially in a review like this. Generally speaking, back and neck pain can be either mechanical or radicular, due to irritation of one of the exiting spinal nerves. Mechanical pain may emanate from the posterior joints or from structures anterior to the transverse process. These structures are the anterior aspect of the dura, the anterior and posterior longitudinal ligament and the capsule of the intervertebral discs, as stressed recently by Bogduk (1983). Radicular pain may be caused by a prolapsed disc or by degenerative bone spurs protruding from the posterior joints or from a degenerated disc.

More mysterious is the role of the sympathetic chain. In many patients with radiating pain, the sympathetic system is obviously more active on the painful side, although we do not know why. On the other hand afferent fibers travelling with the sympathetic system may well be of importance, as witnessed by the effect of prognostic blocks. We know very little about these afferent fibers, except that some of them originate from the capsule of the disc.

To make things more complicated, these pain syndromes are often mixed and appear not to have one single cause. Pain may be a result of too much noxious input from a number of sources.

If one contemplates prolonged neural blockade one has to realize that as a consequence one may have to do more than one block in one specific location. Also, the aim should probably be to decrease noxious input rather than interrupting a nerve tract between one single cause and its effect.

Back and neck pain is a very frequent complaint that usually responds well to conservative treatment. If it does not, the possibility of surgical intervention should be considered. It is only when all these options fail that prolonged neural blockade should be considered.

The anesthetist should be familiar with the anatomy of the exiting spinal nerve and its roots and branches. This anatomy is complex and discrete radiofrequency lesions must be used to avoid untoward effects. Lesions can be made in the following locations:

PERCUTANEOUS FACET DENERVATION

This is the earliest of the procedures available for this type of pain (Shealy 1975). A percutaneous facet denervation is an interruption of the posterior primary ramus of the exiting segmental nerve, or more specifically the medial branch of this nerve serving the posterior joints. The innervation is such that this procedure has to be done at several levels to have a good effect. If properly executed, it is an uncomplicated procedure. If there is radiating pain as well it is often combined with epidural administration of corticosteroids.

The results are good, provided the patient really had mechanical pain emanating from the posterior joints, a so-called posterior compartment syndrome (Sluijter and Mehta 1981). This can be verified by prior prognostic blocks. Even though these are positive, the results in the neck are better than in the back. This may mean that mechanical pain in the neck is often purely of the posterior variety; in the back anterior structures are often involved as well.

ANTEROLATERAL DISC DENERVATION

The innervation of the mechanical structures anterior to the transverse process is much more complex and has many interconnections. Complete interruption is obviously not possible but as has been pointed out this is probably not necessary. Inspired by Bogduk's work one of the authors (M. E. Sluijter) devised a technique to interrupt part of the noxious input emanating from the disc capsule in suitable patients. This procedure was performed in patients suffering from mechanical back pain not responding to a facet denervation. Prognostic injections of the disc capsule are carried out first at various levels. If a prognostic block is completely successful, a 20 SWG 15 cm electrode is introduced into the capsule using a far oblique X-ray projection. After electrostimulation to ensure that the electrode is not in dangerous proximity to the segmental nerve, an 80°C lesion is made. The electrode is then advanced further and the sequence is repeated until the tip of the electrode has reached the anterior level of the vertebral body.

The results are quite promising, 50% of patients being substantially improved or even free of pain. Long-term results will of course have to be awaited.

THERMAL LUMBAR SYMPATHETIC BLOCK

As has been pointed out, the role of the lumbar sympathetic chain in back pain has not been elucidated. Prognostic blocks may be positive, but if these blocks are repeated with 6% phenol in the usual fashion the result is often disappointing. Radiofrequency lesions in the sympathetic chain at the level of the pain have a much better result and this may indicate that in fact the sympathetic fibers do not play a role of any importance but that afferent fibers, carrying impulses from the anterior part of the disc capsule and travelling with the sympathetic system, are the main target when performing this procedure.

PERCUTANEOUS PARTIAL RHIZOTOMY

Radiofrequency thermocoagulation of the dorsal root ganglion was originally suggested by Uematsu (Uematsu et al. 1974) but reintroduced by Sluijter (Sluijter 1981; Sluijter and Mehta 1981). This procedure rests on the assumption that a partial interruption of noxious input is sufficient to relieve pain in many instances and that on the other hand this prevents the occurrence of anesthesia dolorosa, as often happens after surgical rhizotomy. A thermocouple electrode is introduced percutaneously under local anesthesia, to slip into the posterior part of the intervertebral foramen. The position is checked on A-P and lateral X-ray projections and confirmed by response to motor and sensory electrostimulation. When this is satisfactory, a $60-70°C$ lesion is made depending on the sensory stimulation threshold. Temperature measuring equipment should always be used in order to prevent the occurrence of anesthesia dolorosa resulting from a lesion that is too large.

Inserting the electrode is a problem in the sacral area, since the ganglia are covered by bone and an approach through the sacral foramina leads to a position distal to the ganglion. This is solved by visualizing the nerve by injecting a contrast medium and making a small burrhole with a Kirschner wire over the ganglion (Sluijter and Mehta 1981). A percutaneous partial rhizotomy should only be done after preliminary prognostic blocks at several segmental levels. Ideally one of these blocks should be positive while the others are not. Provided the electrostimulation parameters are strictly adhered to this is a safe procedure not causing motor loss. Sensory loss is variable, but if hyperesthesia in the dermatome occurs this tends to disappear in the course of $3-6$ months.

Conclusion

This chapter has indicated the considerable progress which has been made in the treatment of chronic pain, but much remains to be achieved. Nevertheless, it is reassuring for patients, with this severe complaint, to know that the climate of medical opinion has changed and there is no longer complete indifference to their needs or total inability to ameliorate their symptoms.

References

Barnard, D. (1980) The effects of extreme cold on sensory nerves. Ann. R. Coll. Surg. Engl. 62, 180 – 187.

Bates, J. A. V. and Nathan, P. W. (1980) Transcutaneous electrical stimulation for chronic pain. Anaesthesia 35, 817 – 822.

Behar, M., Magora, F., Olshwang, D. and Davidson, J. P. (1979) Epidural morphine in treatment of pain. Lancet 1, 527 – 529.

Bogduk, N. (1983) The innervation of the lumbar spine. Spine 8, 286 – 293.

Bonica, J. J. (1974) Anesthesiology in The People's Republic of China. Anesthesiology 40, 175 – 186.

Bonica, J. J. (1977) Neurophysiologic and pathologic aspects of acute and chronic pain. Arch. Surg. 112, 750 – 761.

Bonica, J. J. (1985) Importance of the problem. In: S. Andersson and M. Mehta (Eds.), Problem of Chronic Pain. IASP Publication for Physicians in Developing Countries.

Boulton, T. B. (1978) Editorial. Anaesthesia 33, 225 – 226.

Bromage, P. R. (1981) Editorial. The price of intraspinal narcotic analgesia: basic constraints. Anesth. Analg. (Cleve.) 60, 461 – 463.

Bromage, P. R. (1984) Epidural therapy. In: P. Wall and Melzack, R. (Eds.), Textbook of Pain. Churchill Livingstone, Edinburgh – London – New York, pp. 558 – 565.

Bromage, P. R., Campores, E. and Chestnut, D. (1980) Epidural narcotics for post-operative analgesia. Anesth. Analg. (Cleve.) 59, 473 – 480.

Budd, K. (1981) Non-analgesic drugs in the management of pain. In: J. Miles and S. Lipton (Eds), Persistent Pain, Vol. III. Academic Press, New York, pp. 223 – 240.

Caron, H. and Litwiller, R. (1975) Stellate ganglion block. Anesth. Analg. (Cleve.) 54, 567 – 570.

Chu, L. S. W., Yeh, S. D. J. and Wood, D. D. (1979) Acupuncture Manual. A Western Approach. Marcel Dekker Inc., New York, Basel.

Cousins, M. J., Mather, L. E., Glynn, C. J., Wilson, P. R. and Graham, J. R. (1979a) Selective spinal anaesthesia. Lancet I, 1141.

Cousins, M. J., Reeve, T. S., Glynn, C. J., Walsh, J. A. and Cherry, D. A. (1979b) Neurolytic lumbar sympathetic blockade – duration of denervation and relief of rest pain. Anaesth. Intens. Care 7, 121 – 135.

Cousins, M. J. and Bridenbaugh, P. O. (Eds.) (1980) Neural Blockade – In Clinical Anaesthesia and Management of Pain. J. B. Lippincott Co., Philadelphia and Toronto.

Davies, G. K., Tolhurst-Cleaver, C. L. and James, T. L. (1980) C.N.S. depression from intrathecal morphine. Anesthesiology 52, 280.

Devoghel, J. C. (1981) Cluster headache and sphenopalatine block. Acta Anaesth. Belg. 32, 101 – 107.

Dimitrijevic, M. R. and Nathan, P. W. (1968) Studies of spasticity in man. 3. Analysis of reflex activity evoked by noxious cutaneous stimulation. Brain 91, 349 – 368.

Duthie, A. M., Ingham, V., Dell, A. E. and Dennett, J. E. (1983) Pituitary cryoablation. The results of treatment using a trans-sphenoidal cryoprobe. Anaesthesia 38, 448 – 451.

Fyfe, T. and Quinn, R. D. (1975) Phenol sympathectomy in the treatment of intermittent claudication. Br. J. Surg. 62, 68 – 70.

Han, J. S. and Terenius, L. (1982) Neurochemical basis of acupuncture analgesia. Ann. Rev. Pharmacol. Toxicol. 22, 193 – 220.

Hannington-Kiff, J. (1974) Intravenous regional sympathetic block with guanethidine. Lancet II, 1020 – 1021.

Hughes-Davis, D. I. and Redman, L. R. (1976) Chemical lumbar sympathectomy. Anaesthesia 31, 1068 – 1075.

Jaffe, J. H. and Martin, W. R. (1980) Opioid analgesics and antagonists. In: A. G. Goodman, L. S. Goodman and A. Gilman (Eds.), The Pharmacological Basis of Therapeutics. MacMillan, New York pp. 494 – 534.

Jannetta, P. J., Abbasy, M., Marvon, J. C. et al. (1977) Observation on the etiology of trigeminal neuralgia, hemifacial spasm, acoustic nerve dysfunction and glossopharyngeal neuralgia. Definitive microsurgical treatment and result in 117 patients. Neurochirurgia 20, 145 – 154.

Kane, K. and Taub, A. (1975) A history of local electric analgesia. Pain 9, 219 – 230.

Levin, A. B., Ramirez, L. F. and Katz, J. (1983) The use of stereotactic chemical hypophysectomy in the treatment of thalamic pain syndrome. J. Neurosurg. 59, 1002 – 1006.

Letcher, F. S. and Goldring, S. (1968) The effects of radiofrequency current and heat on peripheral nerve potentials. J. Neurosurg. 29, 42 – 47.

Liebeskind, J. C., Mayer, D. J. and Akill, H. (1974) Central mechanisms of pain inhibition. Studies of analgesia from focal brain stimulation. In: J. J. Bonica (Ed.), Neurology, Vol IV. Raven Press, New York pp. 261 – 280.

Lipton, S. (1981) Current views on the management of a pain relief centre. In: M. Swerdlow (Ed.), The Therapy of Pain. M.T.P. Press, Lancaster, England, pp. 61 – 86.

Lipton, S. and McLennon, J. (1980) Percutaneous spinothalamic tractotomy. The prototype of neurosurgical pain control. In: M. J. Cousins and P. O. Bridenbaugh (Eds.), Neural Blockade. J. B. Lippincott, Philadelphia, pp. 679 – 690.

Lloyd, J. W., Barnard, J. D. W. and Glynn, C. J. (1976) Cryoanalgesia – a new approach to pain relief. Lancet II, 932 – 934.

160

Loeser, J. D., Black, R. G. and Christman, R. M. (1975) Relief of pain by transcutaneous stimulation. J. Neurosurg. 42, 308 – 314.

Maher, R. M. (1964) Medical treatment of spasticity. Proc. R. Soc. Med. 57, 720 – 724.

Maher, R. M. and Mehta, M. (1977) Spinal (intrathecal) and extradural analgesia. In: S. Lipton (Ed.), Persistent Pain. Modern Methods of Treatment, Vol I. Academic Press, New York and London, pp. 61 – 69.

Mehta, M. (1978) Alternative ways of treating pain. Anaesthesia 33, 258 – 260.

Mehta, M. (1981a) The pain relief clinic. In: N. Williams (Ed.), Symposium on Pain. Int. J. Pharmacol. Ther. 12, 373 – 380.

Mehta, M. (1981b) Recent advances in injection treatment for cancer pain. In: J. Miles and S. Lipton (Eds.), Persistent Pain. Modern Methods of Treatment, Vol. III. Academic Press, London and New York, pp. 265 – 278.

Mehta, M. and Ranger, I. (1971) Persistent abdominal pain. Treatment by nerve block. Anaesthesia 26, 330 – 333.

Mehta, M. and Sluijter, M. E. (1979) The treatment of chronic back pain. A preliminary survey of the effects of radiofrequency denervation of the posterior vertebral joints. Anaesthesia 34, 768 – 775.

Melzack, R. (1975) Prolonged relief of pain by brief, intense transcutaneous somatic stimulation. Pain 1, 357 – 373.

Melzack, R. and Wall, P. (1965) Pain mechanisms, a new theory. Science 150, 971 – 979.

Melzack, R., Stilwell, D. and Fox, E. (1977) Trigger points and acupuncture points for pain. Correlations and implications. Pain 3, 3 – 10.

Merskey, H. and Spear, F. G. (1967) Pain: Psychological and Psychiatric Aspects. Bailliere, Tindall and Cassell, London.

Miles, J. and Lipton, S. (1978) Phantom limb pain treated by electric stimulation. Pain 5, 373 – 375.

Moore, D. C., Busch, W. H. and Burnett, L. L. (1981) Celiac plexus block: a roentgenographic, anatomic study of technique and spread of solution in patients and corpses. Anesth. Analg. 60, 369 – 379.

Moricca, G. (1974) Chemical hypophysectomy for cancer pain. In: J. J. Bonica (Ed.), Advances in Neurology. Raven Press, New York, pp. 707 – 714.

Murphy, T. M. (1980) Neural blockade and the collaborative concept of pain management. In: M. J. Cousins and P. O. Bridenbaugh (Eds.), Neural Blockade – In Clinical Anaesthesia and Management of Pain. J. J. Lippincott Co, Philadelphia and Toronto, pp. 691 – 698.

Nashold, B. S., Jr. and Ostdahl, R. H. (1979) Dorsal entry root zone lesions for pain relief. J. Neurosurg. 51, 59 – 69.

Nathan, P. W. (1978) Acupuncture analgesia. Trends Neurosci. 2, 21 – 28.

Nathan, P. W. and Wall, P. D. (1974) Treatment of post-herpetic neuralgia by prolonged electric stimulation. Br. Med. J. 2, 645 – 646.

Papo, I. and Visca, A. (1979) Phenol subarachnoid rhizotomy for the treatment of cancer pain: a personal account on 290 cases. In: J. J. Bonica and V. Ventafridda (Eds.), Advances in Pain Research and Therapy, Vol. 2. Raven Press, New York, pp. 339 – 349.

Reid, W. J., Watt, J. K. and Gray, T. G. (1970) Phenol injection of the sympathetic chain. Br. J. Surg. 57, 45 – 50.

Rutkowski, B., Niedzialkowska, T. and Otto, J. (1977) Electric stimulation in chronic low back pain. Br. J. Anaesth. 49, 629 – 631.

Schott, G. D. and Loh, L. (1984) Anticholinesterase drugs in the treatment of chronic pain. Pain 20, 201 – 206.

Shealy, C. N. (1975) Percutaneous radiofrequency of spinal facets. J. Neurosurg. 43, 448 – 451.

Simons. D. G. (1976) Muscle pain syndromes. Am. J. Phys. Med. Part I 54, 289 – 309; Part II 55, 15 – 43.

Sluijter, M. E. (1981) Percutaneous thermal lesions in the treatment of back and neck pain. Radionics Instruction Manual, Radionics Inc., Burlington, Mass. U.S.A.

Sluijter, M. E. and Mehta, M. (1981) Treatment of chronic pain in the back and neck by percutaneous thermal lesions. In: J. Miles and S. Lipton (Eds), Persistent Pain, Modern Methods of Treatment, Vol. III. Academic Press, London and New York, pp. 141 – 180.

Smith, H. P., Mc Worther, J. M. and Challa, V. R. (1981) Radiofrequency neurolysis in a clinical model. Neuropathological correlation. J. Neurosurg. 32, 246 – 253.

Stanley, A. (1979) Alternative Medicine. A Guide to Natural Therapies. Macdonald and Jones, London.

Sternback, R. A. (1974) Pain Patients: Traits and Treatment. Academic Press, New York.

Sternbach, R. A. (1981) Chronic pain as a disease entity. Triangle 20, 27 – 32.

Sweet, W. H. and Wepsic, J. G. (1974) Controlled thermocoagulation of trigeminal ganglion and rootlets for differential destruction of pain fibres. J. Neurosurg. 39, 143 – 155.

Swerdlow, M. (1979) Subarachnoid and extradural neurolytic blocks. In: J. J. Bonica and V. Ventafridda (Eds.), Advances in Pain Research and Therapy, Vol. 2. Raven Press, New York, pp. 325 – 337.

Swerdlow, M. (1980) The treatment of shooting pain. Postgrad. Med. J. 56, 159 – 161.

Swerdlow, M. (1983) Relief of Intractable Pain, 3rd edn. Excerpta Medica, Amsterdam.

Swerdlow, M., Mehta, M. and Lipton, S. (1978) The role of the anaesthetist in chronic pain management. Anaesthesia 33, 250 – 257.

Toomey, T. C., Ghia, J. N., Mao, W. et al. (1977) Acupuncture and chronic pain mechanisms: the moderating effects of affect, personality and stress on response to treatment. Pain 3, 137 – 145.

Travell, J. (1976) Muscle pain syndromes. In: J. J. Bonica (Ed.), Advances in Pain Research and Therapy, Vol. 1. Raven Press, New York, p. 919.

Twycross, R. G. and Lack, S. A. (1983) Symptom Control in Far Advanced Cancer. Pain Relief. Pitman Publishing, London.

Uematsu, S., Udvarhelyi, G. B., Benson, D. W. and Siebens, A. A. (1974) Percutaneous radiofrequency rhizotomy. Surg. Neurol. 2, 319 – 325.

Wall, P. D. and Melzack, R. (Eds.) (1984) Textbook of Pain. Churchill Livingstone, London and Edinburgh.

Wood, K. M. (1984) Peripheral nerve and root chemical lesions. In: P. D. Wall and R. Melzack (Eds.), Textbook of Pain. Churchill Livingstone, Edinburgh – London – New York, pp. 577 – 580.

Wensel, L. O. (1980) Acupuncture in Medical Practice. Reston Publ. Co., Reston, Virginia, U.S.A.

Wynant, G. M. (1979) Chronic pain syndromes and their treatment: trigger points. Can. Anaesth. Soc. J. 26, 216 – 220.

Wynn-Parry, C. B. (1980) Pain in avulsion lesions of the brachial plexus. Pain 9, 41 – 53.

Yaksh, T. L. (1981) Spinal opiate analgesia: characteristics and principles of action. Pain 11, 293 – 346.

Burrows/Elton/Stanley (eds.) Handbook of Chronic Pain Management
© *1987 Elsevier Science Publishers B.V. (Biomedical Division)*

19

Drug therapy

GEOFFREY K. GOURLAY, MICHAEL J. COUSINS and DAVID A. CHERRY

Pain Management Unit, Department of Anaesthesia and Intensive Care, Flinders Medical Centre, Bedford Park, South Australia 5042, Australia

Introduction

Significant developments have been made in the understanding of the mechanisms involved in the transmission of nociceptive impulses (Basbaum 1984), the various classes of opioid receptors and endogenous ligands (Rance 1983; Goodman and Pasternak 1984) together with the pharmacokinetic and pharmacodynamic properties of the various classes of drugs used in pain therapy (Gourlay and Cousins 1984; Inturrisi and Foley 1984; Mather and Gourlay 1984). Many of the terms traditionally associated with this area such as pain, narcotics, analgesia, analgesics etc. have various and different meanings to different people and in different settings.

The International Association for the Study of Pain (I.A.S.P.) established a committee on taxonomy which has published a 'Classification of Chronic Pain: Description of Chronic Pain Syndromes and Definitions of Pain Terms', in an attempt to improve clarity and understanding (Merskey 1986). Definitions relevant to this chapter are summarized below. However, the reader is strongly advised to consult the 'Classification' which is published as a complete supplement to the journal 'Pain'.

Pain is defined as an unpleasant sensory and emotional experience associated with actual or potential tissue damage or described in terms of such damage. Thus, all patients complaining of pain should be conceived as having both sensory and psychological components. The difficult clinical decision involves the assessment of the relative contributions of each component which should dictate the emphasis in treatment. It should be noted however, that the minor component cannot be forgotten if effective pain therapy is to be provided.

Analgesia is defined as the absence of pain on noxious stimulation. *Analgesics* should therefore, be defined as therapy which allows the state of analgesia to be realized. It is apparent that the true analgesic drugs are restricted to local anaesthetics and various agents used to induce and maintain general anaesthesia. It is more appropriate to replace the term analgesia with pain relief and analgesics with pain-relieving medication, where possible.

The term *narcotic* is derived from narcosis or a state of sleep or drowsiness. This term has little applicability to the morphine-like and synthetic pharmacological agents used to provide pain relief. Recently, the terms opiate (drugs derived from opium), or opioid (drugs which are not necessarily derived from opium but have morphine-like properties such as pain relief, dependence liability and addiction etc.) have replaced narcotic in the medical literature. The term *narcotic* should be relegated to various regulatory bodies concerned with drafting legislation.

The term *endogenous opioid* refers to any material (peptide or other hormone) which occurs in the brain or other organs that mimic the pharmacological actions of morphine. It should be stated at the outset that the use of drugs in the treatment of chronic pain should only occur after a thorough evaluation of the possible underlying causes of the pain and the effective treatment of any treatable causes. It is also important to characterize the pain very carefully as described elsewhere in this text. In general, somatic pain is well localized whereas visceral pain may have a rather vague distribution and is more often associated with nausea and vomiting. However, deep somatic pain involving bone may be somewhat similar to visceral pain in terms of a more diffuse quality and an association with nausea and vomiting.

It may also be helpful to attempt to further categorize the pain and a number of possibilities have been suggested. One that we have found helpful is as follows.

PAIN THAT IS PREDOMINANTLY DUE TO A PERIPHERAL NOCICEPTIVE FOCUS

It is important to note that this does not preclude a contribution of other factors, including psychological factors. If the nociceptive focus is predominantly of somatic origin, it is useful to commence with non-steroidal anti-inflammatory drugs (NSAIDs). However, there are other measures which may be appropriate in chronic non-cancer pain, such as the injection of trigger points with local anaesthetics (see below). If the nociceptive focus is in a viscus, opioid agents are effective, particularly in patients with cancer. In patients with chronic non-cancer pain, it is preferable to use the so-called 'co-analgesic drugs' or 'adjuvant drugs' such as antidepressants, steroids, anticonvulsants, phenothiazines together with NSAIDs. However, it may sometimes be necessary to use opioid drugs to obtain effective pain relief. Neuropathic pain is due to a disturbance of function or pathological change in a nerve (e.g. due to amyloid or diabetes). Such pain responds poorly to opioids.

PAIN THAT IS PREDOMINANTLY OF 'CENTRAL' ORIGIN

This category includes all pain arising central to the dorsal horn of the spinal cord. Originally, this term 'central pain' was synonymous with pain due to thalamic lesions (i.e. thalamic syndrome). However, it also includes pain due to other lesions in the central nervous system which produce denervation or 'deafferentation' pain as described under the section on Neurogenic pain. It also includes pain which is predominantly of psychologic origin as described below. It would be clearly preferable to manage pain of predominantly psychologic origin by non-pharmacologic techniques whereas pain of central origin is generally not responsive to the opioid drugs.

NEUROGENIC PAIN

This category includes pain which is due to lesions in the peripheral or central nervous system which may produce a neurologic deficit. This includes peripheral neuralgias produced by partial damage in the peripheral nervous system. Trauma or other lesions may produce complete or partial loss of function in a portion of the peripheral nervous system (for example, brachial plexus avulsion) or the central nervous system (e.g. trauma or compression of the spinal cord). This type of lesion can result in a so-called 'deafferentation pain syndrome'. Once patients reach the situation of complete denervation, these syndromes are rarely responsive to the usual pain-relieving drugs (e.g. opioids and NSAIDs). Previously pharmacological approaches to pain relief were extremely disappointing, but it has recently been reported that a combination of tricyclic antidepressant and fluphenazine produces encouraging results (Loeser 1986). Another alternative has been the use of anticonvulsant drugs. Note that a 'peripheral' neuralgic pain may progressively develop into a 'central' pain state as pain persists.

PAIN WITH PREDOMINANT PSYCHOLOGIC AETIOLOGY

It is important to re-emphasize that these patients may have a minor nociceptive focus but that psychological problems are predominant. In such patients it may be appropriate to address simultaneously the physical and psychological basis of the problem, with emphasis on the psychological factors. As discussed in other chapters, there are psychological and psychiatric conditions which may present with pain. The treatment of these conditions may include the pharmacological treatment of anxiety, depression and other problems but often non-pharmacological measures are of equal and greater importance.

The long-term effects of unrelieved pain initiate a vicious cycle involving anxiety, depression, and sleep disturbances as shown in Fig. 1. Chronic pain results in anxiety and frequently depression. Markedly changed sleep patterns occur because of the combined effects of pain, anxiety, and depression which, in turn, reduce the patient's resources to cope with the pain. Under these circumstances, the patient frequently complains of an increase in intensity of pain. It is apparent from Fig. 1 that there are various pharmacological and non-pharmacological options available to practitioners to provide pain relief to patients in acute and chronic pain. The non-pharmacological approaches are detailed elsewhere in this volume. The drug therapy to be discussed throughout this chapter includes centrally acting opioid drugs, peripherally acting NSAIDs, and the previously mentioned 'adjuvant drugs'. Finally, a miscellaneous group including inhalation agents, local anaesthetics, amphetamine and cocaine will also be considered.

Fundamental basis of drug therapy

OPIOID RECEPTORS

Extensive evidence indicates that there are at least four (and probably more) different types of opioid receptors located in the brain and spinal cord (Goodman and Pasternak 1984). Table 1 provides the pharmacodynamic effects obtained when an agonist occupies each of the receptor

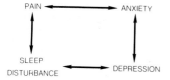

Fig. 1. The relationship between pain, anxiety, depression and sleep disturbance.

subtypes. Morphine is the prototype mu receptor agonist which produces the well documented dose-dependent effects of pain relief, miosis, respiratory depression, sedation, physical dependence and addiction. Many of the older opioid drugs including pethidine, methadone, fentanyl, heroin, codeine, propoxyphene are mu receptor agonists (Table 1).

Ketocyclazocine is the prototype kappa agonist. Animal studies have shown a high localization of kappa receptors in the spinal cord (Gouarderes et al. 1982) leading to the hypothesis that these receptors may be specifically involved in pain relief at the spinal cord level in addition to the usual supraspinal level.

Animal studies (Tyers 1980) have shown that intrathecal kappa agonists demonstrate selective antinociceptive activity against non-heat stimuli resulting in the hypothesis that different populations of opiate receptors could exist on different afferent neuronal types. There are different patterns of respiratory depression, euphoria and abuse liability between kappa and mu receptor agonists. At low doses, kappa agonists show a similar extent of respiratory depression with equivalent pain-relieving doses of mu receptor agonists. However, at higher doses of kappa agonists, the respiratory depression usually reaches a plateau whereas the extent of respiratory depression is much greater with equivalent doses of mu agonists (Romagnoli and Keats 1980). While this respiratory effect appears to be a significant theoretical advantage, the clinical significance has yet to be fully established. For example, the dose associated with plateau effects on respiratory depression may be significantly higher than the normal doses required for pain relief.

TABLE 1

Pharmacodynamic effects obtained when an opioid agonist interacts with the various types of opioid receptor.

Effect	Receptor subtype			
	Mu	Kappa	Sigma	Delta
Pain relief	Yes	Yes, especially at spinal cord level	Yes	Yes
Sedation	Yes	Yes	–	–
Respiratory effects	Depression	Depression but not as much as for mu (may reach plateau)	Stimulation	Depression
Affect	Euphoria	–	Dysphoria	–
Physical dependence	Marked	Less severe than with mu	–	Yes
Prototype agonist other drugs with predominantly agonist activity	Morphine Pethidine Methadone Fentanyl Heroin Cedeine Proxyphene Buprenorphine	Ketocyclazocine Dynorphin Nalbuphine Butorphanol Nalorphine Pentazocine	SKF 10,0 47	Enkephalins D-ala-D-leu enkephalin

The kappa agonists appear to have minimal or no euphoric effects characteristic of the mu agonists (Houde 1979). While physical dependence has been associated with kappa agonists, there are distinct differences in the abstinence syndrome (when compared to mu agonists) which seems to result in a lower level of drug-seeking behaviour (Houde 1979). These findings suggest that the abuse liability of the kappa agonists is less than the mu agonists. However, it is most important to realise that reduced abuse liability does not equate with no abuse liability and physical dependence is highly probable with inappropriate use of the kappa agonists.

The sigma receptor is thought to produce the psychotomimetic side effects associated with the use of the mixed agonist/antagonist opioids such as pentazocine and nalbuphine etc. Other effects include a stimulation of respiratory rate and pain relief.

The endogenous enkephalins show a high affinity for delta receptors whereas morphine demonstrates a low affinity for this receptor. It is difficult to ascertain the pharmacodynamic effects of the delta receptor because the endogenous ligands have a short half-life due to inactivation by peptidase enzymes. At the present time, there are no non-peptide agonists for this receptor.

Current research is directed towards the synthesis of many compounds to act more specifically with a particular receptor, in an attempt to separate the desirable effects of pain relief from the undesirable effects of abuse liability, respiratory depression, sedation, and physical dependence. In this respect, kappa receptor agonists would appear to provide the best option for future development.

Non-steroidal anti-inflammatory drugs (NSAIDs)

The effect of NSAIDs in inhibiting the synthesis of prostaglandins is the mechanism frequently advanced to explain the anti-inflammatory and pain-relieving effects of these drugs (Brune and Lanz 1984; Hart and Huskisson 1984; Huskisson 1984). This inhibition occurs by the inactivation of the enzyme, cyclo-oxygenase, which catalyses the formation of cyclic endoperoxides from arachidonic acid. Prostaglandins are formed in damaged and inflamed tissue and initiate or intensify the oedema, pain and inflammation associated with damaged tissue. Therefore, pharmacological agents which inhibit prostaglandin synthesis should exhibit both anti-inflammatory and pain-relieving activity (see also Chapter 31).

Antidepressants

The neurotransmitter amines, noradrenaline, serotonin, dopamine and gamma-aminobutyric acid (GABA) have been shown to be involved in the transmission and perception of nociceptive impulses (Butler 1984; Potter 1984; Richelson 1984). A more detailed review of this area is provided in Chapter 3 by Messing and Wilcox. Many of the antidepressant drugs block the uptake of noradrenaline and serotonin in the CNS leading to elevated concentrations of these neurotransmitters at the synaptic cleft. It has been suggested that these endogenous amine compounds are also involved in the descending pain-inhibiting pathway which originates in the medulla and terminates in the dorsal horn region of the spinal cord (Basbaum 1984), synapsing with local spinal enkephalin neurons (see Chapter 1). Therefore, activation of the system should result in pain relief (Feinmann 1985).

The following discussion will examine the pharmacokinetics, pharmacodynamics, dosage regimens, side effects and the influences of route of administration for the various classes of drugs used in pain therapy. Drugs used in psychiatry, antidepressants, antipsychotics and benzodiazepines, are considered here, but only briefly. They are also dealt with in Chapter 28.

Classes of drugs

OPIOID DRUGS

Many misconceptions surround the use of opioid drugs in acute and chronic pain, which general-ly results in a marked tendency for inadequate doses at inappropriately long dosage intervals. The net result is that the patient has inadequate pain relief despite the administration of potent pain-relieving medication. Once the decision has been made to treat the pain with opioid drugs, it is both logical and essential to use an effective dosage regimen. The major indications for opioid drugs are in the control of acute pain (e.g. post-operative and trauma) and chronic pain in patients with a terminal disease (e.g. cancer). The use of opioid drugs in non-terminal condi-tions should be avoided and their use is only indicated as a last resort. If, however, opioids are used in such conditions, the practitioner must be prepared to accept and manage the psychological problems that may arise whether or not the patient has adequate pain relief. In this situation, a well organized programme of review is needed to prevent problems of iatrogenic drug dependence and drug abuse.

Pharmacokinetics and pharmacodynamics. Many pharmaceutical companies have invested vast sums into projects searching for the ideal opioid drugs. Over the last decade, an appreciation of the pharmacokinetic characteristics of the opioid drugs and, more particularly, the interaction between pharmacokinetics and pharmacodynamics has resulted in far greater improvements in the treatment of acute and chronic pain than has been obtained with the 'newer' opioid drugs. The concept of a Minimum Effective Concentration (MEC) has been proposed from studies ex-amining the use of pethidine (Austin et al. 1980a, b; Tamsen et al. 1982), morphine (Dahlstrom et al. 1982; Gourlay et al. 1986d), methadone (Gourlay et al. 1982, 1984, 1986d) and fentanyl (Mather 1983; Gourlay et al. 1986c) in the treatment of post-operative pain and for morphine and methadone (Gourlay et al. 1986a) in the treatment of cancer pain. It has been suggested that this relationship occurs because of a proportionality between blood and receptor opioid concen-trations (Gourlay et al. 1986a, d). This concept proposes that continuous pain relief is observed only if the blood opioid concentration is maintained constantly above the MEC. The MEC values for morphine, pethidine, methadone and fentanyl are provided in Table 2. It is apparent that there is at least a 4-fold interpatient variation in MEC. Many factors contribute to this variability including personality factors, depression status, ethnic and cultural factors and 'models' of pain behaviour that the patient experienced as a child. It is therefore difficult to predict an individual patient's MEC value for a particular opioid (Mather and Gourlay 1985).

The clearance (i.e. rate of removal from the body) of the opioid drugs ranges from ultra high (e.g. heroin), high (e.g. fentanyl, morphine, buprenorphine and propoxyphene) through in-termediate (e.g. pethidine, hydromorphone and codeine) to low (e.g. methadone) (Table 2). There are corresponding changes in terminal half-life which range from 10 to 100 hours plus for methadone to 0.05 hours (i.e. $2-3$ minutes) for heroin (Table 2).

The pharmacokinetic characteristic of an intermediate to high clearance results in rapidly fall-ing blood opioid concentrations which explains the relatively short duration of pain relief observed following parenteral doses of these drugs. The only mechanism to provide 'steady state' blood opioid concentrations for these drugs is to administer them frequently. The techniques available for drug input include:

a) Continuous infusion, usually by the intravenous route, but more recently, subcutaneous infusions have become more widespread, particularly in the provision of pain relief in terminal care (Ventafridda et al. 1986).

b) By 'demand analgesia' or 'patient-controlled analgesia' where the pain relief is administered by a micro-processor controlled infusion pump which allows patients to titrate their own pain relief, and

c) By increased surveillance by medical and nursing staff where smaller opioid doses are administered by traditional routes (intravenous, intramuscular and oral) in response to the patients' reporting of pain. In this respect, the nursing and medical staff are acting as the 'infusion pump'.

All of the above techniques should provide relatively constant blood opioid concentrations which can be adjusted to be above a particular patient's MEC thereby providing continuous pain relief.

The alternative approach is to use intermittent doses (usually intravenous or oral) of the low clearance, long half-life opioid drug methadone. The mean half-life of methadone is approximately 30 hours in post-operative and cancer patients (Gourlay et al. 1984, 1986a, d). Therefore, it is possible to maintain a relatively constant blood methadone concentration by using an oral dosage regimen which can vary from one dose every second day to 1 – 3 doses per 24 hours. While the above discussion may appear to relate to the treatment of acute pain, the concepts have direct applicability to the effective treatment of chronic pain (see also Chapter 32).

Route of administration.   The clearance of the majority of opioid drugs (except methadone) combined with the extensive hepatic metabolism has major implications when using the oral route of administration. Drugs are absorbed from the gastrointestinal tract and conveyed by the hepatic/portal blood supply directly to the liver. Therefore, following oral doses, a significant percentage of the dose is metabolized to inactive products prior to the opioid reaching the appropriate receptors in the brain and spinal cord (Mather and Gourlay 1984). This phenomenon is usually referred to as the hepatic 'first pass effect'. Frequently, lack of appreciation of this variable and sometimes poor oral bioavailability is a major factor contributing to the perceived lack of effect from orally administered opioid drugs.

The oral bioavailability ranges from zero for heroin (Inturrisi et al. 1984) to 70 – 95% for methadone (Gourlay et al. 1986a) (Table 2). The effects associated with heroin are mediated via its metabolite morphine following oral doses (Inturrisi et al. 1984) (see also footnote to Table 2).

Since the oral bioavailability of morphine can vary from as low as 10% to as high as 40% indicating extremes in the oral to parenteral ratio of between 2 and 10 (Gourlay et al. 1986a), it is, therefore, not surprising that some patients have inadequate pain relief while others experience unpleasant side effects with oral morphine.

Methadone represents the opposite extreme with a high (70 – 95%) but more importantly, less variable bioavailability. This finding coupled with the low clearance and long terminal half-life indicates that the blood methadone concentration would show much less fluctuation than would be observed with an equivalent dosage regimen of the other opioids.

In summary, the oral route of administration is very effective in the treatment of chronic pain, particularly in patients with cancer, if due attention is given to: 1) the pharmacokinetics of the opioid which is to be administered, and 2) the oral bioavailability of the opioid is taken into consideration, and 3) the dosage regimen implemented is titrated against the severity of the patient's pain and reviewed at regular intervals to ensure efficacy.

Two other routes of administration have been frequently used for opioid drugs, rectal and epidural. Rectal administration of opioid drugs is indicated in patients who cannot swallow or

TABLE 2
Doses, pharmacokinetic parameters, minimum effective concentration and duration of pain relief for various opioid drugs.

Opioid	Dose (mg)		Pharmacokinetic parameters			MEC (ng/ml)	Duration of pain relief (hrs)	Comments
	IM/IV	Oral	Terminal half-life (hrs)	Clearance (L/min)	Bio-availability (%)			
Heroin	5	15	0.05	2 – 2.2	0	*	2 – 3	Very soluble, rapidly converted to 6-mono-acetyl morphine and morphine in vivo. Zero oral bioavailability
Morphine	10	40	2 – 4	0.85 – 1.1	10 – 40	10 – 40	3 – 4	Standard opiate to which new opioids are compared. New sustained release formulation available in some countries – of considerable benefit in treatment of chronic cancer pain
Codeine	30	60	2 – 3	0.6 – 0.8	50	–	3 – 4	Weak opiate, frequently combined with aspirin. Useful for pain with visceral and integumental components
Pethidine (meperidine)	100	300	3 – 5	0.6 – 0.8	30 – 60	200 – 800	2 – 4	Not as effective in relieving anxiety as morphine. Suppositories (200 – 400 mg) have slow onset (2 – 3 hours) but can last for 6 – 8 hours
Methadone	10	10 – 15	10 – 80	0.1 – 0.3	70 – 95	20 – 80	10 – 60	Duration of pain relief ranges from 10 to 60 hours both postoperatively and for cancer pain. Variable half-life. Requires initial care to establish dose for each patient to avoid accumulation. Otherwise of great value

Drug								Comments
Dextromoramide	7.5	10				—	2	Methadone-like chemical structure. Short acting. Useful in covering exacerbation pain. Supposed good oral bioavailability (oral compared to parenteral doses)
Oxycodone	10	30				—	4 – 6	Suppository (30 mg) can provide pain relief for 8 – 10 hours
Hydromorphone	2	4 – 6	2 – 3	0.4	50 – 60	—	4 – 5	More potent but shorter acting than morphine
Fentanyl	0.1	NA	3 – 6	0.7 – 0.9	NA	0.6 – 2	0.5 – 1	Potent opioid. Usually administered by IV injection. Short duration of pain relief. Therefore repeated doses on the basis of pain relieving effects may cause accumulation and respiratory depression. Transdermal 'patch' under evaluation
Propoxyphene	65	130	8 – 24	0.9 – 1.2	40	—	4 – 6	Weak opioid. Unacceptable incidence of side effects
Buprenorphine	0.3	0.8	2 – 3	0.9 – 1.3	30	—	6 – 8	Available as sublingual tablet in many countries which appears useful in treatment of cancer pain
Nalbuphine	10	40	4 – 6	0.9 – 1.5	20	—	3 – 6	Oral form unavailable in many countries. Value in treatment of chronic pain not established

* It has been suggested that heroin has little intrinsic pain-relieving activity and acts as a prodrug for 6-mono-acetyl morphine and morphine at spinal and supraspinal receptor sites.
NA = data not available.

who have a high incidence of nausea or vomiting following oral doses. Studies undertaken with pethidine (200 – 400 mg) in a suppository base have indicated that it can take between 2 and 3 hours to reach the MEC for pethidine (400 – 500 ng/ml) and the rectal bioavailability was approximately 50% (Fig. 2). However, the higher doses (400 mg of pethidine) provided a prolonged duration of pain relief (6 – 8 hours) which probably results from a depot of pethidine in the rectum. Therefore, rectal opioids can be used to provide prolonged pain relief during the night but the time to onset of pain relief can be very slow.

Oxycodone is commercially available in a suppository form (30 mg) and this formulation has been reported to provide pain relief for up to 8 hours. The spinal administration (usually epidural but occasionally intrathecal) of opioids has undergone widespread evaluation following the discovery of opioid receptors in the dorsal horn region of the spinal cord (Yaksh and Rudy 1976). Spinal administration of opioids should only be considered when it is no longer possible to have adequate pain relief without the co-existence of unacceptable side effects with orally administered opioids.

Pethidine (50 – 100 mg) is frequently used epidurally for the treatment of acute pain in opioid-naïve patients and usually provides pain relief for 3 – 4 hours. Although latent (up to 8 hours) and severe respiratory depression has been reported following epidural morphine in patients with no prior exposure to opioid drugs (Gustafsson et al. 1982); pain relief with morphine can last from 12 to 24 hours. Delays in reaching significant morphine concentrations in the respiratory centre via diffusion in the CSF (see Nordberg et al. 1984; Gourlay et al. 1985; Cousins and Mather 1984) are compatible with the delayed onset of respiratory depression observed clinically. However, it is important to emphasize that this phenomenon is most unlikely to occur in patients with recent prior opioid intake: for example, patients with severe cancer pain. This lack of respiratory depression probably occurs because of the acute tolerance that develops to the respiratory depressant effects of opioids following repeated oral or parenteral doses.

Excellent pain relief has been obtained by the repeated administration of epidural morphine by a subcutaneously implanted portal reservoir attached to a conventional epidural catheter, the end of which is tunnelled subcutaneously to the anterolateral chest wall (Cherry et al. 1985a). Morphine doses between 5 and 50 mg at a frequency of 1 – 3 doses per 24 hours have been ad-

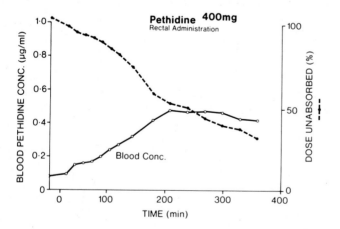

Fig. 2. Blood pethidine concentration (μg/ml) and percent dose unabsorbed as a function of time following the rectal administration of pethidine (400 mg). ———, The blood pethidine concentration; ---, the percent dose unabsorbed.

ministered percutaneously via the portal device by close relatives or nursing staff to treat severe pain in patients with cancer. However, much lower doses (2 – 10 mg) every 12 – 24 hours are recommended in opioid-naïve patients and the possibility of latent and severe respiratory depression must be considered in this patient group.

Dosage regimens. As previously stated, it is essential to use an effective dose at an appropriate dosage interval once the decision to use opioid drugs has been made. Therefore, an effective dose is the lowest dose which provides acceptable pain relief with a low or zero incidence of side effects. The actual dose in milligrams etc. is of much less importance than the balance between pain relief and side effects. Nevertheless, suggested equipotent intravenous or intramuscular doses for the different opioids are given in Table 2. Further, equipotent oral doses taking the oral bioavailability into consideration (vide supra) are also provided in Table 2. These doses are given as an initial guide and it is essential to adjust the dose and dosing interval on an individual patient basis.

A number of other opioid drugs should be considered as they are used intermittently in the treatment of severe pain (see Chapter 32).

Side effects. The major side effects which limit the effectiveness of opioid drugs in chronic pain are sedation, nausea and vomiting and respiratory depression. The incidence and severity of the side effects for different mu receptor agonists are probably similar at doses producing equivalent pain-relieving effects (see e.g. Gourlay et al. 1986a). Tolerance to sedation and the respiratory depressant effects of mu receptor agonists develops rapidly such that sedation is usually not a major problem during long-term therapy.

However, the different profile of respiratory depression of kappa receptor agonists compared to the mu receptor agonists has already been described. There are some side effects reported with epidurally administered opioids such as urinary retention, pruritis as well as the already mentioned latent and severe respiratory depression. The incidence of these side effects is very low in cancer patients referred to our Pain Management Unit.

Chronic pain associated with non-terminal conditions presents a difficult clinical problem in deciding which patients should be placed on long-term opioid therapy. Recent evidence suggests that patients with a predominantly peripheral nociceptive basis to their pain can be successfully treated on a long-term basis with opioids without significant dose escalation (Portenoy and Foley 1986). In contrast, patients with a major psychological focus to their pain can present major management difficulties by requesting frequent dose adjustments on the supposed basis of inadequate pain relief and exhibiting other behavioural manifestations of opioid dependency. Frequently, this type of patient presents to a Pain Clinic and a properly initiated programme of psychological and psychiatric support may be necessary to detoxify the patient from the many different opioid and CNS depressant drugs that are usually administered concomitantly.

Non-steroidal anti-inflammatory drugs

The indications for NSAIDs range from the treatment of minor aches and sprains, dysmenorrhoea, to long-term therapy for rheumatoid and osteo arthritis, as well as degenerative joint diseases (ankylosing spondylitis, gout, etc.) (see Chapter 31). Their anti-inflammatory properties have been shown to result in significant pain relief in cancer patients with bone metastases (see Chapter 32). However, there can be pronounced inter-individual variability in the response to NSAIDs.

Pharmacokinetics and pharmacodynamics. In contrast to opioid drugs, significant relationships between blood NSAIDs concentration and either anti-inflammatory response or pain relief have not been demonstrated at the present time. The pharmacokinetic properties of the more commonly used NSAIDs are given in Table 3. The majority of NSAIDs can be divided into two groups based on their terminal half-lives. The NSAIDs in group 1 have a half-life between 2 and 4 hours. Paracetamol, although it has no anti-inflammatory properties, can be included in this group (Forrest et al. 1982). The recommended frequency of oral doses varies between 4 and 8 hourly for this group of drugs.

The NSAIDs in group 2 have half-lives varying from 6 to 60 hours. Phenylbutazone can also be included in this group (terminal half-life of 60–90 hours) but the regular use of this drug is now contraindicated because of an unacceptable incidence of bone marrow depression. The only legitimate indication for phenylbutazone is in the treatment of ankylosing spondylitis. The frequency of dosage for NSAIDs in group 2 varies from once (piroxicam) or twice daily (fenoprofen, sulindac and diflunisal) to 8 hourly (indomethacin and naproxen). The NSAIDs are generally well absorbed following oral administration and undergo extensive hepatic metabolism.

It has been proposed that patients with renal insufficiency could be at risk because urinary excretion is the major route of elimination of NSAIDs metabolites. However, pharmacokinetic studies for various NSAIDs in renal disease do not indicate that major dosage adjustments are

TABLE 3

Terminal half-life, recommended dose, influence of food on absorption and incidence of erosion gastritis of NSAIDs.

Drug	Terminal half-life (hrs)	Recommended oral dose and frequency (mg/hrs)	Effect of food on absorption	Incidence of erosion gastritis	References
Aspirin[a]	0.2 – 0.3	600 – 900/4	a	+ + +	Needs and Brooks (1985)
Salicylate[a]	2 – 3	600/4	a	+ +	Needs and Brooks (1985)
Diflunisal	8 – 12	500/12	a	+	Brogden et al. (1980)
Diclofenac[b]	1.5 – 2	25 – 50/8	a	+	Willis et al. (1979)
Ibuprofen	2 – 3	200 – 400/8	a	+	Davies and Avery (1971)
Naproxen[b]	12 – 15	250 – 375/12	c	+	Brogden et al. (1979a)
Fenoprofen	2 – 3	400 – 600/6	b	+	Brogden et al. (1977)
Indomethacin[b]	6 – 8	50 – 75/8	a	+ +	Helleberg (1981)
Sulindac[c]	6 – 8	100 – 200/12	b	+	Brogden et al. (1978)
Piroxicam[b]	30 – 60	20 – 30/24	a	+	Brogden et al. (1981, 1984)
Flufenamic Acid	8 – 10	500/6	a	+ +	
Paracetamol	1.5 – 2	500/6	a	–	Forrest et al. (1982)

[a] Also available in various enteric coated and buffered formulations.

[b] Available as suppository to minimize gastric irritation.

[c] Sulindac is reduced to sulindac sulphide and the metabolite has been suggested to be the pharmacologically active species. The half-life of sulindac sulphide is 16–20 hours and will therefore tend to accumulate relative to sulindac on repeated dosing.

+ + + = High incidence; + + = intermediate incidence; + = low incidence of erosion gastritis; a = decrease in rate of absorption, no change in oral bioavailability; b = decrease in rate of absorption and oral bioavailability; c = no change in rate of absorption or oral bioavailability.

indicated. Nevertheless, it is suggested that such patients should be more closely monitored for side effects associated with NSAIDs.

Route of administration. The oral route of administration is the most convenient but is associated with the highest incidence of erosion gastritis (Table 3). The absorption profile can be significantly different if the dose of NSAIDs is taken with food (Table 3). The rate of absorption is generally reduced, but except for a significant reduction with sulindac and fenoprofen concomitant food causes little change in the oral bioavailability.

There are suppository formulations for indomethacin, piroxicam, diclofenac and naproxen (deBoer et al. 1982). Indomethacin is rapidly absorbed following rectal administration with peak blood concentrations usually occurring within one hour (Helleberg 1981). Similar results were obtained with diclofenac, unlike piroxicam which is slowly absorbed after rectal administration with peak concentrations occurring after 5 – 6 hours. There is a sustained release formulation of diclofenac which aims to minimize the frequency of dosing by providing a prolonged release rate following oral administration.

Dosage regimens. The oral dosage regimens for the various NSAIDs are provided in Table 3. These suggested doses will provide near maximal anti-inflammatory and pain-relieving activity and have been derived from studies examining the efficacy of NSAIDs in the treatment of rheumatological disease. Accordingly, these doses are able to be administered on a long-term basis, subject to careful monitoring of possible side effects. The frequency of dosing has some proportionality to the terminal half-life.

Side effects. Gastrointestinal irritation occurs with all NSAIDs and constitutes the major side effect responsible for discontinuation of therapy. Non-buffered or non-enteric coated formulations of aspirin are associated with the highest incidence of erosion gastritis as aspirin has a direct destructive effect on the gastric mucosa. The modified formulations (e.g. buffered, enteric coated) reduce but do not eliminate gastric irritation. In addition, the effects of NSAIDs in inhibiting cyclo-oxygenase result in a reduced amount of prostaglandin present in gastric mucosa. The gastric damage occurs because decreased amounts of prostaglandin result in 1) less mucus production; 2) increased acid secretion and 3) decreased mucosal blood supply. Therefore, rectal NSAIDs may not totally eliminate gastrointestinal side effects. The newer NSAIDs have the lowest incidence of gastric irritation but significant irritation (resulting in gastric haemorrhage) can still occur in some patients.

Inhibition of prostaglandin synthesis has some renal effects resulting in salt and fluid retention. Aspirin and many of the other NSAIDs inhibit platelet aggregation which may result in increased bleeding times. Aspirin has been shown to result in reversible tinnitus and reduced hearing. Paracetamol does not produce the gastric irritant effects of the NSAIDs. However, it can cause fatal hepatic damage when taken in excessive doses.

Antidepressant drugs

The biochemical action of antidepressants by increasing the concentrations of neurotransmitter amines at the synaptic cleft may activate a pain-inhibiting pathway which originates in the medulla and synapses in the spinal cord (see Chapter 1). That is, antidepressants may have an intrinsic pain-relieving effect (Feinmann 1985). Table 4 gives the IC_{50} (i.e. the concentration of antidepressant to provide 50% inhibition of the reuptake of either serotonin or noradrenaline)

TABLE 4

Terminal half-life, recommended daily doses and other properties of antidepressant drugs.

Drug	Amine group	Terminal half-life (hrs)	Inhibitor concentration[a]		Recommended[b] daily dose (mg)
			NA	5-HT	
Amitriptyline	3	20 – 30	4.6	4.4	50 – 150
Nortriptyline	2	18 – 36	0.9	17	50 – 150
Protriptyline	2	50 – 90	–	–	10 – 50
Clomipramine	3	20 – 30	4.6	0.5	50 – 75
Imipramine	3	10 – 24	4.6	4.4	75 – 150
Desipramine	2	12 – 24	0.2	35	75 – 150
Doxepin	3	10 – 25	6.5	20	75 – 150
Dothiepin	3	20 – 30	–	–	50 – 100
Mianserin	3	10 – 20	20	130	20 – 50
Nomifensine	1, 3	2 – 4	2	120	75 – 150
Zimelidine	3	5 – 10	630	14	200 – 300

[a] Inhibitor concentration (IC_{50}) represents the antidepressant concentration ($\times\ 10^{-8}$ m) required to inhibit the uptake of either noradrenaline (NA) or serotonin (5-HT) by 50% using rat mid-brain synaptosomes (adapted from Maitre et al. 1982).

[b] It is generally recommended that the antidepressant be administered as a single dose at night unless significant side effects occur where a night and morning dose (divided dose) may be more appropriate.

1 = Primary amine group; 2 = secondary amine group; 3 = tertiary amine group.

for the commonly used antidepressant drugs. It has been generally proposed that the secondary amines (designated by 2 in the amine group column of Table 4) are more potent blockers of noradrenaline rather than serotonin reuptake. It has been suggested that the tertiary amine antidepressants are more effective in providing pain relief because of their more potent blockade of serotonin reuptake. The serotonin reuptake blocker zimelidine has been shown to be an effective pain-relieving drug (Johansson and von Knorring 1979; Gourlay et al. 1986b). Tertiary amine antidepressants have been shown to be effective in providing pain relief in a variety of non-malignant chronic pain syndromes (see Table 90 in Monks and Merskey 1984).

Pharmacokinetics and pharmacodynamics. The tricyclic antidepressants are well absorbed from the gastrointestinal tract and the oral route of administration is preferred in the treatment of depression. The variability in elimination determines the resultant steady state concentration of antidepressant for a given dosage regimen. The terminal half-lives for the various antidepressant drugs are also given in Table 4. The half-lives for the new agents nomifensine (Brogden et al. 1979b) and zimelidine (Love et al. 1981) are relatively short (mean half-life of 3 – 6 hours) and it is interesting to note that both drugs have been officially withdrawn from the market because of an unacceptable incidence of side effects. There is conflicting evidence in the literature to support the concept of a therapeutic range for antidepressants. Nevertheless, therapeutic ranges for some antidepressant drugs are as follows:

– imipramine: 150 – 250 ng/ml
– desimipramine: 80 – 200 ng/ml

- clomipramine (actually clomipramine and its
  metabolite, desmethlyclomipramine: 250 – 700 ng/ml
- doxepin: greater than 80 – 140 ng/ml
- dothiepin: greater than 90 ng/ml
- protriptyline: 120 – 250 ng/ml
- amitriptyline: 100 – 250 ng/ml
- nortriptyline: 50 – 170 ng/ml

While the above therapeutic ranges apply to optimal antidepressant effects, there is no information available on the equivalent therapeutic range for pain relief using antidepressant drugs. It
is interesting to note that various reports suggest (Monks and Merskey 1984; Gourlay et al.
1986b) that the time taken for the perception of pain relief (between 2 and 7 days) is much shorter
than the usually accepted time of 3 – 4 weeks for near maximal antidepressant activity. These
findings suggest that different mechanisms may be involved in pain relief and antidepressant activity.

Dosage regimens. The normal ranges of acceptable daily doses are also provided in Table 4.
The intermediate half-life antidepressants can be given in a once or twice daily dosage regimen.
The longer half-life agents can be given as a single daily dose (usually at night) unless undesirable
side effects occur with the higher peak antidepressant concentrations associated with the large
size of single doses. Under these circumstances, a divided regimen of two to three doses per 24
hours will reduce the peak but have little effect on the steady state antidepressant blood concentrations. Further information on the clinical use of antidepressant drugs, including details of side
effects, can be found in Chapter 28.

LOCAL ANAESTHETICS

It would seem at first glance that local anaesthetics would have little or no place in the treatment
of chronic pain. Most doctors who are not anaesthesiologists think of local anaesthetics as being
relatively short-acting drugs. In 1963, a new long-acting local anaesthetic, bupivacaine, was introduced. Although this drug produced neural blockade for only one to 2 hours when injected
epidurally and for up to 4 hours by spinal subarachnoid injection, it was able to produce very
long-lasting blockade of up to 24 to 48 hours when injected close to major plexuses such as the
brachial plexus (Cousins and Bridenbaugh 1986). Also detailed pharmacokinetic studies of this
drug provided the necessary information to enable it to be used by prolonged infusion, without
the production of systemic toxicity (Denson et al. 1983; Mather and Cousins 1986). Such infusions have now been carried out via catheters placed in the site of the epidural space, brachial
plexus, lumbar plexus, major peripheral nerves, and lumbar sympathetic chain (Cousins and
Bridenbaugh 1986). This potentially long duration of interruption of sensory, motor and sympathetic function, either alone or in combination, has been important to enable a more effective
contribution of local anaesthetics to chronic pain by means of diagnostic, prognostic and
therapeutic neural blockade.

Diagnostic neural blockade. Nerve blocks with local anaesthetics can be performed in patients
with chronic pain for the following reasons.

  a) To localize anatomically the area of peripheral nociception and the components of the
peripheral nervous system associated with it. For example, in back pain, individual somatic

spinal nerve roots may be blocked to determine which, if any, are involved in the patient's pain. At a more peripheral level, an individual peripheral nerve such as the lateral femoral cutaneous nerve may be blocked to determine if pain is entirely confined to the territory of a discrete peripheral nerve (Cousins and Bridenbaugh 1986). Such blocks inevitably suffer from the problem that the patient experiences an area of loss of sensation (sensory block) or a feeling of warmth (sympathetic block) which will act as a 'cue'. It is then up to the patient to respond to that loss of sensation in whatever manner that they choose. Expectations of secondary gain or other reasons may prompt patients to inappropriate reports.

To overcome this problem, it is useful to use placebo randomized with local anaesthetics of different durations of action. The results of all of these blocks can then be interpreted in terms of the duration of effect, the intensity of effect and the frequency and consistency of response.

Unfortunately, recent evidence has indicated that the situation may be even more complicated than indicated so far. Loh et al. (1981) and Tasker (1986) have reported that patients with central pain may sometimes achieve temporary relief of their pain by peripheral neural blockade. However, pain relief is not sustained if one proceeds to a neurectomy, cryoprobe lesion or other permanent or semi-permanent destruction of peripheral nerves. This is a lesson that has taken a long time for doctors to learn and the literature still abounds with descriptions of neurectomies, neurotomies, rhizotomies and other procedures which have been carried out in patients who clearly had central pain but obtained a brief period of pain relief from temporary interruption of peripheral pathways which was used as a basis for a permanent procedure. Not only do such procedures fail to produce a permanent pain relief, there is a high incidence of intensification of pain or replacement of the original pain by an excruciating dysaesthesia or deafferentation syndromes such as 'anaesthesia dolorosa'. How can these problems be overcome? At the level of the epidural space, it is now commonplace to insert plastic catheters and to leave them in situ for long periods of time. With the availability of excellent peripheral nerve stimulators and needles encased in outer plastic coverings, similar to intravenous cannulae, it is possible to place a fine plastic catheter close to a major plexus, a peripheral nerve or sympathetic chain. Thus it becomes possible to randomize placebo solutions, different local anaesthetics and different strengths of local anaesthetics. Therefore it is now possible to evaluate the patient's response on separate occasions and over a sufficiently long period of time to obtain more precise data. Surprisingly the literature contains very little information about this type of approach for different pain syndromes. There are no controlled studies in the literature on this subject. When such studies are carried out, it will be important to be aware that the local anaesthetic absorbed from the site of local injections into the vascular system may itself have important effects on the perception of pain. These effects may be both peripheral and central (see Cousins and Bridenbaugh 1986).

b) To differentiate pain arising from visceral structures (innervated by sympathetic fibres) from pain arising from somatic structures and innervated by somatic sensory fibres. Since the smallest fibres are sympathetic, medium size are sensory and largest are motor, it has been a classic approach to use various local anaesthetic solutions of increasing strength progressively to block sympathetic, sensory and then finally motor fibres. Recently it has become clear that the sequence of blockade does not necessarily occur in the order of fibre size.

Furthermore, it is now known that there are complex viscero-somatic and somatico-visceral reflexes. The simplest and best known example of this is the patient with visceral pain that is referred to a somatic area corresponding to the spinal segments subserving the visceral nociceptive afferents from that viscus. Surprisingly, it has been found that blocking the somatic referred area of pain with local anaesthetic can at least temporarily relieve the visceral pain (Cousins and Bridenbaugh 1986).

Another complication is that pain arising from a somatic structure may sometimes initiate an increase in reflex activity via interneurons linking dorsal horn cells with sympathetic and anterior horn (motor) cells, resulting in the setting up of noxious impulses in a viscus, for example, by increasing sphincter tone and causing visceral distension. In this situation a sympathetic block may result in a reduction in the patient's pain, even though the original stimulus was of somatic origin (see also Procacci and Zoppi 1983). Thus procedures and interpretations are just as complicated as indicated above for 'Diagnostic neural blockade' (a).

Until further studies are carried out, it must be acknowledged that there are no conclusive data to determine whether 'diagnostic local anaesthetic blockade' can provide reasonably reliable information about the neural pathways involved in chronic pain. In the current authors' opinion, local anaesthetic blockade can provide useful *contributory* information in individual patients, when combined with clinical diagnostic information obtained from the physical examination and physical, psychological and social history.

Prognostic nerve blocks. As mentioned above, it was formerly a common practice to carry out a local anaesthetic block of an appropriate peripheral nerve, nerve root or other neural pathway, prior to making a permanent surgical or neurolytic lesion to relieve pain. In a sense these blocks were both 'diagnostic' and 'prognostic'. All the limitations that applied to the diagnostic use also apply to a purported prognostic application. Today very few neurolytic blocks and surgical lesions are performed, other than for cancer pain. Results obtained, particularly with a single local anaesthetic block of rather short duration, are not always entirely 'prognostic' of the results obtained with a neurolytic solution or other destructive technique. It is possible that better 'prognosis' could be obtained if catheter techniques were employed to produce a more lasting block. There are no published results of correlations between either single injections or catheter techniques prior to destructive procedures.

It has now become clear that sensory loss extending over many days, weeks and then years may become extremely disturbing to patients and may result in a 'deafferentation syndrome'. Thus a patient's report of no discomfort from an anaesthetic area following a nerve block, cannot be interpreted with confidence as a prediction that such a patient will experience no discomfort when that area is denervated on a permanent basis.

Diagnostic use of opioid analgesic drugs via spinal and epidural route. The discovery of opioid receptors in the dorsal horn of the spinal cord (Yaksh and Rudy 1976) opened up the possibilities of more reliable 'diagnostic' spinal blockade in an attempt to separate pain of predominantly peripheral origin from that of predominantly central origin. Epidural or subarachnoid injection of opioid drugs results in blockade of nociception with no discernable change in motor, sensory or sympathetic function (Cousins and Mather 1984). In a preliminary study, Cherry et al. (1985b) reported that a high percentage of patients with pain of predominantly peripheral origin obtained pain relief with epidural fentanyl and this pain relief was antagonized by the intravenous injection of the opiate antagonist, naloxone. On the other hand, patients with pain of predominantly central origin (arising rostrad to the dorsal horn of the spinal cord) did not have their pain relieved by epidural fentanyl and the response was unaltered by the injection of naloxone intravenously. It was stressed that this technique should be used as an aid to determine whether pain was *predominantly* of peripheral or central origin. Further, it was stressed that the technique should be used in a multidisciplinary setting where psychologic aspects of the patient's problem were assessed and the results of the block used as just one piece of the information, together with the other assessments. They also stressed that results indicating a predominant peripheral origin, by no means excluded important contributions of a central nature (Cherry et al. 1985b).

Further development of the 'diagnostic spinal opioid blockade' will depend upon the availability of additional precise pharmacokinetic data.

Therapeutic nerve blocks. The following potential contributions of local anaesthetic nerve blocks to the treatment of chronic pain have been claimed:

a) To relieve muscle spasm, for example associated with a 'trigger point' in myofascial syndromes or in association with somatic lesions which result in muscle spasm.
b) To interrupt reflex sympathetic activity that is increasing the sensitivity of peripheral nociceptors or contributing to pain by reduction in vascular supply.
c) To provide pain relief and motor blockade in order to permit physiotherapy with the aim of increased mobility and an associated reduction in pain.
d) A period of complete pain relief via prolonged 'perineural' infusion of local anaesthetics as described above, in order to build a patient's confidence that pain relief can be obtained, to reduce anxiety and depression and to permit a 'reframing' of the patient's attitude to the pain and ability to cope with family interaction etc.
e) To improve vascular supply in 'acute' or 'chronic' episodes of ischaemia in patients with chronic vascular disease.

The use of local anaesthetic blocks is described in detail in specialized texts on this subject (see Cousins and Bridenbaugh 1986, for a review of the above). In the opinion of the current authors, too little use has been made of local anaesthetic blocks in conjunction with physiotherapy and other modalities which could take advantage of a 'pain-free period' to mount a more positive approach by the patient and family towards the pain problem. Such approaches are only possible when local anaesthetic blocks are used in the context of a multidisciplinary group and in a facility that permits the interaction of those performing nerve blocks with those involved in other modalities of treatment. In the past, it has been assumed that the sensory, motor and autonomic blockade associated with prolonged local anaesthetic block would militate against the use of these drugs for chronic pain. However, specialized pain management units have the staff and facilities to monitor the effects of local anaesthetic block on cardiovascular, respiratory and other important systems. With epidural block it would be necessary for the patient to be carefully monitored and to remain largely in bed. However, with blockade of peripheral nerves and brachial plexus, it may be possible for patients to be ambulatory during treatment. The precise place of long term 'catheter' infusion of local anaesthetics in the treatment of chronic pain is yet to be defined. It is of interest that some patients will respond with a very long period of pain relief to a single injection of local anaesthetic either into a 'trigger point' or close to a major peripheral nerve plexus. Presumably this block breaks up a 'vicious cycle', however, the precise mechanism of prolonged pain relief is yet to be clearly defined.

Local anaesthetic and steroid injection. Recent studies have reported that injection of steroid close to a neuroma, results in decreased neuronal discharge. In clinical practice this type of treatment has produced conflicting results.

Injection of steroid at a peripheral site such as near a major peripheral nerve, close to a tendon insertion or into a joint, may be quite painful. Thus local anaesthetics are usually combined with the steroid for such injections. It is presumed that the steroid reduces inflammation which has been initiated by trauma or degeneration and has increased the sensitivity of peripheral nociceptors. However, such injections are not without hazard, particularly when used at peripheral sites, since steroid solutions can be irritating and some contain neurolytic agents such as benzyl alcohol which may produce necrosis of subcutaneous tissues. The most controversial use of steroids has been in the epidural space for the treatment of back pain. Although some authors have previously advocated the intrathecal injection of steroid, the current authors do not recommend this use, since some steroid preparations have resulted in neurologic deficit when injected into the subarachnoid space (Bogduk and Cherry 1985).

As a result of some concern about the safety and efficacy of the epidural injection of local anaesthetic and steroid, the Australian Pain Society commissioned a major evaluation of the literature on this subject (Bogduk and Cherry 1985). In summary, it was reported that the epidural injection of steroid solutions such as 'depomedrol and prednisolone' appear to be safe. There appeared to be evidence of a beneficial effect of epidural steroid, particularly in patients who had not previously been subjected to surgical procedures and whose pain was predominantly of a 'nerve root irritation' type.

This group of course includes a considerable number of patients who would recover from their pain with conservative measures and precise data are lacking to determine the real contribution of epidural steroid in this patient population. Patients with pain of longer standing, who have previously been subjected to surgery and with symptoms not typical of nerve root irritation, have a much more variable and less clearly defined response. In general, it appears that a favourable response to an initial block warrants repeat of the block in 7 – 10 days if the initial effects subside. There appears little evidence to support the use of multiple and frequent epidural injections of local anaesthetic and steroid and there is no evidence that such injections produce any long term 'cure' of back pain. However, it should be noted that the injection of local anaesthetic and steroid may be used as an aid to mobilization of patients, improvement of posture and thus initiation of a 'preventative programme'. Such approaches are very much in keeping with modern aims of treatment of chronic pain with an emphasis on increased activity (Fordyce et al. 1985).

Intravenous infusion of local anaesthetics.   There is clear evidence, from the treatment of acute pain and from the use of local anaesthetics as an adjunct to general anaesthesia, that intravenous infusion of local anaesthetics may produce some pain relief (Cousins and Bridenbaugh 1986). A small number of reports have indicated that some forms of chronic pain may be effectively treated by a series of brief intravenous infusions of local anaesthetic agents such as lignocaine and 2-chloroprocaine. The agent 2-chloroprocaine has been the most popular since it is the most rapidly metabolized local anaesthetic and thus poses a relatively small risk of systemic toxicity. Boas et al. (1982) reported that infusion of lignocaine resulted in relief of neuralgic pain which was refractory to the usual methods of treatment. However, pain relief was not permanent and it was necessary to repeat the infusion of local anaesthetic. At present, it is unclear as to whether this type of treatment is either practicable or clearly efficacious in patients with chronic pain. One area worth further investigation is the extremely difficult problem of pain due to peripheral neuropathy which currently seems to be refractory to all types of treatment. When such patients are in a terminal phase of their illness and have pain due to severe peripheral neuropathy, it may be reasonable to consider the infusion of local anaesthetics, if the efficacy and safety of such a technique can be confirmed.

INHALATION ANAESTHETICS

There are currently only two inhalation anaesthetics with a powerful pain-relieving effect at subanaesthetic concentrations. Nitrous oxide in a concentration of 50% produces a maximal pain-relieving effect with minimal risk of inducing general anaesthesia. However, it should be stressed that a combination of 50% nitrous oxide and other CNS depressant drugs may indeed produce anaesthesia. Unfortunately, prolonged administration of nitrous oxide results in a block at the level of methionine synthetase, depletion of methionine and a vitamin B12 deficiency syndrome. This is the mechanism of the bone marrow depression that was detected in patients given nitrous oxide pain relief for long periods of time in the course of the treatment of tetanus. Thus, nitrous oxide pain relief should be given for only short periods of time, not to exceed a couple of hours. Nevertheless, this drug may be extremely valuable for carrying out painful procedures in patients with chronic pain or for covering 'acute on chronic episodes' while definitive treatment is being arranged. Nitrous oxide is relatively insoluble in blood and thus has a rapid uptake and also a rapid elimination. Approximately one minute of inhalation should be allowed to provide pain relief and the termination of this effect occurs from 1 to 3 minutes after ceasing inhalation.

Methoxyflurane is a much more potent pain-relieving agent compared to nitrous oxide. At a concentration of approximately 0.1%, which is almost 50% of the concentration required to produce anaesthesia, methoxyflurane produces very potent and long-lasting pain relief. Being more soluble in the blood stream, methoxyflurane continues to produce pain relief after inhalation is ceased. This contrasts with nitrous oxide which produces pain relief only during its inhalation. Methoxyflurane has a potential to produce renal toxicity as a result of its metabolism to inorganic fluoride. However, signs of minimal toxicity arise after 2.5 hours inhalation at an *anaesthetic* concentration and this corresponds to 5 hours of inhalation at a 'subanaesthetic' concentration. Because of the sharp decline in the use of this drug as an anaesthetic agent, it is possible that it may cease to be manufactured. This would be regrettable since the drug is safe, if it is used within the guidelines indicated above. Methoxyflurane is of great value in patients who have no venous access or who are extremely nervous about injections, but require a pain-relieving procedure. The drug was available as a 'whistle' apparatus which contained a wick which was soaked with methoxyflurane prior to its use. This type of apparatus is particularly appealing to children and may be used to cover painful diagnostic or therapeutic procedures. Another attraction of the drug is its rather pleasant odour which contrasts with the odour of most other inhalational anaesthetics. Unfortunately, too little attention is given to the comfort of patients, particularly children, during such procedures.

The more modern inhalation anaesthetics such as halothane, isoflurane and enflurane have rather poor pain-relieving properties at subanaesthetic concentrations and appear to offer very little in the treatment of acute and chronic pain.

CO-ANALGESICS (PAIN-RELIEVING ADJUVANT DRUGS)

A considerable number of drugs are purported to possess 'pain-relieving adjuvant properties' particularly in the treatment of cancer pain. The implication is that these drugs potentiate or add to the pain-relieving effects of opioid and non-opioid pain-relieving drugs (morphine and aspirin-like drugs). Much of the information is anecdotal, but there are reasonably convincing data that pain relief may result from a small number of drugs usually used for purposes other than pain relief.

Steroids. There are a few situations in the treatment of chronic non-malignant pain where parenteral rather than regional administration of steroids may be very valuable. It seems wise to limit these applications because of the side effects of steroid administration.

a) *Non-cancer pain.* It is now generally regarded as being safe to administer parenteral steroids during the acute phase of herpes zoster, if pain is a predominant symptom (Loeser 1986). The use of steroids at this stage appears to minimize the incidence of post-herpetic neuralgia. Unfortunately, there is no evidence that systemic administration (or for that matter administration subcutaneously under the painful area) has any effect on the pain of post-herpetic neuralgia.

b) *Cancer pain.* Corticosteroids have been advocated as 'co-analgesics' or 'adjuvant pain-relieving drugs' in the following situations in association with pain in patients with cancer:

- raised intercranial pressure
- nerve compression
- hepatomegaly
- head and neck tumours
- intrapelvic tumours
- retroperitoneal tumours
- lymphoedema
- metastatic arthralgia

The simultaneous administration of a diuretic may be useful in some of these conditions where lymphoedema is prominent. A special case of nerve compression is spinal cord compression. When this occurs above the level of L1/2, it produces a classic mixed upper and lower motor neuron lesion. Below the level of L1/2, compression is of the cauda equina and thus, is of a lower motor neuron type. Many clinicians now prefer to treat this problem by a combination of radiation therapy and concurrent administration of dexamethasone. The corticosteroid is given as a large initial intravenous dose followed by repeated oral dosing, for example, 100 mg intravenously followed by 24 mg 4 times a day orally for 3 days with a rapid reduction to 4 mg 4 times a day. A similar regimen may be used in the case of cerebral metastases, which may be associated with very severe headaches and thus justify an initial large bolus followed by maintenance steroid therapy. Other situations where steroids have been used in cancer include sub-acute bowel obstruction where a critical reduction in bowel obstruction results in a reduction of abdominal pain.

A side benefit of the use of steroids in cancer pain is an improvement in appetite and an improvement in mood. It is also significant to note that steroids may sometimes have a dramatic effect in reducing the incidence and severity of intractable vomiting which has been unresponsive to other measures. Finally, steroids can be extremely effective in treating itch that may be associated with severe jaundice or other causes in cancer patients. This itch can sometimes be much more distressing to patients than pain.

In summary, the rationale for the use of corticosteroids is thought to be a reduction in perineural oedema, a reduction in the size of viscera with a tight investing fascia, decreased lymphatic oedema or decreased intracranial pressure in the individual situations described above. It should also be remembered that corticosteroids have a membrane-stabilizing effect and probably have a mild effect in reducing the sensitivity of peripheral nociceptors. In addition, their mood-elevating effect undoubtedly contributes to the patient's ability to cope with pain and perhaps alters the patient's perception of pain. In many situations the use of corticosteroids for the treatment of pain is purely empirical. Unfortunately, sometimes pain will become very severe upon the withdrawal of corticosteroids, even if they are tapered rather gradually. Long-term administration of corticosteroids will lead to Cushing's syndrome, adrenal suppression and the potential harmful effects of osteoporosis must be assessed before taking this pharmacological option.

Anticonvulsants.   Anticonvulsant drugs such as carbamazepine, sodium valproate and phenytoin are used for the treatment of certain neuropathic pains which are manifested by superficial dysaesthesias (Maciewicz et al. 1985). They are classically used in trigeminal neuralgia (Loeser 1984). These drugs suppress spontaneous neuronal firing and it is likely that they exert their effects both at a peripheral level and perhaps also at the level of the spinal cord. Carbamazepine is used in a dose of 100 mg/day slowly increasing up to 600 – 1200 mg/day if tolerated. It is useful to monitor blood concentration if this is possible. Unfortunately, side effects are quite frequent and include dizziness, ataxia, drowsiness, blurred vision, gastrointestinal irritation and bone marrow depression. Sodium valproate is a second-line choice because it is capable of producing severe hepatotoxicity and thus it is essential to monitor liver function when this drug is used. A dosage of 200 mg 3 times a day may be required.

Antipsychotic and anti-anxiety drugs.   The phenothiazine methotrimeprazine 15 mg intramuscularly is equivalent to approximately 15 mg of morphine intramuscularly (Stimmel 1983). The drug may be particularly useful in patients who become tolerant to opioid drugs, since it appears that it acts at receptors other than the opioid receptors. Other phenothiazines have been used as 'co-analgesics' in the treatment of pain. However, studies on their pain-relieving effects have yielded highly conflicting results. The most useful study compared the pain-relieving activity of nine different phenothiazines relative to pethidine (Moore and Dundee 1961).

The antihistamine group of drugs is sometimes used as 'co-analgesics'. However, only hydroxyzine has been demonstrated to have definite pain-relieving properties (Stimmel 1983). The mechanism of this 'co-analgesic' effect is unknown. Hydroxyzine also helps to allay anxiety and to relieve nausea and vomiting. Another benefit of adding a phenothiazine to opiate treatment is that it may help to prevent disturbing dreams and hallucinations. These are side effects that are not commonly documented for the opioids but are very disturbing to some patients. It should be restated that the combination of a phenothiazine and tricyclic antidepressant is often the best form of treatment for painful neuropathies.

In this situation, it is important to monitor closely for the occurrence of additive CNS depressant effects particularly in elderly patients. For further details of the use of some antipsychotic drugs (phenothiazines and butyrophenones) and the benzodiazepines, together with their side effects, see Chapter 28.

Central nervous system stimulant drugs.   The amphetamines have been shown to have a definite additive pain-relieving effect, as well as elevating mood and improving alertness. This is particularly so for dexamphetamine. The combination of 10 mg of dexamphetamine with morphine provided pain relief equivalent to twice the morphine dose (Forrest et al. 1977). The situation with cocaine is less clear. Cocaine 30 mg combined with each 10 mg of morphine in the 'Brompton cocktail' was found to be no more effective than morphine alone (Twycross 1979). However, other studies have shown that cocaine has a mild additive pain-relieving effect when combined with morphine. There is some evidence that cocaine produces some mood elevation when added to morphine and increases alertness. However, it seems that the contribution of cocaine is very small. In individual cases, it has been found to be useful in the treatment of intractable hiccups, however, controlled data are not available.

In a recent controlled study from the Sloan-Kettering group, cocaine 10 mg was compared with placebo, cocaine (10 mg) plus morphine (10 mg) and morphine (10 mg). There was no difference in pain-relieving effects when cocaine was combined with morphine, however, the side effects of morphine were decreased. There was less drowsiness, less nausea and mood elevation was superior with the combination. Thus, it seems that it may be beneficial to add cocaine in appropriate doses and it is indicated for the effects as described, rather than for pain relief (Kaiko et al. 1984).

Tetrahydro-aminacrine (THA). In some centres it has been traditional for a mixture of THA and morphine to be used for cancer pain (Mortha). In one study (Simpson et al. 1962), it was reported that a higher dosage of morphine could be tolerated if THA was combined with morphine. However, the pain relief produced by this combination was no better than giving a lower dose of morphine. Thus, it appears that the THA antagonized some of the sedative and respiratory depressant effects of the higher dose of morphine. Unfortunately, it also appeared to antagonize the pain relief. Thus, it would seem logical, if patients experience undue sedation, to attempt to reduce the dose of morphine and if this fails to consider adding a CNS stimulant such as cocaine which has been shown to elevate mood and produce other desirable effects, without adversely effecting the pain relief. In general however, it has been found that appropriate tailoring of the opioid dose results in minimal sedation and that even if sedation does occur, patients rapidly develop tolerance to this effect.

Anti-emetic drugs. Some phenothiazines used for anti-emetic effects are also thought to have mild additive pain-relieving effects. Such drugs include trimeprazine, chlorpromazine and fluphenazine. The new drug domperidone, has proved to be a very promising anti-emetic drug with a much lesser potential for side effects than previously available drugs such as the phenothiazines, since it does not cross the blood-brain barrier. Effective relief of nausea and vomiting may have a secondary effect on the incidence of pain, particularly in patients with pain of abdominal origin. Again, it should be mentioned that the steroids may be a valuable option in the treatment of intractable nausea and vomiting.

NEW HORIZONS FOR DRUG THERAPY

At the level of the spinal cord, a large number of new options are now available. Inhibitory systems that have been proposed include a GABA 2 receptor, an enkephalinergic receptor, a noradrenergic receptor and also mechanisms possibly involving somatostatin and calcitonin. In animal studies, spinal injections of appropriate agonists for all of these systems have now been reported to be antinociceptive: baclofen (GABA 2), morphine (enkephalin), clonidine (noradrenergic), serotonin, somatostatin and calcitonin. Some evidence points to the peptide, substance P, as being the transmitter in the primary afferent system which impinges upon cells in the substantia gelatinosa at the dorsal horn of the spinal cord. Depletion of substance P by injection of the extract of the hot chilli, capsaicin, results initially in intense pain but is then followed by a long period of potent pain relief. Thus, some initial investigation has been carried out in patients with severe arthritic pain where capsaicin has been injected directly into joints with excellent pain relief.

Clinical application of these findings is only just beginning. Cancer patients who had become tolerant to the epidural administration of morphine, obtained pain relief with a modest dose of the alpha agonist clonidine. Preliminary reports have indicated that somatostatin is effective epidurally for cancer pain and has only partial cross tolerance with morphine. Finally, it is now clear that there may be at least two or more populations of opioid type receptors in the spinal cord. There is evidence in animals and also in humans with cancer pain that the peptide, D-ala-D-leu-enkephalin (DADL) produces pain relief by spinal injection which shows no cross-tolerance with morphine (Moulin et al. 1985). A final place of these various agents which are active at a spinal level is yet to be determined in the treatment of severe pain. However, the theoretical frame-work that they have helped to identify poses exciting and wide ranging options for the treatment of severe pain (Fig. 3).

Calcitonin has become available in several different forms. Experiments in animals have indicated that administration of calcitonin both intramuscularly and by spinal subarachnoid injection may result in a potentiation of morphine pain relief. Initial results in the treatment of pain due to spinal metastases and Paget's disease were encouraging (Fraioli et al. 1982). However, subsequent studies have been less enthusiastic and it has become apparent that at best the drug has a potential to reduce the dose of morphine required in the treatment of patients with spinal metastases. Subarachnoid administration of calcitonin appears to have potentially large disadvantages in that studies (Shaw 1982) in dogs reported that the animals refused to eat and became moribund with a calcitonin dose which was not much higher than that known to produce pain relief in man (approximately 200 I.U. per day of salmon calcitonin). A precise mechanism of the pain-relieving effect of calcitonin is unknown.

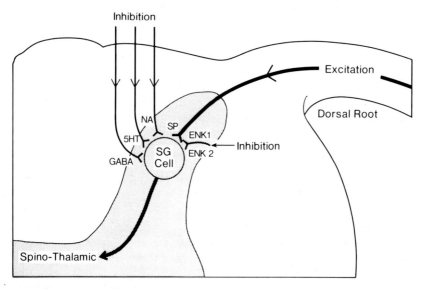

Fig. 3. Model of pain transmission and inhibition in dorsal horn. Proposed excitatory and inhibitory pathways and transmitters are shown. SG cell = cell body in substantia gelatinosa of dorsal horn of spinal cord; SP = substance P; 5-HT = serotonin; NA = noradrenaline (norepinephrine); ENK = enkephalin; GABA = gamma-aminobutyric acid. Primary afferent nociceptive impulses are conducted to spinothalamic and spinoreticular neurons in the dorsal horn with substance P as transmitter. Descending pathways have neurotransmitters, GABA,5-HT, and NA, which inhibit primary afferent transmission. Within dorsal horn there are local enkephalin (opioid) inhibitory systems. These exert both pre-synaptic (ENK$_1$) and post-synaptic (ENK$_2$) inhibition. Morphine acts predominantly presynaptically. (Reproduced with permission from Cousins and Bridenbaugh 1986.)

At a peripheral level, there is also a rapid development of new information (Fig. 4). For example, it is clear that the non-steroidal anti-inflammatory drugs have an important action in decreasing the sensitivity of peripheral nociceptors to painful stimuli (see above). There is also good evidence that increased sympathetic activity may increase the sensitivity of peripheral nociceptors via the release of catecholamines from sympathetic nerve endings. A further mechanism of increased sensitivity of peripheral nociceptors is produced by the vasoconstriction and local increase in hydrogen ion concentration resulting from intense sympathetic nerve activity. A technique of intravenous regional sympathetic block has been developed using the drug guanethidine, which depletes noradrenaline from peripheral sympathetic nerve endings and produces a profound and long lasting regional sympathetic block. This has been shown to be capable of producing pain relief in patients with reflex sympathetic dystrophy of recent onset and in patients with 'acute or chronic' episodes of ischaemia in association with chronic vascular disease.

Finally, it should be emphasized that the precise cause of pain is extremely important in designing the most appropriate primary and 'adjuvant drug' treatment. For example, patients with cancer may develop an infective element to a secondary deposit and this infection may contribute to pain. In some situations it may be appropriate to treat this infection as an aid to the relief of pain. As another example, an isolated secondary deposit in a long bone may be eminently amenable to a brief course of radiotherapy, even if the patient's general condition makes it clear that life expectancy is short. Such radiotherapy may greatly decrease pain and decrease the dose of pain-relieving medication required. In summary, the aim of drug therapy is to tailor it very closely to the individual pain problem or problems in each patient on the basis of a very

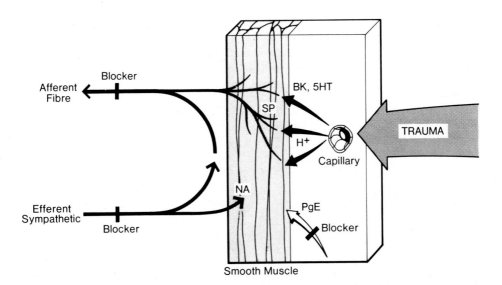

Fig. 4. Peripheral pain receptors and modification of their activity. Note that physical stimuli, the chemical environment (e.g. H^+), algesic substances (e.g. serotonin (5-HT), bradykinin (BK)), and microcirculatory changes may all modify peripheral receptor activity. Note also the important role of efferent sympathetic activity. Substance P (SP) is probably the peripheral pain transmitter. Points of blockade of peripheral pain receptor activity are shown as shaded areas (e.g. sympathetic blockade by local anaesthetic or guanethidine, prostaglandin synthetase blockade by aspirin)

careful diagnosis of the cause of pain. Drug treatment should be used in combination with other methods of pain treatment and often in combination with treatment of the underlying cause. It should be strongly emphasized that, in patients with cancer pain, it is vital to deal with all of the needs of the patient both physical, psychological, social and spiritual. In our experience, careful explanation of the patient's current status, the treatments that can and will be applied, and various other supports that will be made available, will often dramatically reduce the requirement for pain-relieving drugs. In some patients, it becomes apparent that pain has merely been a method of asking for help and when that help is provided the need for pain-relieving medication disappears. Thus in cancer pain, the concept of the 'palliative care team' with a central facility linked to home care services, in patient hospice beds, day care facilities and other resources has made a major impact on the requirements and manner in which pain-relieving therapy is provided. These important areas are covered in other chapters.

THE CONCEPT OF AN 'ANALGESIC LADDER' FOR CANCER PAIN

The World Health Organisation has proposed a series of steps that may be followed in the use of pain-relieving drugs for patients with cancer pain (Fig. 5). It is proposed that treatment starts at step 1 and progresses to step 2 and then to step 3 as further measures are required. It should be noted that at each step the requirement for 'adjuvant drugs' is carefully assessed. An important aspect of this assessment is a careful search for the cause of the pain. Perhaps the most neglected cause of pain in cancer patients is 'deafferentation pain'. Such pain may be associated with brachial plexopathies, paraplegias, large areas of denervation following surgical or other destructive procedures. These patients are usually unresponsive to opioid therapy and require 'adjuvant drugs' as described above.

This 'analgesic ladder' has been field tested in several countries and initial reports indicate that in excess of 90% of patients with cancer pain had their pain effectively relieved simply by following the steps in the 'ladder'. It is of particular interest that the World Health Organisation has recommended that oral morphine be made available in all countries as the first choice for the

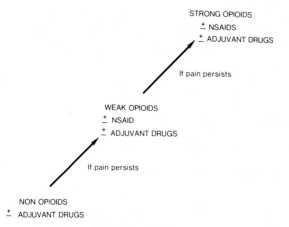

STRONG OPIOIDS
± NSAIDS
± ADJUVANT DRUGS

If pain persists

WEAK OPIOIDS
± NSAID
± ADJUVANT DRUGS

If pain persists

NON OPIOIDS
± ADJUVANT DRUGS

Fig. 5. World Health Organisation recommendation for an 'analgesic ladder' for the treatment of cancer pain. Non-opioids include aspirin, paracetamol and other NSAIDs. Weak-opioids include codeine and dextropropoxyphene. Strong-opioids include morphine, methadone and other mu receptor agonists. Adjuvant drugs include steroids, antidepressants, anticonvulsants, anxiolytics and other drugs discussed in the text.

treatment of severe cancer pain. It is of note that morphine rather than heroin was recommended. It should also be noted that in step 1, NSAIDs can sometimes be effectively used as the sole means of treatment of cancer pain (Stjernsward 1985).

References

Austin, K. L., Stapleton, J. V. and Mather, L. E. (1980a) Multiple intramuscular injections: a major source of variability in analgesic response to meperidine. Pain 8, 422–446.

Austin, K. L., Stapleton, J. V. and Mather, L. E. (1980b) Relationship between blood meperidine concentration and analgesic response: a preliminary report. Anesthesiology 53, 460–466.

Basbaum, A. I. (1984) Anatomical substrates of pain and pain modulation and their relationship to analgesic drug action. In: M. J. Kuhar and G. W. Pasternak (Eds.), Analgesics: Neurochemical, Behavioural and Clinical Perspectives. Raven Press, New York, pp. 97–123.

Boas, R. A., Covino, B. G. and Shahwarian, A. (1982) Analgesic response to I. V. Lignocaine. Br. J. Anaesth. 54, 501–505.

Bogduk, N. and Cherry, D. A. (1985) Epidural corticosteroid agents for sciatica. Med. J. Aust. 143, 402–406.

Brogden, R. N., Pinder, R. M., Speight, T. M. and Avery, G. S. (1977) Fenoprofen: a review of its pharmacological properties and therapeutic efficacy in rheumatic diseases. Drugs 13, 241–265.

Brogden, R. N., Heel, R. C., Speight, T. M. and Avery, G. S. (1978) Sulindac: a review of its pharmacological properties and therapeutic efficacy in rheumatic diseases. Drugs 16, 97–114.

Brogden, R. N., Heel, R. C., Speight, T. M. and Avery, G. S. (1979a) Naproxen up to date: a review of its pharmacological properties and therapeutic efficacy and use in rheumatic diseases and pain states. Drugs 18, 241–277.

Brogden, R. N., Heel, R. C., Speight, T. M. and Avery, G. S. (1979b) Nomifensine: a review of its pharmacological properties and therapeutic efficacy in depressive illness. Drugs 18, 1–24.

Brogden, R. N., Heel, R. C., Pakes, G. E., Speight, T. M. and Avery, G. S. (1980) Diflunisal: a review of its pharmacological properties and therapeutic use in pain of osteoarthritis. Drugs 19, 84–106.

Brogden, R. N., Heel, R. C., Speight, T. M. and Avery, G. S. (1981) Piroxicam: a review of its pharmacological properties and therapeutic efficacy. Drugs 22, 165–187.

Brogden, R. N., Heel, R. C., Speight, T. M. and Avery, G. S. (1984) Piroxicam: a reappraisal of its pharmacological and therapeutic efficacy. Drugs 28, 292–323.

Brune, K. and Lanz, R. L. (1984) Nonopioid analgesics. In: M. J. Kuhar and G. W. Pasternak (Eds.), Analgesics: Neurochemical, Behavioural and Clinical Perspectives. Raven Press, New York, pp. 149–173.

Butler, S. (1984) Present status of tricyclic antidepressants in chronic pain therapy. In: C. Benedetti, C. R. Chapman and G. Moricca (Eds.), Advances in Pain Research and Therapy, Vol. 7, Raven Press, New York, pp. 173–179.

Cherry, D. A., Gourlay, G. K., Cousins, M. J. and Gannon, B. J. (1985a) A technique for the insertion of an implantable portal system for the long term administration of opioids in the treatment of cancer pain. Anaesth. Intens. Care 13, 145–153.

Cherry, D. A., Gourlay, G. K., McLachlan, M. and Cousins, M. J. (1985b) Diagnostic epidural opioid blockade and chronic pain. Preliminary report. Pain 21, 143–152.

Cousins, M. J. and Bridenbaugh, P. O. (1987) Neural Blockade in Clinical Anaesthesia and the Management of Pain, 2nd edn. J. B. Lippincott, Philadelphia (in press).

Cousins, M. J. and Mather, L. E. (1984) Intrathecal and epidural administration of opioids. Anesthesiology 61, 276–310.

Dahlstrom, B., Tamsen, A., Paalzow, L. and Hartvig, P. (1982) Patient controlled analgesic therapy. IV. Pharmacokinetics and analgesic plasma concentrations of morphine. Clin. Pharmacokinet. 7, 266–279.

DeBoer, A. G., Moolenaar, F., deLeede, L. G. and Breimer, D. D. (1982) Rectal drug administration: clinical pharmacokinetic considerations. Clin. Pharmacokinet. 7, 285–311.

Denson, D. D., Raj, P. P., Saldahna, F., Finnsson, R. A., Ritschel, W. A., Joyce, T. H. and Turner, J. L. (1983) Continuous perineural infusion of bupivacaine for prolonged analgesia: pharmacokinetic considerations. Int. J. Clin. Pharmacol. Ther. Toxicol. 21, 591–597.

Feinmann, C. (1985) Pain relief by antidepressants: possible modes of action. Pain 23, 1–8.

Fordyce, W. E., Roberts, A. H. and Sternbach, R. A. (1985) The behavioural management of chronic pain: a response to critics. Pain 22, 113–125.

Forrest, J. A. H., Clements, J. A. and Prescott, L. F. (1982) Clinical pharmacokinetics of paracetamol. Clin. Pharamcokinet. 7, 93–107.

Forrest, W. H., Bronn, B. W. and Brown, C. K. (1977) Dextroamphetamine with morphine for the treatment of postoperative pain. N. Engl. J. Med. 296, 712–715.

Fraioli, F., Fabbri, A., Genessi, L., Moretti, C., Santoro, C. and Felici, M. (1982) Subarachnoid injection of salmon calcitonin induces analgesia in man. Eur. J. Pharmacol. 78, 381–382.

Goodman, R. R. and Pasternak, G. W. (1984) Multiple opiate receptors. In: M. J. Kuhar and G. W. Pasternak (Eds.), Analgesics: Neurochemical, Behavioural, and Clinical Perspectives. Raven Press, New York, pp. 69–96.

Gouarderes, C., Audiger, Y. and Cros, J. (1982) Benzomorphan binding sites in rat lumbo-sacral spinal cord. Eur. J. Pharmacol. 78, 483–486.

Gourlay, G. K. and Cousins, M. J. (1984) Strong analgesics in severe pain. Drugs 28, 79–91.

Gourlay, G. K., Wilson, P. R. and Glynn, C. J. (1982) Pharmacodynamics and pharmacokinetics of methadone during the peri-operative period. Anesthesiology 57, 458–467.

Gourlay, G. K., Willis, R. J. and Wilson, P. R. (1984) Post-operative pain control with methadone: influence of supplementary methadone doses and blood concentration-response relationships. Anesthesiology 61, 19–26.

Gourlay, G. K., Cherry, D. A. and Cousins, M. J. (1985) Cephalad migration of morphine in C.S.F. following lumbar epidural administration in patients with cancer pain. Pain 23, 317–326.

Gourlay, G. K., Cherry, D. A. and Cousins, M. J. (1986a) A comparative study of the efficacy and pharmacokinetics of oral methadone and morphine in the treatment of severe pain in patients with cancer pain. Pain 25, 297–312.

Gourlay, G. K., Cherry, D. A., Cousins, M. J., Love, B. L., Graham, J. R. and McLachlan, M. O. (1986b) A controlled study of serotonin reuptake blocker, zimelidine, in the treatment of chronic pain. Pain 25, 35–52.

Gourlay, G. K., Plummer, J. L., Cherry, D. A., Kowalski, S., Mather, L. E. and Cousins, M. J. (1986c) Blood concentration analgesic response relationships for fentanyl obtained from 'on demand' infusions in post-operative pain control. Anaesth. Intens. Care (in press).

Gourlay, G. K., Willis, R. J. and Lamberty, J. (1986d) A double blind comparison of the efficacy of methadone and morphine in post-operative pain control. Anesthesiology 64, 322–327.

Gustafsson, L. L., Schildt, B. and Jacobsen, K. (1982) Adverse effects of extradural and intrathecal opiates: report of a nationwide survey in Sweden. Br. J. Anaesth 54, 479–486.

Hart, F. D. and Huskisson, E. C. (1984) Non-steroidal anti-inflammatory drugs – current status and rational therapeutic use. Drugs 27, 232–255.

Helleberg, L. (1981) Clinical pharmacokinetics of indomethacin. Clin. Pharmacokinet. 6, 245–258.

Houde, R. W. (1979) Analgesic effectiveness of the narcotic agonist-antagonists. Br. J. Clin. Pharmacol. 7, 297S–308S.

Huskisson, E. C. (1984) Non-narcotic analgesics. In: P. D. Wall and R. Melzack (Eds.), Textbook of Pain. Churchill Livingstone, Edinburgh, pp. 505–513.

Inturrisi, C. E. and Foley, K. M. (1984) Narcotic analgesics in the management of cancer pain. In: M. J. Kuhar and G. W. Pasternak (Eds.), Analgesics: Neurochemical, Behavioural and Clinical Perspectives. Raven Press, New York, pp. 257–288.

Inturrisi, C. E., Max, M. B., Foley, K. M., Schultz, M., Shin, S. U. and Houde, R. W. (1984) The pharmacokinetics of heroin in patients with chronic pain. N. Engl. J. Med. 310, 1213–1217.

Johansson, F. and von Knorring, L. (1979) A double blind controlled study of a serotonin uptake inhibitor (zimelidine) versus placebo in chronic pain patients. Pain 7, 69–78.

Kaiko, R. F., Kanner, R., Foley, K. M., Wallenstein, S. L., Canel, A., Anderson, C., Rogers, A. G. and Houde, R. W. (1984) Cocaine and morphine in cancer patients with chronic pain. Pain (Suppl. 2) S203.

Loeser, J. D. (1984) Tic douloureux and atypical facial pain. In: P. D. Wall and R. Melzack (Eds.), Textbook of Pain. Churchill Livingstone, Edinburgh, pp. 426–434.

Loeser, J. D. (1986) Herpes zoster and post herpetic neuralgia. Pain 25, 149–164.

Loh, L., Nathan, P. W. and Schott, G. D. (1981) Pain due to lesions of the central nervous system removed by sympathetic block. Br. Med. J. 282, 1026–1028.

Love, B. L., Moore, R. G., Thomas, J. and Chaturyedi, S. (1981) Pharmacokinetics of zimelidine in humans – plasma levels and urinary excretion of zimelidine and norzimelidine after intravenous and oral administration of zimelidine. Eur. J. Clin. Pharmacol. 20, 135 – 139.

Maciewicz, R., Bouckoms, A., and Martin, J. B. (1985) Drug therapy of neuropathic pain. Clin. J. Pain 1, 39 – 49.

Mather, L. E. (1983) Clinical pharmacokinetics of fentanyl and its newer derivatives. Clin. Pharmacokinet. 8, 422 – 446.

Mather, L. E. and Cousins, M. J. (1986) Local anaesthetics: principles of use. In: M. J. Cousins and G. D. Phillips (Eds.), Acute Pain Management. Churchill Livingstone, New York, pp. 105 – 131.

Mather, L. E. and Gourlay, G. K. (1984) The biotransformation of opioids: significance for pain therapy. In: W. S. Nimmo and G. Smith (Eds.), Opioid Agonist/Antagonist Drugs in Clinical Practice. Excerpta Medica, Amsterdam, pp. 31 – 47.

Mather, L. E. and Gourlay, G. K. (1985) Rate controlled intravenous administration of analgesics. In: L. F. Prescott and W. S. Nimmo (Eds.), Rate Control in Drug Therapy. Churchill Livingstone, Edinburgh, pp. 220 – 231.

Merskey, H. (1986) Classification of chronic pain: description of chronic pain syndromes and definition of pain terms. Pain (Suppl. 3).

Monks, R. and Merskey, H. (1984) Psychotropic drugs. In: P. D. Wall and R. Melzack (Eds.), Textbook of Pain. Churchill Livingstone, Edinburgh, pp. 526 – 537.

Moore, J. and Dundee, J. W. (1961) Alterations in response to somatic pain associated with anaesthesia. V11. The effects of nine phenothiazine derivatives. Br. J. Anaesth. 33, 422 – 431.

Moulin, D. E., Max, M. B., Kaiko, R. F., Inturrisi, C. E., Maggard, J., Yaksh, T. L. and Foley, K. M. (1985) The analgesic efficacy of intrathecal D-Ala^2-D-Leu^5-enkephalin in cancer patients with chronic pain. Pain 23, 213 – 221.

Needs, C. J. and Brooks, P. M. (1985) Clinical pharmacokinetics of the salicylates. Clin. Pharmacokinet. 10, 164 – 177.

Nordberg, G., Hedner, T., Mellstrand, T. and Borg, L. (1984) Pharmacokinetics of epidural morphine in man. Eur. J. Clin. Pharmacol. 26, 233 – 237.

Portenoy, J. and Foley, K. M. (1986) Chronic use of opioid analgesics in non-malignant pain: report of 38 cases. Pain 25, 171 – 186.

Potter, W. Z. (1984) Psychotherapeutic drugs and biogenic amines – current concepts and therapeutic implications. Drugs 28, 127 – 143.

Procacci, P. and Zoppi, M. (1983) Pathophysiology and clinical aspects of visceral and referred pain. In: J. J. Bonica, U. Lindblom and A. Iggo (Eds.), Advances in Pain Research and Therapy, Vol. 5. Raven Press, New York, pp. 643 – 658.

Rance, M. J. (1983) Multiple opiate receptors – their occurrence and significance. In: R. E. S. Bullingham (Ed.), Clinics in Anaesthesiology, Vol. 1. W. B. Saunders Co. Ltd. London, pp. 183 – 199.

Richelson, E. (1984) The newer antidepressants: structures, pharmacokinetics, pharmacodynamics, and proposed mechanisms of action. Psychopharmacol. Bull. 20, 213 – 222.

Robbie, D. S. (1979) A trial of sublingual buprenorphine in cancer pain. Br. J. Clin. Pharmacol. 7, 315S – 317S.

Romagnoli, A. and Keats, A. S. (1980) Ceiling effect for respiratory depression by nalbuphine. Clin. Pharmacol. Ther. 27, 478 – 485.

Shaw, H. L. (1982) Subarachnoid administration of calcitonin: a warning. Lancet 11, 390.

Simpson, B. R., Seely, E., Clayton, J. I. and Parkhouse, J. (1962) Morphine combined with tetrahydroaminacrine for post-operative pain. Br. J. Anaesth. 34, 95 – 101.

Stimmel, B. (1983) Pain, Analgesia and Addiction: The Pharmacologic Treatment of Pain. Raven Press, New York, pp. 170 – 201.

Stjernsward, J. (1985) Cancer pain relief: an important global public health issue. In: H. L. Fields, R. Dubner and F. Cervero (Eds.), Advances in Pain Research and Therapy, Vol. 9. Raven Press, New York, pp. 555 – 558.

Tasker, R. (1987) Neurostimulation and percutaneous neural destructive techniques. In: M. J. Cousins and P. O. Bridenbaugh (Eds.), Neural Blockade in Clinical Anaesthesia and the Management of Pain, 2nd edn. J. B. Lippincott, Philadelphia (in press).

Tamsen, A., Hartvig, P., Fagerlund, C. and Dahlstrom, B. (1982) Patient controlled analgesic therapy. II. Individual analgesic demand and analgesic plasma concentrations of pethidine in post-operative pain. Clin. Pharmacokinet. 7, 164 – 175.

Twycross, R. G. (1979) The brompton cocktail. In: J. J. Bonica and V. Ventafridda (Eds.), Advances in Pain Research and Therapy, Vol. 2. Raven Press, New York, pp. 291 – 300.

Twycross, R. and Lack, S. (1984) Oral Morphine in Advanced Cancer. Beaconsfield Publ. Ltd., England, pp. 13 – 14.

Tyers, M. B. (1980) A classification of opiate receptors that mediate antinociception in animals. Br. J. Pharmacol. 69, 503 – 572.

Ventafridda, V., Spoldi, E., Caraceni, A., Tamburini, M. and Deconno, F. (1986) The importance of continuous subcutaneous morphine administration for cancer pain control. Pain Clinic 1, 47 – 55.

Willis, J. V., Kendall, M. J., Flinn, R. M., Thornmill, D. P. and Welling, P. G. (1979) The pharmacokinetics of diclofenac sodium following intravenous and oral administration. Eur. J. Clin. Pharmacol. 16, 405.

Yaksh, T. L. and Rudy, T. A. (1976) Analgesia mediated by a direct spinal action of narcotics. Science 192, 1357 – 1358.

Burrows/Elton/Stanley (eds.) Handbook of Chronic Pain Management
© *1987 Elsevier Science Publishers B.V. (Biomedical Division)*

20

The general practitioner and management of chronic pain

ISAAC HENRY JOHN BOURNE

'Richmond', Thorndon Approach, Herongate, Brentwood, Essex, U.K.

Introduction

Treatment of chronic pain in general practice overlaps and is often based on advice from consultant colleagues. The general practitioner has recourse to many methods for treating pain, and is in a special position to offer support and reassurance to the chronic pain patient and the family. This chapter deals with some of the ways in which the physician can improve the patient's situation, whether in dealing with curable or incurable chronic pain. I have mainly emphasized the role of exact palpation of the site of pain and treatment by local injections of corticosteroid. This technique is a useful addition to the general practitioner's therapeutic facilities. Other important approaches to control of chronic pain are dealt with elsewhere in this book.

The patient seeks help from his doctor when he feels that the threshold of his pain tolerance has been crossed. There is no fixed level of the sensation of pain for any person experiencing a given stimulus (Wyke 1981). Chronic pain may be described as a continuous sense of malaise in a localized region of the body, described by the patient as 'pain'. Arbitrarily, the physician may consider the pain to be 'chronic' when it has lasted for more than say 6 weeks, whether or not it has been treated by a professional healer.

Methods of treating pain

The general practitioner has a number of different methods from which to choose (see Table 1). These have been well reviewed by Jayson (1981). They are all concerned with alleviation of pain by drugs, or by stimulating the body to produce substances which counteract pain such as endorphins, or by counter-irritation of nociceptive fibres. Many of these treatments are variations on ancient techniques of analgesia and counter-irritation.

Treatment of pain by rest is open to question, but arm and knee splints may be essential when pain is severe and exacerbated by movement (Barnes 1982). Non-steroid anti-inflammatory drugs are generally prescribed (see Barnes 1982 for side effects). Aspirin remains the drug of first choice and is safe if monitored from the onset of treatment.

All research on results of treatment of pain is bedevilled by the fact that pain at any given site is prone to cyclic remission (Swerdlow 1972). For instance, it has been shown that attacks of 'arthritis' often occur during spring and autumn. Treatment begun during these attacks will have an apparently beneficial effect. Every general practitioner has seen a patient achieve a splendid remission of pain following prescription of the doctor's favourite painkiller, only to be daunted by the patient's confession that he did not take the tablets.

PATIENTS SUFFERING FROM INCURABLE PAIN

In order to focus attention on my suggestion that many so-called 'incurable' chronic pains are rediagnosable and curable, the reader is asked to accept that only patients inflicted with inoperable cancer and certain visceral diseases are suffering from incurable pain. When the general practitioner is asked to care for a patient with terminal cancer he may be aware that surgery, radiotherapy, hormone replacement and chemotherapy have already been given at hospital or refused by the patient. It should be remembered that pain may be present in the early stages of

TABLE 1
Methods which the general practitioner can advise for pain alleviation (modified from Jayson 1981).

Physical methods		Pharmacotherapy	
Rest	– bedrest	See Chapter 19 for analgesics	
	splints and corsets	Chapter 31 for management of rheumatic diseases	
Traction		Chapter 32 for management of the cancer patient	
Local heat	– hot water bottle	Injection therapy	
	flannel pad	Corticosteroids	– local trigger points for:
	radiant heat		fibrositic nodules
	electric pad		torn ligaments
	diathermy		scar tissue
Massage			rheumatic lesions
Exercise	– flexion		pseudo-angina
	extension		pseudo-temporal arthritis
	isometric		pseudo-cervical arthritis
Manipulation	– gentle		– intra-articular
(by physicians,	forced		– epidural
physiotherapists,		Chymotrypsin	– for prolapsed discs
surgeons)		Surgery (see also	– Refer patient to Neurosurgeon
Osteopathy		Chapter 34)	or Orthopaedic Surgeon
Chiropractic			
Spinal supports	– lumbar corsets		
	spinal supports		
	P.O.P. corsets		
Transcutaneous			
nerve stimulation			
(see Chapter 25)			

cancer and that a patient with terminal cancer may have concurrent pain separate from malignant tissue, as occurs in operation scars or infection of a cavity (Hunter 1981).

I treat pain, anxiety, and insomnia from the outset, choosing from the following list of drugs with which I am familiar: acetylsalicyclic acid, ibuprofen, sulindac, soluble aspirin and codeine, piroxicam, indomethacin, mefenamic acid, paracetamol, dihydrocodeine tartrate, ethoheptazine with meprobamate, buprenorphine, dextropropoxyphene, pentazocine, micro-crystalline morphine, papaveretum, methadone, carbamazepine, and lorazepam, diazepam, alprazolam, chlorpromazine, trifluoperazine, prochlorperazine maleate. Every family doctor will have a similar list at his disposal. The *Extra Martindale* devotes two hundred pages to 'pain', and the Monthly Index of Medical Specialties offers a plethora of alternatives to the above list. This *'embarras de richesse'* serves to emphasize that in a way drugs play a secondary role in the treatment of pain. Having decided on the drug regimen for the patient, the doctor may consider other methods of management. Many patients never lose hope of a revision of diagnosis. Physical examination of the site of pain is reassuring to all concerned, and the possibility of finding unrelated treatable lesions adds interest to the situation. The doctor is well qualified to chat to the patient and to support the efforts of the family and nurse to create a pleasant and relaxed atmosphere. A promise to revisit is an insurance against anxiety and alarm if the doctor is called in later when there has been deterioration. The importance of creating a calm, confident and trusting mood in the patient has been stressed by Donald (1977) as being more important than control of pain by drugs. Agitation, despair and a feeling of isolation lower the pain threshold (Wilkes 1977).

PATIENTS WITH CHRONIC PAIN WHICH MAY BE CURABLE

Patients with chronic pain which proves to be curable are a challenge to the practitioner to seek to revise diagnosis and search for new and effective cures. The chronic patient seen for the first time is concerned to be reassured that he has no serious or fatal disease, and hopes to be cured of his pain however long he has suffered. When every effort has been made to diagnose and correct specific ailments, attention is concentrated on the exact site of the patient's pain, with a view to offering local injection treatment as a logical resort. Local injection treatment does not exclude other treatments. I am learning to adopt a tolerant attitude to concurrent fringe or placebo treatment. If the patient feels better, even temporarily, after such treatment, this is the object of the therapeutic exercise.

The rationale of treatment of pain in soft tissues with local injections

Local injection of soft tissue lesions was first used in the treatment of 'tennis elbow'. Since most musculo-skeletal parts of the body are made of the same tissue elements as the elbow, it was not surprising that injection therapy gave the same excellent results as are obtained by accurate injection of tennis elbow.

Inflamed or deranged collagen tissue may be caused by injury, rheumatic disorder, or strain of ligaments near, around or near diseased joints. There is pain due to oedema and irritant metabolites (Simons 1975, 1976). In all these conditions administration of corticosteroid into the affected tissue leads to lysis of collagen to protocollagens. The entrapped nerve endings are normalized. The pain-free pabulum is replaced by normal fibrocytes, collagen fibres and nerve fibrils and is no longer painful when stretched or compressed (Ketchum 1967, 1971). Knee joints of rats were subjected to injury causing disruption of periarticular ligaments, and the lesions were then injected with triamcinolone acetonide. It was found that the steroid degraded collagen to tropocollagen. The liquefied tissue was reorganized by normal fibrocytes and nerve fibrils with the resultant replacement by normal tissue (Ketchum 1967, 1971). This repair occurs when fluocorticosteroid is injected into any lesion of connective tissue whether of recent origin, chronic scarring, or affected by rheumatic disease (Bourne 1979, 1980, 1983, 1984a,b, 1985) (see also Table 2 which shows the results of injection therapy with corticosteroid in 109 back-pain patients).

Clinical aspects of local injection therapy

After routine-history taking and examination is completed attention is focussed on the sites of pain indicated by the patient. Accurate localization of pain calls for expertise in the art of palpation. In a busy pain clinic the use of the fingertips for this purpose is contraindicated for the following reasons: a) the fingers cannot be used for searching for maximum tenderness day after day without risk of pain at the inter-phalangeal joints; b) the width of a finger is 1 cm which is too wide for pin-pointing small lesions such as occur on the postero-lateral aspects of inter-phalangeal joints; c) the clinician instinctively evaluates subjective signs (such as 'tender nodules') instead of objectively noting the patient's feelings of pain; d) in some locations such as the lumbar region and buttock deep pressure requires the use of the thumb, which is too wide for accurate palpation; and finally e) failure to palpate accurately or deeply enough may leave the examiner at risk of diagnosing psychosomatic pain or malingering, with dire consequences for the patient. For these reasons I have abandoned the use of the fingertips in the search for tenderness. I have designed a special prodder (see Fig. 1) which is also used as a skin marker and for writing and sketching.

TABLE 2

Results of the treatment of back pain in 109 patients, using local injection therapy with corticosteroid (adapted from Bourne 1979).

Length of history	No. treated	Results		
		Excellent	Good	Failure
5 – 12 wks	19	8	5	6
4 – 6 mths	3	3	–	–
7 – 12 mths	6	3	3	–
1 – 2 yrs	12	8	3	1
3 – 5 yrs	15	6	4	5
6 – 10 yrs	23	16	5	2
11 – 20 yrs	22	11	5	6
21 – 30 yrs	8	5	3	–
30 + yrs	1	–	1	–

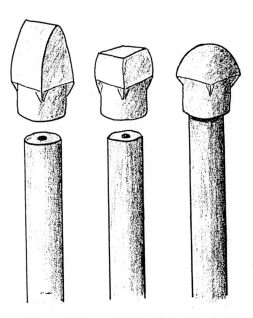

Fig. 1. The prodder: a tool for palpation.

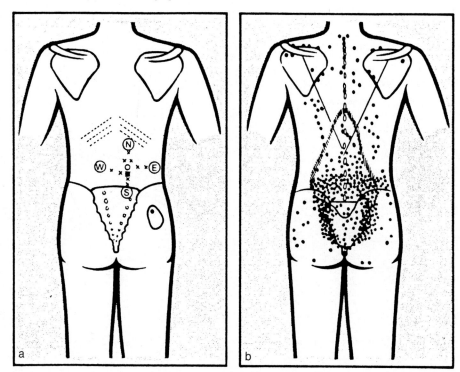

Fig. 2. (a) Location of a tender spot. The point of maximum tenderness is sought by a careful bracketting routine. (b) Composite sketch of the total number of injections for backache in 109 patients. Where locations overlap, the dots have been separated. It is not claimed that they all correspond to the sites of trapped posterior nerve root fibres. It seems probable that many injections were given for muscle and ligament lesions. (From Bourne 1979, with permission.)

LOCALIZATION OF THE SITE OF PAIN

The patient is asked to point to the affected place, and a mark is made on the skin. The examiner starts to prod the skin at 1 cm intervals from a point 10 cm above the mark until a slight pain is felt, when a second mark is made. The prodding is repeated from a point 10 cm below the first mark, then from points to the right and left (see Fig. 2a). The bracketting process is repeated until the most tender spot is found. If the marked-out area is oval a diagnosis of trapped nerve may be confirmed if the most tender spot is found at the junction of the proximal and middle thirds of the area. The depth of the lesion can be provisionally estimated by pinching the tender site. Figure 3 illustrates diagrammatically possible sites of lesion and the differential diagnosis of chronic pain in the soft tissues of the back.

TECHNIQUE OF INJECTION

I use a mixture of 1 ml triamcinolone acetonide suspension (10 mg/ml) and 1 ml of 2% ligno-caine suspension, in a 2 ml syringe with a one inch 23 gauge or half-inch 28 gauge needle; the latter for tiny lesions over small joints. The lesion is sought by advancing the needle tip slowly through the most tender spot until the patient experiences maximum pain. I warn the patient that this pain is an essential part of successful treatment and that they should not bear the pain in silence. When muscle tissue is involved, the needle is advanced with a side-to-side motion until

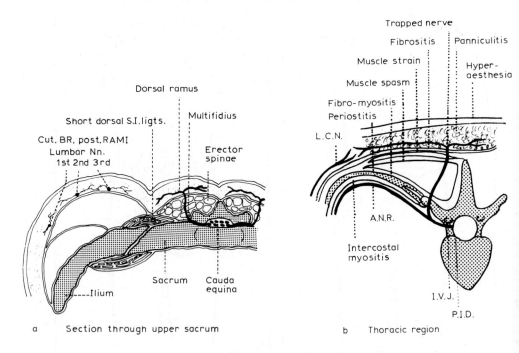

Fig. 3. Possible sites of the lesion in patients with backache. (a) Section of sacral area to illustrate the tissues liable to injury or disease. (b) Section through the dorsal region to illustrate the various types of lesion which may cause chronic backache. (From Bourne 1984a, with permission.)

the tip is caught in the deep fascia. Injection into the muscle on the underside of the deep fascia will usually cure the pain. Trapped nerves are also located by this method. All tender lesions are noted on a sketch of the affected part. Where there is more than one tender spot the two most tender spots are injected at the first session, and other spots at weekly intervals. It is my impression after years of follow-up assisted by careful drawings of affected parts, that pain does not recur at the sites of injection but only in adjacent tissue. This is encouraging for with persistence all painful sites can be cured.

SIDE EFFECTS OF LOCAL INJECTION THERAPY

The patient is given a leaflet (see Advice to patients, below) to reassure him or her that there are no serious side effects such as may be seen when cortisone tablets are taken daily over long periods. Female patients are warned that the injection may cause an extra period which is harmless. Diabetic patients are assured that transient glycosuria after an injection is of no importance. After 10,000 injections I have seen only one instance of pitting of the skin, and that disappeared after 3 months. I have never seen a case where injection therapy of ligaments caused weakness of a muscle or joint due to overstretching or rupture of the injected tissues. Patients with a history of fainting are treated in the recumbent position, especially in hot weather. The pamphlet warns the patient of feelings of discomfort for a few days after the injection. He is advised to continue with normal activities after the injection. In my opinion, this encourages the regrowth of normal fibrocytes in the corticosteroid-induced pabulum along normal lines of stress.

When the patient is symptom-free or the pain is controlled by minimum doses of his favourite analgesic drug he is advised to return if severe chronic pain returns after months or years.

Advice to patients. The patient is presented with a leaflet containing the following information concerning treatment of pain with adcortyl injections:

1) The injection is of small amounts of cortisone mixed with a short-acting local anaesthetic.
2) One injection may be sufficient to cure each tender area. Sometimes a second or third injection at weekly intervals is needed.
3) The pain may return after months or years. The injection may then be repeated.
4) There may be discomfort for a day or two after the local anaesthetic wears off. Aspirin or other tablets may be taken during this period.
5) Each painful spot needs a separate injection.
6) There are no side effects such as may be seen when cortisone tablets are taken over a long period.
7) If the treatment is successful, there will be no need to take painkilling tablets.
8) The injection may cause extra menstrual periods but this is not harmful in any way.

FEAR OF INJECTIONS

I am aware that many patients are terrified of injections of any sort, and especially of injections into certain parts of the body such as the scalp, front of neck, presternal area, jaw joint and pubic arch. Confidence, patience, tact and a sense of humour are necessary in such cases. If injection therapy is refused, the patient at least has the knowledge that his pain has been localized to an exact, usually small site, that the site is not deep in the body, neither is it a figment of the imagination. It should be mentioned that many patients are seen who are afraid of 'tablets' and other treatments for pain. Apart from the many patients who are terrified of injections there are those who by the acquisition of a little knowledge, have developed 'cortisone phobia'. Someone – who knows someone – has warned them that cortisone is a dangerous drug. Unfortunately the source of this advice is often a doctor or nurse. The memory of the catastrophic effects of large daily oral doses of cortisone dies hard. Most patients will see the analogy of comparing the effects of drinking a tot of whisky once a week with the results of drinking a bottle of whisky each day for a year. For those patients who dread the thought of injections I prescribe diazepam 2 – 5 mg, and distalgesic tablets one hour before the injection.

Clinical trials to evaluate the effectiveness of local injection therapy

In a series of 250 patients seen in general practice, cure of chronic soft tissue pain was achieved in 75% of cases (Bourne 1979). Similar results were recorded in a prospective controlled hospital-based trial in a series of 57 patients suffering from chronic backache (Bourne 1984a). Treatment of chronic pain in patients suffering from pain in the abdomen, head and neck, thigh and foot gave similar results. The effect of treatment was assessed as follows: *Excellent result* – a rapid and complete disappearance of pain from each site within 2 weeks and lasting for at least 5 months; *Good result* – alleviation of pain within 2 weeks but requiring further injections during the following 3 months, with relief for at least 5 weeks before relapse; *Failure* – no benefit from injections, or a refusal to continue treatment despite benefit from the first injection. The following examples have been published in *'The Practitioner'* and *'The Physician'*, and are reproduced here for illustration by kind permission of the Editors of these journals.

ASPECTS OF TREATMENT

Head and neck. When intracranial disease, high blood pressure, migraine, arteritis and neuritis have been ruled out, a search should be made for tender spots in the scalp or pericranium, the forehead, temples, or sub-occipital region. Patients who complain of neck pain should not be treated for degenerative disease of cervical vertebrae based on radiological evidence until soft tissue lesions have been excluded (Bourne 1984b).

Tennis and golfer's elbow. These conditions were the starting point of modern injection therapy. There is no classic injection site since recurrence seldom occurs at exactly the same place.

Case history: Mrs A., a housewife aged 51, fell downstairs in January 1982. She had intractable back pain until November when the backache was cured by local injection. In February 1983 she requested an injection for a left tennis elbow that had been present since the accident. She also mentioned pain in the right big toe joint, which had been operated on some years previously for hallux valgus. There was tenderness over the plastic replacement toe joint. The elbow and toe joints were injected with excellent results (Bourne 1984b).

Abdominal wall. In a series of 98 patients with localized lesions of the abdominal wall, treatment with local injection of triamcinolone acetonide and xylocaine was successful in more than 80% of cases. The patients were grouped as follows: 1) stress lesions of fibrous and muscle tissue and nerves, due to accident, occupation or sport; 2) lesions of the linea alba – strains and fatty epigastric hernia; 3) post-operative and post-injury strain of scars; 4) '*maladie d'amour*' – lesions of muscle due to active intercourse (Bourne 1984b).

Thigh. The lateral cutaneous nerve of the thigh has many branches; each one emerges through a separate aperture in the deep fascia where it may be 'trapped'. When this occurs, oval areas of hyperaesthesia are found, corresponding to the distribution of the emergent nerve (Bourne 1984b).

Foot. Almost any chronic pain in any part of the foot can be cured by local injection of corticosteroid.

Case history. Mr M., aged 60, had a life-long pain in a left club foot. This had become much worse since he trod on a nail 2 weeks previously. Palpation (with the fingertip and prodder) revealed a neuroma at the site of pain, injection into which resulted in a cure. He also suffered from chronic abdominal pain that was cured by injection into the linea alba (Bourne 1984b).

Table 3 shows some results of injection therapy as performed by the author. Sketch plans showing location of sites of maximum tenderness and sites of injection can be seen in the published reports as cited in this chapter. Two such sketch plans are shown in Fig. 2.

SOLUBLE VERSUS INSOLUBLE CORTICOSTEROIDS IN INJECTION THERAPY

Soluble cortisone is useless for treatment by local injection of diseased collagen tissues. It is washed out of the injected site into the blood stream before it can have the desired effect of

TABLE 3
Results of local injection treatment of pain (adapted from Bourne 1979, 1980, 1984).

Area of lesion	No. in group	Results n (%)		
		Excellent	Good	Failure
a) *Results of treatment of backache patients (n = 115)*				
Sacro-iliac region	82	42(51)	23(28)	17(21)
Other regions	33	17(52)	8(24)	8(24)
Disc degeneration	22	9(41)	4(18)	9(41)
b) *Results of treatment of non-backache patients (n = 216)*				
Abdominal wall group:				
Accident and stress	57	36(63)	14(25)	7(12)
Scar pain	16	10(62)	2(13)	4(25)
Linea alba strain	9	5(56)	4(44)	0
Maladie d'amour	16	14(87.5)	2(12.5)	0
Other areas of treatment				
Head and neck	34	15(44)	15(44)	4(12)
Hand	14	8(57)	5(35)	1(8)
Chest wall	19	11(58)	5(26)	3(16)
Thigh	23	13(56)	8(35)	2(9)
Foot	28	19(68)	7(25)	2(7)

reducing diseased collagen to its protocollagen constituents. Its use has led to disillusion with the method among some practitioners.

Pain associated with disease or injury to joints

Many patients will indicate the region of a joint as the site of pain. In my experience, the pain is almost always outside the joint, often localized in ligaments on the antero-lateral aspects of the knees or the dorsolateral aspects of the interphalangeal joints.

The fallacy of intra-articular injection of corticosteroid

Articular cartilage is insensitive to pain (Currey 1982). Injection of corticosteroid into a joint gives short-term relief only (Barnes 1982). By contrast, the joint capsule and associated ligaments, tendons, and periosteum are highly sensitive. Strain of vulnerable fibrous joint structures may be an important cause of symptoms (Currey 1982). When temporary relief from pain occurs after intra-articular injection it is probably because the corticosteroid is squeezed out of the joint space into the surrounding tissues (Barnes 1982; see also Sedgwick et al. 1984).

Chronic pain associated with walking on concrete pavements with leather shoes

Animal studies show that repetitive impulse loading in rabbits and exercising sheep on concrete causes arthritic changes in knee joints (Radin et al. 1978, 1982). Pain in the spine and locomotor system can be minimized if compliant visco-elastic, shock attenuating pads (viscolast) are incorporated into footwear (Voloshin and Wosk 1981, 1982; McLellan et al. 1982).

Conclusion

Local injection therapy with insoluble corticosteroid into painful soft-tissue lesions wherever they are found outside the body cavities is a useful addition to the General Practitioner's therapeutic facilities. The technique is simple but by no means easy. The search for the tender lesions should be methodical, painstaking, and persistent. The rewards of successful treatment are considerable.

References

Barnes, C. G. (1982) Rheumatoid arthritis. In: H. L. F. Currey (Ed.), Mason and Currey's Clinical Rheumatology, 3rd edn. Pitman, London, pp. 30 – 62.
Bourne, I. H. J. (1979) Treatment of backache with local injections. Practitioner 222, 708 – 711.
Bourne, I. H. J. (1980) Treatment of painful conditions of the abdominal wall with local injections. Practitioner 224, 921 – 925.
Bourne, I. H. J. (1983) The treatment of pain with local injections. Practitioner 227, 1877 – 1883.
Bourne, I. H. J. (1984a) Treatment of chronic back pain, comparing corticosteroid-lignocaine injections with lignocaine alone. Practitioner 228, 333 – 338.
Bourne, I. H. J. (1984b) Local injection therapy. Physician, Nov. 185 – 188.
Bourne, I. H. J. (1985) Injecting painful knees with triamcinolone. Practitioner 229, 33 – 34.
Currey, H. L. (1982) Osteoarthritis. In: H. L. Currey (Ed.), Mason and Currey's Clinical Rheumatology, 3rd edn. Pitman, London, pp. 96 – 105.

Donald. I. (1977) Pain – a patient's view. In: A. W. Harcus, R. Smith and B. Whittle (Eds.), Pain. New Perspectives in Measurement and Management. Churchill Livingstone, Edinburgh, pp. 1 – 4.

Hunter, R. D. (1981) Current views on the management of pain in the cancer patient. In: M. Swerdlow (Ed.), The Therapy of Pain, Current Status of Modern Therapy. M.T.P. Lancaster, England, pp. 191 – 214.

Jayson, M. I. V. (1981) Back Pain. The Facts. O.U.P. Oxford, pp. 60 – 119.

Ketchum, L. D. (1971) Effects of triamcinolone on tendon healing and function. Plast. Reconstr. Surg. 47, 471 – 482.

Ketchum, L. D., Robinson, M. D. and Masters, F. W. (1967) The degradation of mature collagen: a laboratory study. Plast. Reconstr. Surg. 40, 89 – 91.

McLellan, G. E., Platts, R. G. S. and Miles, H. (1982) The use of a shock absorbing heel construction on degenerative hip disease. J. Bone Joint Surg. 64B, 384.

Radin, E. L., Ehrlich, M. G., Chernack, R., Abernethy, P. and Paul, I. L. (1978) Effect of repetitive impulse loading on the knee joints of rabbits. Clin. Orthop. Related Res. 131, 288 – 293.

Radin, E. L., Orr, R. B., Kelman, J. L., Paul, I. L. and Rose, R. M. (1982) Effect of prolonged walking on concrete on the knees of sheep. J. Biomechanics 15, 487 – 492.

Sedgwick, A. D., Sin, Y. M., Moore, A. R., Edwards, J. C. W. and Willoughby, D. A. (1984) Effects of local administration of hydrocortisone on cartilage degradation in vivo. Ann. Rheum. Dis. 43, 418 – 420.

Simons, D. G. (1975) Muscle pain syndromes. 1. Am. J. Phys. Med. 54, 289 – 311.

Simons, D. G. (1976) Muscle pain syndromes. 2. Am. J. Phys. Med. 55, 15 – 42.

Swerdlow, M. (1972) Problems in the clinical evaluation of pain. In: J. P. Payne and R. A. P. Burt (Eds.), Pain. Basic Principles, Pharmacology, Therapy. Churchill Livingstone, London, pp. 49 – 51.

Voloshin, A. and Wosk, J. (1981) Influence of artificial shock absorbers on human gait. Clin. Orthop. 160, 52 – 56.

Voloshin, A. and Wosk, J. (1982) An in vitro study of low back pain. Shock absorption in the human locomotor system. J. Biomechanics 15, 20 – 27.

Wilkes, E. (1977) Doctors and the dying patient. In: A. W. Harcus, R. Smith and B. Whittle (Eds.), Pain. New Perspectives in Measurement and Management. Churchill Livingstone, Edinburgh, pp. 129 – 137.

Wyke, B. D. (1981) Neurological aspects of pain therapy. In: M. Swerdlow (Ed.), The Therapy of Pain. Current Status of Modern Therapy, Vol. 6. M.T.P. Lancaster, England, pp. 1 – 30.

Burrows/Elton/Stanley (eds.) Handbook of Chronic Pain Management
© *1987 Elsevier Science Publishers B.V. (Biomedical Division)*

21

The management of chronic pain in children

PATRICIA A. McGRATH

Department of Paediatrics, Faculty of Medicine, The University of Western Ontario, London, Canada

Introduction

The topics that are included in this chapter reflect the multiplicity and diversity of approaches that are essential for a comprehensive understanding of the phenomena of chronic pain. As reviewed in individual chapters, an exciting array of knowledge about the complexity and plasticity of nociceptive systems, the nature of endogenous pain modulating systems, and the variety of factors that can modify pain perception, has accrued during the last decade (for additional review, see Beers and Bassett 1979; Katz et al. 1982; Sjolund and Bjorklund 1982; Bonica et al. 1983; Basbaum and Fields 1984; Wall and Melzack 1984). The wealth of new information on nociceptive processing has led to revisions in our conceptualization of chronic pain mechanisms and in our approach to chronic pain management, as demonstrated by the development and refinement of pharmacological, neurosurgical, behavioural and psychological methods for alleviating chronic pain (Twycross 1985; Bradley et al. 1981; Newburger and Sallen 1981; Fordyce 1982; Hall 1982; Turner and Chapman 1982; Bond 1984).

However, recent advances in pain control have been confined almost exclusively to adults, with the consequence that our understanding about both the experience of chronic pain in children and also the efficacy of various pain control methods is limited (Eland and Anderson 1977; Lollar et al. 1982; Varni et al. 1982; Barr 1983; Jeans 1983; Ross and Ross 1984; Schechter 1985). Three reasons may account for the current lack of empirical data on pain management in children. First, the scientific investigation of pain is relatively young and initial basic research focussed logically on either adults, who could communicate their subjective experience of pain, or animals, in which nociceptive mechanisms could be directly monitored. Second, much information on the development of valid methods for pain measurement, on the relationship between attributes of a noxious stimulus and the perception of pain, and on the efficacy of different techniques for pain control, has been obtained in studies in which experimental pain is induced in healthy volunteers. Since ethical concerns limit the use of children in such studies, there has been a lack of basic research on paediatric pain. Third, clinical studies on pain control in children have been frequently confounded by a lack of objective and consistent criteria for assessing pain or by the investigator's unidimensional concept of pain. Recently, basic and applied investigations on pain measurement and pain control in infants and children have increased (Beyer et al. 1983; Gaffney and Dunne 1986; Menahem 1983; Craig et al. 1984; Johnston and Strada 1984; Katz et al. 1984; Owens 1984; Piquard-Gauvain 1984; Pothman and Goepel 1984; McGrath et al. 1985). New attention is focussing on how pain perception, pain behaviour, and pain attitudes vary throughout childhood as a function of sex, age, learning and previous pain experience, as well as on how to improve existing programmes for controlling acute and chronic pain in children.

Although observational, behavioural, projective, interview, and direct scaling techniques have been used to measure pain in children (Shultz 1971; Scott 1978; Jay and Tomasi 1981; Lollar et al. 1982; Savedra et al. 1982, 1984; Jeans 1983a, b; McGrath et al. 1983; Unruh 1983; Ross and Ross 1984; Savedra et al. 1984), there has been little systematic study on method reliability, the consistency of the pain scores across different testing times, between sexes, and among different age groups, and method validity, the extent to which pain scores represent actual estimates of the strength or unpleasantness of a child's pain. The reliability and validity of paediatric pain measures are particularly important to establish because many factors such as, developmental level, sex, age, birth order, previous pain experience, and parental attitudes about pain expression, may influence not only how accurately children use a particular pain measure but also how children perceive or respond to a noxious stimulus (Woodrow et al. 1972; Vernon 1974; Poznanski 1976; Craig 1978; Gaffney and Dunne 1986; Thompson and Varni 1986).

Both indirect and direct pain measures may be validated for use with children. Indirect pain measures, in which a child's pain is inferred from his/her behaviour, must be used when children are too young to understand scaling instructions. However, direct measures, in which a child scales the strength, unpleasantness, quality or duration of his/her pain, potentially provide the most comprehensive information on the child's experience of pain. Recent research has shown that children above 5 years of age can reliably use Visual Analog Scales to rate the strength of pain and affective face scales to rate the unpleasantness of their pain (McGrath et al. 1983, 1984, 1985). These methods have also been used to evaluate the efficacy of techniques for management of chronic paediatric pain (McGrath 1987).

Most of the studies on paediatric pain have assessed only one dimension of pain, intensity. Yet, an adequate description of pain, particularly chronic pain in which the source of noxious stimulation may not be precisely identified, requires information on many dimensions of the sensation such as, quality, location, duration, or frequency. In addition, the design of a comprehensive pain management programme requires information on the emotional, motivational and situational factors that can modify the perception of pain (Johnson 1973; Melzack and Wall 1982; McGrath 1983; Bond 1984; Price 1984; Wall and Melzack 1984). Consequently, a systematic multidimensional approach to the evaluation and management of chronic pain in children, in which the situational and psychological factors that can modify children's pain are assessed, is described in this chapter following the sections on specific categories of chronic pain in children.

Chronic pain in children

Many of the distinct differences in aetiology, mechanisms and therapy between acute and chronic pain, that have been described for adults, may be assumed to be similar for children. Acute pain, defined as pain of relatively short duration that is evoked by some well-defined noxious or tissue damaging stimulus, usually has an important biological function in that the pain provides a warning signal that something is wrong. Chronic pain, defined as a persistent pain that lasts beyond the usual time period required for healing, often has no biological warning function, even when it is associated with an underlying disease process. Psychological and environmental factors rather than injury or disease, frequently play a prominent role in the aetiology of chronic pain. Since chronic pain may be considered a disease state in its own, the physiological, psychological and behavioural responses are quite different from those of acute pain (Bradley et al. 1981; Fordyce 1982; Bonica et al. 1983; Webb 1983; Lavigne et al. 1986).

While chronic debilitating pain is a serious problem for adults, the incidence of chronic pain in children is generally low (Dunn and Jannetta 1973; Apley 1978; Beales 1979; Varni 1984). However, in view of the lack of basic research on pain in children and the usual inconsistency in clinical investigations regarding the criteria for assessing children's pain perceptions, the reported incidence and prevalence of chronic pain in children may be low. Children may experience chronic pain that is either not reported for fear of invasive medical treatment or that is not recognized by medical professionals. As yet, there have been no comprehensive surveys on the comparative incidence of different types of chronic pain for children. Descriptive studies on the pain produced by specific diseases often consist of retrospective, rather than prospective, studies so that information is inferred from medical charts rather than documented using objective criteria. Pending systematic investigation in prospective research designs, it may be premature to state that the incidence of chronic pain in children associated with disease or injury is significantly less than that for adults with similar disease or injury (Cornaglia et al. 1984; Hahn and McLone 1984).

Like adults, children and adolescents may experience chronic pain that is evoked by injury or disease (carcinoma, arthritis, sickle cell anaemia, haemophilia, neuralgia, accident trauma, severe burns), as well as chronic pain that is evoked primarily by psychological factors. Pain problems associated with a functional aetiology may develop as a consequence of anxiety, emotional distress related to chronic illness, or environmental factors that exacerbate an existing acute pain state. However, a major difference between adults and children may be that children experience significantly less of the constant debilitating pain that has a primary psychological origin.

As demonstrated by both literature review and frequency of presenting pain problems for the paediatrician, the most prevalent conditions of chronic pain in children and adolescents are chronic-like recurrent pain syndromes (Oster 1972; Apley 1976; Liebman 1978; McGrath 1983; Gascon 1984; Varni 1984; Greene et al. 1985; McGrath 1987). Children experience a variety of recurrent headaches, abdominal pain, and aching limb pains, in which pain constitutes the predominant symptom in an otherwise healthy child. Although these recurring syndromes do not represent classic chronic pain states, they represent chronic conditions in which the provision of adequate pain relief is a major concern. Since the aetiology and mechanisms for these recurring pains presumably differ from those associated with acute pain in the head, stomach, or limbs, the recurring pain syndrome may constitute a special type of chronic pain in children. Consequently, this chapter will describe three categories of paediatric chronic pain: pain evoked by disease or injury, pain associated primarily with psychological aetiology, and chronic recurrent pain syndromes.

Chronic pain evoked by disease or injury

Like adults, children's perceptions of chronic pain are not simply and directly related to the extent of their physical injuries or to the severity of their diseases. Instead, a variety of psychological and situational factors can modify the strength or unpleasantness of the pain that is evoked by injury. Children perceive a noxious stimulus, such as arthritic joint pain associated with haemophilia, in relationship to a certain context. The context is defined by their frame of reference, that is, their age and cognitive level, their previous pain experiences against which they evaluate each new pain, the significance of the pain-producing stimulus or disease to their lives, their expectations for obtaining eventual pain relief, and their ability to control the pain by themselves. Children's emotional responses to chronic pain are also not determined solely by the intensity or quality of the noxious stimulus, but are determined by the context in which they experience that pain. A variety of emotions such as, anger, fear, frustration, depression, or anxiety may result from the same noxious stimulus presented in different contexts. Certain emotions, such as fear or anxiety regarding the outcome of an amputation to prevent metastases of a tumour, may subsequently alter children's perceptions so that any pain after amputation is exacerbated. Consequently, it is essential to evaluate the contextual factors and emotional responses that may modify chronic pain in children.

Major contextual factors that may modify the perception of chronic pain evoked by disease include the life-threatening potential of the disorder, the potential for disfigurement, and the potential for physical disabilities. Although the importance of these factors for the psychological, social and familial welfare of children with chronic disorders has been well documented (Grogan et al. 1977; Frydman 1980; Drotar 1981), there has been little specific study on their impact for modifying the pain that is associated with the disorder (Beales 1979; Beales et al. 1983). Most studies of children with life-threatening illness have focussed on the control of acute pain and anxiety, since acute pain produced by repeated medical procedures is often a greater problem than chronic pain (Katz et al. 1980; Jay et al. 1983; Hilgard and LeBaron 1984; McGrath and deVeber 1986).

It is essential to recognize that the psychological and situational factors for children who experience chronic pain that is evoked by life-threatening disorders such as cancer, are quite different from those for children who experience chronic pain that is evoked by disorders that are not life threatening. Consequently, optimal pain management for children with chronic pain evoked by disease requires not only medical treatment for the disease including symptomatic pain relief, but also evaluation of the factors that can progressively influence the pain. These factors will necessarily differ in relation to the type of disease and the child's and family's response to the diagnosis and prognosis. Reliance on information about the psychological, situational, and emotional factors that exist for a particular child rather than sole reliance on the nature and severity of the physical disorder is important for the provision of comprehensive pain control.

A similar multidisciplinary approach should be used for the management of chronic pain evoked by injuries such as, burns or those sustained in automobile accidents. Burn pain represents a special pain problem in children because burns cause more pain, discomfort, and disability over a longer period of time than many other injuries or illnesses (LaBaw 1973; Ravenscraft 1982; Szyfelbein and Osgood 1984). The burn pain and extensive medical treatment required for therapy represents a well-defined source of pain, similar to acute pain, but with a special set of psychological and emotional consequences, similar to chronic pain. For burn children, there are many factors that can potentially affect the strength or unpleasantness of both the pain evoked by the burns and also the pain evoked during necessary treatments. These include separation, loss, denial, anxiety, depression, uncertainty about potential disfigurement, fear, and general feelings of passivity or lack of control.

The pain management problems associated with burn children are typical of those that are frequently encountered for children hospitalized with serious injuries. The use of medication to reduce pain may be problematic since complete analgesia may only be achieved by high doses of narcotic analgesics that may necessitate longterm reliance on medication. The focus of much of the research on burn pain in children has been similar to that in acute pain in cancer patients, that is, to provide adequate pain control without sole reliance on medication and to minimize distress and anxiety (LaBaw 1973; Ravenscraft 1982; Szyfelbein and Osgood 1984).

In addition to the pharmacological methods that are used to treat specific diseases and injuries, various non-pharmacological techniques have been successfully used for children with cancer, sickle cell anaemia, arthritis, haemophilia, burns, and serious injuries, to alleviate their chronic pain. Hypnotherapy has been the most documented method used to reduce pain (LaBaw 1973, 1975; Cioppa and Thai 1975; LaBaw 1975; LaBaw et al. 1975; Gardner 1976; Zeltzer et al. 1979; Ellenberg et al. 1980; Elkins and Carter 1981; Hartman 1981; Olness 1981a,b; Hilgard and LeBaron 1984), but progressive relaxation techniques (Richter 1984; McGrath and deVeber 1986; Richter et al. 1986), behavioural programmes (Varni et al. 1980, 1982; Varni 1981), electroacupuncture (Leo 1983) and individual or group pain programmes in which relevant situational factors are modified (Guenthner et al. 1980; Newburger and Sallen 1981) have also proven effective. These techniques share a common focus by altering psychological and situational factors that can modify pain, such as improving the child's understanding of their disease and medical procedures, increasing their control over painful procedures, and providing them with age-appropriate strategies that help them to cope with any pain that will be produced. Some coping strategies that have been adapted from adult research include distraction, absorption techniques, and guided visual imagery. The child learns to concentrate on a positive coping mechanism, rather than to concentrate on the fear or pain that he/she may experience. Parents also receive instructions on how to reassure and support the child so that the children can learn to choose among available techniques of pain management.

The treatment of pain associated with a disease process begins with the identification and specific treatment of the disease and with the symptomatic relief of the pain. Good analgesic regimens require adequate doses at appropriate intervals, as determined by the child's response. The classic PRN model of narcotic administration, that is contingent upon a child's pain complaints, requires periodic suffering and makes the drug a positive reinforcer of pain and pain behaviour in a drug-dependent behavioural pattern. This situation may pose special pain management difficulties for children who are hospitalized with pain from either a disease or injury. Children may learn to ask for medication at progressively shorter intervals for fear of pain and they may learn to develop certain pain behaviours to prove their need. Although pharmacological administration may be the primary method prescribed for pain control, situational factors may exert a powerful role for enhancing or reducing the analgesic efficacy of the selected pharmacological treatment. The same principles of pain management, that have been used to enhance pain relief for children with acute pain evoked by medical treatments (Katz et al. 1980; Melamed and Siegel 1980; Jay et al. 1983; McGrath and deVeber 1986), may be modified and used for hospitalized children with chronic pain. These include: providing the child with age-appropriate information about the pain source and prescribed treatments; encouraging the child to learn some coping strategies to enhance the efficacy of prescribed analgesic interventions, rather than inadvertently encouraging him/her to rely solely on medication; allowing the child to make choices when possible; and providing adequate psychosocial support to enable the child to adjust to the trauma of the disease and concomitant pain. In this manner, some of the major contextual and psychological factors, that have been demonstrated in adult and animal studies to modulate nociceptive mechanisms, will be modified to promote optimal chronic pain management.

Chronic pain associated with psychological aetiology

Chronic paediatric pain in which there is a predominant psychological aetiology may be defined as pain that develops as a consequence of an emotional state that is either not recognized or not resolved such as, anxiety, fear, depression or anger. Pain may develop as a conversion reaction for a child who demonstrates emotional trauma, with no evidence of organic pathology. Pain of psychological origin may also develop for a child with disease such as, cancer, as a consequence of the child's concerns about the effects of the disease. Children may develop pain in body sites that are distal to those that are affected by a disease because they are unable to identify, understand or communicate effectively their emotions. The pain provides a signal that the child requires appropriate psychological or psychiatric therapy. Pain management requires identification and resolution of the source of emotional conflict by individual and family counselling. Concurrent with therapy, a behavioural management programme may be used to discourage pain behaviours and encourage healthy behaviour.

Pain of psychological origin may also develop for children as a consequence of learning or operant conditioning by parents, family, or teachers. A child may receive positive reinforcement when he/she experiences acute pain, by increased attention from significant others and decreased demands for performance. The quality and pattern of reinforcement may lead children to develop exaggerated pain behaviours associated with pain of organic aetiology or to develop new pains. Accurate pain assessment requires the differentiation of pain behaviour from pain experience by evaluation of children's subjective descriptions of pain and the relevant psychological and situational factors that contribute to their perception. Children who exhibit pain as a consequence of reinforced pain behaviours may not require extensive therapy; instead, they may require only a brief behavioural management programme to reduce their learned pain responses.

Recurrent pain syndromes

Unlike chronic pain evoked by disease or psychological factors, the prevalence of recurrent headaches, abdominal pain, and limb pains in children and adolescents is high, varying in reported incidence from 7 to 30% for school children (Oster 1972; Christensen and Mortensen 1975; Deubner 1977; Apley 1978; Rothner 1979; Galler et al. 1980; Bille 1982; Barr 1983; McGrath 1983; Farrell 1984; Schechter 1984; McGrath 1987). Several features are common to all three recurrent pain syndromes: children experience intense pain episodes in the absence of a well-defined organic aetiology; pain episodes may be triggered by a variety of external and internal factors, particularly events that provoke stress; children are usually healthy and pain-free between episodes; and there is frequently a history of similar pain for one of the children's parents.

After the absence of organic disease has been established by appropriate medical examination, treatment has frequently consisted of the provision of reassurance to parent and child that 'nothing is wrong' or 'your child will grow out of it'. However, reassurance alone has disadvantages in that the child still has painful episodes, the parents may remain anxious about the source of the pain, familial and situational factors that may precipitate pain episodes are not identified or treated, and children may not 'grow out of it' (Apley 1978; Barr 1983; Hodges et al. 1985). The incidence of children who continue to experience recurrent pain or who develop new pains has been estimated at 33% for abdominal pain (Apley 1978; Barr 1983) and 40−60% for headaches (Jay and Tomasi 1981; Bille 1982). A recent study indicates that children with recurrent headaches experience significantly more general pains (abdominal, back, limb) as well as headaches than a matched group of healthy children and that they rated their pains as significantly stronger and more unpleasant. In addition, the longer children have endured recurrent headaches, the more likely they are to develop other recurrent pains and to manifest psychological problems (McGrath 1987). There is a need for definitive longitudinal studies in order to determine the prognosis for children who have recurrent pain syndromes, as a function of their age of onset, frequency of episodes, severity of pain and the type of pain treatment that they received.

Unless an organic aetiology is established as for certain types of headaches (Lai et al. 1982) or abdominal pain (Barr 1983), pharmacological methods may reduce the pain during an episode but have not been found particularly effective for reducing the frequency of episodes (Forsythe et al. 1984). Non-pharmacological methods such as, hypnosis, relaxation training, biofeedback, and operant conditioning, have proven successful for reducing pain and for reducing the frequency of painful episodes (Michener 1981; Labbe and Williamson 1983; Farrell 1984; Hoelscher and Lichstein 1984; Werder and Sargent 1984; Larsson and Melin 1986; Richter et al. 1986). However, comprehensive pain management requires evaluation of the factors (environmental and psychological) that precipitate painful episodes, as well as application of specific methods to reduce the painfulness of episodes.

A multidisciplinary approach to pain control

Since the management of pain in children requires a multidisciplinary approach, a Pediatric Pain Research Program and Pain Clinic were initiated at the Children's Hospital of Western Ontario to provide an integrated and comprehensive programme for the control of acute, chronic and recurrent pain in children and adolescents. Physicians refer children with a variety of pain problems to this programme for evaluation of the relevant psychological, situational and emotional factors that may modify the child's pain perception and for design of individual pain management programmes to supplement required medical treatment.

Pain assessment includes a structured interview with parents, child, and medical staff (when appropriate) in which information is obtained on the type of pain experienced, the child's pain behaviour, children's and parental pain histories, parents' criteria for evaluating the presence and intensity of their child's pain, and the usual methods that have been used by a child to reduce the pain and their efficacy. The child completes a Comprehensive Pain Questionnaire (CPQ), that has been adapted from adult research on chronic pain, and a Pain Perception Inventory (PPI) (McGrath, submitted for publication). The CPQ includes Visual Analog and Verbal Descriptor Scales to provide information about: the sensory dimensions of the child's pain, such as intensity, quality, duration, frequency and location; the child's emotional responses to the pain, such as fear, anxiety, depression, frustration, and anger; the effects of the pain on the child's life with respect to the three major effects for adults with chronic pain, interference with daily lives, difficulty of enduring the pain on a continuing basis, and fear that the pain is signalling future physical harm; and the child's expectations and desires for future pain relief (Price 1984). The Pain Inventory is used to evaluate the child's previous pain experiences and to provide information on the child's pain attitudes. It depicts 30 situations, consisting of both familiar events (toothache) and medical treatments (injection in the arm) that vary in intensity and affect. The child uses Visual Analog Scales and a Facial Affective Scale to rate the intensity and unpleasantness of these events. The child's data is compared with the pain profiles that have been obtained for other children of the same sex, age, and diagnosis, as well as for normative samples for children with other disorders (for example, headache, arthritis, or pain associated with a psychological aetiology). Each child also completes standardized age-appropriate psychological tests to provide some basic descriptive information on the child's anxiety, depression, and personality characteristics.

This type of pain assessment provides the framework for evaluating the environmental, psychological, and situational factors that may affect the child's pain perception. These factors may modify the intensity, unpleasantness or duration of pain, trigger specific pain episodes, or create maladaptive pain behaviours. Recommendations from the assessment vary according to the needs of a particular child and family. They may include: participation in a 4 to 6-week programme in which the child learns strategies for coping with the pain such as, hypnosis or relaxation exercises; an operant conditioning programme in which medical staff and the family participate; or psychological therapy with the child and parents. The efficacy of each approach is evaluated by monitoring the child's pain and pain behaviour with self-completed pain logs, objective behavioural rating scales, and re-assessment with the CPQ.

In summary, after children have received the medical examinations necessary for diagnosis and treatment for their disorders, they may be referred to the Pain Program for assessment and management of their specific pain complaints. A variety of non-pharmacological approaches are effective for reducing different components of chronic pain in children such as, strength, unpleasantness, duration or frequency of pain episodes. Multi-strategy treatments which combine biofeedback, relaxation training, assertiveness training, systematic desensitization, and cognitive coping strategies for pain may be used successfully for a variety of chronic and recurrent pain syndromes.

Proposed directions

Future research on pain in children should include an integration of cross-sectional and longitudinal investigations on developmental aspects of pain perception, pain attitudes, and pain behaviour in order to provide comprehensive information about the effects of sex, age, cognitive level, previous pain experience, parental attitudes, and culture on the perception and expression of pain. There is a special need for both basic and applied studies on paediatric pain control that integrate the results of animal and adult studies of pain modulation in order to develop multidisciplinary programmes for controlling acute, chronic and recurrent childhood pain.

Research on the control of chronic pain in children must continue with a thorough evaluation of the pain experience in children and an adaptation of the principles of pain management (both pharmacological and non-pharmacological) that have been shown to successfully reduce pain in adults. The efficacy of non-traditional methods for pain control such as acupuncture and TENS, should be investigated for certain types of paediatric chronic pain. A major focus for improving chronic pain management for children consists of the design of multidisciplinary programmes for the evaluation and treatment of prevalent chronic and recurrent pain problems. Perhaps, more comprehensive multidisciplinary approaches to pain in childhood would minimize the frequency of chronic debilitating pain in adulthood.

References

Apley, J. (1976) Pain in childhood. J. Psychosom. Res. 20, 383 – 389.

Apley, J. (1978) The Child and His Symptoms. Blackwell Scientific Publ., Oxford.

Barr, R. B. (1983) Pain tolerance and developmental change in pain perception. In: M. D. Levine (Ed.), Developmental-Behavioral Paediatrics. W. B. Saunders, Philadelphia, pp. 505 – 511.

Basbaum, A. and Fields, H. (1984) Endogenous pain control systems: brainstem spinal pathways and endorphin circuitry. Ann. Rev. Neurosci. 7, 309 – 338.

Beales, J. G. (1979) Pain in children with cancer. In: J. J. Bonica and V. Ventafridda (Eds.), Advances in Pain Research and Therapy, Vol. 2. Raven Press, New York, pp. 89 – 98.

Beales, J. G., Keen, J. H. and Holt, P. J. (1983) The child's perception of the disease and the experience of pain in juvenile chronic arthritis. J. Rheumatol. 10, 61 – 65.

Beers, R. F. and Bassett, E. G. (Eds.) (1979) Mechanisms of Pain and Analgesic Compounds. Raven Press, New York.

Beyer, J. E., DeGood, D. E., Ashley, L. C. and Russell, G. A. (1983) Patterns of postoperative analgesic use with adults and children following cardiac surgery. Pain 17, 71 – 81.

Bille, B. (1982) Migraine in Childhood. Panminerva Med. Eur. Med. 24, 57 – 62.

Bond, M. R. (1984) Pain: Its Nature, Analysis and Treatment. Churchill Livingstone, Edinburgh.

Bonica, J. J., Lindblom, U. and Iggo, A. (Eds.) (1983) Advances in Pain Research and Therapy: Proceedings of the Third World Congress on Pain, Vol. 5. Raven Press, New York.

Bradley, L. A., Prokop, C. K., Gentry, W. D., Van der Heide, L. and Prieto, E. J. (1981) Assessment of chronic pain. In: C. K. Prokop and L. A. Bradley (Eds.), Medical Psychology – Contributions to Behavioural Medicine. Academic Press, New York, pp. 91 – 117.

Christensen, M. F. and Mortensen, O. (1975) Long-term prognosis in children with current abdominal pain. Arch. Dis. Child. 5, 110 – 114.

Cioppa, F. J. and Thai, A. D. (1975) Hypnotherapy in a case of juvenile rheumatoid arthritis. Am. J. Clin. Hyp. 18, 105 – 110.

Cornaglia, C., Massimo, L., Haupt, R., Melodia, A., Sizemore, W. and Benedetti, C. (1984) Incidence of pain in children with neoplastic disease. Pain (Suppl. 2) S28.

Craig, K. D. (1978) Social modeling influences on pain. In: R. A. Sternbach (Ed.), The Psychology of Pain. Raven Press, New York, pp. 73 – 110.

Craig, K. D., McMahon, R. J., Morison, J. D. and Zaskow, C. (1984) Developmental changes in infant pain expression during immunization injections. Soc. Sci. Med. 19, 1331 – 1337.

Deubner, D. C. (1977) An epidemiologic study of migraine and headache in 10 – 20 year olds. Headache, Sept. 1977, 173 – 179.

Drotar, D. (1981) Psychological perspectives in chronic childhood illness. J. Pediatr. Psychiatry 6, 211 – 228.

Dunn, D. K. and Jannetta, P. J. (1973) Evaluation of chronic pain in children. Cur. Prob. Surg. 64 – 72.

Eland, J. M. and Anderson, J. E. (1977) The experience of pain in children. In: A. K. Jacox (Ed.), Pain: A Source Book for Nurses and Other Health Professionals. Little, Brown, and Co., Boston, pp. 453 – 473.

Elkins, G. R. and Carter, B. D. (1981) Use of a science fiction-based imagery technique in child hypnosis. Am. J. Clin. Hyp. 23, 274 – 277.

Ellenberg, L., Kellerman, J., Dash, J., Higgins, G. and Zeltzer, L. (1980) Use of hypnosis for multiple symptoms in an adolescent girl with leukaemia, J. Adol. Health Care 1, 132 – 136.

Farrell, M. K. (1984) Abdominal pain. Pediatrics (Suppl. 74) 955 – 957.

Fordyce, W. E. (1982) A behavioral perspective on chronic pain. Br. J. Clin. Psychiatry 21, 313 – 320.

Forsythe, W., Gillies, D. and Sills, M. A. (1984) Propanolol ('Inderal') in the treatment of childhood migraine. Dev. Med. Child Neurol. 26, 737 – 741.

Frydman, M. (1980) Perception of illness severity and psychiatric symptoms in parents of chronically ill children. J. Psychosom. Res. 24, 361 – 369.

Gaffney, A. and Dunne, E. A. (1986) Developmental aspects of children's definitions of pain. Pain 26, 105 – 117.

Galler, J. R., Neustein, S. and Walker, W. A. (1980) Clinical aspects of recurrent abdominal pain in children. In: L. A. Barnes (Ed.), Advances in Pediatrics, Vol. 27. Year Book Medical Publ., Inc., Chicago, pp. 31 – 53.

Gardner, G. G. (1976) Childhood, death, and human dignity: hypnotherapy for David. Int. J. Clin. Exp. Hyp. 24, 122 – 139.

Gascon, G. G. (1984) Chronic and recurrent headache in children and adolescents. The Pediatric Clinics of North America, 31, 1027 – 1052.

Gracely, R. H. (1979) Psychophysical assessment of human pain. In: J. J. Bonica, J. C. Liebeskind and D. G. Albe-Fessard (Eds.), Advances in Pain Research and Therapy. Raven Press, New York, pp. 805 – 824.

Greene, J. W., Walker, L. S., Hickson, G. and Thompson, J. (1985) Stressful life events and somatic complaints in adolescents. Pediatrics 75, 19 – 22.

Grogan, J. L., O'Malley, J. E. and Foster, D. J. (1977) Treating the pediatric cancer patient: a review. J. Pediatr. Psychiatry 2, 42 – 48.

Guenthner, E. E., Hilgartner, M. W., Miller, C. H. and Vienne, G. (1980) Hemophilic arthropathy: effect of home care on treatment patterns and joint disease. J. Pediatr. 97, 378 – 382.

Hahn, Y. S. and McLone, D. G. (1984) Pain in children with spinal cord tumours. Child's Brain 11, 36 – 46.

Hall, W. (1982) Review: psychological approaches to the evaluation of chronic pain patients, Aust. N.Z. J. Psychiatry 16, 3 – 9.

Hartman, G. A. (1981) Hypnosis as an adjuvant in the treatment of childhood cancer. In: J. J. Spinetta and P. Deasy-Spinetta (Eds.), Living with Childhood Cancer. C. V. Mosby, Toronto, pp. 143 – 152.

Hilgard, J. R. and LeBaron, S. (1984) Hypnotherapy of Pain in Children with Cancer. William Kaufman, Inc., Los Altos.

Hodges, K., Kline, J. J., Barbero, G. and Flanery, R. (1985) Depressive symptoms in children with recurrent abdominal pain and in their families. The Journal of Pediatrics, 107, 622 – 626.

Hodges, K., Kline, J. J., Barbero, G. and Woodruff, C. (1985) Anxiety in children with recurrent abdominal pain and their parents. Psychosomatics, 26, 859 – 866.

Hoelscher, T. J. and Lichstein, K. L. (1984) Behavioral assessment and treatment of child migraine: implications for clinical research and practice. Headache, 24, 94 – 103.

Jay, G. W. and Tomasi, L. G. (1981) Pediatric headaches: a one year retrospective analysis. Headache 21, 5 – 9.

Jay, S. M., Ozolins, M., Elliott, C. H. and Caldwell, S. (1983) Assessment of children's distress during painful medical procedures. Health Psychiatry 2, 133 – 147.

Jeans, M. E. (1983a) The measurement of pain in children. In: R. Melzack (Ed.), Pain Measurement and Assessment. Raven Press, New York, pp. 23 – 37.

Jeans, M. E. (1983b) Pain in children – a neglected area. In: P. Firestone, P. J. McGrath and W. Feldman (Eds.), Advances in Behavioural Medicine for Children and Adolescents. Lawrence Erlbaum Associates, New Jersey.

Johnson, J. E. (1973) Effects of accurate expectations about sensations on the sensory and distress components of pain. J. Pers. Soc. Psychiatry 27, 261 – 275.

Johnston, C. C. and Strada, M. E. (1984) Pain responses in infants: vocalization and heart rate. Pain (Suppl. 2) S24.

Katz, E. R., Kellerman, J. and Siegel, S. E. (1980) Behavioral distress in children with cancer undergoing medical procedures: developmental considerations. J. Consult. Clin. Psychiatry 48, 356 – 365.

Katz, E. R., Sharp, B., Kellerman, J., Marston, A. R., Hershman, J. M. and Siegel, S. E. (1982) β-Endorphin immunoreactivity and acute behavioral distress in children with leukemia. J. Nerv. Ment. Dis. 17, 72 – 77.

Katz, E. R., Varni, J. W. and Jay, S. M. (1984) Behavioral assessment and management of pediatric pain. Progress in Behavior Modification, 18, 163 – 193.

Kruger, L. and Liebeskind, J. C. (1984) Neural mechanisms of pain. In: Advances in Pain Research and Therapy. Raven Press, New York.

LaBaw, W. L. (1973) Adjunctive trance therapy with severely burned children. Int. J. Child Psychother. 2, 80 – 92.

LaBaw, W. L. (1975) Autohypnosis in haemophilia. Haematology 9, 103 – 110.

LaBaw, W., Holton, C., Tewell, K. and Eccles, D. (1975) The use of self-hypnosis by children with cancer. Am. J. Clin. Hypn. 17, 233 – 238.

Labbe, E. E. and Williamson, D. A. (1983) Temperature biofeedback in the treatment of children with migraine headaches. J. Pediatr. Psychiatry 8, 317 – 326.

Lai, C.W., Ziegler, D. K., Lansky, L. L. and Torres, M. D. (1982) Hemiplegic migraine in childhood: diagnostic and therapeutic aspects. J. Pediatr. 101, 696 – 699.

Larsson, B. and Melin, L. (1986) Chronic headaches in adolescents: treatment in a school setting with relaxation training as compared with information-contact and self-registration. Pain, 25, 325 – 336.

Lavigne, J. V., Schulein, M. J. and Hahn, Y. S. (1986) Psychological aspects of painful medical conditions in children. I. Developmental aspects and assessment. Pain, 27, 133 – 146.

Lavigne, J. V., Schulein, M. J. and Hahn, Y. S. (1986) Psychological aspects of painful medical conditions in children. II. Personality factors, family characteristics and treatment. Pain, 27, 147 – 169.

Leo, K. C. (1983) Use of electrical stimulation of acupunture points for the treatment of reflex sympathetic dystrophy in a child. Phys. Ther. 63, 957 – 959.

Liebman, W. M. (1978) Recurrent abdominal pain in children: a retrospective survey of 119 patients. Clin. Pediatr. 17, 149 – 153.

Lollar, D. J., Smits, S. J. and Patterson, D. L. (1982) Assessment of pediatric pain: an empirical perspective. J. Pediatr. Psychiatry 7, 267 – 277.

McGrath, P. A. (1983) The role of situational factors in pain perception. Anesthesia Progress, 30, 137 – 146.

McGrath, P. A. (1987) The multidimensional assessment and management of recurrent pain syndromes in children. Journal of Behavior Research and Therapy.

McGrath, P. A. and deVeber, L. L. (1986) The management of acute pain evoked by medical procedures in children with cancer. Journal of Pain and Symptom Management, 1, 145 – 150.

McGrath, P. A., de Veber, L. L. and Hearn, M. T. (1983) Modulation of acute pain and anxiety for pediatric oncology patients. Am. Pain Soc. (Abstr.) 93.

McGrath, P. A., de Veber, L. L. and Hearn, M. T. (1984) Multi-dimensional pain assessment in children. Pain (Suppl. 2) S26.

McGrath, P. A., de Veber, L. L. and Hearn, M. T. (1985) Multidimensional pain assessment in children. In: H. L. Fields, R. Dubner and F. Cervero (Eds.), Advances in Pain Research and Therapy: Proceedings of the Fourth World Congress on Pain, Vol. 9. Raven Press, New York, pp. 387 – 393.

McGrath, P. J. (1983) Migraine headaches in children and adolescents. In: P. Firestone, P. J. McGrath and W. Feldman (Eds.), Advances in Behavioral Medicine for Children and Adolescents. Lawrence Erlbaum Associates, New Jersey, pp. 39 – 58.

McGrath, P. J., Johnson, G., Goodman, J. T. and Schillinger, J. (1984) The development and validation of a behavioral pain scale for children. Pain (Suppl. 2) S24.

Melamed, B. G. and Siegel, L. J. (Eds.) (1980) Behavioral Medicine: Practical Applications in Health Care, Vol. 6. Springer Publ., New York.

Melzack, R. and Wall, P. D. (1982) The Challenge of Pain. Penguin Books, New York.

Menahem, S. (1983) Understanding the management of the child with pain. Med. J. of Aust. 1, 579 – 582.

Michener, W. M. (1981) An approach to recurrent abdominal pain in children. Primary Care 8, 277 – 283.

Newburger, P. E. and Sallen, S. E. (1981) Chronic pain: principles of management. J. Pediatrics 98, 180 – 189.

Olness, K. (1981a) Hypnosis in pediatric practice. Curr. Prob. Pediatr. 12, 1 – 47.

Olness, K. (1981b) Imagery (self-hypnosis) as adjunct therapy in childhood cancer: clinical experience with 25 patients. Am. J. Pediatr. Haematal./Oncol. 3, 313 – 321.

Oster, J. (1972) Recurrent abdominal pain, headache and limb pains in children and adolescents. Pediatric 50, 429 – 436.

Pantell, R. H. and Goodman, B. W. (1983) Adolescent chest pain: a prospective study. Pediatrics 71, 881 – 887.

Piquard-Gauvain, A., Rodary, C., Razvani, A. and Lemerle, J. (1984) Establishment of a new rating scale for the evaluation of pain in young children (2 – 6 years) with cancer. Pain (Suppl. 2) S25.

Pothman, R. and Goepel, R. (1984) Comparison of the visual analog scale (VAS) and a smiley analog scale (SAS) for the evaluation of pain in children. Pain (Suppl. 2) S25.

Poznanski, E. O. (1976) Children's reactions to pain: a psychiatrist's perspective. Clin. Pediatr. 15, 1114 – 1119.

Price, D. D. (1984) Role of psychophysics, neuroscience, and experimental analysis in the study of pain. In: L. Kruger and J. C. Liebeskind (Eds.), Advances in Pain Research and Therapy, Vol. 6. Raven Press, New York, pp. 341–355.

Ravenscraft, K. (1982) The Burn Unit. Psychiatr. Clin. North Am. 5, 419–432.

Richter, N. C. (1984) The efficacy of relaxation training with children. J. Abnorm. Child Psychiatry 12, 319–344.

Richter, I. L., McGrath, P. J., Humphreys, P. J., Goodman, J. T., Firestone, P and Keene, D. (1986) Cognitive and relaxation treatment of migraine. Pain, 25, 195–203.

Robertson, W. O. (1981) Managing pain in children. J. Am. Med. Assoc. 245, 2429–2430.

Ross, D. M. and Ross, S. A. (1984a) The importance of type of questions, psychological climate and subject set in interviewing children about pain. Pain 19, 71–79.

Ross, D. M. and Ross, S. A. (1984b) Childhood pain: the school-aged child's viewpoint. Pain 20, 179–191.

Rothner, A. D. (1979) Headaches in children: a review. Headache 19, 156–162.

Savedra, M., Gibbons, P., Tesler, M., Ward, J. and Wegner, C. (1982) How do children describe pain? a tentative assessment. Pain 14, 95–104.

Savedra, M., Tesler, M., Ward, J. and Wegner, C. (1984) Adolescents' description of the pain experience. Pain (Suppl. 2) S27.

Schechter, N. L. (1984) Recurrent pains in children: an overview and an approach. The Pediatric Clinics of North America, 31, 949–968.

Schechter, N. L. (1985) Pain and pain control in children. Current Problems in Pediatrics, 15, 1–67.

Scott, R. (1978) It hurts red: a preliminary study of children's perception of pain. Percept. Motor Skills 4, 787–791.

Shultz, N. (1971) How children perceive pain. Nurs. Outlook 19, 670–693.

Sjolund, B. and Bjorklund, A. (Eds.) (1982) A Brainstem Control of Spinal Mechanisms, Elsevier Biomedical Press, Amsterdam.

Szyfelbein, S. K. and Osgood, P. F. (1984) The assessment of analgesia by self-reports of pain in burned children. Pain (Suppl. 2) S27.

Thompson, K. L. and Varni, J. W. (1986) A developmental cognitive-biobehavioral approach to pediatric pain assessment. Pain, 25, 283–296.

Turner, J. and Chapman, C. (1982) Psychological interventions for chronic pain: a critical review. Pain 12, 1–46.

Twycross, R. G. (1975) Diseases of the central nervous system – relief of terminal pain. Br. Med. J. 4, 212–214.

Unruh, A., McGrath, P., Cunningham, S. J. and Humphreys, P. (1983) Children's drawings of their pain. Pain 17, 385–392.

Varni, J. W. (1981) Self-regulation techniques in the management of chronic arthritic pain in hemophilia. Behav. Ther. 12, 185–194.

Varni, J. W. (1984) Pediatric pain: a biobehavioral perspective. Behav. Ther. 7, 23–25.

Varni, J. W., Bessman, C. A., Russo, D. C. and Cataldo, M. R. (1980) Behavioral management of chronic pain in children: case study. Arch. Phys. Med. Rehab. 61, 375–379.

Varni, J. W., Katz, E. R. and Dash, J. (1982) Behavioral and neurochemical aspects of pediatric pain. In: D. C. Russo and J. W. Varni (Eds.), Behavioral Pediatrics – Research and Practice, Plenum Press, New York, pp. 177–224.

Vernon, D. T. (1974) Modeling and birth order in responses to painful stimuli. J. Pers. Soc. Psychiatry 20, 794–799.

Wall, P. D. and Melzack, R. (Eds.) (1984) The Textbook of Pain. Churchill Livingstone, Edinburgh.

Webb, W. L. (1983) Chronic pain: psychosomatic illness review. Psychosomatics 24, 1053–1063.

Werder, D. S. and Sargent, J. D. (1984) A study of childhood headache using biofeedback as a treatment alternative. Headache, 24, 122–126.

Wiley, F. M. and Rhein, M. (1977) Challenges of pain management: one terminally ill adolescent. Pediatr. Nurs. 3, 26–27.

Woodrow, K. M., Friedman, M. D., Siegel, M. S. and Collen, M. D. (1972) Pain-tolerance: differences according to age, sex, and race. Psychosom. Med. 34, 548–556.

Zeltzer, L. K., Dash, J. and Holland, J. P. (1979) Hypnotically induced pain control in sickle cell anemia. Pediatrics 64, 533–536.

Burrows/Elton/Stanley (eds.) Handbook of Chronic Pain Management
© *1987 Elsevier Science Publishers B.V. (Biomedical Division)*

22

Social work management of chronic pain

RANJAN ROY

School of Social Work and Faculty of Medicine, Headache Clinic, Psychological Services Centre, University of Manitoba, Winnipeg, Canada

Introduction

There are many types of chronic pain attributable to a variety of disorders. The type of chronic pain under consideration here is what has been described as chronic intractable benign pain syndrome (Pinsky et al. 1979). This syndrome presents a complex picture that includes these common factors: a) mood and affect changes that tend to be dysphoric; b) drug dependency, and CNS side effects; c) multiple surgical and pharmacological treatments; d) increasing psychosocial withdrawal; e) inter-personal conflict with significant others; f) loss of self-esteem; g) depression and anhedonia; h) increasing physical incapacity, and i) conflict with medical personnel. This is indeed one of the more comprehensive descriptions of chronic benign pain syndrome and draws its strength from the fact that it takes into account the multi-dimensional nature of the problem which includes biological, psychological, and social factors.

Psycho-social problems among chronic pain sufferers

It can be confidently stated that while the neurological, psychiatric and psychological aspects of chronic pain syndrome have come under considerable scrutiny, the social variables, by and large, still remain under-researched. Nevertheless, the significance of psycho-social parameters in understanding behavior of patients with chronic pain has been acknowledged (Roy 1981). Bonica (1973) recognized that social work assessment provided pertinent information about the family, the work environment and other factors that could significantly contribute to the behavior of patients with chronic pain. Similarly, Melzack and Chapman (1973) acknowledged the importance of social factors in the affective experience of pain. Sternbach (1974) identified a number of social variables affecting the outcome of intervention with pain victims. He found that married people with good premorbid sexual adjustment, and people who continued to work despite the pain improved more than patients without these attributes.

Depression and anxiety are indeed common among sufferers of chronic pain although there is some confusion and controversy about the rate of prevalence of clinical depression among this population (Roy et al. 1984). There is, however, no debate whatsoever that the patients with chronic pain assume invalid status within a relatively short period of time, and demonstrate a whole host of psychologically and socially maladaptive behaviors (Sternbach 1973; Violon 1982). On the Minnesota Multiphasic Personality Inventory (MMPI) they evidence elevation on depression, hysteria and hypochondriacal scales (Sternbach 1974). Pilowsky (1969) has developed the concept of abnormal illness behavior which lends further credence to the concept of clinical observation that chronic pain sufferers experience a host of psychological difficulties. According to Pilowsky et al. (1976, 1979), they demonstrate a heightened level of hypochondriasis, disease conviction, somatic preoccupation, affective inhibition, affective disturbance, irritability and also a tendency to deny psychological difficulties (see also Chapter 16).

From a social perspective, the single most important issue which has been subjected to consistent scrutiny is the loss of occupational role for the pain patient (Roy 1984a). Another way of stating the problem is to recognize that restoration of the occupational role has been viewed as the most significant measure of positive treatment outcome (Tunks and Roy 1982). Loss of the occupational role is interpreted by patients and unfortunately by many clinicians as a global loss of roles and functions. Several years ago, Fordyce (1973) warned against such generalizations. He observed that physical impairment in many chronic patients resulted from the operations they had to undergo to alleviate the pain. Sternbach (1974) agreed that the return to work was a crude measure of success and rehabilitation and perhaps too strong an application of the work ethic. Despite the emphasis on the occupational role, there is relative poverty of information concerning other major social roles, particularly with respect to the chronic pain patient. This paucity of research interest is obvious in a majority of studies concerned with the outcome of treatment. The outcome is usually measured in terms of analgesic intake, levels of activity, and reported change of pain severity; all obviously related to functioning, but they portray only a partial view of the overall role functions of patients (Roy 1984a).

Maintenance of activities

It has been argued elsewhere that the rehabilitation of chronic pain sufferers necessarily consists of reconstitution of weakened defenses, restoration of lost roles, and resumption of normal family life (Roy and Tunks 1982). From the point of view of social work, the focus has to be on a critical examination of the consequences of chronic pain on the patient himself and as it affects all the other systems with which the patient has to necessarily interact. Generally speaking, these systems consist of the family, the world of work, the health-care system and other social systems which serve a variety of social, religious, recreational and health needs. With a view to unravelling the consequences of chronic pain on the patient's role functions, a study was conducted at McMaster University (Roy and Bellissimo 1980). A questionnaire was developed to assess role functioning in the area of social, occupational, leisure, home, family and illness-related activities. Forty subjects with intractable pain and a group of 34 normal subjects completed the questionnaire and the findings were in the predictable direction. Overall, the mean number of activities performed by the pain group, on a regular basis, as compared to the adult normals, was lower in every area except the scale on illness-related activities, where the pain group predictably demonstrated considerably more activities than the normal group. On the other hand, in the area of family-related activities there was only a nominal difference between the two groups. In terms of occupational, social, leisure and illness-related activities, the differences between the normal and the pain groups were quite dramatic. The most revealing finding in the study was that individual patients do give up many of their activities, but attempt to maintain important functions, especially as they relate to home and family. To reiterate, the occupational, social and leisure activities were the major casualties of chronic pain.

The individual-environment fit

Given that situation, it is imperative that considerable attention needs to be paid to what can be described as the individual-environment fit which is significantly disrupted as a result of chronic pain. Before proceeding to some case examples, it may be instructive to further review the literature to determine the extent to which psycho-social problems encountered by chronic pain sufferers have been studied. The area that has come under somewhat close examination is the marital and family issues in patients with chronic pain (Roy 1982a, b). Marital and sexual difficulties are common and there is indeed mounting evidence that spouses of chronic pain patients tend to become victims of various kinds of emotional disorder themselves (Maruta and Osborne 1978; Mohamed et al. 1978; Roberts and Reinhardt 1980; Maruta et al. 1981; Shanfield et al. 1979). Unfortunately, there is virtually no information about the effect on children when a parent is a victim of chronic pain. However, there is ample clinical evidence that the impact on the family system in the presence of a chronic pain patient is far-reaching (Roy 1982a, b, 1984b). Given the magnitude of the suffering experienced by the families of chronic pain patients, it stands to reason that, in the first place, a very thorough understanding is required of the family dynamics and secondly, intervention is imperative with the whole family and related systems.

Social support network

From the point of view of social work, another commonly observed problem is the rapid disappearance of the patients' social support network. Again it should be stated that while there is limited direct empirical evidence for this phenomenon, clinical evidence is indeed powerful (Roy 1980). Research findings have consistently demonstrated the inter-relationship between availability of social support and the individual's ability to cope with stressors (Cobb 1976; Caplan 1981; McFarlane, et al. 1983). Nevertheless, from time to time patients are seen who present a very complex picture of pain. By and large, this group of patients sustains only minor injuries (some of them work-related) and within a relatively short period of time they tend to decompensate to the point of becoming almost totally dysfunctional. Barros-Ferreira (1976) reported similar findings in a group of immigrant Portugese workers in France. In the absence of organic pathology, close attention has to be paid to the psychological, social, and personality factors. Again the premorbid history for many of these individuals is characterized by adequate coping. Strictly from a psychiatric point of view, they do not easily fit into any diagnostic categories.

These patients manifest a degree of helplessness which is somewhat incongruous with their past history of coping. They take on a strictly dependent posture and the message clearly is that the whole situation is beyond their control. They demonstrate a pervasive sense of loss of autonomy and their inter-personal relationships are characterized by a certain amount of paranoia, i.e. they tend to see themselves as victims of circumstances which are almost designed to perpetuate their state of helplessness. They also find themselves in a massive struggle with the rest of the environment (Tunks and Roy 1982).

A careful review of the social support network of these patients reveals that some of the individuals are single or married with very young families. The scope of their social support network is extremely limited. Whatever formal and informal network of relationships these patients had prior to the onset of the pain problem, at the time of their arrival to the clinic, they are socially isolated. Even for those individuals who have families, their relationship with the family members changes for the worse and systematic assessment of the family situation time and time again reveals considerable collusion on the part of the family members to help maintain the patient's angry, hostile, dependent and helpless posture. It is noteworthy that many of these families consist only of very young children and the spouses are socially very isolated.

The following is an approximate expression of the sentiment of this group of individuals. 'Through no fault of our own, we get hurt and now we are finding out that no one cares.' The message is clearly that they feel abandoned and trapped. They perceive their environment as non-caring and callous. Their experience with the world of medicine is almost totally negative. The physicians, in the patient's judgement, not only fail to cure the pain but significantly add to their hurtful feelings by directly and indirectly suggesting that they are either faking the pain or the pain is 'in their head'. This is too readily interpreted by the patients to mean that they are lying or imagining the pain.

Retrospective analysis of these patients' help seeking behavior indicates that, among other factors, lack of an adequate and acceptable explanation for their pain launches them into a long and costly search for a cure. Maintaining ongoing contact with doctors, hospitals and clinics, assumes enormous significance for them as these activities give legitimacy to their sick role. Their search for a cure, in effect, makes them almost totally dependent on the health-care system and the impersonal nature of the health-care system allows the dependency to grow almost totally unchecked.

Absence of adequate social support for this group of patients results in their human needs being met through interaction with the health-care system. The health-care system, or more specifically the pain clinic, quite often becomes the patient's reference group.

Loss of social roles

To summarize the overall nature of social problems encountered by many chronic pain sufferers, it would seem, that they experience loss of many of the major social roles including the occupational ones. In addition, family conflicts are inordinately common in this group of patients and sexual difficulties arise with almost clockwork regularity. Patients are totally dependent on the health-care system and view themselves as victims of the system (Roy 1980). From a social work perspective, restoration of roles, reintegration of patients with the community at large, and sorting out the family relationships, are areas of primary interest.

In the section that follows three cases will be discussed to illustrate efficacy of social work interventions to ameliorate many of the problems discussed in the preceding paragraphs.

Case 1: Mr. A, age 28. This young man was referred to a pain clinic following a rear-end collision which resulted in whiplash injury. He suffered immediately the expected discomfort in the back and neck, but it did not abate and instead was followed by progressive disability and anxiety, some depression and elaboration of physical complaints which included indigestion and insomnia. He found himself preoccupied with his misfortune to the point that he could not concentrate well during the day and he was very worried about his future. He was unable to carry on with his work and was laid off. His family history was quite unremarkable. He lived alone and over a relatively short period of time became devoid of any close friendships. At the time of his inception into the pain clinic, he was involved in a variety of struggles which included the landlord, Workmen's Compensation Board, family physician, his lawyer and the only person he could think of as his friend was his employer, who, interestingly enough, had terminated his employment. Mr. A was single and had a higher professional degree.

Intervention in this case involved taking a task-centered approach. This meant working out with the patient a rational and acceptable explanation for both the pain and dysfunction. It was agreed that pain would mainly be a non-negotiable issue. Getting control of the medication intake, instituting a step-wise rehabilitation program, utilizing activities of daily living and mustering whatever social support could be made available within the health-care system to provide reinforcement were additional goals. All this was done simultaneously with any indicated physical treatment, which in the case of Mr. A included physiotherapy and tricyclic antidepressant medication, which proved ineffective.

Eventually, the strategy involved creating an environment where the patient began to develop a feeling of being understood. It served an additional purpose of giving recognition that he had a series of identifiable problems which needed intervention. The social worker emphasized, from the very outset, that the treatment was designed to create a need for him to resume normal living which necessitated an equal partnership between the clinic and the patient and mutual agreement was sought and reached on deciding what tasks had to be accomplished. From a psychological perspective, recognition was given to the patient's sick role which also meant that he would need to assume some responsibility for improving his situation. The overall objective of the intervention was to stir the patient's sense of autonomy and give him a sense of mastery over his environment. Specifically, interventions included individual counselling, advocacy on behalf of the patient with various organizations and enabling the patient to link up with friends and social organizations. The approach was pragmatic and active, requiring an intense inter-disciplinary cooperation. It took Mr. A nearly a year before he was able to resume normal living which included returning to his profession, reactivation of his social activities, resolution of legal and W.C.B. related problems, moving home and finally termination with the pain clinic.

The task-centered approach used in this case derives its strength from the knowledge that individuals have a high level of investment in maintaining their social roles, and that while certain circumstances might jeopardize those roles, individuals remain primarily invested in regaining them (Reid 1977). This became apparent in the case of Mr. A. While he gradually abandoned all his roles and became enormously invested in maintaining his chronic sick role, once his sick role was legitimized and his level of distress acknowledged, he was willing to enter into negotiations with the social worker to begin to examine his difficulties and explore ways of resolving them. Space does not permit a detailed account of some of the very critical issues of assessment of these cases, but suffice it to say that a comprehensive psycho-social assessment is imperative before this kind of approach can be adopted (Roy 1981). In the second place, getting the trust of the patient, who has learned to distrust hospitals, clinics and health-care professionals, is an absolute necessity for any kind of therapeutic venture, but especially in this kind of contractual arrangement where his motivation is of paramount importance. The very essence of task-centered approach is predicated mainly on the patient's motivation to alleviate his distress and 'help clients move forward with psycho-social problems that they define and hope to solve' (Reid 1978).

Case 2: Mr. B, age 36. This man was referred to the pain clinic with a prolonged history of headache. He had reached a point where he was unable to continue his work as an office manager and spent most of his time in bed. He was married with two young children. He complained bitterly about the inability of the medical profession to cure his 'simple headache'. He further complained of anhedonia, pervasive loss of interest and general dissatisfaction with his way of life. He also felt that he was greatly misunderstood by his wife. He claimed that she had no understanding of his pain problem. And yet he contradicted himself by stating that she 'babied' him when he was in pain, which, usually made him feel even worse. Since he was unable to continue in his employment and was on sick leave, his wife, in effect, became the bread winner of the family which was a further blow to Mr. B's self-esteem. An agreement was reached between the social worker and Mr. B that on his next visit he would bring his wife as many of the problems seemed to implicate his wife in one way or another.

The next session attended by Mr. and Mrs. B, revealed that Mr. B tended to be somewhat impulsive and was not particularly responsible about managing the financial affairs. In addition, he had an extremely bad temper of an unpredictable nature which kept Mrs. B pretty much on edge. Their financial situation was in such a precarious state that Mrs. B suggested taking over the family finances which of course was rejected by Mr. B. Their sexual relationship had virtually ended and Mrs. B expressed a great deal of frustration about her inability to please her husband. Therefore, she was inclined to infantilize him when he had pain. She mentioned that during severe bouts of pain he was in fact a nicer man and was quite repentant about his day-to-day conduct. Clearly, she was engaging in actively reinforcing his pain behavior and from his point of view the pain was serving a clear purpose assuaging his feelings of guilt. Functions of pain in this particular marriage have been described elsewhere (Roy 1984c).

At the completion of this session, an agreement was reached between the couple and the therapist that in the first place, Mrs. B would take over the family finances, and as soon as possible they would try and engage in making joint decisions. Secondly, Mrs. B was not to pay undue attention to her husband while he had these serious bouts of head pain, but rather they would try to do things together when he felt well. They were encouraged to resume their normal physical intimacies and again, as in the preceding case, a specific agreement was reached about these tasks and Mr. B was to resume his employment. The couple was seen altogether for seven sessions at the end of which they had resolved a great deal of their difficulties and Mr. B's head pain was much improved.

From a theoretical point of view, the rationale for marital therapy was derived from the initial data presented by Mr. B and there was further evidence that there was a marked exacerbation of his headache at a point when Mrs. B commenced paid employment. The task was to reframe the problem of his headache into the context of marital conflict and his head pain was seen primarily as serving two functions: 1) to assuage his guilt for his generally unpredictable and aggressive behavior and 2) to seek succor and nurturance in the only way he knew how. There was also a third element, that could be interpreted as a form of protest against his wife's desire to become independent. For a man who was heavily invested in his macho image, this constituted a serious threat.

The focus of intervention was to bring about a realignment of roles and help them develop more acceptable ways of seeking and receiving nurturance. The intervention was of a short-term nature and Mr. and Mrs. B were seen on seven occasions, spread over a period of some 20 weeks. This model of family therapy intervention is based on the problem-centered system family therapy of Epstein and his colleagues (1981, 1982). The use of this model to treat families of chronic pain patients has been described in detail elsewhere (Roy 1984b, 1986). This model of family therapy is predicated on some of the same principles as the task-centered approach. They are rooted in systems theory, subscribe to a clear definition of problems, require patients' and family members' active participation in defining the issues and setting practical ways of resolving them. Both these methods advocate short-term therapy.

Case 3: Mr. C, age 54. Mr. C was involved in a motor vehicle accident and sustained back injury. Extensive radiological, neurological and orthopedic investigations failed to reveal any damage. Nevertheless, Mr. C embarked on the career of a chronic pain patient which culminated in the total loss of his business, major disruption in his family relationships, depression and in the final analysis, an invalid status. Along with a variety of interventions which included, transcutaneous nerve stimulation (TNS), relaxation therapy, antidepressant medication and analgesics, the family approach was adopted.

The family of Mr. C consisted of his wife and three children, two of whom were grown up and living away, leaving a teenage daughter at home.

The essential findings in the family were as follows. Predictably, the roles in this family were drastically altered. As Mr. C sank deeper and deeper into his sick role, Mrs. C had to take on the major responsibilities, including going out to work for the first time in her life. The daughter became tremendously isolated and depressed. In a very real sense she lost both her parents. Her mother was not around and for the most part too tired to give her any attention, and her father was irritable and unpredictable most of the time. As Mrs. C put it, she not only lost a partner and a friend, but she gained a man who was in pain a great deal of the time, irritable most of the time, and unpredictable all of the time. The emotional side of this family underwent dramatic change over a period of some 18 months. From being a well-functioning family where there was considerable evidence of give and take and caring for one other, there was a great deal of expression of what Epstein et al. (1981) have described as emergency feelings, i.e. negative emotions such as anger, hostility and sadness. With regard to communication, once again this family demonstrated a major shift from being able to communicate openly and directly to indirect and masked forms of communication, i.e. messages were unclear to the point that they never said to each other what they meant and at the same time it was never clear for whom the message was intended. In short, this family became, for all practical purposes, a chaotic one. All three members experienced a great deal of isolation and frustration and were at a total loss as far as any resolution was concerned.

Following a detailed assessment of the problems, an agreement was reached with the family in the following areas. Mr. C was to spend a few minutes each day talking to his daughter about her school and generally sharing information; secondly, the three of them were to have their dinner together following which there was to be time set aside for a family-type discussion; Mr. C agreed to undertake certain chores in the house which he could perform without aggravating his pain problem; Mrs. C agreed that once a week they would go out on their own to visit with friends and relatives or for a meal etc.; Mr. C also agreed that his daughter should come and talk to him any time she wanted to about any of her problems; Mr. and Mrs. C agreed to resume sleeping together and gradually resume normal sexual activities; finally they all agreed that if either Mrs. C or the daughter found Mr. C's irritability or inexplicable anger unacceptable, they were to openly let him know and deal with it on the spot.

The problem-centered systems family therapy was utilized to treat this family. This family was seen on nine occasions over a period of 6 months. Mostly the couple was seen together without the child and at the point of termination they had successfully achieved all of the tasks that they had set for themselves. It is noteworthy that Mr. C's pain problem did not substantially change and he continued to receive other kinds of treatment through the pain clinic, but the family issues were significantly improved as was his role performance in many areas. There was marked improvement in the overall morale of the family.

Summary

It has to be acknowledged that the case discussions, of necessity, are somewhat sketchy due to limited space. Hopefully, they convey adequately the role and function a social worker is required to perform in a pain clinic. Germain (1984) has succinctly summarized the social work process in health care as follows: 'In general the major social work function in face to face practice is to help patients and their families deal with social and emotional needs and problems that may accompany or predate illness and disability. Attention is given to person-environment relationship by easing the associated stress and enhancing internal and external coping resources for dealing with associated stress.' As was stated at the beginning of this chapter, what seems to suffer most as a direct consequence of chronic pain is the individual-environment fit. Regardless of the size of the system, the objective of social work intervention is to facilitate the family or individuals to reorganize their lives whereby they can begin to resume a semblance of normal living. This can be achieved frequently in spite of the pain problem. In this chapter an attempt has been made to demonstrate the efficacy of social work interventions. With an individual it is proposed that a short term, task-centered approach is effective and economical and provides the patient with a clear sense of direction and an opportunity for him to assume responsibility for his own actions.

Adopting a family approach must be viewed as imperative. The presence of a chronic pain patient in the family system is enormously disruptive as has been demonstrated by the two case examples. Theoretical orientations for treating couples and families are rooted in systems theory, are usually of short duration, behaviorally oriented and mostly effective. The strength of social-work interventions in treating chronic pain has to be seen in its commitment to treating the patient in the context of the larger society. Social work is not primarily concerned with psychopathology, but rather with identifying strengths in individuals and families and enabling the patient and family members to begin to use their inherent strengths to cope with the vicissitudes of living. In the context of chronic pain patients where the notion of disease in still elusive, incorporation of social work strategies into the overall treatment and management plan of these patients has to be viewed as essential.

References

Barros-Ferreira, de M. (1976) Hysteria et fait psychosotique chez l'immigrant portugais. Acta Psychiatr. Belg. 76, 551 – 578.
Bonica, J. (1973) Fundamental considerations of chronic pain therapy. Postgrad. Med. 53, 81 – 85.
Caplan. G. (1981) Mastery of stress: psychosocial aspects. Am. J. Psychiatry 138, 413 – 420.
Cobb, S. (1976) Social support as moderator of life stress. Psychosom. Med. 38, 300 – 314.
Epstein, N. and Bishop, D. (1981) Problem-centered systems therapy of the family. In: F. Gurman and D. Kniskern (Eds.), Handbook of Family Therapy. Brunner/Mazel, New York, pp. 444 – 482.
Epstein, N. B., Bishop, D. and Baldwin, L. (1982) McMaster model of family functioning: a view of the normal family. In: Froma Walsh (Ed.), Normal Family Process. Guilford Press, New York, pp. 115 – 141.
Fordyce, W. (1973) Operant conditioning in the treatment of chronic pain. Arch. Phys. Med. Rehab. 54, 399 – 408.
Germain, C. B. (1984) Social Work Practice in Health Care: An Ecological Perspective. The Free Press, New York, pp. 57 – 86.
Maruta, T. and Osborne, D. (1978) Sexual activity in chronic pain patients. Psychosomatics 19, 531 – 537.
Maruta, T., Osborne, D., Swenson, D. W. and Holling, J. M. (1981) Chronic pain patients and spouses: marital and sexual adjustment, Mayo Clinic Proc. 56, 307 – 310.

225

McFarlane, A., Norman, G., Streiner, D. and Roy, R. (1983) The process of social stress: stable, reciprocal, and mediating relationships. J. Health Soc. Behav. 24, 160 – 173.

Melzack, R. and Chapman, C. R. (1973) Psychologic aspects of pain. Postgrad. Med. 53, 69 – 75.

Mohamed, S. N., Weisz, G. M. and Waring, E. M. (1978) The relationship of chronic pain to depression, marital adjustment and family dynamics. Pain 5, 285 – 289.

Pilowsky, I. (1969) Abnormal illness behaviour. Br. J. Med. Psychol. 42, 347 – 351.

Pilowsky, I. and Spence, N. D. (1976) Is illness behaviour related to chronicity in patients with intractable pain? Pain 2, 167 – 173.

Pilowsky, I., Murrell, T. G. C. and Gordon, A. (1979) The development of a screening method for abnormal illness behaviour. J. Psychosom. Res. 23, 203 – 207.

Pinsky, J. J., Griffin, S. E., Agnew, D. C., Kamdar, M. D., Crue, B. C. and Pinsky, C. H. (1979) Aspects of long-term evaluation of pain unit treatment program for patients with chronic intractable benign pain syndrome treatment outcome. Bull. Los Angeles Neurol. Soc. 44 (1 – 4 special edition), 53 – 69.

Reid, W. J. (1977) Task-centered treatment and trends in clinical social work. In: W. J. Reid and L. Epstein (Eds.), Task Centered Practice. Columbia University Press, New York, pp. 1 – 18.

Reid, W. J. and Epstein, L. (Eds.) (1978) The Task-Centered System. Columbia University Press, New York, pp. 12 – 19.

Roberts, A. H. and Reinhardt, L. (1980) Behavioural management of chronic pain: long term follow-up with comparison groups. Pain 8, 151 – 162.

Roy, R. (1980) Social support and chronic pain. Presented at the annual meeting of Canadian Pain Society, Montreal, Canada.

Roy, R. (1981) Social work and chronic pain. Health Soc. Work 6, 54 – 62.

Roy, R. (1982a) Marital and family issues in patients with chronic pain. Psychother. Psychosom. 37, 1 – 12.

Roy, R. (1982b) Chronic pain and family dynamics. In: D. Freeman and B. Trute (Eds.), Treating Families with Special Needs. C. A. S. W., Ottawa, pp. 219 – 232.

Roy, R. (1984a) Pain clinics: reassessment of objectives and outcome. Arch. Phys. Med. Rehab. 65, 448 – 451.

Roy, R. (1984b) Chronic pain: a family perspective. Int. J. Fam. Ther. 6, 31 – 43.

Roy, R. (1984c) The phenomenon of 'I have a headache': functions of pain in marriage. Int. J. Fam. Ther. 6, 165 – 176.

Roy, R. (1986) A problem-centered family systems approach in treating chronic pain. In: A. D. Holzman and D. Turk (Eds.), Pain Management: A Handbook of Treatment Approaches. Pergamon Press, New York, pp. 113 – 130.

Roy, R. and Bellissimo, A. (1980) Role functions and illness behaviour of chronic pain patients and a group of normal subjects (unpublished research report, McMaster University, Hamilton).

Roy, R. and Tunks, E. (Eds.) (1982) Chronic Pain: Psycho-social Factors in Rehabilitation. Williams & Wilkins, Baltimore.

Roy, R., Thomas, M. and Matas, M. (1984) Chronic pain and depression: a review. Comp. Psychiatr. 25, 96 – 105.

Shanfield, S. B., Heiman, E. M., Cope, D. M. and Jones, J. R. (1979) Pain and marital relationship: psychiatric distress. Pain 7, 343 – 351.

Sternbach, R. (1973) Chronic low-back pain: the low-back loser. Postgrad. Med. 53, 135 – 138.

Sternbach, R. (1974) Pain Patients: Traits and Treatment. Academic Press, New York, pp. 79 – 93.

Tunks, E. and Roy, R. (1982) Chronic pain and the occupational role. In: R. Roy and E. Tunks (Eds.), Chronic Pain: Psychosocial Factors in Rehabilitation. Williams & Wilkins, Baltimore, pp. 53 – 67.

Violon, A. (1982) The process involved in becoming a chronic pain patient. In: R. Roy and E. Tunks (Eds.), Chronic Pain: Psychosocial Factors in Rehabilitation. Williams & Wilkins, Baltimore, pp. 20 – 35.

Burrows/Elton/Stanley (eds.) Handbook of Chronic Pain Management
© *1987 Elsevier Science Publishers B.V. (Biomedical Division)*

23

The role of the nurse in chronic pain management

LAUREL ARCHER COPP

Carrington Hall, University of North Carolina, Chapel Hill, NC 27514, U.S.A.

The role of the nurse in chronic pain management

The role of the nurse is critical to the successful management of the patient experiencing chronic pain. Whereas that role may vary in the choice and options of treatment, the responsiveness and sensitivity of the nurse to the treatment goals facilitate or block effective pain management.

Patient's role perception

Who is the nurse to the patient in pain? In viewing that role from the pillow, patients tell us (Copp 1974) the nurse is seen in the following ways.

1) *Controller* – pain relief is in the purview and power of the nurse. Hence the nurse chooses to attend to or inattend to pain.
2) *Transporter* – although the nurse may feel she is doing only routine things when putting the patient on the cart and taking him to the treatment room, the patient sees her as transporting him to pain; and upon return, helping him escape from pain.
3) *Communicator* – the nurse is seen to tell others about the patient's pain, to interpret it, to validate if it is reasonable, and to give a judgemental commentary on the appropriateness of his bid for relief.
4) *Informant* – the pain patient decides if the nurse can be trusted with sensitive data related to his pain and his personal privacy. He reveals pain reluctantly which may be misread and interpreted as having no pain.
5) *Judge* – the nurse is seen to 'rule' if, in her opinion, the patient's pain is reasonable, timely, and stated in appropriate terms related to quality and quantity. The nurse is even seen as to go so far as to make verbal value judgements about the appropriateness of the patient's pain language and pain behavior.

6) *Avoider* – patients perceive staff to literally avoid patients who cannot report pain relief or appreciation for the care given.

7) *Empathizer* – the nurse lets the patient know she really understands because she too has had pain. In some cases the nurse may upstage his pain by self-report of those recalled experiences.

8) *Barterer* – like physicians and other therapists, nurses often are perceived to trade good care, quick attention to pain management relief in exchange for desired patient behavior.

Just as patients are stereotyped by nurses, the patient in pain may ascribe to nurses role perceptions not intended. Yet in perception there is a reality which may not be conductive to therapeutic pain management.

In a study of role perceptions of patients to nurses and nurses to patients some implications for care of the patient in pain are worthy of thought. In a sample of nurses ($n = 165$), they perceived the patient to be frightened dependent/complaining questioner; worried questioner/demanding protester/and bewildered endurer/asserting decision maker. Patients ($n = 101$) saw nurses as preoccupied medication givers/reassuring professionals; stern supervisors/controlling teacher-explainers; and concerned record keepers and firm medicine givers (Copp 1971). The seeds of power politics are evident.

'Inattending' to chronic pain

Because pain is subjective and experienced only by the sufferer, the nurse must infer pain. These inferences have been studied in various settings and during the process of nursing education (Davitz and Davitz 1981). In a series of studies it has been demonstrated that through their clinical curriculum nurses learn to attend to pain and a year later have learned to inattend to it. This is not a part of the agreed-upon regime to be followed by the staff as behavioral methods for chronic pain (Fordyce 1976). Rather it is a learned response more valued than maintaining the sensitive state required for responding to the patient in pain.

How to account for attention or inattention to pain? Researchers in this area urge investigation into a) nurses' beliefs regarding the degree to which patients are responsible for their illnesses; b) nurses' beliefs about what patients are capable of doing and; c) nurses' beliefs about the effectiveness of various therapeutic measures (Davitz et al. 1980).

Pain as stimulus

Traditionally, therapists interested in cure think of pain as stimulus and therefore are concerned with symptoms, measurements, diagnosis, treatment, and cure. The nurse may have come to see the role of pain in only these terms as well. If so, nurse behaviors focus on observation and careful reporting of symptoms, making sure that measurements are carefully recorded, and that lab tests are available for the physician making rounds. But, nurses may perceive themselves as facilitators of therapy, therefore arranging treatment rather than providing it. To the nurse involved in pain management of the patient with chronic pain, the purview of the pain experience and the nurse's role must be expanded.

Pain as response

As one studies the reponse the patient makes to pain, the larger dimensions of the pain experience and the meaning it holds for the patient is revealed. Assessment is in a broader context. Descriptors, pain language, pain history, pain coping history are all important ingredients. Pain management is the goal. To achieve this the nurse attempts to learn more about the experience through attempting to understand 'the view from the pillow'. Nurses do not tell patients how pain is to be manifested − they listen to those experiencing it, learn from it, and base their practice on the report of this subjective experience with re-validation from the source.

Reacting and responding

Reacting to the patient in pain is quite different from responding to him − to his experience − to his needs. A nurse reacting to the patient in pain may decide on an injection without ever assessing the pain or associated needs and problems. In so doing the nurse absents herself from the patient almost immediately after concurring with the presence of pain. Instead of asking about its nature, how long it has been present; without noting if there is concomitant stress, anxiety, or fear, the order sheet is sought and the pain medication delivered in a type of knee-jerk reaction. Even a moment spent in responding to the sufferer may provide data equally vital for pain relief and pain management. Nor are the alternatives mutually exclusive. There is assessment, therapeutic communication and touch, empowering transmission of concern and empathy, simultaneously with administration of medications.

The primary method of responding is to hear and analyze the nature of the pain patient's question. What is he really asking for? It may or may not be medication. It may be medication and more. Is it going to hurt? For how long? Where? How badly? What will the pain be like? Am I safe? Will the pain be unbearable? Can pain kill you? Can you be damaged for life from pain just as you can from a disease? What causes the pain? What does the pain mean? Am I in safe hands? What if I can't talk to describe the pain? What if nobody notices me? What if nobody comes? Can I stand it? What are the limits of my endurance? Will I be called upon to face that test? What kind of relief is available? What kind of relief is possible? Relief at what price?

Bellissimo states 'Patients regularly arrive in therapy demoralized, frightened, confused, and bankrupt of measures to sort out the problem themselves. They are not looking for a university education, but rather for someone to help make sense out of the problem and suggest a clear plan of action'. (Bellissimo and Tunks 1984).

Chronic pain differences

One might assume that pain relief is the presenting request of the patient in pain over time. The health team is committed to that goal. These special patients, however, may be fairly realistic in view of their long quest. What are they really asking? The Johnson assessment guide (Johnson 1977) reveals an important difference between assessment of acute and chronic pain which is especially helpful. What are the patient's expectations in relation to the pain? Does he want complete relief or just enough control to be able to pursue certain activities. What activities have a high priority for him?

In interpreting results of assessment and evaluation, we learn (McCaffery 1983) one must make some choices: i.e. comfort versus a pain-free state. Additionally the nurse is urged to recall the declining success of the chronic pain patient, the need to revise goals, and to confront the possibility of the patient's refusal to use effective pain-relief methods which might be offered. Chronic pain elicits what is thought by some to be patients who try one's patience. The nurse must recognize the no-win competition between patient's needs and nurse's needs. For both, important energy is sapped and effectiveness lessened. There may be overriding depression and hopelessness. A patient said, 'Suppose that you had an abcessed tooth and every dentist in the world had just died . . . that's what chronic intractable pain is like' (Hancock 1978).

Variety of roles

The nature of the role played by the nurse is determined by many things: setting, experience, academic credentials and license to practice, culture, community, administrators, fellow health team members (nurses, doctors, social workers, clergy, and a host of specialized therapists), as well as expectation of the sufferer and the family.

Rather than dwell on the constraints which some settings dictate, let us look at the functioning roles of nurses which are available in many countries. In settings where the expanded role of the nurse is accepted, the chronic pain patient, the family, and the health team benefit.

Nurse as therapist

In the generic sense one might ask if the nurse is not a therapist in all situations whether or not the designated therapist to which we will refer. Certainly any nurse relationship is therapeutic or has the potential to be so. But in some settings the nurse is indeed the designated therapist. This role may take its form in the Nurse Practitioner or Nurse Specialist − a role which requires extra study, testing, and credentials, and clinical study perhaps with a mentor or preceptor in the learning phase. A nurse with such preparation may work in the structured hospital, in clinics, in an office where multi-disciplinary therapists combine their practices. The range of settings in which nurses work as primary therapists varies from Cancer Centers to rural health. The nurse may be trained in relaxation techniques, imagery, biofeedback procedures, suggestion and hypnosis, and individual and group therapy.

Nurse as implementor of therapy

More traditional roles dictate the nurse as the implementor of therapy designed and designated by other therapists. For such a role to be therapeutic the therapist must communicate extensively about the goals of the therapy and the optimum conditions for success. Imperative as well is the nurse's skill in assessment, interpreting therapeutic goals, practicing nursing skills effectively, motivating nursing staff, learning the individual pain patient's needs, expectations, reactions, and repsonses to the therapy.

Nurse as evaluator of therapy

In the same manner the nurse assesses her own effectiveness and that of the staff; responses of patients to their therapy are data collected by those sharing the day's 24 hours with the client. This evaluation is intra-disciplinary and extra-disciplinary. As nurses report to each on-coming nursing staff at change of shift, evaluative data regarding the therapy and its effect is gathered for multidisciplinary sharing. A part of this data is feedback from the patient's point of view.

But evaluation must include more than corresponding through notes on the chart to doctors and others. Evaluation must be live, dynamic dialogue between doctor, nurse, and other members of the health care team. Such discussion will at times be confirming, validating, estimating, and represent consensus. Since the chronic pain patient is cared for over time it would be expected that there will be times when the interaction will consist of speculating, questioning, even challenging. Because patients with chronic pain may have already been at the mercy of a contradictory society and a progression of abandoned therapies and therapists, effective management will only come as a result of nurse-doctor consensus.

Nurse as negotiator

Because the management of the person in persistent pain often involves what may be perceived as too many individuals, the nurse is in a privileged position as negotiator. This is more than the 'go-between transmitting the latest message'. In settings where literal contracts are arrived at between therapist, staff, and sufferer, the basis for these contracts must be arrived at initially, evaluated, and perhaps modified at various phases of treatment. The patient may be unable or unwilling to speak for himself until trustable relationships are evolved. Arriving at such is as much a part of the nurse's responsibility and care plan as is delivering correct medications on time. And, it could have equally dramatic effects related to management of the patient experiencing chronic pain.

Nurse as advocate

Often the nurse is patient advocate which may have the effect of empowering and enabling the patient through careful building of his own skills in communicating his real feelings. The nurse may also be the doctor's advocate, the family's advocate, the therapist's advocate, etc. Such advocacy should not suggest taking sides or politicizing the environment. Rather it should be a voice for the vulnerable and in long-term care of the person in pain, every participant may at one time or another find himself in that situation and its attending powerlessness. In addition to the tyranny of the pain, there is the tyranny of the system, the setting, and/or the situation.

Nurse as care planner/giver

Professional nursing perceives its realm of practice as that of nursing care planning and nursing care giving. The terms are not in the care/cure dichotomy. Nurses professionally address the regretful practice contributed to neglectfully by many other health professionals – that of custodial care or warehousing.

Modern nursing rejects cues given to nurses to play roles which are not patient-centered and by which patients do not profit. Contrary to the prescriptive roles and dictates given it, nursing service is not a traffic coordinator, room service, a phone answering service, professional secretary and record-keeping service, or custodian. Nursing is responsible and accountable for nursing care on a 24 hour basis. In dealing with patients with problems of chronic pain, nurses plan and coordinate nursing care which is based on a therapeutic plan with goals and means of evaluation of the effectiveness of nursing care. Whether therapeutic goals are reached or not, nurses are accountable and may not evade responsibility to the patient in pain. If evaluation indicates nursing goals are not met, that care can be made more individualized, more effective, more therapeutic, it must be made so. Not to do so is considered by McCaffery (1983) and Copp (1985) to be unethical.

The nursing process

For those nurses educated in the nursing process, the implications for the client in pain are obvious. Using the work of Yura and Walsh (1973) the process includes assessing, planning, implementing, evaluating. Nursing care assessing is the act of reviewing a situation for the purpose of diagnosing the client's problems. Planning means to determine what can be done to assist the client perhaps involving setting goals, judging priorities, and designing methods to resolve problems. Implementation involves action − it is the phase in which the nurse initiates and completes the actions necessary to accomplish defined goals. Evaluation means to appraise the client's behavioral changes due to the actions of the nurse.

Nursing assessment

Nursing assessment of the patient in pain consists of obtaining a pain history and better understanding of the following important aspects of the chronic pain experience:

1) Previous pain experiences
2) Expectations of the nursing staff
3) Self-perceived and stated needs
4) Choice of pain language
5) What the client expects of the staff
6) Self-image and self expectation
7) Pain-coping strategies and practices
8) Effect of people on the pain
9) Dependency and need for empowering
10) Existence and strength of significant others
11) Perception of outcomes
12) Perception of the nurse's role

Assessment of the pain at this point in time may be a limited concept of pain assessment. The nurse is urged to keep in mind what is hypothesized by some to be a process of becoming a chronic pain patient (Roy and Tunks 1982). Assessment of the present situation should be put in a three tense context. What factors in the patient's past may be influencing the present pain picture? (early suffering, distortion of body perception, child abuse, or pain as a method of communication). What implications do today's pain situation have for the future? (depression, deinvestment in life, suicide).

Nursing intervention

Successful management will only result if the nurse considers the question 'Nursing intervention for what?' Important is not only the in-advance consideration of the variety of interventions available, but the probability of success of the outcomes. Intervention may include: pain relief, reinforcement, stress reduction, pain reduction, patient education, and other options.

A pain-free state may be an assumed goal. Will the intervention enhance relief? The unintended and unthinkable is that pain relief will be diminished, or delayed, or barriers to relief will be constructed.

Reinforcement of therapeutic behaviors is another desired intervention. But careful speculation of the desired outcome of the plan of the nursing staff must be thought through. What of the failure to reinforce therapeutic behaviors? What of the reinforcement of old counterproductive attitudes and approaches? Too often inadequate attention is given to the reinforcement of staff behaviors and staff revert to non-therapeutic habits, behaviors, opinions, and judgements. Only challenging ward politics and staff bias will provide conditions for reformulation of non-therapeutic attitudes and practices.

Stress reduction is a particularly salient approach to pain reduction. What is more, the nurse has a great deal of power to control stress. By failing to do so, the milieu may be most non-therapeutic to pain control. Two representative examples are pertinent.

1) *Waiting time*. Whether it be be waiting for a bus or waiting in a hospital waiting room, time fuels stress. Pressures of work, child care, or negative response to the environment seem to come to a focus. The nurse can see stress manifest itself in the patient kept waiting – and can attest to the complaints of increasing pain by those in the grip of time and powerlessness.

2) *Fear*. Also fueling stress, and pain, is fear. Though few pain patients may admit to fear, it seems an insidious process. Louis Evely states:

'What is unbearable is not to suffer, but to be afraid of suffering. To endure a precise pain, a definite loss, a hunger for something one knows – this is possible to bear. One can live with this pain. But in fear there is all the suffering in the world: to dread suffering is to suffer an infinite pain since one supposes it unbearable.'

Pain reduction is well within the nurse's power in most cases. There may be standing orders for relief. The nurse must know the patient as an individual, tailoring the dose, the timing, and the method of administering his medications. Nurses often do not appreciate they have both authority and responsibility to manage the patient in pain. By being too passive and compliant the patient's interest may not be best served. Cohen (1980) illustrated a research finding that whereas physicians tend to under-medicate surgical patients, hence not managing their pain, nurses tended to give less than permitted doses of pain reduction medication. We challenge nurses to see their role and responsibility in pain management. They are given an armamentarium they may not use adequately, appropriately, or fully. How many patients go home without ever knowing they had a pain medication ordered although they could have received something for their pain? Why did they not know? The nurse may not have told them. When queried why not, the nurse often answers 'Well, he didn't say he was in pain – he didn't ask for anything'.

In an opposite circumstance, nurses often state their feelings of helplessness. The patient is begging for something for pain 'but the doctor hasn't left any orders'. In addition to assertive behavior which may produce the order from the doctor, the nurse may well be reminded of the many other alternatives available apart from and in addition to medications. If, as we have suggested, stress, fear, and anxiety can worsen the pain experience, the nurse can plot counter-strategies to reduce pain by stress reduction and the allaying of fear.

Patient education should be a natural extension of nursing intervention. Included in factors to consider (Miller 1983) are work on self-concept improvement (integrate body image change into positive concept of self); develop patient's knowledge about the health problem and treatment; explore how the problem and treatment will affect the patient's life; provide patient-specific instruction; and collaborate with the patient on tailoring the regimen. There is a growing number of nursing research studies which demonstrate the effect of patient teaching. The skillful transmission of information is seen as a prescription against pain (Hayward 1975).

Vital continuing education for nurses is updated knowledge of current pain-reducing drugs and their many proprietary names. There is a need for constant review of approximate equivalent doses of narcotics and analgesics. Safety indicates study of common combinations of drugs. Beyond safety is the understanding of compatibility and/or synergistic effect of medications which maximize pain relief. Nurses may well question and revise timing of medications if the basis for time of administration is arbitrary or ward ritual. Unnecessary interruption of the pain patient for convenience of the staff is intolerable and often is not intentional yet goes unanalyzed and uncorrected.

Pain bias and misconception

There seems to be a great deal of stress building in the frustrating process of not being believed. Nurses in pain experience tremendously similar feelings when they are patients. These include guilt and anger. One nurse said, 'I felt helpless, angry, embarrassed. Nurses aren't supposed to get sick much less hurt. I felt guilty to bother people. I felt resentful because the condescending attitude that was shown me told me they really didn't believe the pain was as bad as I had reported. If they didn't want to believe me why did they ask for my description of the nature and intensity of the pain?. I felt diminished as a person'.

Fifteen years ago Hackett posed the question 'Why do we doubt that the patient is in pain?' (Hackett 1971). He addressed our pre-judgement of the patient in pain regarding the issues of addiction, placebos, and malingering. In addition to these points we ask nurses who are interested in assessing and changing their nursing practice of pain patients to consider what effect have their opinions and resultant actions related to the following myths and biases:

As a nurse too you believe that:

1) Males or females have predictable pain behaviors by virtue of gender?
2) The acute pain model is the only criterion for assessment of the patient in pain?
3) Every patient is a potential addict?
4) To be legitimate pain must be evidenced by a measurable or demonstrable change (lab test, X-ray, cell change, etc)?
5) Patients tend to lie about their pain (exaggerate or deny)?
6) The same dose of medication over the same time frame (i.e. 100 mg every 4 hours) applies to most patients?

7) Pain transcends individual differences?
8) Pain relief by demand is a better care plan than consistent pain medication?
9) Consistent, repeated doses of pain medication are more dangerous than a p.r.n. mode of drug administration?
10) Patients cannot be trusted to take their own medications?
11) In general, physicians tend to over-medicate patients?
12) Children to not feel pain or cannot express pain trustably?

Each of the above is a distortion of the truth. In most cases a reliable amount of data exists to refute the point of view. In many cases there is extensive writing on the points. For example, Eland (1985) writes of the role of the nurse in children's pain. In what has been called 'Old Nurses' Tales' (Eland and Anderson 1977) mis-assumptions and mis-conceptions about a child in pain include the following:

a) Children's nerves aren't the same as adults.
b) If you give narcotics to children they will become addicted.
c) Narcotics always depress respiration.
d) Children cannot tell you where they hurt.
e) Active children cannot hurt.
f) Children tell the truth about pain.
g) Shots aren't such a bad thing.
h) Parents know all the answers about their children's pain.
i) If they won't cooperate − use restraint.

In each case, Eland disputes these mis-conceptions by giving evidence and data. For example, in a recent study (Porter and Jick 1980), it was reported out of 11,882 adults and children being treated for pain, only four became addicted.

Bases for comparison

Therapeutic nursing practice is jeopardized when bases for comparing patients in pain cannot be justified. There are basic assumptions, years in the making, that nudge nurses into believing that one diagnosis hurts more than another. In breaking these perceptions it is a useful exercise to ask nurses to list in rank order what diagnoses urge emergency consideration of narcotics in their practice settings. Just as interesting as those commanding diagnoses are the rankings near the bottom of the list. Once this de-valued pain is identified nurses sheepishly admit to thinking 'I don't know why she is making such a fuss, she only suffers from . . .'. Yet, this hierarchy of 'allowable pain' is learned by emulation, through studying prescribing behaviors of physicians, and non-questioning attitudes due to social pressure.

Another non-justified comparison is that of two patients with the same diagnosis. After more careful thought we realize that the diagnosis, migraine for example may be the least thing two migraine patients have in common. They may vary in: length and frequency of hospitalization, prescriptions, behavior, presenting complaints, age, culture, education, work, economic status, roles, etc.

Most conducive to productive pain assessment is comparing one pain experience to another in the same individual. This can be done while taking a pain history and the patient is able to put the present pain experience in context. Advantages in comparing the patient to himself are that one is dealing with one sensorium, one life experience, one value system, one culture, one personality, one socio-economic status, etc. After exploration of the various apects of pain experience, the nurse learns the dimensions of the experience including patient-valued coping mechanisms.

Pain coping and the nurse's role

We use Lipowski's definition of a coping style as an individual's enduring disposition to deal with challenges and stresses with a specific constellation of techniques and coping strategies as the techniques actually used by the individual to deal with illness and its consequences (Lipowski 1970). We have examined several hundred patients' self reports of coping mechanisms (Copp 1974). In subsequent years, and expanding the sample to include chronic pain patients, we learned that patients describe their coping as having external and internal foci.

External foci include:

1) the use of counter-pain (my word to denote the inflicting of additional pain or pressure by the sufferer in a nearby site or related area, i.e. pounding, biting, rubbing);
2) other muscle use such as rocking, pacing;
3) use of the presence of people to play such roles as witness, strength-lender, runner-reporter, verbal monitor, etc;
4) the use of comfort and pain objects, i.e. chair, clothing, food, etc.

Internally focused copers seem to use many variations on the concept of vigilant focusing. In this sample the most used in rank order included: 1) mathematics or counting; 2) memorized words, or words repeated many times; 3) mental visualization. These consisted of such strategies as reviewing routes of travel, replay of conversations, mental needlepoint, household chores done mentally, etc.

One woman this author interviewed reported 'when the pain becomes intolerable I concentrate on taking my husband to work'. When asked to share verbally with this researcher what that entailed she agreed to do so. When the pain increased she stated:

'I see my husband standing in the middle of the room, getting ready to leave the house. First he checks his back pocket to be sure he has his keys. Then he closes the front door firmly and walks down the steps toward the bus stop. He waits there several minutes. When the bus arrives, he steps up one step, two steps, and reaches into his pocket. Today he has four coins and puts them in the container. He finds a seat in the third row on the aisle. Now the bus is passing the intersection of Main and 74th street, 73rd street, 72nd street; 71st street, 70th street . . .'

In all ill-timed and unfortunate interruption, I said to the patient in pain, 'My, that must take you a long time!' The patient opened her eyes, and said confidently, 'Oh, yes, and if the pain is still there I bring him home again!'

That interaction taught that pain patients who must tolerate pain over time not only dip into a rich well of personal resources in order to cope, but those very coping mechanisms are 'expandable' and 'contractable'. They can be fashioned to the current pain experience. Whereas upon admission, patients may be asked to give up their clothing, their dentures, their jewelry, the pain-coping mechanism is gratifyingly internal, portable and personal.

Other internal focus coping mechanisms manifested by patients in pain include visualization of mind-body separation. They also report spatial relationships with pain. 'I am here − the pain is over there . . . sometimes I get so tired of it chasing me'. Another patient explained, 'Sometimes I can't get relief until I just submit to pain − it's like a cloud between me and relief. It is only when I go through it and come out the other side, I can finally relax'.

A number of patients exhibited something this author refers to as tropistic yearning. Some patients in pain seem to have an inordinate need to 'feel the sun on my back − then I could stand the pain' or to touch earth or growing things or 'just to hear the sea'. Patients also reported a change in their dream patterns and often wanted to discuss the dreams with nurses.

Implications for nursing care and management

It is obvious if the patient copes using the external mode, the very circumstances of a busy ward − people, attention, interruption, conversation, movement, all present types of distraction the patient may choose to use in his coping. He may fix upon some aspect of ward routine, his neighbor, the passing parade of health professionals, patients, and visitors and find therapeutic distraction from the presence of pain.

But to the internally focused patient experiencing pain, the hospital or busy clinic may intensify his pain, may exacerbate it, may push him past his endurance. Vigilant focusing requires concentration, control of the setting, management of space, traffic and visitor control. In order to insure pain management, the nurse's role is enlarged, therapeutically to protect the environment, to influence the milieu. Having some power over the setting, but inadequate for complete control, the nurse must assess the pain patient's methods of coping and coping needs. The vigilant focuser finds interruption a barrier to the use of internal resources he could otherwise utilize. Protecting his privacy is vital. Even inquiring about the pain is a substantial interruption, inviting pain rather than the well-intentioned concern and caring.

Pain-coping model

Pain is an individual and private experience. One is loath to compartmentalize or make generalizations. Yet, for the understanding of nurses attempting to deal with large numbers of patients, only some of whom are in chronic pain, the pain-coping model shared here has seemed to present some assistance.

Over years of observation and attempting to match pain language, self image, and coping styles, the following types of pain/sufferer postures have evolved (Copp 1985, see Table 1)

POSTURE NO. 1

The pain is perceived by the patient to be all-powerful. Its authority is evidenced both in severity and duration. The sufferer perceives himself to be a victim and is increasingly passive. Implications to the nursing staff are many. He may use coping strategies flaccidly, if at all − is skeptical, engages in magical thinking, some ritualistic behavior, and believes he is fated for pain. Nursing staff are often rebuffed when trying to support through the teaching of coping strategies which seem to be effective for other pain patients. Since he feels fragile, helpless, abandoned, and alone, the nurse may try methods of empowering and supporting him. But when the pain returns he often reinforces himself by making sure it is understood 'See . . . it didn't help'. Pain is interpreted as merciless, overwhelming, continuous.

POSTURE NO. 2

The pain is perceived as invading. Therefore the patient fashions himself as a combatant – he analyzes, strategizes, confronts, and fights the pain. Oddly, and conversely, he may take a stoic posture – waiting pain out – holding it at bay. Usually he takes inventory of his armamentarium, uses counterpain, assigns pain tasks to himself and delegates to 'his army' – the nursing staff, of course. He is not pleased with insubordination – just as the nurse may be unwilling to literally 'let him call the shots'. In those cases where patient and nurse join forces, overcoming pain together builds a strong alliance.

TABLE 1
Copp-coping model (from Copp 1985 with permission).

Posture	Language	Self-situation	Coping
No. 1 Pain = powerful Coper = passive victim	Merciless Cosmic Overwhelming Continuous Irrevocable Irreparable Irrational	Fragile Helpless Dread-filled Abandoned Alone Suffering	Skepticism Fate Ritual Magic
No. 2 Pain = invading Coper = combatant	Episodic Strong Sharp Dominating Testing	Fighter Coper Survivor Soldier Confronter	Counterpain Muscle language Delegates Assigns tasks Armamentarium
No. 3 Pain = reality Coper = responsive	Testing Demanding Mysterious Hidden Cosmic	Confronter Endurer Suffering Analyzing Strategizing	Meditating Focusing Searching for meaning
No. 4 Pain = cunning Coper = reactive	Hidden Faceless Sneaky Sly Invading Degrading	Watcher Waiter Monitor Vigilant Ready	Anticipating Rehearsal Review Early warning Not risking Avoidance
No. 5 Pain = demanding Coper = consumer	Intense Persistent Sharp Probing Treacherous Ill-tempered Strong	Cooperator Collaborator Communicator Contractor Dependent Reporter Consumer	Contractual Arrangement Permission Compliant Bonding Rule keeper Sets limits

Posture no. 3

Pain is not perceived as a problem but a mystery, a reality. The sufferer attempts to be responsive to it, to understand its present and potential and perhaps even its perennial meaning. He confronts and endures. He meditates on the pain as well as the meaning of the pain experience. He searches for meaning of it long after he is pain free.

Posture no. 4

Pain is seen to be cunning. It may evidence itself in sly and sneaky ways. It is hidden and faceless. Therefore the sufferer must be ready to react to it — the patient in pain must watch, wait, be always ready. Even pain medication is rejected because it clouds the sensorium and makes him ripe for invasion. He asks others to help him rehearse for pain, anticipate it. He will give nurses early warning in a strong attempt to avoid full-blown pain. His face signals pain with a look of alarm, super-alertness, and impending panic. Nursing staff must empower him and realize even a suggestion of things to try for relief will be viewed as risky in time of danger.

Posture no. 5

Pain is seen as demanding and the sufferer does not so much interact with pain as with the staff. Pain is very sharp, intense, persistent. He views himself as a reasonable individual making rational and reasonable requests of the nursing staff. He is most willing to keep his word, carry out his end of the bargain, if they too will enter in to a pain pact and keep their contracts. He sets limits and keeps the rules. He expects the staff to enter into arrangements with him that will reduce pain. He is a consumer and believes that he has the right to ask for this type of nursing care and pain management. When he and the staff carry out a plan to mutually agreeable ends he is appreciative, bonds with them, and may even introduce them with pride as 'my nurse' and 'my doctor'.

In the pain model, grouping should not be seen as mutually exclusive or as predictable. The model is to assist the nurse in the understanding of the the patient's perception of pain and his ability to deal with it. It is intended to reveal patient and staff opportunities for understanding and cooperation toward the therapeutic goals of care.

Types of pain experiences

Looking at various types of pain provides a nursing context for chronic pain. The nurse may wish to consider the variety of pain he/she has attended, and see the salient features of chronic pain.

It is unlikely that either nurse or client have experienced life without some prior pain experience. Types may include the following.

Life pain

The nurse as well as the client may be experiencing some life pain . . . loss, grief, divorce, disillusionment, abuse, abandonment . . . all thought to play some part in 'pain proneness' (Roy et al. 1982). If such life pain is significant in the nurse's life, there are unexplored but we hypothesize crucial effects on the nurse-patient relationship.

DISEASE ASSOCIATED PAIN

Pain as an effect of disease process figures largely in the curriculum of health professionals. Learning which may serve well in acute illness becomes somewhat a barrier to understanding when the nurse has no working diagnosis as a base for the nursing care plans of chronic pain patients. The concept of algopathia is confounding and chronic pain syndrome requires a new type of learning.

THERAPY INITIATED PAIN

When the chemotherapy, radiation, or manipulation is over, it is the nurse who is confronted with a patient who may suffer from the effects of the therapy in addition to the pain associated with the disease. Bedside attendance to that pain throughout the evening and night requires special nursing skills and complicates pain management. Further, this type of pain has a commonality with chronic pain, namely, the variable of time.

TERMINAL PAIN

In caring for the terminally ill patient, the fruitlessness of therapy, the torture of care, and the prolongation of the dying process are expressed freely by patients. Changing the goals, modifying the regime, curtailing procedures planned as part of learning in teaching centers are suggestions often initiated by the nurse in order to reach pain control. Enhanced will be conditions for a good death, open communication with loved ones, and a clear sensorium to conduct business, meditate, or appreciate beauty.

NURSING CARE INITIATED PAIN

In the same way that therapy may initiate pain, something both patient and nurse may wish to avoid, the nurse may be perceived as the bringer of pain. Interpreting nursing care as preventative in the larger view may bring little comfort to those who struggle with what must be done, and quiescent pain, pain held at bay, rushes in. Nursing management of that pain requires anticipation, skill and interpretation. The most simple requests may seem overwhelming to the patient, i.e. ambulation, turning, or treatments. In many cases the nurse must lend energy to a depleted patient through timing, encouragement, and adapting nursing care to his speed and wishes.

RESEARCH RELATED PAIN

Many health professions teaching centers have large programs of ongoing research. Therapy is experimental and acknowledged to be so. Informed consent includes assisting the patient to know what to expect. However, when he asks 'Will it hurt?', or 'Will it hurt more?' even the most conscientious investigator may just not know. To state otherwise spoils the milieu and encourages feelings antithetical to trust and pain management – fear, blame, and distrust associated with perceived deception. Pain and hope are studied in balance.

FOREGOING TREATMENT

'No treatment' certainly does not mean 'no pain'. Actually, it may mean increased pain, delayed pain, unattended pain. The client who elects not to participate in available treatment is unstudied and often misunderstood. He may not appear at the pain clinic assuming that he has been written off as ineligible for treatment since he declined offered treatment. As a result he often is a missing client – and only in crisis is the health team forced to confront his legitimate right to pain management.

ACUTE PAIN

Using the acute pain model so routinely it subtly is assumed by the nurse to be the only pain model, and becomes a barrier to therapeutic care of the patient exhibiting other types of pain – chronic, persistent, terminal, etc. As a result the nurse caring for patients with chronic pain may have to adjust, alter, modify, and change nursing practice. A re-examination of the assumptions on which the nursing practice is based must be entered into with the possible risk and the discomfort of inevitable, self-initiated change.

CHRONIC PAIN

Patients themselves often ask us to use another word to substitute for chronic. For the care-giver the word is technical and not judgemental. However, as one patient writes 'Never use the word chronic – persistent is better' (Wolf 1977). She tells with the emotion of experience the feelings associated with being labeled 'a chronic' by doctors and nurses.

Fortunately nurses are coming to see rewarding professional potential in electing chronic pain settings and patients as their life's work. These nurses work in hospitals, in home care, in pain clinics, or with specific therapists. They extend their assessment expertise to addressing the pain of specific populations: the elderly, children, war veterans and war victims, the prisoner, minorities, the abused, and those whose specific afflictions (patients with migraine, trigeminal neuralgia, back pain, etc) have yet to be successfully addressed and managed. Some nurses elect to work with patients who can find no relief. They intentionally take on this pain.

References

Anderson, M. (1977) Assessment of clinical pain. In: A. Jacox (Ed.), Pain: a Sourcebook for Nurses and other Health Professionals. Little, Brown, Boston, pp. 159 – 160.

Bellisimo, A. and Tunks, E. (1984) Chronic Pain: The Psychotherapeutic Spectrum. Praeger Scientific, New York.

Cohen, F. (1980) Postsurgical pain relief: patient status and nurse medication choices. Pain 9, 265 – 274.

Davitz, L. and Davitz, J. (1981) Inferences of patients' pain and psychological distress. Springer, New York, pp. 119 – 132.

Davitz, L., Davitz, J. and Rubin, C. (1980) Nurses' Responses to Patient's Suffering. Springer, New York, pp. 131 – 132.

Copp, L. A. (1971) A projective cartoon investigation of nurse-patient psychodramatic role perception and expectation. Nursing Res. 20, 100 – 112.

Copp, L. A. (1974) The spectrum of suffering. Am. J. Nursing 74, 63 – 67.

Copp, L. A. (1985) Chapter 1: Pain coping, p. 19; Chapter 9: Pain, ethics, and the negotiation of values, p. 138. In: Perspectives on Pain. Churchill Livingstone, Edinburgh.

Eland, J. (1985) The role of the nurse in children's pain. In: Perspectives on Pain. Churchill Livingstone, Edinburgh, pp. 34 – 40.

Eland, J. and Anderson, J. (1977) The experience of children's pain. In: A. Jacox (Ed.), Pain: A Sourcebook for Nurses and Other Health Professionals. Little, Brown, Boston, pp. 453 – 473.

242

Evely, L. (1967) Suffering. Herder and Herder, N.Y., pp. 152–153.

Fordyce, W. (1976) Behavioral methods for chronic pain and illness. Mosby, St. Louis, p. 105.

Hackett, T. (1971) Pain and prejudice: why do we doubt that the patient is in pain? Med. Times 99, 130–141.

Hancock, E. (1978) I didn't want to face another day of pain. Johns Hopkins Magazine, Baltimore, Maryland, 14–24.

Hayward, J. (1975) Information – a prescription against pain. Royal College of Nursing, London.

Johnson, M. (1977) Assessment of clinical pain. In: A. Jacox (Ed.), Pain: A Sourcebook for Nurses and Other Health Professionals. Little, Brown, Boston, pp. 159–160.

Lipowski, Z.J. (1970) Physical illness, the individual and the coping process. Psychiatry Med 1, 91–101.

McCaffery, M. (1983) Pain: A Nursing Approach to Assessment and Analysis. Appleton-Century-Crofts, Norwalk, Connecticut, pp. 353–355.

Miller, J. (1983) Coping with Chronic Illness: Overcoming Powerlessness. F. A. Davis, Philadelphia, p. 244.

Porter, J. and Jick, H. (1980) Addiction rare in patients treated with narcotics. N. Engl. J. Med. 302, 123.

Violon, A. (1982) The process involved in becoming a chronic pain patient. In: R. Roy and E. Turks (Eds.), Chronic Pain – Psychosocial Factors in Rehabilitation. Williams & Wilkins, Philadelphia, pp. 20–35.

Wolf, B. (1977) Living with Pain. Seabury Press, N.Y., pp. 23–24.

Yura, H. and Walsh, M. (1973) The Nursing Process, 2nd edn. Appleton-Century-Crofts, N.Y., pp. 26–31.

Burrows/Elton/Stanley (eds.) Handbook of Chronic Pain Management
© 1987 Elsevier Science Publishers B.V. (Biomedical Division)

24

The role of the physical therapist in chronic pain management

JO CLELLAND[1], EMILY SAVINAR[2] and KATHERINE F. SHEPARD[3]

[1]Division of Physical Therapy, School of Community and Allied Health, The University of Alabama at Birmingham, Birmingham, AL 35294, [2]Department of Physical Therapy, Kaiser Permanente Medical Center, Oakland, CA 94611, and [3]Division of Physical Therapy, Stanford University School of Medicine, Stanford, CA 94305, U.S.A.

Introduction

Patients are often referred to physical therapists (physiotherapists) by physicians for evaluation and treatment of chronic pain. The physical therapist may be providing care in a physical therapy outpatient clinic or be one of many health care providers in a multidisciplinary pain management program. Often before the physical therapist sees the patient, the patient has already been evaluated and treated by many health care practitioners. The patient may have several different diagnoses which have been treated with an array of surgeries, medications, psychotherapies, physical modalities and acupuncture or chiropractic treatments. The purposes of this chapter are to present the role of the physical therapist in evaluation of patients with chronic pain, briefly discuss treatment interventions which have proven successful and comment on the role of the physical therapist in chronic pain research.

Evaluation

The evaluation of each patient in chronic pain is vital to determining whether there is a specific mechanical pathology present which may be amenable to physical therapy interventions such as mobilization, friction massage or acupressure. Alternatively, and more commonly, chronic pain is present in the generic sense and the physical therapist will work closely with the patient and other health care team members to help the patient live a more pain-free life through the use of relaxation training, general physical conditioning programs, and education directed at decreasing sedentary lifestyles.

The physical therapy evaluation process consists of three components: assessment of musculoskeletal, neuromuscular and related systems dysfunction, identification of specific goals for the patient, and selection of a treatment plan to achieve the specific goals. The evaluation also yields valuable information concerning the patient's willingness to participate in his or her health care.

The physical therapy evaluation consists of a subjective (history) and objective (physical) exam. The subjective exam is a patient interview which generally takes between 15 and 30 minutes (see Fig. 1). Data are collected regarding the area of pain, the behavior of the pain and general health information which may affect the patient's complaint or the treatment of the complaint

PHYSICAL THERAPY RECORD

1. Age, Sex, Occupation: _____

   _____

2. Behavior of Pain: (see *Body Chart*) _____

   _____

   What aggravates symptoms _____

   _____

   What eases symptoms _____

   _____

   How does pain change over 24 hours ___

   _____

   Sleep Behavior _____

   _____

3. Medical Data:

   X-rays _____ General Health _____

   Medication _____ Steroids _____

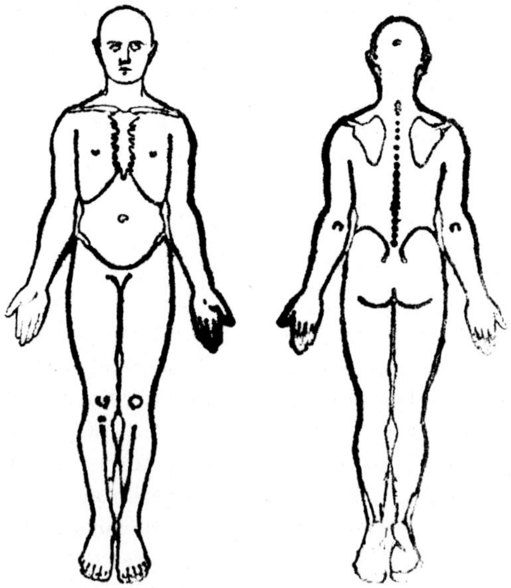

4. Special Questions:

   Cauda Equina (bowel/bladder dysfunction) _____

   _____

   Cord (bilateral numbness hands or feet) _____

   Unexplained weight loss _____

5. History (date of onset, progression of symptoms, intervention)

   Present Hx _____

   Past Hx _____

Body Chart: Record area of pain or complaint, area of paresthesias, anesthesias. Describe the quality of pain (e.g. intermittent or constant, sharp, burning, ache).

Fig. 1. Subjective musculoskeletal/neuromuscular and related systems exam.

including current and past health history, current medications and radiographic findings. A chronological history of the complaint, which includes the perceived cause and the progression of symptoms, is recorded. All treatment given to the patient since the onset of the complaints and the benefit the patient received from each type of treatment is also noted. The patient's medical records should be reviewed before proceeding with the objective exam to verify and add to the subjective exam. Any contraindications or precautions relating to the physical therapy exam or treatment are noted at this time. At the end of the subjective exam, the therapist knows the patient's perception of the severity, irritability and nature of the complaint as well as evaluative information recorded by other health care personnel. The objective exam will be modified according to this data base.

The musculoskeletal objective exam is a physical examination of the painful site and the structures that may refer pain and/or paresthesia to the site (Fig. 2). The exam begins with an observation of the patient. Posture, musculoskeletal asymmetries, structural deformities and the patient's willingness to move are noted. Active, passive and active resisted movements of relevant trunk and limb joints are performed and the patient's range of motion, strength and subjective response to these movements are recorded. Based on the area of pain and/or paresthesias, deep tendon reflexes, sensation and plantar responses are assessed and recorded. Relevant structures are palpated for muscle spasm, joint and soft tissue stiffness, tenderness and atrophy.

The patient's ability to relax during the objective exam is also recorded. Often the patient with chronic pain exhibits constant muscle tension in selected muscle groups and an inability to 'let go' and generate a relaxation response. Other specific tests may be added to the evaluation if

1. Observation (posture, willingness to move, atrophy)	7. Passive movements – (physiological and accessory)
2. Active movement	
3. Static tests (resistive tests of specific muscles)	8. Palpation (temperature, soft tissue mobility)
4. Clear other joints (active and static tests of joints and soft tissues that may refer to the painful site)	9. Blood pressure, H.R., pulses
5. Dural tension signs (e.g. leg raises, prone knee bend)	10. Fitness level (duration of walking with HR and BP guidelines)
6. Neurological exam (DTR, strength, sensation, Babinski)	11. Special tests

ASSESSMENT

PROBLEM LIST

GOALS

PLAN

Fig. 2. Objective musculoskeletal and related systems exam.

indicated such as dura tension tests, ligamentous laxity tests, blood flow assessment and gait analysis.

A neuromuscular objective exam will be performed if the patient has residual neuromuscular dysfunction secondary to a neurologic insult such as cerebrovascular accident, spinal cord injury, head trauma, or multiple sclerosis (see Fig. 3). The primary focus of this exam is to assess voluntary motor control and level of independence in functional activities. Often a patient who has suffered a cerebrovascular accident has a complaint of chronic shoulder pain and it is necessary to assess both the musculoskeletal and neuromuscular dysfunction in order to select a treatment that affects the appropriate structures involved in generating pain. For example, treatment of adhesive capsulitis of the shoulder is quite different from treatment for a subluxed humeral head secondary to lack of motor control following a stroke.

In addition to the musculoskeletal and neuromuscular exam, the chronic pain patient is often suffering from poor cardiovascular fitness secondary to a lack of physical activity. Blood

1. Observation	11. Weight bearing and posture
2. Cognition (orientation to person, place, time)	12. Ambulation and gait deviation
3. Vision (gross visual fields deficits)	
4. Speech (gross speech dysfunctions)	13. Strength
5. Cardiopulmonary (blood pressure, heart rate and fitness level)	14. Sensation (pain/temp., proprioception, touch)
6. Pain (complete musculoskeletal exam)	
7. Passive ROM	15. Cerebellar (rapid alternating movements)
8. Tone and deep tendon reflexes	
9. Primitive reflexes	16. Righting and equilibrium
10. Motor control/synergies/selected voluntary movement	
17. Functional activities (e.g. rolling, supine <--> sit, sit <--> stand, transfers)	
18. Skin (e.g. breakdown)	19. Cranial/bulbar (mastication and deglutition)

ASSESSMENT

PROBLEM LIST

GOALS

PLAN

Fig. 3. Objective neuromuscular and related systems exam.

pressure and heart rate are part of the objective exam as well as a functional cardiovascular fitness test.

GOALS

Physical therapy goals are based on the patient's status as determined by objective and subjective exams and the patient's expressed needs. Mutually agreeing on realistic, functional measurable goals provides a contractual relationship that helps to ensure mutual responsibility for outcome. It is helpful to communicate with other health care team members who have evaluated the patient's physical and psychological health before setting goals with the patient in order to insure that the goals are realistic.

Specific changes in subjective and objective findings which are measurable are used in setting goals. A patient who states on subjective exam that he can sit only 5 minutes or walk only one block due to back pain, may agree to goals of increasing sitting endurance to 30 minutes and walking eight blocks. Increased range of motion, strength, or improved cardiovascular fitness may be used as objective goals. Specific short-term goals (measured in weeks) are necessary for the patient to achieve in order to realize long-term goals (measured in months) such as returning to work. Depending on the patient's ability to achieve a succession of short-term goals, long-term goals are modified accordingly. The patient who has been unable to work for one year secondary to constant back and leg pain is being unrealistic to expect to participate in downhill ski competition after 2 months of treatment. To encourage unrealistic goal setting is setting up the patient for failure and setting up the therapist for frustration and burn out.

TREATMENT PLAN

Based on the subjective and objective evaluation, the physical therapist identifies the pain and concomitant musculoskeletal and neuromuscular dysfunction which may be responsive to physical therapy interventions. Problems of dysfunction may include pain, selected joint and soft tissue stiffness, selected weakness, muscular instability and imbalance, muscle spasm, abnormal gait, abnormal posture, decreased selective voluntary movement and decreased independence in functional activities. Poor cardiovascular fitness and the inability to generate a relaxation response may also be recorded as problems. Although these secondary problems may not be causing the patient's pain, they may be contributing to poor pain management.

The treatment plan addresses the problems listed in the assessment and is specifically directed towards achieving the patient's goals. Selection of a particular treatment modality, for example, mobilization, heat or cold, biofeedback, exercise, or acupressure is dependent upon the needs of the patient and the therapist's expertise. Certain treatment techniques require a great deal of patient-therapist interaction and individual instruction. Other interventions require an initial patient contact followed by independent work done by the patient that is periodically monitored by the therapist. In addition, some treatment techniques require elaborate equipment that may or may not be available to the physical therapist.

It is important to allow the patient to realize his ability to manage his pain. If the patient who needs fitness training is convinced that coming into a physical therapy department and riding a stationary bicycle is the only way that he can train aerobically, he becomes dependent on the health care system to maintain his optimal level of fitness. If on the other hand, the same patient learns how to train aerobically by vigorous walking and monitoring his own heart rate he can 'own' this skill and take responsibility for managing this aspect of his personal health.

Occasionally, it is difficult to identify the source of pain in a patient. The subjective and objective exams may be incongruent or the patient's pain may not be reproduced during the physical examination. The patient may, in fact, be free of musculoskeletal or neuromuscular dysfunction and the complaint of pain may come from other physical or psychological sources. For this type of patient, emphasis on pain management through cardiovascular fitness, instruction in posture and activities of daily living and relaxation training are strongly emphasized.

We should note that some patients with chronic pain will not benefit at all from physical therapy intervention. These patients often have a combination of characteristics that lead therapists to predict an unfavorable outcome. These characteristics include:

1) The subjective and objective exams are inconsistent.
2) The patient demonstrates an unwillingness to follow through with home exercises and posture instructions.
3) The patient's goals are unrealistic and vary greatly from the physical therapist's.
4) Litigation is pending.
5) The patient is not willing or interested in returning to work.

Patients who demonstrate several or more of these characteristics should be identified early and short-term goals assessed weekly. If any patient does not achieve his or her short-term goals, the physical therapy plan should be reviewed. The therapist may need to re-evaluate the patient to verify the initial assessment of the patient's status. The patient's lack of success with physical therapy intervention may also be due to the therapist's lack of expertise in performing a particular treatment, limited repertoire of treatment techniques or poor communication with the patient and family. A consultation on the patient's physical therapy management by another physical therapist is often useful at this point. If the physical therapist has used all her or his skill and a consulting physical therapist has no further suggestions, termination of physical therapy should be considered and discussed with the referring physician.

Treatment

Physical therapists employ a variety of techniques in the treatment of chronic pain. Physical therapy approaches to management of pain secondary to identifiable pathology are based, for the most part, on the premise that the treatment procedure will alter the vicious cycle of pain. For example, an injury that causes pain in a specific joint leads to protective muscle spasm; the spasm will lead ultimately to partial occlusion of the vessels in the area with a build-up of metabolic end products and eventual ischemia; both lack of oxygen and increased metabolites are stimuli for pain receptors; as the pain increases, the spasm increases, and the vicious pain cycle ultimately leads to dysfunction.

Based on their subjective and objective findings, physical therapists may attempt to treat the dysfunction directly or attempt to relieve pain phenomena. Some techniques attempt to reverse the pain cycle by increasing the blood supply to the area. Use of heat for increasing blood supply, decreasing pain, and increasing relaxation is widely accepted. Heat is most often applied via moist hot packs, paraffin baths, whirlpool baths, infrared radiating sources, ultrasound, microwave and shortwave diathermy. The application of cold generally elicits the same physiologic effects as heat except for the initial phase of vasoconstriction. Cryotherapy may be given via ice packs, ice massage, cold baths and vapocoolant sprays such as ethyl chloride and fluorimethane. Lehmann and DeLateur (1982) have discussed the uses of therapeutic heat and cold in detail.

Soft tissue massage is another approach to pain management and the effectiveness also is attributed, in part, to the increase in circulation to an area. Stroking massage movements elicit a direct effect on circulation (Wood and Becker 1981). Friction massage usually is aimed toward restoration of mobility and extensibility of specific soft tissues (Kessler 1983) (see Fig. 4). However, an increase in extensibility may also allow for a secondary increase in circulation. The effects of massage on pain also may be related to sensory input along the large diameter fibers that transmit tactile input which may inhibit the smaller pain fibers via the 'gate' in the region of the dorsal horn of the spinal cord as proposed by Melzack and Wall (1965). Massage movements that are limited to skin overlying acupuncture points may be referred to as acupressure which presumably elicits some of the same beneficial effects as acupuncture and acupuncture-like transcutaneous electrical nerve stimulation (TENS) (Tappan 1978; Chan 1982; Yao 1984) which will be discussed in the next few pages. Tappan (1978) has discussed in detail the variations of massage techniques. Mechanical vibration is another form of sensory stimulation that has been reported to relieve both acute and chronic pain (Melzack 1983; Hansson and Ekblom 1981, 1983; Ottoson et al. 1981; Lundeberg et al. 1983, 1984; Melzack and Wall 1983; Lundeberg 1984). Recent research indicates that vibration may successfully alleviate chronic low back pain, orofacial pain, central pain, myalgia, pain from rheumatoid arthritis, tendinitis, epicondylitis, and phantom limb (Russell and Spalding 1950; Hansson and Ekblom 1981, 1983; Ottoson et al. 1981; Lundeberg et al. 1983, 1984; Lundeberg 1984). Although heat and massage have been used since ancient time, few experimental studies have been reported for either the

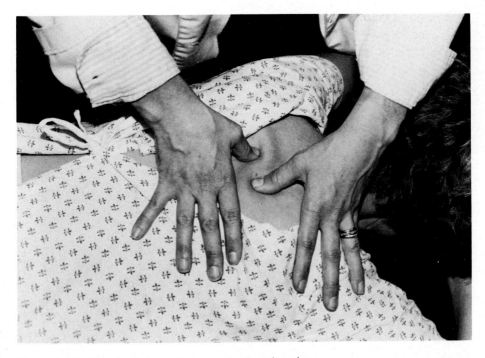

Fig. 4. Application of soft tissue massage to the thoracic region.

efficacy of use of these treatments or for the underlying physiological basis for their effectiveness (Wood and Becker 1981; Lehmann and DeLateur 1982).

In addition to soft tissue massage, other passive movement techniques are used by physical therapists. For example, joint mobilization is used to restore full painless joint function by the application of rhythmic, repetitive, passive movements (Maitland 1977; Grieve 1981) (see Fig. 5). The therapist performs these movements to the patient's tolerance, in voluntary or accessory range. These movements are graded according to objective and subjective evaluation findings and are performed within the control of the patient so that he can prevent the movement if he so chooses. Stretching of shortened soft tissue and manual or mechanical traction of a body part are also passive movement techniques used to treat musculoskeletal dysfunction with accompanying pain. Assessment of these techniques is evaluated during and after treatment by examination of the patient's objective complaint and comparison of these findings with initial and subsequent evaluations.

A relatively new approach to the management of pain, TENS, has been studied extensively during the past 10 – 15 years. TENS is a form of peripheral conditioning stimulation which is non-invasive and non-addictive, does not cause severe side effects, uses the body's own mechanism for pain relief, and can be a self-treatment with proper instruction. TENS may be applied in a variety of ways. The two most common techniques are often referred to as 'conventional' and 'acupuncture-like'. The 'conventional', or traditional, approach consists of a high-frequency, narrow pulse width, and low-to-moderate intensity stimulation; while 'acupuncture-like', or low-rate, consists of a low-frequency, narrow to wide pulse width, and high intensity stimulation.

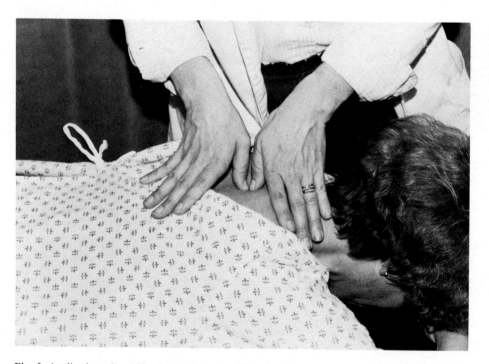

Fig. 5. Application of mobilization to the upper thoracic spine.

Although the same instrument is used, characteristics of the electrical stimulus, electrode placement, and neurophysiologic bases differ. The electrode placement for conventional TENS is any one of the following: over or surrounding the painful area, proximal or distal to the pain site, or along the related peripheral nerve or spinal cord segments (see Fig. 6). The treatment may be given for long periods of time up to many hours per day, and is a comfortable sensation often described as tingling or vibrating in nature. Conventional TENS is founded in the 'gate' theory of pain, i.e. the high frequency-low intensity electrical stimuli selectively activate larger myelinated fibers which close the gate to, and thus inhibit, the smaller unmyelinated fibers which transmit pain impulses. Relief from pain may be immediate but the duration is often short-lived after removal of the stimulation (see also Chapter 25).

Acupuncture-like TENS is applied over specific acupuncture points that are selected according to the patient's diagnosis and symptoms. The stimulation is at a low frequency and the intensity is sufficient to produce visible muscle contractions. The intensity of treatment is at a point just under the pain threshold level within the tolerance level of the patient. Treatment is given for

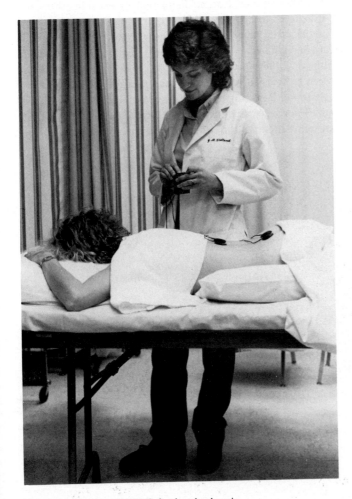

Fig. 6. Application of TENS for low back pain.

approximately 30 minutes. Pain relief does not occur as fast as with conventional TENS but the duration usually is longer than following conventional TENS. This technique developed as a variation of standard acupuncture techniques and is based on the same postulates, i.e. that endogenous opiates such as enkephalins and endorphins are released to inhibit pain (Sjolund and Eriksson 1976, 1979; Sjolund et al. 1977). Recent studies give reasons to question this explanation (Chapman et al. 1983; O'Brien et al. 1984).

Both techniques for TENS have been used to treat acute and chronic pain: headache, postherpetic neuralgia, pain from arthritis, low back disorders, phantom limb, reflex sympathetic dystrophy, labor and various other syndromes (Melzack et al. 1983; Mannheimer and Lampe 1984). Conventional high frequency TENS is used routinely by many to treat post-operative pain (Solomon et al. 1980; Mannheimer and Lampe 1984). The use of TENS is discussed in detail by Joseph Yao (1984), Mannheimer and Lampe (1984), and Gersh and Wolfe (1985).

The term auriculotherapy, a component of acupuncture, refers to various methods of stimulation of the external ear for therapeutic purposes (Huang 1974; Wexu 1975; Oleson and Kroening 1983; Yao 1984). When trauma or pathological change occurs in internal organs or in other parts of the body, this traumatic insult is believed to be reflected by a change at the specific related points on the auricle. The change on the auricle may be manifest through tenderness, erythema, papules, desquamation, or a decrease in resistance to electrical stimuli (Huang 1974; Wexu 1975; Oleson et al. 1980; Oleson and Kroening 1983; Yao 1984). Oleson (1980) and his colleagues reported a 75% concordance between established medical diagnosis and auricular diagnosis.

According to Chinese acupuncturists and Paul Nogier, M. D., a French neurologist, stimulation of appropriate auricular points by massage, needling or other methods has healing effects. Recently, clinical success has been reported supporting the use of acupuncture-like TENS at

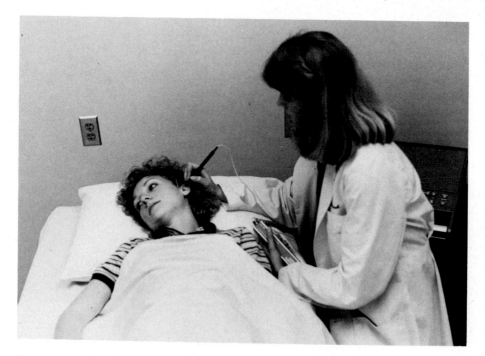

Fig. 7. Application of auricular TENS.

points on the auricle of the ear. Auricular TENS, applied with a pencil electrode point stimulator of approximately 2 mm diameter, has been shown to increase pain thresholds in normals (Oliveri et al. 1985) (see Fig. 7). In addition, auriculotherapy has resulted in a decrease in the pain of migraine headaches and a variety of chronic pain syndromes (Chun and Heather 1974; Leung and Spoerel 1974; Kajdos 1976). Auricular TENS in conjunction with TENS to body acupuncture points also has been effective in the treatment of ankle sprains and reflex sympathetic dystrophy (Leo 1983; Paris et al. 1983).

Physical therapists can affect the pain cycle by employing techniques that directly elicit relaxation and gain secondary effects of an increase in circulation and a decrease in pain. Stress and tension influence strongly the perception of pain and pain tolerance. According to Chapman (1983),

'Reduction of tension occurs in several ways: letting go of increased tension in a muscle allows that muscle to assume a more relaxed state; concentration on breathing slower and deeper calms autonomic functions; and clearing the mind of distracting thoughts by focusing instead on internal sensations and on imagery enhances a mental state of calm.'

Physical therapists have long been involved in techniques for muscle relaxation; the use of imagery is a relatively recent adjunct to physical therapy techniques. Progressive relaxation, developed by Edmund Jacobson, is probably one of the most widely used methods for enhancing muscle relaxation. This procedure entails training one to relax muscles by first asking the patient to tense and hold and then release tension in a series of muscles in the body, that is, the patient learns to discriminate and control muscle tension (Chapman 1983; Hertling and Jones 1983). Another effective relaxation procedure is autogenic training, devised by Schultz and Luthe. The emphasis in this technique is on the patient's achieving autonomic balance and reduced sympathetic outflow by performing two sets of mental exercises, i.e. standard exercises and meditative exercises (Chapman 1983; Hertling and Jones 1983). The six standard exercises are physiologically oriented and focused on somatic attention, e.g. specific systems and areas of the body. The meditative exercises are more cognitive in nature and focus primarily on imagery and single-focus mental concentration. These techniques are discussed in detail by Schultz and Luthe (1969) and by Hertling and Jones (1983).

Biofeedback training is often used to help produce relaxation and thus contribute to the management of chronic pain. Electromyography (EMG), galvanic skin response (GSR), skin temperature and heart rate are all useful measures of sympathetic output (arousal) and can be used to guide the patient in achieving relaxation. Use of EMG biofeedback has been effective in decreasing the severity of pain, for example, in whiplash syndrome, headache, low back pain and temporomandibular joint (TMJ) pain (Chapman 1983; Mannheimer and Lampe 1984; Finneran 1985). Biofeedback is recommended to be used in conjunction with progressive relaxation, sensory modulation procedures, other physical therapies and/or other psychological methods (Chapman 1983; Kessler 1983; Melzack and Wall 1983).

Exercise may be one of the most important treatments offered by physical therapists to patients with chronic pain. Sarno (1984), in discussing therapeutic exercise for back pain, lists multiple purposes of exercise.

1) It counteracts ischemia by stimulating local circulation.
2) It restores strength to muscles weakened by prolonged inactivity.
3) It increases mobility and flexibility.

4) It provides patients with a practical demonstration of their recovery.

5) It builds patient confidence in the integrity of their backs (Sarno 1984).

Patients suffering from chronic pain avoid normal movements and the inactivity ultimately leads to loss of flexibility, strength, endurance, and possibly coordination (Siracusano 1984; Arnheim 1985). Considering this loss of normal function and the fact that many persons who have chronic pain have tended to focus continuously on their pain for months or years, the physical therapist should direct the patient's attention away from the pain and toward exercise, increasing function, and decreasing pain behaviors (Blossom 1983; Siracusano 1984). The patient's program should include exercises for increasing range of motion, strengthening areas of weakness, and enhancing endurance and coordination. In addition, braces and external support devices should be eliminated when appropriate (Blossom 1983; Siracusano 1984; Arnheim 1985). Other general benefits of exercise have been discussed by many authors (Exercise and Health 1984; Sarno 1984; Sharkey 1984; Arnheim 1985). The tranquilizer effect of exercise, as described by de Vries in Exercise and Health (1984) for anxious elderly subjects, may be another important benefit of exercise, i.e. to combat the anxiety usually found in patients who have chronic pain.

As with all patients, the exercise program for chronic pain patients should be designed for the individual patient. Since most chronic pain patients have a sedentary lifestyle, a change in attitude toward exercise and physical function may need to be aggressively promoted via patient education regarding exercise theory, body mechanics, posture, and the need for daily exercise. In addition, having the patient monitor and document his own progress is beneficial in that it shows him how he is progressing; it teaches him to monitor his progress by objectively looking at function rather than pain; and it teaches him to assume some responsibility for his own health (Blossom 1983; Siracusano 1984).

In summary, Melzack (1983) states, 'Two therapies, each with slight effects that do not reach statistical significance, may produce significant reduction in pain when given together'. There are many physical therapy techniques/procedures for pain relief, with advocates for each. However, even the most staunch advocate for a particular procedure will recommend a combination/integration of techniques for maximum effect (Hertling and Jones 1983; Kessler 1983; Melzack and Wall 1983; Wolf and Vaddai 1983; Wood and Becker 1981). In addition, the most effective approach for treating patients with chronic pain is a multidisciplinary approach. Therefore, the physical therapy program must be consistent with the philosophy and objectives of all other disciplines involved.

A case study of a patient referred for chronic pain to a physical therapy outpatient setting is illustrated in the following case study.

Case study: A 50-year old female secretary with a diagnosis of whiplash secondary to auto accident one year ago. She complains of constant pain at base of skull, post-cervical spine and both shoulders. She is unable to sleep through the night and is not working due to pain. Patient reports neck pain is aggravated with head rotation left, stress, poor posture and eased with change of position. General health is not remarkable. X-rays of cervical spine are normal. Patient treated in physical therapy for 2 months with hot hot packs, ultrasound and massage with no significant improvement. Patient also treated with anti-inflammatory and analgesic medication and acupuncture without success. Patient currently taking aspirin daily for pain.

The patient sits with a rounded back and forward head. Active movements of cervical spine are limited in the cervical spine to rotation L secondary to pain and stiffness. Palpation reveals tight upper trapezius and paracervical muscles, and joint stiffness in the upper cervical spine and the cervical-thoracic junction. Neuromuscular evaluation is normal, shoulders and thoracic spine are not dysfunctional. Patient unable to relax upon command and demonstrates a poor fitness level.

ASSESSMENT – CERVICAL SPINE DYSFUNCTION

Problem list
1) Constant cervical spine pain
2) Neck rotation left – 50% normal range of motion
3) Unable to sleep secondary to pain
4) Inability to generate a relaxation response
5) Deconditioned – poor fitness level

Short-term goals
1) Patient able to generate a relaxation reponse as measured by lowering EMG and GSR output during relaxation exercise
2) Range of motion of cervical spine to 60% L rotation
3) Patient participates in exercise regime daily and performs at 'good' fitness level as measured by a standardized fitness scale
4) Patient can demonstrate proper posture in sitting, lying down, sit <--> supine
5) Constant cervical spine pain intensity has decreased and varies as measured by subjective pain scale
6) Patient able to sleep through night

Plan
1) Relaxation training with EMG biofeedback and Jacobson's Relaxation Exercises
2) Joint mobilization of upper cervical spine and cervical-thoracic junction
3) TENS application
4) Posture and activities of daily living instruction
5) General conditioning program (flexibility, strength, aerobic activity).

Physical therapists in pain management centers

In a review of the role of physical therapists at pain treatment centers in the United States, Doliber (1984) reports that the most common types of pain treated were cervical pain, low back pain, headache, nerve root injury, myofascial syndromes. Physical therapy treatments most commonly cited were individualized exercise programs (82%), instruction in body mechanics (75%), relaxation training (69%), TENS (65%), biofeedback (54%) and group exercise (51%). Ninety percent of the physical therapists were also involved in behavior modification as a fundamental part of the patient's program and 66% were involved in family education. Roesch and Urich (1980) provide a detailed report of physical therapy management at one pain management center. From this literature, it is obvious that therapists at these centers are working with teams of health care professionals primarily to enhance the patient's functioning despite chronic pain rather than directly intervening in musculoskeletal dysfunctions. This use of simultaneous interventions from a variety of health care disciplines supports the philosophy that chronic pain should be treated as a biosocial phenomenon. In turn, although 'success' can be documented by patients demonstrating decreased pain behaviors and increased physical functioning, it is impossible to say which of the many simultaneous interventions are most effective.

Research

Physical therapy evaluation and treatment techniques provide many baseline measures against which short and long-term outcomes can be assessed: specific musculoskeletal findings such as muscle strength, joint range of motion and postural asymmetries; neuromuscular findings recorded by EMG on the ability to initiate relaxation responses; cardiopulmonary findings such as pulse rate and minute ventilation after controlled exercise periods; and activities of daily living findings such as ambulation endurance, stair climbing and standing/sitting tolerance. These findings provide researchers with many non-invasive dependent and independent variables for chronic pain research.

Physical therapy clinicians are currently participating in many different kinds of clinical research studies. Doleys et al. (1982) used a multiple baseline design to demonstrate that patients responded to a structured exercise quota system accompanied by positive reinforcement with a significant level of sustained increase in physical activity. Fordyce et al. (1981), in a study of 25 chronic pain patients who performed to tolerance, found a consistent relationship between increased exercise and fewer pain complaints or visible/audible expressions of pain. Jones and Wolf (1980) demonstrated the effectiveness of 15 sessions of EMG biofeedback training to retrain low back musculature of a patient with chronic pain while the patient was engaged in painful upright activities.

Unfortunately, little experimental research is available on the short and long-term effectiveness of many widely used physical therapy interventions such as heat and cold modalities, massage and acupressure. In addition, chronic pain studies which are currently being conducted often suffer from methodological problems, such as lack of validated evaluation tools, lack of baseline assessment measures, and lack of significant follow-up to determine long-term effects of intervention (Cinciripini and Floreen 1982; Doliber 1984; Gersh and Wolf 1985).

Doliber (1984) points out that 45% of physical therapists in the pain treatment centers in her study were involved in research and that 26% of these reported conducting independent research. As physical therapists become more actively involved in research as primary or co-investigators, two undeniable side benefits will occur – increased reliability and validity of their evaluation techniques and expanded knowledge and skill in the application of their treatment techniques. Physical therapists, working closely with other members of the health care community, have an important role and growing responsibility for the care of patients with chronic pain and their families.

References

Arnheim, D. D. (1985) Modern Principles of Athletic Training. Times Mirrow/Mosby College Publishing, St. Louis.

Blossom, B. M. (1983) The role of the physical therapist. In: S. F. Brena and S. L. Chapman (Eds.), Management of Patients with Chronic Pain. S. P. Medical and Scientific Books, New York, pp. 211 – 216.

Chan, P. C. (1982) Finger Acupressure. Price/Stern/Sloan Publishers, Inc., Los Angeles, California.

Chapman, C. R., Benedetti, C., Colpitts, Y. H. and Gerlach, R. (1983) Naloxone fails to reverse pain thresholds elevated by acupuncture: acupuncture analgesia reconsidered. Pain 16, 13 – 31.

Chapman, S. L. (1983) Relaxation, biofeedback, and self-hypnosis. In: S. F. Brena and S. L. Chapman (Eds.), Management of Patients with Chronic Pain. S. P. Medical and Scientific Books, New York, pp. 161 – 172.

Cinciripini, P. and Floreen, A. (1982) An evaluation of a behavioral program for chronic pain. J. Behav. Med. 5, 375 – 389.

Chun, S. and Heather, A. J. (1974) Auriculotherapy: micro-current application on the external ear – clinical analysis of a pilot study on 57 chronic pain syndromes. Am. J. Chin. Med. 2, 399–405.

Doleys, D., Crocker, M. and Patton, D. (1982) Response of patients with chronic pain to exercise quotas. Phys. Ther. 62, 1111–1114.

Doliber, C. (1984) Role of the physical therapist at pain treatment centers. Phys. Ther. 64, 905–909.

Exercise and Health (1984) American Academy of Physical Education Papers no. 17. Human Kinetics Publishers, Inc., Champaign, IL.

Finneran, J. (1985) A biofeedback program for the patient with pain. Clin. Mgt. Phys. Ther. 5, 6–9.

Fordyce, W., McMahon, R., Rainwater, G., Jackins, S. Questad, K., Murphy, T. and DeLateur, B. (1981) Pain complaint – exercise performance relationship in chronic pain. Pain 10, 311–321.

Gersh, R. G. and Wolf, S. L. (1985) Applications of transcutaneous electrical nerve stimulation in the management of patients with pain. Phys. Ther. 65, 314–322.

Grieve, G. (1981) Common Vertebral Joint Problems. Churchill Livingstone, New York.

Hansson, P. and Ekblom, A. (1981) Acute pain relieved by vibratory stimulation. Letter. Br. Dent. J. 151, 213.

Hansson, P. and Ekblom, A. (1983) Transcutaneous electrical nerve stimulation (TENS) as compared to placebo TENS for the relief of acute orofacial pain. Pain 15, 157–165.

Hertling, D. and Jones, D. (1983) The revival of relaxation techniques and the development of related techniques. In: R. M. Kessler and D. Hertling (Eds.), Management of Common Musculoskeletal Disorders. Harper and Row, Philadelphia, pp. 202–230.

Huang, H. L. (1974) Ear Acupuncture. Rodale Press, Emmaus, PA, pp. 1–52, 78–104.

Jones, A. and Wolf, S. (1980) Treating chronic low pack pain: EMG biofeedback training during movement. Phys. Ther. 60, 58–63.

Kajdos, V. (1976) Experiences with auricular acupuncture. Am. J. Acupunc. 4, 130–136.

Kessler, R. M. (1983) Friction massage. In: R. M. Kessler and D. Hertling (Eds.), Management of Common Musculoskeletal Disorders. Harper and Row, Philadelphia, pp, 192–201.

Lehmann, J. F. and DeLateur, B. J. (1982) Therapeutic heat. In: J. E. Lehmann (Ed.), Therapeutic Heat and Cold, 3rd edn. Williams and Wilkins, Baltimore, pp. 404–562, 563–602.

Leo, K. C. (1983) Use of electrical stimulation at acupuncture points for the treatment of reflex sympathetic dystrophy in a child. Phys. Ther. 63, 1287–1288.

Leung, C. Y. and Spoerel, W. E. (1974) Effect of auriculo-acupuncture on pain. Am. J. Clin. Med. 2, 247–260.

Lundeberg, T. (1984) Long-term results of vibratory stimulation as a pain relieving measure for chronic pain. Pain 20, 13–23.

Lundeberg, T., Ottoson, D., Hakansson, S. and Myerson, B. A. (1983) Vibratory stimulation for the control of intractable chronic orofacial pain. In: J. J. Bonica, U. Lindblom and A. Iggo, (Eds.), Advances in Pain Research and Therapy, Vol. 5. Raven Press, New York, pp. 555–561.

Lundeberg, T., Nordemar, R. and Ottoson, D. (1984) Pain alleviation by vibratory stimulation. Pain 20, 25–44.

Maitland, G. (1977) Peripheral Manipulation, 2nd edn. Butterworth and Company, London.

Mannheimer, J. S. and Lampe, G. N. (1984) Clinical Transcutaneous Electrical Nerve Stimulation. F. A. Davis Co., Philadelphia.

Melzack, R. (1973) The Puzzle of Pain. Basic Books, Inc., New York, pp. 110–111.

Melzack, R. and Wall, P. D. (1965) Pain mechanisms: a new theory. Science 150, 971–979.

Melzack, R. and Wall, P. D. (1983) The Challenge of Pain. Basic Books, Inc., New York, pp. 306, 338–355.

Melzack, R., Vetere, P. and Finch L. (1983) TENS for low back pain. Phys. Ther. 63, 489–493.

Mirabelli, L. (1985) Pain management. In: D. A. Umphred (Ed.), Neurological Rehabilitation. C. V. Mosby Co., pp. 600–615.

O'Brien, W. J., Rutan, F. M., Sanborn, C. and Omer, G. E. (1984) Effect of transcutaneous electrical nerve stimulation on human blood β-endorphin levels. Phys. Ther. 64, 1367–1374.

Oliveri, A. C., Clelland, J., Jackson, J. and Knowles, C. (1985) The effects of auricular transcutaneous electrical nerve stimulation on experimental pain threshold. Phys. Ther. 66, 12–16.

Oleson, T. D. and Kroening, R. J. (1983) A comparison of Chinese and Nogier auricular acupuncture points. Am. J. Acupunc. 11, 205–223.

Oleson, T. D., Kroening, R. J. and Bresler, D. E. (1980) An experimental evaluation of auricular diagnosis: the somatotopic mapping of musculoskeletal pain at ear acupuncture points. Pain 8, 217–229.

Ottoson, D., Ekblom, A. and Hansson, P. (1981) Vibratory stimulation for the relief of pain of dental origin. Pain 10, 37–45.

Paris, D. L., Baynes, F. and Gucker, B. (1983) Effects of the Neuroprobe in the treatment of second degree ankle inversion sprains. Phys. Ther. 63, 35–40.

Roesch, R. and Ulrich, D. (1980) Physical therapy management in the treatment of chronic pain. Phys. Ther. 64, 53–57.

Russell, W. R. and Spalding, J. M. K. (1950) Treatment of painful amputation stumps. Br. Med. J. 68, 68–73.

Sarno, J. E. (1984) Therapeutic exercise for back pain. In: J. V. Basmajian (Ed.), Therapeutic Exercise, 4th edn. Williams and Wilkins Co., Baltimore, pp. 441–463.

Schultz, J. H. and Luthe, W. (1969) Autogenic methods. In: W. Luthe (Ed.), Autogenic Therapy, Vol. 1. Grune and Stratton, New York, pp. 1–255.

Sharkey, B. J. (1984) Physiology of Fitness, 2nd edn. Human Kinetics Publishers, Inc., Champaign, IL.

Siracusano, G. (1984) The physical therapist's use of exercise in the treatment of chronic pain. J. Ortho. Sports Phys. Ther. 6, 73–75.

Sjolund, B. H. and Eriksson, M. B. (1976) Electro-acupuncture and endogenous morphines. Lancet 2, 1085.

Sjolund, B. H. and Eriksson, M. B. (1979) The influence of naloxone on analgesia produced by peripheral conditioning stimulation. Brain Res. 173, 295–301.

Sjolund, B. H., Terenius, L. and Eriksson, M. B. (1977) Increased cerebrospinal fluid levels of endorphins after electroacupuncture. Acta. Physiol. Scand. 100, 382–384.

Solomon, R. A., Viernstein, M. C. and Long, D. M. (1980) Reduction of postoperative pain and narcotic use by transcutaneous electrical nerve stimulation. Surgery 87, 142–146.

Tappan, F. M. (1978) Healing Massage Techniques: A Study of Eastern and Western Methods. Reston Publishing Co., Reston, VA.

Wexu, M. (1975) The Ear Gateway to Balancing the Body: A Modern Guide to Ear Acupuncture. ASI, Publisher, New York, pp. 1–39, 65–70.

Wolf, S. L. and Vaddai, R. (1983) Transcutaneous electrical stimulation. In: S. F. Brena and S. L. Chapman (Eds.), Management of Patients with Chronic Pain. S. P. Medical and Scientific Books, New York, pp. 185–194.

Wood, E. C. and Becker, P. D. (1981) Beard's Massage, 3rd edn. W. B. Saunders Co., Philadelphia.

Yao, J. (1984) Acutherapy: Acupuncture, T.E.N.S. and Acupressure. Acutherapy Postgraduate Seminars. Libertyville, IL.

Burrows/Elton/Stanley (eds.) Handbook of Chronic Pain Management
© *1987 Elsevier Science Publishers B.V. (Biomedical Division)*

25

Transcutaneous nerve stimulation

JOAN MERRILYN McMEEKEN and BARRY CHARLES STILLMAN

Lincoln Institute of Health Sciences, School of Physiotherapy, Carlton, Victoria, Australia

Introduction

Whilst the term 'transcutaneous nerve stimulation' is relatively new, this method of analgesia has existed for several hundred years. Transcutaneous nerve stimulation (TNS) describes all modalities whose neural effects are achieved by transmission of a therapeutic force through the skin. Transcutaneous electrical nerve stimulation (TENS) refers to transmission through the skin of an electric current capable of stimulating excitable tissue.

The focus on TENS throughout this chapter reflects the research predominance into electroanalgesia; partly because TENS dosage allows for more rigid quantification than that for other forms of TNS. Nevertheless, the theory of TENS closely parallels that for TNS.

Physiological mechanisms

The basis for TENS analgesia is somewhat speculative, but stems from the capacity of electric current to modulate the discharge of action potentials along peripheral nerve fibres.

Diminished or blocked conduction along peripheral nerve fibres by sustained stimulation with current of adequate frequency is one of the peripheral mechanisms. This requires > 10 Hz for group IV nociceptive afferents and > 50 Hz for larger diameter afferents (Torebjörk and Hallin 1974). However, our research shows that pain can be perceived by normal human volunteers during stimulation using frequencies up to 40 kHz because many nociceptive afferents continue to fire given sufficient current intensity. Another form of blocking involves hyperpolarization or subthreshold depolarization during application of continuous direct current (Campbell and Long 1982).

TENS increases microcirculation and vascular permeability by: 1) axon reflexes from group IV afferent stimulation; 2) activation of sympathetic vasodilator fibres; and 3) release of vasodilator substances (including vasoactive intestinal peptide) (Kaada and Eielsen 1983a). A resulting enhanced tissue healing and diminished circulatory stasis may indirectly relieve pain, particularly that of the ischaemic type.

260

Spinal mechanisms of electroanalgesia appear to be mediated by gate control processes, invocation of which subsumes an ability to selectively stimulate large diameter non-nociceptive afferents. We investigated this in normal human subjects using rectangular and sinusoidal pulses of duration 5 μs – 100 ms and frequencies 1 Hz – 40 kHz. Intensity – time graphs were obtained for thresholds of non-painful sensation (S), muscle contraction (M) and pain (P).

Figure 1 shows results using 7 cm² bipolar electrodes (over the brachioradialis muscle motor point) and rectangular pulses of frequency 1 Hz. At all durations the threshold order from low to high was S, M and P. This shows that threshold is inversely proportional to nerve fibre

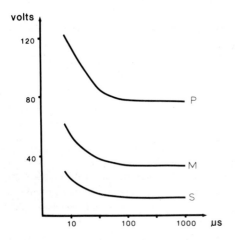

Fig. 1. Intensity – time graphs for thresholds of non-painful sensation (S), muscle contraction (M) and pain (P).

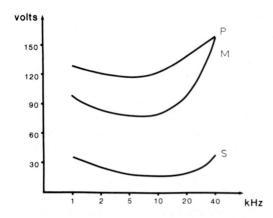

Fig. 2. Thresholds of non-painful sensation (S), muscle contraction (M) and pain (P) at frequencies 1 Hz – 40 kHz.

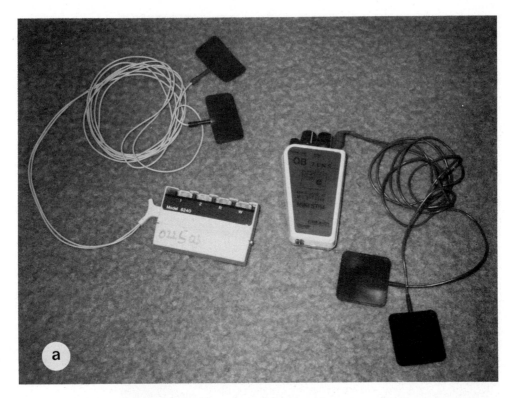

Fig. 3. Examples of TENS apparatus: (a) battery-powered units; (b) mains-operated conventional stimulator; (c) mains-operated interferential unit.

diameter. Selective stimulation of large afferents was most readily achieved with pulse widths < 50 μs. However, any gating effect from 1 Hz current is minimal because the large afferents are only discharging at the current frequency. Current at 100 Hz reduces the thresholds (P $>$ M $>$ S). As with 1 Hz current, non-painful sensation from 100 Hz is more readily achieved at pulse widths < 50 μs.

At frequencies $50 - 100$ Hz, temporal and spatial summation should ensure maximum or near maximum discharge from the activated afferents. Additionally, post-tetanic potentiation should cause the evoked effects to persist maximally after termination of the stimulus.

Figure 2 indicates S, M and P thresholds using rectangular pulses at frequencies up to 40 kHz. Maximum separation of S and M from P occurs at $8 - 10$ kHz; a factor relevant to the efficacy of interferential apparatus (see 'Apparatus'). At all frequencies, use of small electrodes increases thresholds (M $>$ P$>$ S), and their order changes from S-M-P to S-P-M.

The stimulation site is relevant to gating mechanisms. Lee et al. (1984) recorded from monkey spinothalamic tract neurons during TENS application. Maximum inhibition of these neurons occurred with TENS application over skin with the same cord segment as that giving rise to the inhibited spinothalamic neurons. This suggests that for maximum gating, stimulation should be of afferents with the same segmental innervation as the tissue from which pain originates. Ot-

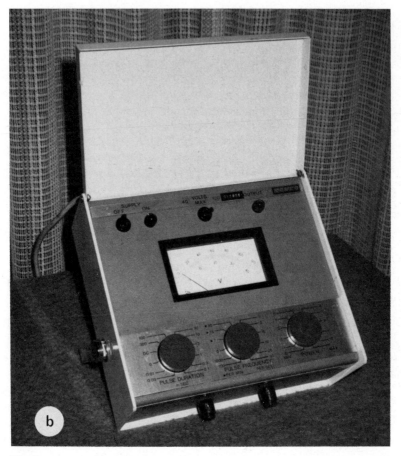

Fig. 3b.

toson et al. (1981) showed that mechanical vibration is most effective for pain suppression when applied segmentally. Stimulation of afferents one or two segments above and below that/those corresponding to the painful tissue may reinforce gating effects. Simultaneous application of TENS over the corresponding contralateral afferents may also be indicated. This requires further research.

Supraspinal systems for analgesia are divisible into two groups. The first involves modulation of nociceptive information as it ascends to, or on arrival at sensory areas of the brain. The second employs descending pathways which modulate transmission of nociceptive information through the dorsal horn. These systems may be activated by non-noxious and noxious stimulation; the latter falling under the heading 'stress-induced analgesia'. Mechanisms of supraspinal pain modulation are elaborated elsewhere in this volume. The following supplementary observations are pertinent.

Vascular and analgesic effects from TENS are closely linked. Kaada and Eielson (1983b) showed that TENS causes descending sympathetic inhibition and vasodilation via a serotonergic pathway. Kenins (1981) proposed that cutaneous vasodilation is a 'physiological defense

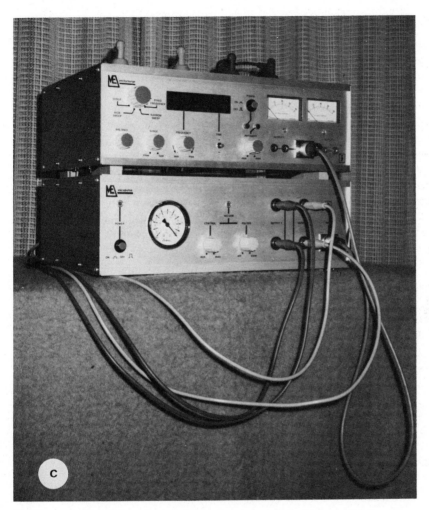

Fig. 3c.

response to localized cutaneous damage'. Also, Omura (1975) found a direct correlation between acupuncture analgesia and cutaneous vasodilation.

Duggan (1984) presents a cogent argument, supported by experimental findings, clarifying the biological purpose of pain and analgesia. Acute injuries do not always produce pain, at least for up to 4 hours after the injury (Melzack et al. 1982). An intense descending inhibition from the region of the periaqueductal gray is the principal analgesic mechanism employed. Duggan showed that stimulating the periaqueductal gray also produces cardiovascular responses which seem part of the 'fight-or-flight' response, and that opioid peptides are not essential for this reaction. Duggan argues that release of endogenous opiates, associated with and triggered by pain, suppresses mobility through effects on motorneurons and their associated reflexes. In this 'post-fight-or-flight' response immobility and facilitated healing are thought to take precedence. This hypothesis implies that stress-induced analgesia may not involve release of significant amounts of endogenous opiates, and that accompanying vascular reactions are to be expected.

Apparatus

TNS encompasses many different forms of therapy employing mechanical, thermal, electrical, chemical and psychobehavioural effects. Examples are massage, manipulation, exercise, vibration, laser, acupuncture, shortwave, ultrasound, ice and low frequency electric current.

TENS apparatus includes more than the small battery-powered devices to which the term 'TENS' has heretofore been exclusively assigned. The essence of TENS is the current and TENS current can be derived from a variety of sources (Table 1).

Medical galvanism (Category 1) is one of the earliest approaches to electroanalgesia. This current may also be used for the deliberate introduction of ions such as salicylates through the skin ('iontophoresis'). The use of medical galvanism and iontophoresis in management of chronic pain has been superseded by safer, simpler and apparently more effective methods.

A wide range of pulse widths (10 μs – 1 s) and frequencies (0.5 Hz – 2 kHz) is available from apparatus in Category 2. Rapid developments in the field obligate the clinician to check the output from each type of apparatus. The name of the apparatus may give little indication of the type(s) of current provided.

TABLE 1
TENS apparatus.

Category		Types of apparatus
Category 1:	Continuous direct current	Conventional stimulation units
Category 2:	Low frequency current up to 2 kHz	Conventional stimulation units, battery-powered 'TENS' units, 'high voltage' units, 'Russian faradism' units
Category 3:	Low frequency current > 2 kHz	'Interferential' units

TABLE 2
Properties of electrodes.

	Metal	Carbonized silicone rubber	Pre-gelled
Interface	Saline pad, electrode gel	Saline pad, electrode gel, water (electrodes with rough surfaces only)	Adhesive gel (gel may require moistening with water)
Impedance	Low	Medium	High
Contiguity	Fair	Fair	Good
Durability	Poor	Good	Fair
Cost	Low	Medium	High

Interferential apparatus (Category 3) uses two (sometimes three) alternating 'carrier' currents of up of to 10 kHz. These are cross-fired so as to produce a modulated ('interference') current at their point of intersection. The interference current can be caused to 'beat' at frequencies of 0 – 250 Hz. Details of the apparatus listed in Table 1 can be found in Ward (1986).

For treatment of pain TENS apparatus should produce: 1) pulse widths < 50 μs and > 50 μs; 2) at least 50 Hz frequency; 3) a zero nett ionic effect (see 'Dangers'); and 4) continuous and modulated current. Apparatus meeting these specifications is, at present, uncommon. Some battery-powered TENS units, high voltage units and 10 kHz interferential units have the smallest pulse widths (50 μs); but only a few interferential units have modulated power output.

Figure 3 shows examples of TENS apparatus. Figure 4 is a diagrammatic representation of the controls available in a majority of all types of TENS apparatus. Coupling of the apparatus to the patient is summarized in Fig. 5.

Electrodes are of three main types (Table 2). Electrode fixation may be by adhesive gel,* adhesive patches, adhesive tape, cloth or rubber bandages, open-weave elasticized bandages and suction devices. Given appropriate connections, all suction devices, leads and electrodes may be interchanged between different types of TENS apparatus.

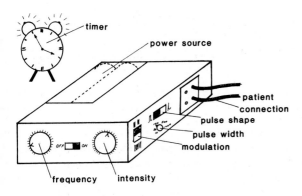

Fig. 4. Controls of TENS apparatus.

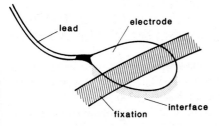

Fig. 5. Electrode coupling.

---

* Karaya gel, a viscous hydrophilic product of a tree indigenous to the Indian sub-continent, is commonly used.

Indications

TENS should be viewed as the physical equivalent of non-steroidal anti-inflammatory agents. Its prescription is appropriate in virtually all circumstances where these drugs would be indicated for analgesia. The availability of TENS for patient use outside the clinical environment is particularly important.

Although TENS usually only provides symptomatic relief, at times it may affect the cause of pain. Examples are stimulated healing of chronic skin ulcers and enhanced circulation in patients with ischaemic pain. The most common forms of chronic pain are headache and spinal, arthritic and cancer pain. In all instances best results follow use of TENS as early as possible. Success from TENS has been achieved with neuritis, neuralgia, post-amputation pain, arthritic and spinal pain (Gersh 1981). TENS appears least successful for peripheral neuropathies and pain of central origin (Campbell and Long 1982). TENS is appropriate in managing cancer pain but, as is also true of simple medication, it may have only limited value (Avellanosa and West 1982).

Many disorders manifest acute exacerbations, so producing indications for TENS similar to those for treatment of acute disorders. TENS has value following accidental or surgical trauma (Jameel et al. 1981) and may reduce the need for narcotic analgesics. TENS is also indicated before, during and/or after painful therapeutic procedures such as wound dressing and joint mobilization (Mannheimer and Lampe 1984).

The indications for TNS are similar to those for TENS. Han and Terenius (1982) suggested that TENS and acupuncture are equally effective in treatment of pain; Melzack et al. (1980) indicated that ice may be as effective as TENS; and Lundberg (1984a, b) showed that vibration may be more effective.

Technique

Electrode placement may be: 1) segmental — over the source of pain and/or anywhere between the source and the spinal cord along the path of nerves with the same segmental innervation as the tissues producing the pain; and 2) elsewhere.

The segmental method presumes gating mechanisms, for which a non-noxious stimulus is required. TENS application elsewhere is justifiable if delivered as a noxious stimulus; that is stress-induced analgesia. Noxious stimulation may also be applied over the segmental field, in which instance the effects should be stress-induced rather than a result of gating.

Since acupuncture is noxious, it may also be applied anywhere on the body. There is no anatomical or physiological justification for believing that acupuncture points have any unique value as a site for stimulation (Perl 1980).

'Myofascial trigger points' commonly reside in sclerotomes related to the source of pain and may be the site of secondary pathological changes. Application of TENS over these local tender spots may form a useful part of segmental field TENS application.

With single channel apparatus, one or both leads may be bifurcated to allow an increase in electrode size and/or application of electrodes over more than two locations. Further combinations are possible from dual and multiple channel apparatus. Where the current is such that the electrodes have polarity, reversing the positions of the anode and cathode has no effect on the outcome. Practical considerations include positioning electrodes over areas where complete and constant contact can be maintained, and where the skin is intact. Positioning electrodes, leads and power source so that they are not visible may be an aesthetic consideration.

Noxious and non-noxious stimulation may be obtained using any electrode size provided current intensity is adjusted appropriately. However, large electrodes offer less risk of burns. The maximum surface area of the electrodes is limited by the power output of the apparatus.

Care should be taken in skin preparation and electrode application. The patient should be questioned about any history of skin disorders, the site checked for disorders, and the skin washed and dried after each treatment.

Metal electrodes are separated from the skin by pads soaked in 1% saline. Saline pads may also be used with carbonized silicone rubber (CSR) electrodes. These options are only suitable for treatments up to 30 minutes. This is also true for roughened CSR electrodes moistened with water. Pre-gelled electrodes and CSR electrodes covered with gel are suitable for prolonged treatments. The entire surface of the CSR electrodes should be evenly covered with gel. 'Disposable' pre-gelled electrodes may be re-used with care if re-moistened with water. Fixation should provide even pressure over the entire electrode, but should not be so great as to displace gel or water. CSR electrodes and pads should be thoroughly washed after each use.

Dosage

The optimum dosage for non-noxious and noxious TENS analgesia is given in Table 3. Justification for the parameters in Table 3 was given under 'Physiological mechanisms'. Note that the given frequency may produce some blocking, hence for stress-induced analgesia the pulse train should be interrupted ('burst mode'). This provides the small afferents an opportunity to recover from the blocking effect.

For acute or chronic pain TENS should only be used when the pain is troublesome, or during procedures/activities where such pain is anticipated. Where TENS is effective there should be no limit set on its use. TENS should be interrupted after 30 minutes to 1 hour to determine the duration of relief. TENS may be recommenced as and when necessary. Some clinicians seem unduly concerned about overuse of TENS. TENS does not produce dependency or addiction and there is little evidence suggesting that the 'true' (non-placebo) effects from TENS are self-limiting. Any diminution in benefit during the first 6 weeks of use is likely to be the result of a weakening placebo response.

TABLE 3
Dosage for TENS.

	Non-noxious	Noxious
Mechanism	Gating	Stress
Wave form	Optional – preferably rectangular	Optional – preferably rectangular
Pulse width	Optional – preferably < 50 μs	Optional – preferably > 50 μs
Frequency	50 – 100 Hz	50 – 100 Hz
Modulation	Optional	Yes
Intensity	Low	High

Since patients prefer non-noxious TENS, this method should be tried first. If after 30 minutes to 1 hour there is no benefit, the noxious mode should be considered along with other variations in technique. If this fails, additional or alternative forms of treatment should be considered.

Dangers

Electric shock is a potential hazard with all mains operated apparatus. This risk is minimized by: 1) only using properly functioning apparatus; 2) regular service; 3) using the apparatus distant from earthed objects; and 4) installing protective equipment such as core-balanced relays. Passage of current through the *vagus nerve, stellate ganglion* or *heart* is potentially dangerous.

Skin reactions may follow prolonged TENS use. Skin care should be meticulous, pads and electrodes regularly washed and electrode positions regularly changed. Allergic dermatitis and chemical irritation are uncommon. They may be traced to the adhesive tape, gels, pads or electrodes (Fisher 1978). More frequent is mechanical irritation from skin traction following improper application of adhesive tape. Bruising may result from excessive suction, particularly when the skin is friable. Most people safely and comfortably tolerate up to 0.2 bars of suction.

Burns may be chemical or thermal. Chemical burns are caused by concentration of acid and alkali beneath the anode and cathode, respectively, when using a stimulus with a nett ionic effect. Thermal burns may occur using any type of current. Aside from the above difference the causes of burns are the same: too much current flowing through too small an area with too much resistance, and/or for too long. Accordingly current intensity should be the minimum necessary to achieve the desired effect and electrodes should be as large as practical.

Even large electrodes may cause problems if their effective surface area is reduced by inadequate or uneven gel thickness, dry pads, metal resting on the skin, electrodes too close to each other, broken skin or uneven contact. Incorrect coupling agents are particularly dangerous. Burns have resulted from the use of ultrasound gel with stimulation equipment. Even slight variations in ultrasound gel thickness will cause marked current concentration (Ward 1984). Another cause of burns is increased impedance from dry and thickened skin, chronic oedema or fibrosis. Interference from high frequency electrical apparatus (microwave and shortwave) also causes burns. The electromagnetic field associated with high frequency generators induces current in any nearby conductor, including the leads and electrodes of TENS apparatus. At least 3 m distance should be maintained between operating high frequency apparatus and all TENS machines attached to patients.

Passage of current through a *gravid uterus* should be avoided. Current is known to influence tissue growth by increasing cellular metabolism and mitotic rates.

During TENS use for analgesia the clinician and patient should be sensitive to inadvertently produced muscle contractions. Associated joint movement may cause exacerbation of the pathology and sustained low grade muscle contraction may produce unwanted consequences of fatigue. There is no evidence supporting the contention that TENS analgesia depends on, or is improved by accompanying muscle contractions. Where TENS is effective in relieving pain, care must be taken to avoid exacerbating the pathology by excesses of treatment or activity.

Contraindications

Dosage and safety are based on the patient's skin sensations. Therefore, TENS should be avoided: 1) with patients who are unable to understand or adequately communicate; and 2) over areas of anaesthetic or analgesic skin. Electrodes should not be placed over broken skin or skin with allergic or other reactions.

The danger of current and normal hearts has been mentioned. *Cardiac disease* and *pacemakers* constitute even greater risks. Implanted metal will distort and concentrate current. If the current has a nett ionic effect, electrolytic reactions may occur in and adjacent to the implant.

Overview

Chronic pain is characterized by the varied physical, psychological, social and economic factors which serve to create and sustain it. Hence assessment must be of the person, the pathology and the pain. This combined information is necessary to establish the most appropriate management. Treatment should first be of the cause, however this is often difficult when pain is chronic. Here management of the pain becomes mandatory. 'TENS treatment' is a misnomer. TENS is a technique which therefore forms but one part of the management of chronic pain.

Through contrived and incidental behaviour modification, patients may develop greater functional capacity and less externalization of pain, whilst actually tolerating the same or an increased magnitude of pain. Therefore in assessing the results from TENS, evaluation should be extended beyond simple clinically derived test results into the sphere of everyday function. 'Restoration of these functions must be a clearly stated objective of the programme as they represent true meaures of the success or effectiveness of the intervention strategies' (Roy 1984).

There is much remaining to be discovered about TENS outside the laboratory as well as within, and the clinician should seek to learn from every patient. The only remaining responsibility is to communicate with one's peers.

The optimum analgesic technique should be effective, safe, simple to use, inexpensive and readily available to both clinician and patient. In chronic pain management TNS is not the answer, but does appear to be part of it.

References

Avellanosa, A. M. and West, C. R. (1982) Experience with transcutaneous electrical nerve stimulation for relief of intractable pain in cancer patients. J. Med. 13, 203 – 213.

Campbell, J. N. and Long, D. M. (1982) Transcutaneous electrical stimulation for pain: efficacy and mechanisms of action. In: N. H. Hendler, D. M. Long and T. N. Wise (Eds.), Diagnosis and Treatment of Chronic Pain. Wright, Boston, pp. 90 – 91.

Duggan, A. W. (1984) The suppression of pain. Proc. Aust. Physiol. Pharmacol. Soc. 15, 25 – 54.

Fisher, A. A. (1978) Dermatitis associated with transcutaneous electrical nerve stimulation. Current Contact News 21, 24, 33, 47.

Gersh, M. R. (1981) Applications of transcutaneous electrical nerve stimulation in the treatment of patients with musculoskeletal and neurologic disorders. In: S. L. Wolf (Ed.), Electrotherapy. Churchill Livingstone, New York, pp. 155 – 177.

Han, J. S. and Terenius, L. (1982) Neurochemical basis of acupuncture analgesia. Ann. Rev. Pharmacol. Toxicol. 22, 193 – 220.

Jameel, A., Yotte, C. S. and Serette, C. (1981) The effect of transcutaneous electrical nerve stimulation on post-operative pain and pulmonary function. Surgery 89, 507 – 512.

Kaada, B. and Eielsen, O. (1983a) In search of mediators of skin vasodilation induced by transcutaneous nerve stimulation. I. Failure to block the response by antagonists of endogenous vasodilators. Gen. Pharmacol. 14, 623 – 633.

Kaada, B. and Eielsen, O.   (1983b)   In search of mediators of skin vasodilation induced by transcutaneous nerve stimulation. II. Serotonin implicated. Gen. Pharmacol. 14, 635 – 641.

Kenins, P.   (1981)   Identification of the unmyelinated sensory nerves which evoke plasma extravasation in response to antidromic stimulation. Neurosci. Lett. 25, 137 – 141.

Lee, K. H., Chung, J. M. and Willis, W. D.   (1984)   TENS inhibits spinothalamic tract cells. Pain (Supplement 2) S50.

Lundberg, T.   (1984a)   Long-term results of vibratory stimulation as a pain relieving measure for chronic pain. Pain 20, 13 – 24.

Lundberg, T.   (1984b)   Pain alleviation by vibratory stimulation. Pain 20, 25 – 44.

Mannheimer, J. S. and Lampe, G. N.   (1984)   Electrode placement techniques. In: Clinical Transcutaneous Electrical Nerve Stimulation. F. A. Davis, Philadelphia, pp. 331 – 495.

Melzack, R., Jeans, M. E., Stratford, J. G. and Monks, R. C.   (1980)   Ice massage and transcutaneous electrical nerve stimulation: comparison of treatment for low-back pain. Pain 9, 209 – 217.

Melzack, R., Wall, P. D. and Ty, T. C.   (1982)   Acute pain in an emergency clinic: latency of onset and description patterns related to different injuries. Pain 14, 33 – 43.

Omura, Y.   (1975)   Patho-physiology of acupuncture treatment: effects of acupuncture on cardiovascular and nervous system. Acupunc. Electro-Ther. Res. 1, 51 – 140.

Ottoson, D., Ekblom, A. and Hansson, P.   (1981)   Vibratory stimulation for the relief of pain of dental origin. Pain 10, 37 – 45.

Perl, E. R.   (1980)   Pain and nociception. In: J. M. Brookhart and V. B. Mountcastle (Section Eds.), Handbook of Physiology, Vol. III, Part 2, Section I. American Physiological Society, Bethesda, pp. 915 – 975.

Roy, R.   (1984)   Pain clinics: reassessment of objectives and outcomes. Arch. Phys. Med. Rehabil. 65, 448 – 451.

Torebjörk, H. E. and Hallin, R. G.   (1974)   Responses in human A and C fibres to repeated electrical intradermal stimulation. J. Neurol. Neurosurg. Psychiatry 37, 653 – 664.

Ward, A. R.   (1984)   Electrode coupling media for transcutaneous electrical nerve stimulation. Aust. J. Physiother. 30, 82 – 85.

Ward, A. R.   (1986)   Electrical stimulation of nerve and muscle. In: Electricity, Fields and Waves in Therapy, 3rd edn. Science Press, Marrickville (in press).

Burrows/Elton/Stanley (eds.) Handbook of Chronic Pain Management
© *1987 Elsevier Science Publishers B.V. (Biomedical Division)*

26

The psychologist and management of chronic pain

DIANA ELTON and GORDON STANLEY

Department of Psychology, University of Melbourne, Australia

Introduction

As understanding of the mechanisms of pain developed, and as greater awareness of the psychological variables which affect the pain experience occurred, psychologists became more involved in the treatment of pain (Degood et al. 1979; Parker et al. 1983). Their role in the psychological approaches to pain management is not exclusive, as other professions are also involved in holistic approaches to pain patients. Some hospitals and pain clinics still do not include psychologists in their interdisciplinary teams, and treatments by relaxation are often carried out by nurses and occupational therapists, while treatments by biofeedback are sometimes carried out by doctors and physiotherapists, or neglected. Family therapy may be handled by psychiatrists and/or social workers.

There is often a lack of awareness of what a psychologist can contribute to the pain team. This is probably due to the fact that psychology is a broad discipline, and includes many interests, only a few of which are directly relevant to psychosomatic conditions. These differences seem extreme in theory, but in practice many psychologists adopt a relatively eclectic attitude and include in their therapeutic approach whatever seems to be of most benefit to the patient, rather than following rigid outlines and dogmatic approaches.

This chapter only covers a few of the techniques developed and used by psychologists. The role of the psychologist in assessment will be discussed briefly, followed by discussion of relaxation, biofeedback and hypnosis as clinical treatments. Finally case studies using these procedures in an adjunctive way are presented.

Recent resesarch indicates that psychological interventions are associated with greater coping abilities by the patients, greater well-being, and a decrease in the intake of medication (Olbrisch 1977; Elton et al. 1983). Psychologists have various functions from assessment to the treatment of pain.

Assessment

Accurate assessment of pain is essential if the complaint and therapeutic outcomes are to be evaluated. While this area is covered in detail in another chapter (Chapter 7), an overview of some of the available approaches will be pertinent.

PERSONALITY SCALES

To examine the relationship between personality and chronic pain, various personality questionnaires have been used. Many workers employ the Minnesota Multiphasic Personality Inventory (MMPI), or the California Personality Inventory (CPI). These inventories are lengthy and provide personality profiles which relate to various areas of function, only some of which are useful in the interpretation of pain. For instance, Sternbach (1978) and Merskey (1986) concentrated on the measurement of depression, hypochondriasis and hysteria from the MMPI and have shown that there are usually elevated profiles on these scales in chronic pain sufferers. The use of the MMPI scales enabled some understanding of the personality variables affecting the pain experience. While Merskey (1987) has pointed out certain dangers of an unthinking interpretation of the scales, these measures are popular with many researchers in the field.

Other approaches involve use of specific scales, including Depression, Anxiety, Introversion-Extroversion, etc. Elton et al. (1978) used a Self-Esteem scale to differentiate between pain-prone patients and other groups (see Chapter 11). The use of personality and mood scales has important implications for the treatment of pain, as it highlights the complexity of the variables operating to produce changes in the intensity and duration of pain, and in behaviour.

MEASUREMENT OF PAIN

As mentioned in other chapters (Chapters 7 and 8) there are many ways to measure the pain experience. Among these are the Analogue Scale (Elton et al. 1979), Melzack's McGill Pain Assessment Questionnaire (1975), and the Budzynski et al. self-report scale (1973). Although some scales have been used for years, there tends to be little agreement on a standard procedure. This creates difficulties in the multiple assessment of the patients' states and in the interpretation of results by other practitioners. Psychologists are skilled in the administration of scales and their evaluation. Discussion when pain measures are being used can assist communication between the practitioner and the patient, and can provide a useful index of improvement, thereby increasing motivation for self-regulation. If there is no improvement, the charts point to the need to alter the treatment, or to add other interventions.

Relaxation

The use of relaxation in the treatment of medical conditions is not new. Formerly, doctors prescribed 'rest' which could be variously interpreted, but which basically included relaxation. The difference here is that 'rest' involved passive use of relaxation, while modern approaches prefer dynamic self-regulation. Jacobson (1938) attempted to place relaxation on a scientific basis and to make it a standard form of medical treatment. He has shown clinically and experimentally the usefulness of relaxation in the treatment of many conditions. While the medical profession has been slow in adopting these approaches, there has been a growing interest in relaxation as a means of dealing with tension and anxiety and of generally improving the patients' well-being.

Jacobson (1938) stated that neuromuscular patterns are an essential part of the mental and emotional activities of an individual. The energy expended in a neuromuscular activity is identical with and not a transformation of the energy of the corresponding mental and emotional activity. There are muscular tensions associated with all mental processes, such as imagery, attention, cognition and so on. When an organ is active, the muscles which control it are also active. Relaxation, that is, the lowering of tension, brings with it a diminution of emotional or mental processes. Jacobson has provided both clinical and experimental evidence for his theory. Elton and Stanley (1976) have tested the effectiveness of relaxation techniques in an empirical study. Further evidence to support Jacobson's views comes from behavioural scientists. Wolpe (1969) showed that relaxation was an essential part of systematic desensitization, because it was antithetical to tension states. Hay and Madders (1971) demonstrated that relaxation therapy coupled with a discussion group was successful in relieving migraine headaches (presumably partly due to tension) in 69 out of 98 patients. Rachman (1965) argued that therapeutically the most useful component of relaxation was the resultant 'mental calmness'. Mental calmness can be achieved even without muscular relaxation, by the use of pleasant imagery, or by concentration on words such as 'calm, calm' or 'relax, relax'. Further evidence of the importance of mental relaxation comes from studies of Yoga, Transcendental Meditation and other forms of mental self-control.

Davison (1966) has shown that subjects who were injected with curare, a substance which produces complete relaxation of all the skeletal muscles, experienced a great deal of anxiety during this procedure. Jacobson did not consider the importance of suggestion in the relaxation procedures, yet it is vitally important, as shown by the studies of hypnotic analgesia (Hilgard 1969; Elton et al. 1979).

Some of the effectiveness of hypnosis is attributed to the placebo effect. Placebo treatment cannot be viewed in isolation, but rather as a 'situation' associated with childhood memories of comfort, love and caring by mother and significant others (Elton et al. 1977). A dependency on doctors, nurses and others in an 'illness situation' may constitute a form of regression to childhood. The trust in the members of the 'helping professions' may in itself be sufficient to allay anxiety and produce improvement (Sternbach 1968). Anxiety is antagonistic to relaxation. Both placebos and relaxation techniques appear to relieve anxiety and pain. It is therefore assumed that placebo effects are correlated with and inherent in relaxation techniques, just as they are in other forms of therapy.

Jacobson's progressive relaxation focussed initially on the dominant arm only. Differentiation was stressed. The patient was asked to become aware not only of maximum and minimum tensions, but also of the range of tensions in between. For example: The patient was trained to consider a total lack of tension as 0, and the highest possible level of tension as 10. He was then asked to produce in his dominant arm a tension of level 8, then 5 and so on. Jacobson used both isotonic and isometric exercises to facilitate the learning of tension levels by the patient. Only after the relaxation of the dominant arm was achieved, were the other parts of the body given relaxation training.

Differentiation of tension levels required in this method is useful, particularly for patients who are not aware of their own tension, since it has become a habitual state to them. It is equally important for patients who have continuing tension in one or more muscle groups, for example, the shoulder girdle muscles. Constant awareness of the level of tension is valuable therapeutically. The treatment extended up to 200 hours of training, over a long period of time. No imagery techniques or breathing exercises were included. Jacobson's techniques are still used at present, as many patients enjoy the easily observable experience of muscles tensing and untensing, particularly when first learning about relaxation.

Farmer (1967) partially adopted Jacobson's techniques. He also commenced training with the use of the dominant arm only, and used differential relaxation in conjunction with breathing. When the patient breathed out, he was asked to say the word 'relax'. When he breathed in, he was asked to say the word 'tense'. When the dominant arm was relaxed, other parts of the body received relaxation training. Usually the patient was asked to imagine his own calm, happy, sedative scene. This technique is useful because of its emphasis on different degrees of relaxation and the introduction of breathing and imagery.

Mitchell (1980) argued that the human brain cannot recognize muscle consciousness, but can recognize the sensory messages from joints and skin. Therefore, training in relaxation must be based on joint and skin consciousness. To relax one needs to adopt patterns opposite to those habitually associated with tension. Mitchell's instructions are rather strict. For instance, to relax the shoulders, she states: 'Pull your shoulders towards your feet. When you cannot pull them down any further, stop. Register your new position of ease.' This pattern elongates the joints and stretches the muscles: a tension pattern involves pulling up of the shoulders, and shortening of the muscle groups. Similarly, separating and stretching out of fingers and thumb is opposite to the tension pattern of clenched fists. Mitchell included the use of positive imagery and pleasant thoughts in her procedures. Her methods are particularly popular with physiotherapists, as they are effective in dealing with pain and spasm. This latter condition makes voluntary tension as required by Jacobson's technique rather difficult for the patients.

Kleinsorge and Klumbies (1964) asked the patient to repeat a combination of both physical and mental relaxation instructions: e.g. 'I am very much at rest. My right arm is very heavy. My left arm is very heavy. My heart is beating strong and well. My breathing is very relaxed. My head feels pleasantly cool.' This method, originally based on the principles of autogenic training (Schultz and Luthe 1959) requires a great deal of concentration by the patient, and the therapist. It appears too taxing for many of the patients requiring treatment. On the other hand, the repetitive instructions promote deep relaxation in some patients, where other methods are less successful.

Boome and Richardson (1931) emphasized the role of colour: e.g. 'Divide the body into a rainbow of colours, such as a red head, orange shoulders, yellow arms and chest, a green waistline, blue thighs, purple legs and feet'. Instead of mentioning only the parts of the body, the therapist trains the patient to learn the 'colour scheme', and then just quotes them. For instance, 'concentrate on the colour of your head and notice your relaxed breathing'. This method requires longer time, it may be difficult for the colour blind and the unimaginative patient, and may be too complex. It is very popular with patients who are weak on their knowledge of anatomy, but strong on colour visualization, and produces good results.

Another approach is relaxation involving standing and moving and teaching the patient to relax in all positions and circumstances. The patient is asked to stand with feet wide apart and to transfer weight from one leg to another, while relaxing the shoulders. The instruction given is 'tell your shoulders to have a holiday, and let them go'. While the body sways, the patient breathes in and out, and with the third breath makes a deep sound. Benson (1973) argued that swaying is an important form of relaxation and it is known from early childhood development. Mothers rock their babies, to soothe them, autistic children sway when distressed, and swaying is part of some religious ceremonies. Relaxation in swaying has been useful in treatment of individuals and groups.

Schultz and Luthe (1959) instructed patients as follows: 'Think of the space between the outer borders of your feet . . . make it empty . . . make it empty and relaxed . . . Now, think about the space between the outer borders of your knees . . . make it empty and relaxed . . . Now, the space between the outer borders of your waist . . . make it empty and relaxed . . . Now, the space between the outer borders of your shoulders . . . make it empty and relaxed . . . Now, the space between the outer borders of your ears . . . make it empty and relaxed, empty and relaxed . . .'

This technique is enjoyed by many patients, who would have found it more difficult to 'empty their minds'. When given such an instruction, many state either that 'there is nothing there anyway' or 'I can't do it, there are too many thoughts there'. Concentration of empty space between feet and then moving upwards, creates a positive set in the patient, as initially it validates the real experience of distance between the feet. It is therefore easier to adapt it to the other parts of the body, where imagery is required.

Elton et al. (1983) use an 'awareness' relaxation, based upon Ericksonian techniques. Some patients have difficulties in concentrating on the therapist's voice. As other thoughts come to their minds, they get irritated with themselves for their inability to shut them out, and therefore feel worse, rather than better during the procedure of relaxation. A useful technique to utilize this difficulty instructs: 'This is an awareness exercise . . . focus on your feet touching the floor . . . now, experience the light touch of shoes on your feet . . . clothing on your knees, position of your body in the chair. You may listen to the sound of my voice or listen to your thoughts or a blend of both. You can't go wrong because whatever you listen to, or are aware of can be used by you to relax even more. Give yourself the permission to relax.'

Imagery techniques may enhance the experience of relaxation. Some practitioners use a form of meditation, and advocate blanking out of the mind (Meares 1968). This is difficult for some patients. Other therapists use unstructured imagery, where patients are instructed to focus 'on something pleasant', based upon their past experience, or wish fulfillment fantasy. A semi-structured imagery involves guiding the patients part of the way, and then letting them take over (Elton and Burrows 1978). Finally, a structured imagery provides the patient with a detailed account of the pleasant experience. Some patients prefer to follow the therapists' imagery, while others like to do what seems most appropriate within their frame of reference. There are specific imagery techniques which may be used in the relief of pain. These are often designed for treatment by hypnosis, but are also successful if used with relaxation procedures.

Some people relax best when moving and jogging. Dancing and sport indicate the beneficial affects of physical activity. Rhythmic movements may be combined with music. Music therapy is gaining acceptance in the treatment of various conditions, and has been used to good advantage in the treatment of chronic pain.

In summary, there are many relaxation techniques. All of them are useful for some, but not for all patients. The efficacy of the technique depends not only on the patient's suitability for it, but also on the belief in its merit by the therapist. Individual attention is needed for the patient who does not benefit from a particular technique. If audio tapes are to be used, they should be made individually for each patient.

RELAXATION IN GROUPS

At present, many practitioners give training in relaxation in group situations. Group relaxation has both advantages and disadvantages. Some of the advantages are that more patients may be treated in a limited space of time; groups provide friendship and social network links for the patients. Meeting others, and hearing of their problems may help the patient feel less isolated. Groups may be used as a catalyst for discussion, and the members of a group may provide a support system for each other. Finally, modelling is easier in groups where the more capable members act as models for the others.

Among the disadvantages are that the space given to each patient is not always adequate in a group. A group does not always cater to the individual needs of the patient, as it is aimed at the 'mythical average'. Homogeneity of a group is difficult to attain. A therapist handling several group members may find it difficult to observe deleterious effects of the programme on one of the participants. The more severely disturbed the patient, the more need for individual attention.

All the above disadvantages are augmented if audio-cassettes are used. Lately there has been growing interest in the use of these cassettes (Sherman 1982). It was believed that this saved the therapist's time, providing uniform instructions and permitting training of patients by semi-skilled personnel. This had led in some instances to their inappropriate use. If tapes are to be used in group therapy for relaxation, certain guidelines need to be observed: initial detailed patient screening is essential. This may include an interview, a careful taking of history, and the use of psychological questionnaires. Other important aspects to be considered are the degree of motivation for change by the individual, the ability to persevere and to understand the instructions. Imagination greatly adds to successful therapy.

The first session should be individual, so that the patient may assess whether he or she can benefit from that particular cassette. Patient responses are also assessed by the therapist. The programme of training should be discussed with each individual, to ensure co-operation, a contractual arrangement and an integrated treatment regimen. An immediate follow-up after the group session should be used to assess the effect of the group practice on each individual.

Clinical biofeedback

Biofeedback is a procedure in which an external sensor provides an indication of the state of a bodily process, usually in an attempt to effect a change in the measured quantity of that state. Historically, it evolved out of the behaviourist tradition in psychology.

The improvement of symptoms by biofeedback therapy is not just dependent on the person's ability to control their own biological processes, but also on the motivation to give up the gains achieved by the unconscious use of the symptoms and substitution of alternative methods of goal achievement (Linkenhoker 1983). Given the uncertainty about the mechanisms by which biofeedback operates, it is essential to consider the possible contribution of placebo effects to the therapeutic outcome derived from biofeedback training.

Biofeedback, along with hypnosis is seen as an 'active' method for the treatment of pain. Both require the patient to participate actively in their own therapy, and depend on autogenic training and practice for their lasting effect. Hilgard and Hilgard (1975) pointed out that in biofeedback training the person learns to become acutely aware of changes in bodily functions, as physiological responses are amplified by the machine, in the form of easily discernible signals.

door. She was asked to use the 'bear' imagery on biofeedback, and to shrink it as the needle went down. This was partially successful and the pain showed mild improvement. In one of the following sessions the therapist suggested that the bear is only a blown up balloon and that she could pull the plug out, and deflate it. She was greatly surprised at that notion, but followed the suggestion. Her pain gradually abated.

In the 6 months of follow-up, Noreen continued improving. She was able to work full-time and a tendon transplant removed the need for a caliper. She became active in attempting to provide pain relief programmes for other unfortunate sufferers. Her positive, practical approach to life returned and she reported considerable life satisfaction. She still wanted to continue with monthly biofeedback sessions as she felt much better after them and was able to implement the other techniques if she had biofeedback as well. Transfer of training was taught, but she preferred the experience of the machine.

Case 2: Anne was a 38-year-old married woman with two children. She was injured whilst at work, lifting a heavy filing cabinet and since then reported severe pain in her neck, shoulders and hands, frequent headaches, inability to sleep and anxiety and depression. She attempted to return to work, but was unable to perform any duties and had been on workers' compensation for 2 years. She stayed at home, but because of pain she was unable to perform even minor household duties and could not drive the children to school. She could not read because of her headaches and she did not enjoy television. She did not have many friends and the few who visited her were sent away as 'they could not understand how tough life was'. Her husband and her employers were very supportive, but she still felt isolated and lonely. She was taking 14 pain tablets per day, with no effect. All standard medical treatment had been attempted, without success. Her history revealed that she was one of two children. She was an anxious reserved child, who did not make friends easily. She was a perfectionist and everything she did had to be of highest quality. She drove herself relentlessly both at home and at work. At the same time she was considered kind-hearted, and would always help others and take over their duties if they needed it. She was a good scholar, but she did not attempt tertiary training, having married early. Her relationship with her husband was good, and she was very concerned about the children.

She was given EMG biofeedback training, but was very anxious about a band around her forehead, feeling that this might be a form of shock treatment. Because of her anxiety, she was given literature and explanation prior to the treatment. After two sessions on biofeedback, machine relaxation was introduced, but it was not successful as the patient stated that she wanted to 'get the needle down to where I want it to be' before she tried anything else. This was complied with. At the sixth session, she stated that she was ready for relaxation. She enjoyed the colour relaxation, but after a week reported that relaxation was better if she imagined the needle of the biofeedback going down. Transfer of training procedures was given and she felt very comfortable about lowering her rate of breathing and pulse, to reduce anxiety and pain. At the same time training was given in intra- and interpersonal coping skills. She was asked to read *'A new guide to rational living'* by Ellis and Harper, and to underline the parts which she identified with. Slowly she realized that her anxiety and perfectionism made her life difficult and that her low self-esteem made her shy of making new friends as she was afraid of rejection. She decided to attempt using her newly acquired coping skills and tentatively rang a few friends and met them during the day. She found this pleasant. As her pain and anxiety abated she decided that she was very bored at home and returned to work, at first in a part-time capacity. A discussion with her employers assured her that she would not be given heavy lifting.

A 2 year follow-up showed that she was still relatively pain-free and continued to work. She reported much greater life satisfaction and still used biofeedback techniques by herself.

Behavioural approaches in the treatment of pain

As pointed out by Turk and Meichenbaum (Chapter 10), we need a multicomponent approach to the treatment of pain particularly in the treatment of chronic pain patients. Turk and Meichenbaum focus on the need to conceptualize pain, before there is willingness to attempt self-regulation. The patients' attitudes and beliefs are crucial to the outcome of treatment.

Treatments by biofeedback, relaxation and hypnosis may be considered a treatment by behavioural techniques, since the approach to the patients is based upon learning theory principles, and there is an attempt to tailor broad outlines of treatment to the specific needs of the individual (Turner 1982; Turk et al. 1983).

The major difference between this and the standard medical approaches to patient care is that the patients learn to take over responsibility for their own conditions, and therapeutic outcomes. This is a growth experience for many patients, as it gives them increased self-esteem, and the coping abilities which generate to other problem areas of life.

Treatment of pain sometimes fails because of many personal and interpersonal problems causing stress and potentiating the pain experience. Therefore, attention to self-esteem of the individual has been one of the cornerstones of treatment of pain by the present authors. Psychological treatment of pain is not successful with all individuals. Some patients feel very angry at the thought that they need to take over the responsibility for their pain. They believe that just as a mechanic does not ask them to crawl under the car and take over the repairs, when they come for assistance, the members of the helping professions should be able to 'fix' their pain without their participation and strenuous effort. The anger grows, when they feel that they are 'blamed' for their pain. Educational programmes, demonstrating to patients the maladaptiveness of anger may be necessary, before pain control treatment is attempted. Such programmes have been conducted at Macquarie University, Sydney, Australia, with considerable success (Elton et al. 1983).

Often, treatment is directed at the area of weakness of the patients which can result in panic reactions when things go wrong, and consequently increase the pain experience itself. It is important to find the areas of strength of individuals and to use them to increase life satisfaction, prior to attempting the difficult work of self-education. The authors asked some patients to enjoy sitting out in the sun (with pain), or listening to their favourite music, and saying to themselves 'at this point, I feel pleasure', before learning how to deal with life's problems.

Other problems involve primary and secondary gains derived from pain, and they have powerful implications for possible success of treatment. A patient who is expecting monetary compensation for pain and disability, may focus on these feelings more than someone whose pain is not compensatable. A person who finds work distasteful, or even just bearable, may cling to disability and pain more than someone who enjoys work, and looks forward to returning to normal duties as quickly as possible. Unless these aspects are considered, the usefulness of pain management may be limited. Families need to be considered at all times, as they are powerful sources of support or sabotage of pain management. Sometimes, if pain becomes the focal point of the family's life, it is difficult to give up an established equilibrium. At that point, attention to all members of the family may be crucial to produce positive changes.

Summary

This chapter attempted to highlight the role of the psychologist in the treatment of pain. It was demonstrated that they are useful members of interdisciplinary teams, where they can take part both in the assessment and the treatment of pain. They can also be used as individual consultants, who deal with difficult cases. Psychologists working in the area of pain are particularly useful if they are familiar with behavioural techniques of pain management, understand the placebo effects, and use relaxation, biofeedback and hypnotherapy techniques. The technical skills in all these areas is augmented by attempts to understand the patients in pain, and all the negative forces operating upon the situation in which they find themselves, when suffering from pain and disability.

References

Benson, H. (1975) The Relaxation Response. William Morrow, New York.

Boome, E. J. and Richardson, M. A. (1931) Relaxation in everyday life. Methuen, London.

Budzynski, T. H., Stoyva, J. M. and Adler, C. S. (1970) Feedback-induced muscle relaxation: application to tension headache. J. Behav. Ther. Exp. Psychiatry 1, 205 – 211.

Budzynski, T. H., Stoyva, J. M., Adler, C. and Mullaney, P. M. E. (1973) E.M.G. biofeedback and tension headache: a control outcome study. Psychosom. Med. 484 – 496.

Davison, G. C. (1966) Anxiety under total curarization. J. Nerv. Ment. Dis. 143, 443 – 448.

Degood, D. E. (1979) A behavioral pain-management program: expanding the psychologist's role in a medical setting. Prof. Psychol. Res. Practice 10, 491 – 502.

Elton, D. and Burrows, G. D. (1978) Specific use of imagery in treatment by hypnosis: the secret room. Aust. J. Clin. Hypnosis 6, 17 – 25.

Elton, D. and Stanley, G. V. (1976) Relaxation as a method of pain control. Aust. J. Physiother. 22, 121 – 123.

Elton, D., Burrows, G. D. and Stanley, G. V. (1977) Psychological control of pain. Aust. J. Clin. Hypnosis 5, 12 – 24.

Elton, D., Stanley, G. V. and Burrows, G. D. (1978) Self-esteem and chronic pain. J. Psychosom. Res. 22, 25 – 30.

Elton, D., Burrows, G. D. and Stanley, G. V. (1979) Clinical measurement of pain. Med. J. Aust. 1, 109 – 111.

Elton, D., Stanley, G. V. and Burrows, G. D. (1983) Psychological Control of Pain. Grune and Stratton, Sydney.

Farmer, R. C. (1967) Technique for the development of rapid relaxation of the skeletal musculature: combatting anxiety in the real-life situation. La Trobe University Manual, Psychology Clinic, Melbourne, Australia.

Hay, K. M. and Madders, S. (1971) Migraine treated by relaxation therapy. J. R. Coll. Gen. Pract. 21, 664 – 669.

Hilgard, E. R. (1969) Pain as a puzzle for psychology and physiology. Am. Psychologist 24, 103 – 113.

Hilgard, E. R. and Hilgard, J. R. (1975) Hypnosis in the Relief of Pain. William Kaufman Inc., Los Altos, CA.

Hurrell, M. (1976) Biofeedback: clinical promise, theoretical problems. New. Sci. September 9, 532 – 534.

Jacobson, E. (1938) Progressive Relaxation. University of Chicago Press, Chicago.

Kleinsorge, H. and Klumbies, G. (1964) Technique of Relaxation. John Wright & Sons, Bristol.

Meares, A. (1968) Relief without Drugs. Doubleday, London.

Melzack, R. (1975) The McGill Pain Questionnaire: major properties and scoring methods. Pain 1, 277 – 299.

Merskey, H. (1965) Psychiatric patients with persistent pain. J. Psychosom. Res. 9, 299 – 309.

Merskey, H. (1987) Pain, personality and psychosomatic complaints. In: G. D. Burrows, D. Elton and G. V. Stanley (Eds.), Handbook of Chronic Pain Management. Elsevier Science Publishers, Amsterdam, pp. 137 – 146.

Miller, N. E. (1978) Biofeedback and visceral learning. Ann. Rev. Psychol. 29, 373 – 404.

Mitchell, L. (1980) Simple Relaxation. John Murray, London.

Olbrisch, M. E. (1977) Psychotherapeutic interventions in physical health. Effectiveness and economic efficiency. Am. Psychol. 33, 761 – 777.

Parker, J. C., Karol, R. L. and Doerfler, L. A. (1983) Pain unit director: role issues for health psychologists. Prof. Psychol. Res. Practice 14, 232 – 239.

Rachman, S. (1965) Studies in desensitization. Behav. Res. Ther. 3, 245 – 251.

Schultz, J. H. and Luthe, W. (1959) Autogenic Training. Grune & Stratton, New York.

Sherman, R. (1982) Home use of tape-recorded relaxation exercises as initial treatment for stress-related disorders. Military Med. 147, 1062 – 1066.

Sternbach, R. A. (1968) Pain: A Psychophysiological Analysis. Academic Press, New York.

Sternbach, R. A. (1978) Clinical aspects of pain. In: R. A. Sternbach (Ed.), The Psychology of Pain. Raven Press, New York.

Turk, D. C. and Meichenbaum, D. (1987) Behavioral approaches in pain management. In: G. D. Burrows, D. Elton and G. V. Stanley (Eds.), Handbook of Chronic Pain Management. Elsevier Science Publishers, Amsterdam, pp. 85 – 89.

Turk, D. C., Meichenbaum, D. and Genest, M. (1983) Pain and Behavioral Medicine: A Cognito-Behavioral Perspective. Guilford Press, New York.

Turner, J. A. (1982) Comparison of group progressive-relaxation training and cognitive-behavioral group therapy for chronic low back pain. J. Consult. Clin. Psychol. 50, 757 – 765.

Wickramasekera, I. (1976) Biofeedback, Behavior Therapy and Hypnosis: Potentiating the Verbal Control of Behavior of Clinicians. Nelson-Hall, Chicago.

Wolpe, J. (1969) The Practice of Behavior Therapy. Pergamon Press, New York.

Burrows/Elton/Stanley (eds.) Handbook of Chronic Pain Management
© 1987 Elsevier Science Publishers B.V. (Biomedical Division)

27

Hypnosis and chronic pain management

FREDERICK J. EVANS

Carrier Foundation and The University of Medicine and Dentistry of New Jersey, Robert Wood Johnson Medical School, Belle Mead, New Jersey, U.S.A.

Introduction

The aims of this selective review are to a) highlight the role of hypnosis in understanding pain mechanisms; b) review methodological issues relevant to research in this area; c) review a few representative studies examining the role of both specific and nonspecific components of hypnotic analgesia, supporting the conclusion that, at least for some people, hypnosis may provide unique opportunities to develop cognitive and self-mastery experiences over pain; and d) review clinical guidelines for the use of hypnosis in the management of chronic pain.

Hypnosis and pain

Although the modern history of hypnosis is generally considered to begin with Franz Anton Mesmer, a Scottish physician, Esdaile (1850, 1957) gave prominence to the use of hypnosis in the control of pain. In 19th century India, just prior to the development of chemical anesthesia, Esdaile used hypnosis as the only form of anesthesia in amputations, tumor removals, and complex surgical procedures.*

There are well-documented clinical reports that hypnosis can be used as an effective technique to control chronic pain (e.g. Sacerdote 1970), and to assist in the management of the chronic or terminally ill, suffering patient (e.g. Domangue and Margolis 1983). However, there are relatively few controlled empirical studies of the efficacy of hypnosis in pain management (Turner and Chapman 1982). The evidence suggests that about 50% of terminal cancer pain pa-

---

* Overlooked in Esdaile's reports was the fact that most of his patients survived surgery — a rare event in those days because of hemorrhage, shock, and post-surgical infection. Apparently hypnosis had autonomic and/or immunological effects that transcended the usual complications of the surgical techniques of the time.

tients (Hilgard and Hilgard 1975) and 95% of dental patients (Barber 1977) can be helped by the judicious use of hypnotic techniques.

ACUTE AND CHRONIC PAIN: RELEVANCE TO HYPNOSIS

Significant contributions to understanding the nature of acute pain have been made in the hypnosis literature, particularly the meticulous psychophysical studies of experimental pain conducted by Ernest R. Hilgard (Hilgard 1969, 1974, 1977). Under controlled experimental conditions, Hilgard and his colleagues have shown that there is a lawful relationship between the intensity of the noxious stimulation and the subjective experience of transient, acute pain. This relationship has been shown to be lawful both for normal conditions, and for the reduction of pain following hypnotic analgesia in subjects differing in hypnotic susceptibility (Hilgard 1969).

Experimental studies of acute pain have been conducted in situations where the significance of the stimulation is not psychologically meaningful beyond the confines of the transient noxious stimulation (Beecher 1959). In these studies, anxiety about the meaning of the painful stimulation has been minimized or eliminated. It is doubtful whether such studies are particularly helpful to the clinician confronted with patients in pain, although they are important for understanding pain mechanisms. In his later work, Hilgard (1977) recognized this issue. His elaboration of pain control within the context of neodissociation theory, particularly using the method of the 'hidden observer', helps document that pain perception may take place at different levels of awareness. Multiple cognitive pathways are readily accessible to the hypnotized subjects enabling them to experience minimal pain at a conscious level, even though at another cognitive level (or an observing ego), they are able to report the actual intensity of the painful stimulation. Complex and subtle techniques have been developed to study pain control capitalizing on the highly hypnotizable subject's ability to maintain this dissociative control − remaining comfortable with suggestions of hypnotic analgesia while 'experiencing' pain. The multiple cognitive controls implicit in the 'hidden observer' procedure are not especially different from our own subjective experiences under dental analgesia, for example, when we experience that the drill does not hurt, even though we maintain awareness of the level of painful stimulation that we would be experiencing without the chemical intervention.

THE HIDDEN MESSAGE OF PAIN

It is important to make explicit the assumptions affecting the use of hypnotic techniques in pain management. Rational clinical applications of hypnosis for pain management must differentiate the typical sequence of events involved in acute versus chronic pain. The laboratory assumption of a one-to-one correlation between the intensity of short-lasting, noxious stimulation and reported pain does not hold true for chronic pain. With most chronic pain patients, the intensity of the pain is not as significant as its psychological meaning, especially when a specific organic basis to the pain cannot be documented. This suggests that a careful evaluation of the pain process itself must be made before hypnotic techniques can be employed as an adjunct in its management and control (see Chapter 11).

TRANSITION FROM ACUTE TO CHRONIC PAIN: ANXIETY TO DEPRESSION

The management of acute pain primarily involves the management of anxiety. The growing anxiety about the short- and long-term consequences of the injury which accompanies the increasing intensity of the noxious stimulation is usually relieved by adequate treatment (e.g. pain medication, hypnosis, or other interventions to reduce anxiety).

When the pain is not relieved satisfactorily, a different set of dynamics arises as another pattern becomes established. Although pain intensity may have increased initially, it tends to abate gradually, but the fear of continued suffering remains. The anticipatory feelings of future pain give way to the frightening awareness that a painful injury or lesion may have a more permanent, residual effect. Despair and despondency gradually develop as the suffering remains partially unrelieved, and activities remain restricted. Hypnotic intervention based on anxiety reduction will only frustrate the patient and the therapist, and will usually be unsuccessful. The use of hypnosis in these patients may be helpful, but different strategies are needed. While using hypnosis for pain control it is necessary to address simultaneously the depression and secondary gain as psychotherapeutic issues.

THE NATURE OF HYPNOSIS: RELEVANCE TO PAIN CONTROL

There is controversy concerning the nature of hypnosis, and one's theoretical stance will influence research design and the strategies used in hypnotic treatment programs. Some theorists emphasize motivation and social psychological interaction as the main components of hypnotic behavior. Hypnosis involves motivated striving to play the role of the good hypnotic subject or an intensification of an interpersonal relationship. The experience of hypnosis is operationally defined as a response to the induction process. Representative statements of this position, applied to discussions of hypnotic analgesia, can be found in Barber (1969); Chaves and Brown (1978); Sarbin and Coe (1972); Spanos (1982); and Wagstaff (1981). Solutions to pain problems are presented in terms of interpersonal processes or self-generated cognitive and motivational strategies, such as the reallocation and focusing of attention away from the pain, distraction, imagery, convincing oneself that the pain really isn't very severe, denial, and anxiety reduction. Specific management strategies utilizing hypnosis are presumably facilitated by the hypnotic relationship or induction procedure. In general, these strategies involve implementations of approaches like Meichenbaum's stress inoculation (1977) or other behavioral methods (Fordyce 1976) within the hypnotic context.

The other dominant view of hypnosis is that it reflects a stable capacity of the individual. The hypnotic experience may entail an ability to readily change levels of consciousness, or states of awareness, that may be either interpersonally- or self-induced (e.g. Hilgard 1965, 1974, 1977; Bowers 1976; Evans 1983). This view is supported by data showing very stable individual differences in hypnosis (Morgan et al. 1974). Thus, an important research issue is to show how differences in pain control strategies relate to measured individual differences in hypnotic ability.

Hilgard formulates this approach in terms of a neodissociation view of multiple cognitive pathways. Evans (1983) views hypnosis as a manifestation of a more general ability involving cognitive flexibility, or a switching mechanism that allows one to change psychological, cognitive, or physiological processes, or readily access different levels of consciousness. Hypnotizability correlates with: the ability to utilize imagery effectively; napping and the ease of falling asleep; the ability to become absorbed in other engaging experiences, such as becoming 'lost' in a movie or novel and experiencing some of the emotions of the characters; occasional lateness for appointments; the ease with which patients will give up psychiatric (and possibly medical) symptoms (Evans 1983).

If empirical data confirmed that measured hypnotizability correlates highly with pain control, or if situational and/or relationship variables were found to be better predictors of pain control, then the controversy would not survive. In fact, the correlation between measured hypnotizability and pain control in a variety of experimental situations has been reported by Hilgard and Morgan (1975) to be only a moderate 0.5, significantly less than the joint reliabilities of either the pain reports (analogue scale or behavioral measures) or the hypnotizability measures. When data falls somewhere between two extreme sets of predictions, the most compelling conclusion is that both views have some degree of truth. The existing data highlights the fundamental paradox in hypnotic pain control – clinicians claim that most of their patients can benefit from hypnotic intervention techniques, while empirical data suggests that only relatively few people have sufficient (dissociative) capacity to experience the profound sensory and cognitive skills that eliminate pain. The resolution of this paradox, discussed below, has important implications for the application of hypnotic techniques in chronic pain management.

Methodological issues in hypnotic analgesia research

Significant effects of hypnotic intervention on experimental pain tasks have only been shown over the last two decades. Unfortunately, most earlier studies (see reviews by Shor 1962; Hilgard 1974; Elton et al. 1980) used transient painful stimulation such as electric shock and radiant heat – procedures which share neither the enduring qualities of chronic pain, nor the debilitating anxiety of acute pain. Indeed, early studies deliberately minimized anxiety and stress. The deliberate attempt to minimize anxiety in early experiments obscured the problem that many of the pain stimulation procedures used are not affected by standard analgesic drugs such as morphine, and therefore may not be useful analogues of clinical pain.

Partly for reasons of subject welfare, many of these early studies were restricted to measuring pain threshold, or the point at which pain first becomes noticeable. Clinically, patients do not report that they have a problem with their pain threshold! Meaningful studies are restricted to those in which protracted measurements approaching pain tolerance and endurance levels are made. For the most part, the only viable experimental pain induction methods satisfying such criteria are the cold pressor and ischemic pain tasks. Both tasks measure severe, protracted pain, and are sensitive to analgesic medications, and therefore reflect some of the qualities of chronic pain.*

Screening for hypnotizability must be done carefully in studies of hypnotic pain control. Many studies do not carefully select extreme high and low hypnotizable subjects. If hypnosis involves a unique set of skills, then subjects who have been selected for high hypnotizability will have the best opportunity to experience hypnotic analgesia. Even in an experimental setting, it is difficult to get stable measures of hypnotizability without using two or three scales because the initial session tends to be contaminated by preconceptions, curiosities and anxieties about the meaning of hypnosis.** This is even more complicated in the clinic because a hypnotized patient may respond well to hypnosis during a screening session, but because of an unreadiness to give up the pain symptom, may refuse to experience hypnosis in a subsequent therapeutic context.

---

* The adequacy of other current methods, including pressure pain and dental tooth stimulation remains open to future investigations.

** There are now several well standardized, objective scales measuring hypnotic ability. The scales most widely used are the Harvard Group Scale of Hypnotic Susceptibility (Shor and Orne 1962), and the Stanford Hypnotic Susceptibility Scale, Form C (Weitzenhoffer and Hilgard 1962). For a useful discussion of these measurement issues, see Kihlstrom (1985).

Therefore it is critically important to evaluate hypnosis in the clinic independently of the treatment session so that hypnotic ability will not be confounded with the desire to be helped, or the impact of any lack of readiness to get better (Frankel et al. 1979).

Representative studies of hypnotic analgesia

Instead of reviewing the experimental literature on hypnosis and pain (see Hilgard 1977; Hilgard and Hilgard 1979), key studies helping to illustrate the methodological and conceptual issues raised above will be reviewed briefly.

In a marked deviation from the methods used in prior hypnotic analgesia studies, McGlashan et al. (1969; see also Orne 1974; Evans 1977, 1985) tested 12 extreme high and 12 extreme low hypnotizable subjects, using the ischemic pain task, during three sessions: 1) highly motivated baseline conditions; 2) following the induction of hypnotic analgesia; 3) after ingesting a placebo capsule. The capsule was presented as an experimental pain-killing drug serving as a control procedure against which to evaluate the effects of hypnosis. In this session, the experimenter believed subjects were randomly given placebo or Darvon compound in double-blind fashion, although all subjects received placebo.

It is difficult to motivate low hypnotizable subjects to participate in hypnotic procedures, such as analgesia, because they are convinced it will not work with them. A simple but compelling deception was used with the low hypnotizable subjects to legitimize an expectancy of analgesia. Prior to the experimental hypnosis session, an independent experimenter induced a glove analgesia using a hypnotic relaxation induction geared to each subject's description of his prior minimal hypnotic experiences. This was tested by administering a brief electric shock to the fingers. These low hypnotizable subjects experienced the analgesia — because the experimenter surreptitiously turned down the shock intensity from the pre-analgesic test level!

The logic of this study was to maximize variables influencing the placebo effect, as is done in the clinic, rather than to control or eliminate them, as is done in traditional experimental studies. No attempt was made to minimize and control critical variables (demand characteristics) that might affect the results, such as expectations, anxieties, order effects, etc. Instead, a deliberate attempt was made to maximize the effect of confounding variables that might influence changes in (ischemic) pain tolerance. A conservative test was set up to evaluate whether the hypnotic analgesia achieved by deeply hypnotized subjects would exceed the pain relief produced in hypnotically unresponsive subjects who were set up to respond to nonspecific aspects of the hypnotic treatment context and to placebo medication. A similar test of the effects of hypnotic analgesia was conducted, using the subject as his own control, after he ingested what was thought to be powerful pain-killing medication.

The improved ability to tolerate excruciating ischemic muscle pain for these extremely hypnotizable and unhypnotizable subjects after suggestions of hypnotic analgesia, and subsequently after ingesting a placebo, is shown in Fig. 1. Three aspects of the results should be noted:

a) There was a dramatic increase in pain tolerance for deeply hypnotizable subjects during hypnotically-induced analgesia. This is directly attributable to the dissociative aspects of the hypnotic condition when it occurs in highly responsive hypnotic virtuoso subjects.

b) The much smaller but significant placebo-induced change in ischemic pain tolerance was equal in magnitude for both highly hypnotizable and unhypnotizable subjects.

c) The hypnotic analgesia suggestions significantly improved tolerance of ischemic pain even

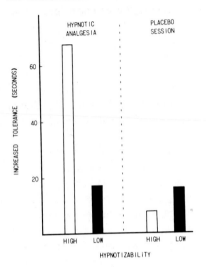

PAIN TOLERANCE INCREASE WITH HYPNOSIS AND PLACEBO

Fig. 1: Increase in ischemic pain tolerance (from baseline) for high and low hypnotizable subjects following the induction of hypnosis and the ingestion of placebo medication (n = 12 high, and 12 low, hypnotizable subjects).

for unhypnotizable subjects who do not have the ability to enter hypnosis. This can be labeled as the 'placebo' component of the hypnotic induction procedure. Indeed, for these hypnotically unresponsive subjects, the pain relief produced by the placebo component of the hypnotic context and the placebo component of ingesting a pill are about equal, and highly correlated (0.76, n = 12). The expectation that hypnosis can be helpful in reducing pain produces similar significant reductions in pain as the expectation derived from taking a pain-killing pill, particularly in those individuals who otherwise have no special hypnotic skills. This somewhat manipulative and deceptive study indicated that hypnosis has both specific and nonspecific effects, just as the administration of medication has specific drug effects and nonspecific placebo effects.

In contrast to studies in which attempts were made to minimize the nonspecific or placebo effects of the hypnotic context, they were maximized and allowed to run free in this study. Significant pain relief was achieved under both the placebo analgesia and placebo hypnosis conditions, even though this relief was not nearly as great as that obtained with hypnotic analgesia in hypnotizable subjects. In drug research, for example, it has been shown that for patients who respond to a placebo injection 95% will also respond to a standard dose of morphine to reduce pain. However, in those patients who did not respond to the placebo trial, only 54% responded to morphine (Lasagna et al. 1954). The expectation of relief that presumably mediates the placebo response is a powerful therapeutic effect. Evans (1977, 1985) reviewed double-blind medication pain reduction studies and showed that the relative effectiveness of placebo compared to a standard dose of morphine is about 56%. The placebo is also from 50 to 60% as effective as aspirin, Codeine, Darvon, and Zomax, as well as nonpain procedures including the pharmacological and behavioral treatment of insomnia and the double-blind use of lithium in psychiatric patients. This is a remarkable finding, because it implies that the nonspecific factors arising from the treatment milieu are important clinical variables to the extent that the therapist communicates his enthusiasm and expectation of success to the suffering patient.

The study by McGlashan et al. (1966; Evans 1977, 1983) documented that the mechanisms by which a placebo pill and hypnosis produced analgesia were different in subjects with high hypnotic capacity. Knox et al. (1981) compared acupuncture with hypnosis and found similar results to those reported above comparing placebo with hypnosis. The pain reduction with acupuncture was similar in high and low hypnotizable subjects, but the pain response of highly hypnotizable subjects was significantly greater with hypnosis than with acupuncture.* The independence of hypnotic analgesia from nonspecific pain reduction methods was also demonstrated in a recent study (Miller and Bowers, in press) that involved cold pressor pain in three groups, each preselected for high and low hypnotizability: a) Meichenbaum's (1977) stress inoculation procedure; b) the same procedure defined as a hypnotic intervention (without any hypnotic induction); c) hypnotic analgesia. They argued that the two stress inoculation groups captured the essential features of interventions used by Spanos (1982) and others from the social contextual approach to hypnosis. Not surprisingly, the results were quite clear-cut, and directly comparable to the hypnotic versus placebo (McGlashan et al. 1969) and acupuncture (Knox et al. 1981) studies. High and low hypnotizable subjects gained significant and equal pain relief from the stress inoculation procedures. However, the pain reduction of highly hypnotizable subjects with hypnotic analgesia surpassed the degree of relief from all subjects where hypnosis was not involved.

In summary, these studies and others show that hypnosis can facilitate a number of cognitive strategies that can be helpful in alleviating pain. Specific interventions such as acupuncture, attention/distraction, placebo, relaxation, stress inoculation, all have a significant effect on pain, but these effects are independent of individual differences in hypnotic capacity. The use of the label 'hypnosis' produces a strong, almost magical, connotation that *change* is expected. This expectation of therapeutic success may be strong in the therapist as well as in the patient. The communication of confidence and the message to the patient that help is on its way is a powerful therapeutic intervention that cannot be overlooked in treating chronic pain. The magical connotations and ritual of the hypnotic induction process produce powerful nonspecific therapeutic elements that may lead to effective pain control in many patients, even those with limited hypnotic capacity. In this sense, hypnosis may work for everybody except the treatment-resistant patient, even though the clinical effects are produced by the context of hypnosis rather than the hypnotic condition itself.

On the other hand, these studies show that at least for some highly selected individuals, hypnosis produces a means of controlling and mastering pain that is different from procedures such as placebo, acupuncture, stress inoculation, and naloxone-induced biochemical changes. The critical point in clinical management is that, just like the studies on the interaction between

---

* The independence of the mechanisms of acupuncture and hypnosis has been confirmed in studies reporting that the opiate antagonist, Naloxone, reverses the pain alleviation of acupuncture, but does not affect the pain reduction produced by hypnosis (Goldstein and Hilgard 1975; Spiegel and Albert 1983). Strictly correlational studies are likely to be misleading when comparing different techniques. For example, a clinical study by Katz et al. (1974) found a correlation between treatment by acupuncture and treatment by hypnosis. The correlational analysis failed to reveal the nonlinear relationship between the two variables. There was a group of pain patients who responded to neither hypnosis nor acupuncture – equivalent to the chronic pain patient who remains unresponsive to any intervention. However, at the successful end of the treatment scale, there was no relationship between those who responded to hypnosis and those who responded to acupuncture.

placebo response and morphine response, these interpersonal and individual trait aspects of hypnosis cannot be separated. However, only the trait components depend on measured hypnotic skill. Therefore it is not surprising that many patients with moderate to low hypnotizability will be responsive to hypnotic manipulations, particularly if they are ready to respond at that time. The fact that there are two interacting mechanisms involved helps to explain why clinicians often see compelling pain relief in patients who otherwise seem unhypnotizable. The capacity to experience hypnosis may be at best a bonus. Careful diagnosis of the nature of the pain will often suggest that the nonspecific components of the hypnotic situation may provide powerful therapeutic leverage. If hypnosis is useful with chronic pain cases where depression and secondary gain are the key therapeutic issues, it is most likely to involve these nonspecific aspects of the hypnotic context rather than hypnotic capacity.

Hypnosis and chronic pain management

CLINICAL ASSESSMENT OF CHRONIC PAIN

The average chronic pain patient will have unsuccessfully attempted an average of five previous types of treatment before coming to a therapist who uses hypnosis. These will often have included neurologists and neurosurgeons ('when in doubt, cut it out'), manipulative procedures by orthopedic and chiropractic specialists ('when in doubt, pound it out'), psychological intervention ('when in doubt, talk it out'), and extensive pharmacological intervention ('when in doubt, medicate'). The typical chronic pain patient will often be simultaneously taking many different medications. In addition, they will have typically been involved in psychological and psychiatric treatment, and other well-meaning sources including the local hairdresser, spouse, lover, and friends. Given the background of depression and internalized anger, it is usually discouraging to the clinician that the initial confrontation is often an adversarial one. The patient's demand to 'help poor me, doc' (when the implicit meaning is 'I know you can't'), 'fix me up' ('you're probably another quack'), 'at least write me another prescription' ('I need to maintain my addiction'), are not conducive to a meaningful therapeutic relationship (Sternbach 1974). For many of these patients, the demand, 'hypnotize me and get rid of my pain' is often an invitation to failure. When the burden of cure is abrogated to the implicit magic of the technique, any initial attempt to use hypnosis would, at best, be unsuccessful, and at worst, precipitate an early termination of the therapeutic encounter.

The importance of the initial therapeutic contract must be emphasized when hypnosis is to be used with the chronic pain patient. Many of these patients will require a confrontational style in order for the therapist to evaluate the secondary gain issues rather quickly, because it will be these issues that will determine the focus of the treatment plan. Three direct questions are often sufficient to help do this.

1) 'What difference would it make to your life if suddenly you had no pain?' The response to this is often hedged with anger and impatience. It will quickly reveal hints about the psychic utility of the pain as a reinforcing system. For example, the implications are quite clear from the response: 'Oh, I would have to go back to my goddamned traveling salesman job and be away from my family most of the time.'

2) 'Do you want to get better?' Patients with chronic pain masking depression will rarely give an unequivocal 'yes' to this question. An angry 'What do you mean? Of course I want to get

better' is a typical response. I will repeat this question three times with some patients, giving them the opportunity to give a simple 'yes' response. Failure to obtain a sincere 'yes' usually indicates poor prognosis.

3) 'Are you willing to work hard to get better?' This question is useful to explain to the patient that the therapist has no magical cure, and that certainly hypnosis does not guarantee dramatic results. The emphasis is on the ability of the patient to work at getting better rather than expecting the therapist to produce some magical, effortless 'quick fix'.

If the answers to these direct questions are unsatisfactory, it may be necessary to tell patients who cannot accept the basic therapeutic contract that this approach may not be right for them, and perhaps they should seek help elsewhere. The clinician has to make a difficult decision as to whether continuing therapy with a case with poor prognostic outcome is better than dismissing the patient who may then seek help from one who may actually do him harm.

These three questions also provide a useful transition to discuss two additional areas. The first is to ensure that the patient can accept as a therapeutic contract that total pain relief will probably not be possible. In fact, it is desirable to establish reduction of the pain to about half its current maximum intensity as a realistic goal: better results than that are presented as a bonus for being skilled and hard-working at the task at hand. This will also lead to a discussion of misconceptions about hypnosis and to indicate that the responsibility for improvement rests with the patient rather than with the hypnotist. The hypnotist's role as a special and powerful teacher or facilitator must be emphasized.

Finally, the manner in which the patient is asked to describe his pain may be very useful for the selection of appropriate imagery and cognitive strategies when it is time to use hypnotic interventions. Many patients find it difficult to describe their pain verbally, but can complete written instruments such as the McGill Pain Questionnaire (Melzack 1975). Techniques such as asking about the 'color' and 'shape' of the pain, drawing the pain, and exploring conditions under which it is more or less intense (heat, cold, sitting), may be relevant to later treatment strategy.*

HYPNOTIC TECHNIQUES IN PAIN MANAGEMENT

The nature of the hypnotic interaction will largely depend on the evaluation of co-existing masked depression and secondary gain components to the pain, or if the pain is primarily a residual of a clearly localized or well-documented somatic process. The extreme clinical examples are low back pain, or injury that is involved in litigation, versus terminal cancer pain. The patient involved in compensation or litigation cannot easily give up the pain until the legal proceedings are resolved. Although initially hypnosis will not usually be very successful, when gradually introduced with supportive psychotherapy, hypnosis may still be the adjunctive treatment of choice. Similarly, the low back pain patient who is masking depression will not easily relinquish his symptom with hypnotic intervention, unless the depression is also treated. The symptom is too important to relinquish with simple hypnotic interventions such as posthypnotic suggestion. Where there is the possibility of unmasking depression due to too rapid removal of the pain symptom, complications, including suicide risk, must be carefully considered.

---

* Particularly in outpatient settings, chronic patients do not react well to extensive psychological testing. I find that elevations on the Somatic, Depression and possibly Hysteria scales of the short Crown-Crisp Experiential Inventory (1979) to be as helpful as a clinical indicator of somatic depression as the elevated Hs, D, and Hy scales of the much longer Minnesota Multiphasic Personality Inventory (Sternbach 1974).

THE INITIAL HYPNOSIS SESSIONS

After careful assessment, the initial work with hypnosis (in a first or later treatment session) will usually not entail work related to the pain problem. This session will need to explore the patient's expectation about the nature of hypnosis, to allow the patient to find out about his own hypnotic skills, and to become familiar with the hypnotic procedures. No attempt should be made to evaluate the depth of hypnosis because it is largely irrelevant to the treatment plan.* Whether progress is capitalizing on the nonspecific components of the relationship, or the patient's special hypnotic skills, is not important clinically.

This initial hypnotic experience should gradually build upon relatively easy suggestions that are based on subtle physical manifestations (e.g. eye fixation procedures based on eye strain and fatigue leading to suggestive eye closure and relaxation). Such procedures yield successes that can be easily reinforced, as are any suggestions for which an end point defining success is not obvious to the patient. For example, suggestions that the arm is light and floating up are appropriate as long as the patient does not find out how far up is 'up'. It is easy for the therapist to reinforce a partial response, but it is very difficult for the suffering patient to recover from a clear-cut perception of failure if his hypnotic response cannot be positively reinforced.

In the subsequent hypnosis experience a delicate balance is required between the initial, somewhat authoritarian and manipulative approach by the hypnotist as he teaches the patient mastery experiences, and the nondirective cognitive discovery of success and mastery in areas that the patient will see as related to pain control. At the same time, this progress must be sufficiently slow so that the patient can be drawn into the therapeutic alliance to handle the psychological issues that are more relevant than the pain experience (e.g. 'What are the alternative career opportunities?', 'What if I don't win the compensation case?', 'How do I handle my spouse's sexual advances and the children's behavior?').

SPECIFIC HYPNOTIC PROCEDURES – SOME EXAMPLES

Suggested glove analgesia can be induced in almost all patients. In fact, a failure to induce a glove analgesia is more likely to involve resistance than lack of responsivity. Glove analgesia can be induced with a variety of suggestions directed at localized physical sensations including those focusing on the sensations in the hand, any movement or twitching response, breezes blowing on the hand, the sensation of pressure against clothing or the chair, or feelings of warmth or coolness as one continues to focus and experience the eyestrain, etc. The inclusion of relevant images is helpful to patients who have good imagery. The unusual experience of focusing on such limited physical experiences in itself is surprising to the patient, and fortunately most patients will attribute any noted changes to the therapeutic suggestions, rather than to the natural physiology of the event. This may be facilitated if the wrist is positioned over a sharp edge of the chair's armrest, or the therapist applies mild pressure to an artery, thereby inducing an ischemic numbness that can be tested by pinching the numb hand (somewhat less than the control hand). Done with care, the patient gradually begins to become impressed that he can control a physiological experience in a part of his body. Obviously, repeated experience with this kind of

---

* Depth of hypnosis should not normally be evaluated in a clinical session, although standardized scales should be used during psychological evaluation and assessment, in a setting where performance has no immediate implication for treatment (Frankel et al. 1979). Preconceived notions about a patient's hypnotizability may lead to a change in the therapist's expectations about treatment success.

analgesia can eventually be transferred to the pain-afflicted area, but this should be done cautiously.

Hallucinating pain, which can then be taken away (e.g. with the analgesic hand), may be useful. These techniques should be integrated with ego-strengthening suggestions, and with extensive use of imagery, including utilization of places or feelings or people that are exceptionally pleasurable and/or important to the patient. A suggested haven chosen by the patient (a special room, or garden, or beach) that the patient can escape to under stress can be very important later when self-hypnosis procedures are introduced. The imagery need not be especially vivid, and sometimes nonvisual modalities are useful or preferred.

Relaxation procedures are often important to the patient, particularly when anxiety is also present. However, some patients, especially those with clear organic or cancer pain, are so involved in marshalling their own resources to help control their pain that relaxation experiences can sometimes intensify, rather than reduce the pain. The use of relaxation techniques based on Jacobsonian procedures, or the Benson relaxation response (1974), or the eye roll method (Spiegel and Spiegel 1978), may increase the experience of self-mastery, and provide a method for teaching self-hypnotic procedures which the patient will eventually learn and use at home. Especially useful is a modification of Spiegel's procedure involving the simultaneous rolling up the eyes while taking in a deep breath, 'feeling the relaxation surge down through your body as you breathe out and close your eyes and relax and let yourself float away to one of your very special places where you can enjoy the experience'. The upgaze of the eye roll simultaneously performed with deep inhalation is a tension-inducing maneuver, and quickly leads to deep relaxation as the eyes close with exhalation. Related strategies including clenching and opening the fists with the breathing exercise can heighten the tension/relaxation cycle, and later allow the transfer of pain (or anger) into the clenched fist, so that it can be 'given away' as the fist is released, or crushed. Metaphors based on imagery are often helpful, including changing the color of the pain, e.g. from intense red to a relatively mild pastel tone (blue, red, and purple are often associated with pain in depressed patients – changes to bright colors such as green or yellow are often helpful). Another variant is visualizing changes in pain intensity as corresponding to different sizes so that it can shrink away as the pain dissipates. Many out-of-body dissociative floating experiences, and Sacerdote's Magical Mountain (1977) can also be effective in learning self-control and mastery. Two outstanding books (Gardner and Olness 1981; Hilgard and LeBaron, 1984) on hypnosis in children describe many creative techniques to control pain and most of them can be adapted to adults.

It is the melody rather than the lyrics that are important in hypnotic techniques, and the procedures need to be a comfortable mix of the patient's abilities and the therapist's style. The emphasis of these hypnotic interventions is on the learning of mastery experiences, and allowing the patient to discover that he has the ability to gain mastery over the pain. However, it is especially important that the patient has permission not to use these mastery techniques in all situations. For example, in a litigation case a contract can be established (usually while under hypnosis) that the pain can be controlled using hypnosis, but the patient will remain free to decide when and where to use these mastery techniques. Thus, the tactic of allowing the patient complete choice as to when to control pain, not as a therapeutic issue, is an important way to handle the problems associated with the exposure to psychological threat, and the removal of the pain as a defensive reaction. The thrust of the hypnotic intervention is simply to teach the patient that he/she is capable of controlling pain, but not to become involved in the ethical and moral issues as to *when* the patient should use these techniques. Such contracts are often the keys to success with this kind of patient. They allow the patient to manipulate pain when it is psychologically necessary, progress at his own pace, provide time to develop a therapeutic alliance, and to treat the depression, either with antidepressant medication or psychotherapeutic techniques.

Finally, hypnosis may be the method of choice when, for whatever psychological reasons, the patient is ready to give up the pain. Hypnosis provides a face-saving procedure for the patient who needs an excuse to give up a long-lasting symptom when it no longer has any functional utility. If the patient is able to give up the pain, he is confronted with a hostile family — 'Why can you do it now, and not thousands of dollars ago with all of your therapists?'. If the patient is allowed to capitalize on the magical label of hypnosis as a more powerful technique than other therapists have tried in the past, and if he can attribute the change to the hypnosis, rather than to himself, the need for face-saving strategies for giving up a symptom is thereby successfully eliminated.

HYPNOSIS WITH ORGANIC, SOMATIC AND CANCER PAIN

While many of the techniques described will be the same with patients for whom there is a clear-cut organic basis to the pain, the treatment process will often be shorter and much simpler. For these patients, success is more likely to be dependent upon hypnotic skill than on the hypnotic relationship. It is helpful to relate hypnotic techniques to natural experiences that help the person alleviate their pain (e.g. warmth or cold, movement, distraction, fantasy, etc.), and gear hypnotic suggestions around any warning signals of pain onset. Thus, lying on a warm beach is a fine substitute for a heating pad, but only if warmth rather than coldness helps reduce the patient's pain. While this point seems obvious, inexperienced hypnotists will often not bother to check the appropriateness of a specific set of images with the patient, and not allow the patient to choose the imagery and the kinds of suggestions that might work best. The patient must always remain in control of the pain experience — he/she controls what will work and what will not be helpful.

While the first session will follow the evaluation procedures and initial hypnotic contact described above, it is possible to begin direct hypnotic intervention more quickly with these patients, as the psychological risk is minimized. There is no need for concern about the effects of a too rapid alleviation of the symptom. The direct therapeutic focus is to find the 'magic formula' that will work for that particular patient. Self-hypnosis exercises should be introduced as quickly as possible. The patient should be required to practice these exercises both when pain is and is not present. By being able to use self-hypnosis when there is no need for it, it becomes much easier to remember the self-hypnotic procedure and to have it available automatically when there is need for it. The utilization of active imagery techniques, e.g. scenarios in which patients select good images which devour the cancer-producing cells, using a blatant immunological metaphor, may be effective. Attention to the nausea, vomiting and discomfort of these patients is also very relevant.

For the patient with terminal illness, the techniques will vary depending on the stage of illness. In the early stages, emphasis will be on relaxation, the control of anxiety, and the handling of medication side effects. The middle stages will be concerned more with the meaning of life and death, and the ability to suffer and die with dignity. The terminal phase will focus on maintaining enough control over the pain and treatment side effects in order to maintain good social relationships with family, etc., during the final period. In all cases, the application of hypnotic intervention techniques will almost certainly result in a reduction of the amount of medication needed to control pain, though, particularly in the terminal case, there should be little concern over addiction, as opposed to patient comfort, until such time as there is evidence of remission of the illness and the pain.

Particularly in terminal cases, the availability of the therapist is more important than the regularity or length of treatment sessions. 'Booster shots' of hypnosis to help counteract any temporary failure of the mastery experience (due to uncontrollable factors, such as a family argument, change in medication, course of illness, etc.) should be used when needed. If appropriately set up, these 'boosters' can even be conducted over the telephone.

Summary

Some of the ways in which hypnosis is relevant and useful in the management of chronic pain have been summarized. Differences in the theoretical understanding of hypnosis were highlighted, particularly as they relate to pain control. Important conceptual and methodological factors that are relevant to the design of meaningful research in the area of hypnosis and pain control were reviewed. Although research on hypnotic analgesia has contributed to existing knowledge about pain mechanisms, they have had relatively few implications for the management of chronic pain. Available studies support the conclusion that for highly hypnotizable subjects, hypnosis can effectively reduce pain. In selected individuals such pain reduction differs from that produced by a variety of psychological (placebo, distraction, stress innoculation) and physiological (acupuncture, naloxone reversal) methods of pain reduction. The dissociative advantages of deep hypnosis cannot be overlooked, but may not be available to many patients. However, hypnosis occurs in a special context that maximizes nonspecific components of expectation, trust, and belief in cure, similar to the placebo response that occurs with medication. The combination of the specific and nonspecific components of hypnosis provides a powerful clinical tool even though the nonspecific components are independent of hypnotic capacity. The specific applications of hypnosis in pain management will be different depending on the nature and history of the patient's pain.

Acute pain is best managed by anxiety-reducing strategies, particularly those having to do with interpersonal interactions which minimize the importance of the pain. Relaxation procedures can be designed which are incompatible with anxiety, and therefore will be pain reducing.

Chronic pain which has gradually become a weapon in the control of contingencies in the sufferer's interaction with the external world will require strategies that deal with handling one's psychological environment effectively. In such cases, the pain has no clear organic basis, even though from the patient's viewpoint 'it hurts'. The difficulties in using hypnosis with chronic pain patients, particularly in those whose pain masks depression and who use pain instrumentally to reinforce psychological processes and behaviors (secondary gain) were highlighted, particularly as they apply to the initial stages of treatment. The use of several hypnotic strategies − relaxation, imagery, dissociation, self-hypnosis − was summarized.

For the patient whose pain is due to a chronic or *terminal* condition, where there is clear evidence of organic pathology (e.g. terminal cancer pain), hypnosis can be used extremely effectively, avoiding issues related to reactive depression. For these patients, hypnosis may be the method of choice to teach the patient to control and manipulate pain levels, as well as to reduce medication and to minimize side effects of simultaneous treatment, including chemotherapy.

Further research and controlled clinical trials will be necessary to evaluate which of these approaches will be most helpful to individual patients with both acute and chronic pain. However, as each patient suffers in his/her own private way, clinical sensitivity must always take priority over general guidelines and prescriptions for these difficult and misunderstood pain patients.

Acknowledgment

Supported in part by the Carrier Foundation. I wish to thank Richard K. Goodstein, Kenneth S. Mathisen, Helen M. Pettinati, and Carmine E. Salierno, for their many helpful contributions, and Amy Kight-Law, Julie Staats, Julie Wade and Jean Balcom for their helpful comments and technical assistance. Several of the clinical procedures discussed were stimulated by discussions over several years with Martin T. Orne.

References

Barber, J. (1977) Rapid induction analgesia: a clinical report. Am. J. Clin. Hypnosis. 19, 138–147.

Barber, T. X. (1969) Hypnosis: A Scientific Approach. Van Nostrand, New York.

Beecher, H. K. (1959) Measurement of Subjective Responses: Quantitative Effects of Drugs. Oxford University Press, New York.

Benson, H. (1975) The Relaxation Response. William Morrow, New York.

Bowers, K. S. (1976) Hypnosis for the Seriously Curious. W. W. Norton & Co., New York.

Chaves, J. F. and Brown, J. M. (1978) Self-generated strategies for the control of pain and stress. Paper presented at the Annual Meeting of the American Psychological Association, Toronto, Canada.

Crown, S. and Crisp, A. H. (1979) Manual of the Crown-Crisp Experiential Index. Hoddard Stoughton, London.

Domangue, B. B . and Margolis, C. G. (1983) Hypnosis and a multidisciplinary cancer pain management team: role and effects. Int. J. Clin. Exp. Hypnosis. 31, 206.

Elton, D., Burrows, G. D. and Stanley, G. V. (1980) Chronic pain and hypnosis. In: G. D. Burrows and L. Dennerstein, (Eds.), Handbook of Hypnosis and Psychosomatic Medicine. Elsevier/North-Holland Biomedical Press, Amsterdam.

Esdaile, J. (1957) Hypnosis in Medicine and Surgery. Julian Press, New York. (Originally titled Mesmerism in India, 1850).

Evans, F. J. (1977) The placebo control of pain: a paradigm for investigating non-specific effects in psychotherapy. In: J. P. Brady, J. Mendels, W. R. Reiger and M. T. Orne (Eds.), Psychiatry: Areas of Promise and Advancement. Spectrum, New York, pp. 129–136.

Evans, F. J. (1983) The hypnotizable subject: the hypnotizable patient. Presidential Address presented at the 35th Annual Meeting of The Society for Clinical and Experimental Hypnosis, Boston.

Evans, F. J. (1985) Expectancy, therapeutic instructions, and the placebo response. In: L. White, B. Tursky and G. Schwartz (Eds.), Placebo: Clinical Phenomena and New Insights. The Guilford Press, New York, pp. 215–228.

Fordyce, W. E. (1976) Behavioral Methods for Chronic Pain and Illness. C. V. Mosby, St. Louis.

Frankel, F. H., Apfel, R. J., Kelly, S. F., Benson, H., Quinn, T., Newmark, J. and Malmaud, R. (1979) The use of hypnotizability scales in the clinic: a review after six years. Int. J. Clin. Exp. Hypnosis. 27, 63–73.

Gardner, G. G. and Olness, K. (1981) Hypnosis and Hypnotherapy with Children. Grune and Stratton, New York.

Goldstein, E. and Hilgard, E. (1975) Failure of opiate antagonist naloxone to modify hypnotic analgesia. Proc. Natl. Acad. Sci. U.S.A. 72, 2041–2043.

Hilgard, E. R. (1965) Hypnotic Susceptibility. Harcourt, Brace & World, New York.

Hilgard, E. R. (1969) Pain as a puzzle for psychology and physiology. Am. Psychol. 24, 103–113.

Hilgard, E. R. (1974) Toward a neo-dissociation theory: multiple cognitive controls in human functioning. Perspect. Biol. Med. 17, 301–316.

Hilgard, E. R. (1977) Divided Consciousness: Multiple Controls in Human Thought and Action. John Wiley & Sons, New York.

Hilgard, E. R. and Hilgard, J. R. (1975) Hypnosis in the Relief of Pain. William Kaufman, Inc., Los Altos, CA.

Hilgard, J. R. and LeBaron, S. (1984) Hypnotherapy of Pain in Children with Cancer. William Kaufman, Inc., Los Altos, CA.

Katz, R. L., Kao, C. Y., Spiegel, H. and Katz, G. J. (1974) Acupuncture and hypnosis. Adv. Neurol. 4, 819 – 825.

Kihlstrom, J. F. (1985) Hypnosis. Ann. Rev. Psychol. 36, 385 – 400.

Knox, V. J., Gekoski, W. L., Shum, K. and Mclaughlin, D. M. (1981) Analgesia for experimentally induced pain: multiple sessions of acupuncture compared to hypnosis in high- and low-susceptible subjects. J. Abnorm. Psychol. 90, 28 – 34.

Lasagna, L., Mosteller, F., von Felsinger, J. M. and Beecher, H. (1954) A study of the placebo response. Am. J. Med. 16, 770 – 779.

McGlashan, T. H., Evans, F. J. and Orne, M. T. (1969) The nature of hypnotic analgesia and the placebo response to experimental pain. Psychosom. Med. 31, 227 – 246.

Meichenbaum, D. H. (1977) Cognitive-Behavior Modification: An Integrative Approach. Plenum Press, New York.

Melzack, R. (1975) The McGill Pain Questionnaire: Major properties and scoring methods. Pain. 1, 277 – 299.

Miller, M. E. and Bowers, K. S. (1986) Hypnotic analgesia and stress inoculation in the reduction of pain. J. Abnorm. Psychol. 95, 6 – 14.

Morgan, A. H., Johnson, D. L. and Hilgard, E. R. (1974) The stability of hypnotic susceptibility: a longitudinal study. Int. J. Clin. Exp. Hypnosis. 22, 249 – 257.

Orne, M. T. (1974) Pain suppression by hypnosis and related phenomena. Adv. Neurol. 4, 563 – 572.

Sacerdote, P. (1970) Theory and practice of pain control in malignancy and other protracted or recurring painful illnesses. Int. J. Clin. Exp. Hypnosis. 18, 160 – 180.

Sacerdote, P. (1977) Applications of hypnotically elicited mystical states to the treatment of physical and emotional pain. Int. J. Clin. Exp. Hypnosis. 25, 309 – 324.

Sarbin, T. R. and Coe, W. (1972) Hypnosis: A Social Psychological Analysis of Influence Communication. Holt, Rinehart & Winston, New York.

Shor, R. E. (1962) Physiological effects of painful stimulation during hypnotic analgesia under conditions designed to minimize anxiety. Int. J. Clin. Exp. Hypnosis. 10, 183 – 202.

Shor, R. E. and Orne, E. C. (1962) The Harvard Group Scale of Hypnotic Susceptibility, Form A. Consulting Psychologists Press, Palo Alto, CA.

Spanos, N. P. (1982) A social psychological approach to hypnotic behavior. In: G. Weary and H. L. Mirels (Eds.), Integration of Clinical and Social Psychology. Oxford, New York, pp. 241 – 271.

Spiegel, D. and Albert, L. H. (1983) Naloxone fails to reverse hypnotic alleviation of chronic pain. Psychopharmacology 81, 140 – 143.

Spiegel, H. and Spiegel, D. (1978) Trance and Treatment: Clinical Uses of Hypnosis. Basic Books, New York.

Sternbach, R. A. (1974) Pain Patients: Traits and Treatment. Academic Press, New York.

Turner, J. A. and Chapman, C. R. (1982) Psychological interventions for chronic pain: a critical review. II. Operant conditioning, hypnosis, and cognitive-behavioral therapy. Pain 12, 23 – 46.

Wagstaff, G. F. (1981) Hypnosis, Compliance and Belief. St. Martin's Press, New York.

Weitzenhoffer, A. M. and Hilgard, E. R. (1962) Stanford Hypnotic Susceptibility Scale, Form C. Consulting Psychologists Press, Palo Alto, CA.

Burrows/Elton/Stanley (eds.) Handbook of Chronic Pain Management
© *1987 Elsevier Science Publishers B.V. (Biomedical Division)*

28

The psychiatrist in the management of chronic pain

FIONA K. JUDD[1], GRAHAM D. BURROWS[1] and BRENDAN J. HOLWILL[2]

Department of Psychiatry, University of Melbourne, [1]Austin Hospital, Heidelberg, Victoria, and [2]Repatriation General Hospital, Heidelberg, Victoria, Australia

Introduction

The management of patients with chronic pain requires a multidisciplinary team approach. What is the unique role of the psychiatrist in a team comprising physicians, surgeons, physiotherapists and occupational therapists, psychologists, social workers and nursing staff? The psychiatrist has a firm biomedical base and a knowledge of psychosocial issues and is able to conceptualise ways in which these varying approaches can be synthesised (German 1980).

The clinical method of the psychiatrist differs from that of other medical practitioners. The psychiatric examination includes the mental status examination, the physical examination and examination of the doctor-patient relationship. The psychiatrist's skill in mental status examination distinguishes him from both his medical and non-medical colleagues (Kalucy 1980). Aspects of both phenomenology (descriptive) and psychodynamics (explanatory) are examined. Observed phenomena include not only the patient's behaviour, but also that of his family, the psychiatrist and other staff.

All this data is used to generate explanatory hypotheses. The psychiatrist is also skilled in neurochemical and neuropharmacological concepts important both for explanation of behaviour and for treatment of specific disturbances.

The role of the psychiatrist in the management of the patient with chronic pain varies according to the type of patient referred and the treatment situation. In general, the psychiatric aspects of management of chronic pain patients can be sub-divided to the broad areas of assessment and treatment.

Assessment

The major aims of psychiatric assessment of the patient with chronic pain are identification of the causes and sequelae of the pain. All patients with chronic pain have some emotional disturbance. This may be the cause of the pain itself or may be a secondary effect. Psychological factors may evoke pain by a number of different mechanisms. The first is represented by pain due to muscle tension, where tension itself results from psychological causes. Secondly, pain may occur as part of a hysterical conversion reaction. Pain may be associated with, or be the presenting symptom of a depressive illness, e.g. 'burning tongue syndrome' (Gerschman et al. 1981). Rarely pain may occur as a hallucination in either schizophrenia or severe depression.

Commonly the psychiatrist assesses the patient with chronic pain in his role as consultation-liaison psychiatrist, in the psychiatric inpatient unit or the specialist pain clinic. The reported prevalence of psychiatric morbidity among patients with chronic pain varies depending upon how the evaluation of mental illness is made. Recent surveys have shown that 30 – 50% of patients have measurable psychiatric disturbances (Tyrer 1985). Two thirds of these patients have a major depressive disorder (DSM-III criteria). Other diagnoses include personality disorder, anxiety states, hysteria, drug dependence and organic brain syndrome.

Main areas of assessment in relation to the psychiatric aspects of management include personality predisposition, the role of psychodynamic and interpersonal factors and whether or not an overt diagnosable psychiatric diagnosis is present.

PSYCHIATRIC ILLNESS

Chronic pain and psychiatric illness are frequently linked. Depression, whether neurotic or psychotic is often associated with pain. Fifty to sixty percent of patients with a depressive illness complain of pain (Merskey and Spear 1967). Some specific chronic pain syndromes, e.g. atypical facial pain, are particularly likely to be the presenting symptom of a depressive illness (Lascelles 1966). Many patients with chronic pain due to physical illness, develop a secondary depressive syndrome (Le Shan 1964).

Generalised anxiety and muscle tension may produce muscular pain and referred pain from muscular action. Common examples include tension headache, 'fibrositis' and the abdominal pains accompanying irritable colon. Pain is the most common misdiagnosed somatic symptom in patients with panic disorder (Katon 1984). Chronic pain as a major complaint is infrequent in schizophrenia. Somatic delusions and the hallucination of pain have been reported (Watson et al. 1981). Chronic pain may be the central feature of monosymptomatic hypochondriacal psychosis. Chronic pain as a hysterical conversion symptom is well recognised. Walters (1961) has criticised the term 'hysterical pain' emphasising that the psychiatric background of most patients extends well beyond hysteria to include most other psychiatric states.

PERSONALITY FACTORS

The Minnesota Multiphasic Personality Inventory (MMPI) has been widely used in the assessment of patients with chronic pain. Most often patients show the pattern of the 'conversion triad', i.e. elevated hypochondriasis, depression and hysteria scales (Sternbach 1974). Alexithymia (Flannery 1978), disease conviction, somatic focussing and denial of life problems (Pilowsky and Spence 1976) have commonly been reported. We have found depression, hypochondriasis and obsessionality to be common.

Interpersonal and social factors

Interpersonal factors may contribute to the development/maintenance of chronic pain. Hirschfeld and Behan (1967) described the 'accident process' in which unacceptable psychological disability was converted to acceptable physical disability. Where chronic pain is the result of injury, several factors may maintain the disability. These include the psychological impact of the accident or injury, cultural factors related to illness behaviour, interpersonal and family dynamics, the litigation process and monetary compensation (Ellard 1970; Mendelson 1981; Stagoll 1981).

Psychodynamic factors

Psychodynamic theorists generally view pain as a form of hysteria and emphasise the association of pain with resentment and guilt. Engel (1959) described a group of 'pain-prone patients' in whom he suggested psychological factors played a primary role in the genesis of pain. These patients generally described a background characterised by aggression, pain and suffering. Guilt was an invariable factor in the choice of pain as a symptom. He suggested pain occurred when external circumstances failed to satisfy the unconscious need to suffer, in response to real, threatened or fantasied loss, or when intense aggressive or sexual feelings occurred.

Organic factors

The organic aspects of various chronic pain disorders are discussed in detail in other areas of this book.

The family

Chronic pain not only affects the patient, but also the patient's family. Spouses of chronically ill patients often report physical symptoms and a high role of tension (Klein et al. 1967). Chronic pain may mean the family and not simply the individual is disabled. Many aspects of family functioning including sexual activity, income, and social and leisure activity may be disrupted. Secondary depression resulting in social withdrawal, irritability and dependence may exacerbate these problems. Problems may occur when developmental issues within the family are neglected because priority is given to the family's adjustment to chronic illness (Steinglass et al. 1982). The families of chronic pain patients often break down, or may establish a new equilibrium, at times less stable and adaptive than that prior to illness (Bruhn 1977).

Diagnostic classification

The principal role of psychiatrists has been in assessment and management of patients variously diagnosed as suffering from chronic pain syndrome (Black 1976; Chapman 1977), the learned pain syndrome (Brena and Chapman 1981) operant pain (Fordyce 1976) and psychogenic regional pain (Walters 1961). More recently, the term 'psychogenic pain disorder' has been used (A.P.A 1980) (Table 1).

These terms all imply that psychological factors are prominent in the maintenance of pain. These descriptive classifications are inadequate as they do not emphasise the need to elucidate the degree to which depression, anxiety, personality and interpersonal factors and various interpersonal and social gains may contribute to continued pain.

TABLE 1
DSM-III criteria: psychogenic pain disorder.

A) Severe and prolonged pain is the predominant disturbance
B) The pain presented as a symptom is inconsistent with the anatomic distribution of the nervous system; after extensive evaluation, no organic pathology or pathophysiological mechanism can be found to account for the pain; or, when there is some related organic pathology, the complaint of pain is grossly in excess of what would be expected from the physical findings
C) Psychological factors are judged to be aetiologically involved in the pain, as evidenced by at least one of the following:

　　1) a temporal relationship between an environmental stimulus that is apparently related to a psychological conflict or need and the initiation or exacerbation of the pain
　　2) the pain's enabling the individual to avoid some activity that is noxious to him or her
　　3) the pain's enabling the individual to get support from the environment that otherwise might not be forthcoming.

D) Not due to another mental disorder

CONSULTATION-LIAISON PSYCHIATRY

Patients with chronic pain are commonly referred for liaison psychiatry assessment. The most usual presentation is with somatic complaints for which no organic cause can be found or where presented symptoms are out of proportion to organic pathology. In the assessment and management of these patients, both the roles of 'consultation' and 'liaison' must be filled. 'Consultation' requires the provision of expert diagnostic opinion and management advice. 'Liaison' involves both interpretation and mediation (Lipowsky 1974). The attitude and behaviour of patients and those treating them must be considered. Conflict and contentious attitudes must be identified. The psychosocial consequences of the patients' illness, and the influence of his disability and illness behaviour on his family must be assessed. Hospitalisation often occurs at times of psychosocial stress.

THE PAIN CLINIC

The psychiatrist must fulfill three major roles in the pain clinic. He must persuade other members of the treatment team that not all pain is psychogenic. He must determine the psychological and interpersonal factors contributing to the patient's pain and plan appropriate management taking these into account (Pilowsky 1976). In addition, the psychiatrist must convey to other members of the clinic what the multidisciplinary approach entails and how it may be used. This should include an explanation of the way in which many variables influence pain and the way in which various treatment programmes can be initiated simultaneously.

Patients treated in the pain clinic have commonly consulted a wide variety of doctors and paramedical health professionals prior to consulting members of the multidisciplinary pain team. Frequently this results in a plethora of medical opinions, diagnoses and management plans. As a result, patients may be bewildered and frightened, feeling there is no coherent or effective treatment of their condition. Alternatively, patients may use this situation in a manipulative manner to defend their continued illness behaviour. Such behaviour may 'split' team members and cause difficulties in management of the chronic pain behaviour.

The psychiatrist is involved in the management of both situations. The first requires that the psychiatrist has a sound knowledge of other medical specialities and their various investigations and procedures such as CT scanning, myelography, discography, electromyography (EMG) and thermography. The psychiatrist is the team member able to offer a coherent explanation of conflicting opinions and management plans, as a result of his medical background and objective distance from physical management. The second situation requires that the psychiatrist assist the team to formulate a consistent, practical approach to the patient, preventing manipulative behaviour and splitting of the team.

Chronic pain patients frequently make excessive demands on team members for support, explanation and care. This, coupled with the difficult nature of patients' problems, causes stress amongst staff. Staff morale requires constant monitoring by the psychiatrist who must help team members maintain realistic goals and expectations of patients, preventing the development of negative attitudes and feelings of hopelessness.

The psychiatrist has a specialised knowledge of psychotropic drugs and their pharmacokinetics. These drugs are frequently used in the management of chronic pain, both for the treatment of specific symptoms of anxiety and depression and for their analgesic properties.

The psychiatrist and pain management

Psychiatric management of the patient with chronic pain is based on the true psychosomatic approach. The relative contribution of psychological, biological and social factors to the development course and outcome of the patients' pain complaints must be assessed. This is best done in a multidisciplinary pain centre (see Chapter 36). The psychiatrist is particularly concerned to elucidate and treat the psychological and interpersonal factors contributing to the pain.

Treatment can be divided into the main groupings of psychotherapy and pharmacotherapy. Where pain is a symptom of a distinct psychiatric disorder such as depression, anxiety or psychosis, treatment is primarily directed towards that illness. More often several factors contribute to the maintenance of chronic pain complaints.

For most patients, management strategies include some or all of cognitive therapy (Chapter 9), behavioural modification (Chapter 11), relaxation therapy (Chapters 24 and 26), hypnosis (Chapter 27), biofeedback (Chapters 24 and 26), family, marital and sex therapy (Chapters 13, 22 and 29) and the use of psychotropic drugs (Table 2). As patients with chronic pain often have difficulty expressing their feelings and are often unable to accept psychologically-based explanations of their pain, individual psychotherapy is less often used. Group therapy may be of value (see Elton et al. 1983; see also Chapter 26).

TABLE 2
Psychiatric management of chronic pain.

Psychotropic medication
Individual and group psychotherapy
Cognitive therapy
Behaviour modification
Relaxation therapy
Hypnosis
Biofeedback
Family and marital therapy

Antidepressant medication

Pain may be the presenting symptom of a depressive illness. Alternatively depression may develop in response to physical disease and may subsequently reduce tolerance to pain. Antidepressants have increasingly been used to treat chronic pain. Pain relief has been associated either with or without relief of depressive symptoms.

Antidepressants have been shown to be effective in a wide range of chronic pain conditions including arthritis (McDonald Scott 1969; Gringas 1976), postherpetic neuralgia (Woodforde et al. 1965; Taub 1973, Watson et al. 1982), diabetic neuropathy (Davis et al. 1977; Turkington 1980), migraine (Gomersall and Stuart 1973; Couch et al. 1976, 1979; Noone 1977), tension headache (Lance and Curran 1964; Diamond and Balter 1971; Sherwin 1979), facial pain (Lascelles 1966; Gessel 1975) and back pain (Hameroff et al. 1982). A summary of these studies is provided in Table 3. Most studies have used tricyclic antidepressants. Doses found to be effective have varied from as little as 10 mg/day to 200 mg/day.

Mode of action. Several possible explanations for the effectiveness of antidepressants have been suggested. The antidepressant may alleviate depressive symptoms associated with or secondary to chronic pain. Some studies demonstrating the efficacy of antidepressants in the relief of pain have specifically excluded depressed patients (McDonald Scott 1969; Gomersall and Stuart 1973; Gringas 1976) or noted the improvement in pain independent of change in depressive symptoms (Hughes et al. 1963; Lance and Curran 1964; Taub 1973; Johansson and Von Knorring 1979; Watson et al. 1982; Pilowsky et al. 1982; Feinmann et al. 1984) (Table 4). These researchers have concluded the beneficial effects are not simply due to a reduction in depressed mood.

TABLE 3
Studies demonstrating the efficacy of antidepressants, in particular chronic pain conditions.

Investigator	Drugs (mg)	Depression
McDonald Scott (1969)	Imipramine 75	Excluded
Gringas (1976)	Imipramine 75	Excluded
Woodforde et al. (1965)	Amitriptyline 100	Included
Taub (1973)	Amitriptyline 25 – 100	Included
Watson et al. (1982)	Amitriptyline 75	Included
Davis et al. (1977)	Amitriptyline and phenothiazine	
Turkington (1980)	Amitriptyline 100	
	Imipramine 100	Included
	Diazepam 5	
Couch et al. (1976)	Amitriptyline 75	Included
Couch and Hassanein (1979)	Amitriptyline 100	Included
Noone (1977)	Clomipramine 30	Not examined
Gomersall and Stuart (1973)	Amitriptyline 10 – 60	Excluded
Sherwin (1979)	Amitritpyline 100 – 200	Not examined
	Perphenazine 8 – 64	
Diamond and Balter (1971)	Amitriptyline 10 – 25	Not examined
Lance and Curran (1964)	Amitriptyline 30 – 75	
	Imipramine 30 – 75	Not examined
	other	
Lascelles (1966)	Phenelzine 45	Not examined
Hameroff et al. (1982)	Doxepin 2.5 mg/kg	Not examined

The dose of tricyclic antidepressants used has often been well below those generally required for the relief of depressive illness.

Secondly, antidepressants may alter neurotransmitters involved in the control of pain transmission. 5-Hydroxytryptamine (5-HT) is the primary transmitter in the inhibitory projection from the nucleus raphe magnus (NRM) of nociceptive neurons in the dorsal horn (Fields and Basbaum 1978). Direct stimulation of the NRM elicits a potent inhibition of nociceptive neurons in the dorsal horn (Fields and Basbaum 1978). This is attenuated by pharmacological agents that reduce 5-HT mediated neurotransmission (Anderson and Proudfit 1981). Pain perception can be reduced by giving a serotonin precursor such as L-tryptophan (King 1980). Antidepressants increase synaptic serotonin, noradrenaline and dopamine.

Thirdly, antidepressants may interact with the endogenous opioids and their receptors in the brain. Enkephalin-containing neurons and nerve terminals are concentrated in laminae I and II of the dorsal horn (Hökfelt et al. 1977), the periaqueductal gray region (PAG) and in the NRM. Administration of opiates leads to excitation of neurons in PAG and to enhancement of activity of NRM neurons (Gebhart 1982). Biegon and Samuel (1980) demonstrated the specific binding of tricyclic antidepressants to opiate receptors in the brain and suggested this may be the basis for their analgesic effect.

Choice of drug. Most tricyclic antidepressants have been tried in chronic pain. Studies to date have not demonstrated any differential efficacy. Few studies reporting the use of monoamineoxidase inhibitors are available. If antidepressants are effective as a result of increased availability of serotonin, clomipramine, a more potent inhibitor of serotonin uptake, may be the drug of choice. Drugs such as mianserin and maprotiline whose main effect is to increase the amount of noradrenaline in the synapse may be less likely to benefit patients with chronic pain.

All the tricyclics have similar capacity to bind to opiate receptors. The non-tricyclics including mianserin have lower affinity (Biegon and Samuel 1980).

Dosage. Pain relief has been achieved with doses of antidepressants well below those used to treat depressive illness. The dose chosen will be determined by clinical response and side effects. Most often doses of 75 – 150 mg/day have been used. Higher doses may be required.

TABLE 4
Studies demonstrating pain relief independent of antidepressant effect.

Investigator		Drug
Hughes et al. (1963)	Terminal cancer ($n = 118$)	Imipramine
Lance and Curran (1964)	Tension headache ($n = 27$)	Amitriptyline
Taub (1973)	Postherpetic neuralgia ($n = 5$)	Amitriptyline Perphenazine
Watson et al. (1982)	Postherpetic neuralgia ($n = 24$)	Amitriptyline
Johansson and Van Knorring (1979)	Various sites ($n = 20$)	Zimelidine
Pilowsky et al. (1982)	Various sites ($n = 52$)	Amitriptyline
Feinmann et al. (1984)	Facial pain ($n = 93$)	Dothiepin

TABLE 5
Side effects of tricyclic antidepressant drugs.

Site of action	Effect	Management
Autonomic nervous system	Dry mouth, blurred vision, urinary retention, excessive perspiration, erectile dysfunction	Reassure patient and/or decrease dosage, usually tolerated in a few weeks
Cardiovascular system	Postural hypotension ECG abnormalites	Advise patient to get up slowly Decrease dose, cardiological examination in patients with pre-existing abnormalites
Endocrine system	Weight gain	Diet
Central nervous system	Agitation, insomnia, convulsions, sedation, confusion (elderly)	Lower dose
Gastrointestinal system	Nausea, vomiting Constipation	Reassurance, lower dose Exercise, mild laxative
Dermatological system	Skin rash	Usually disappears on further treatment
Haematological system	Leucocytosis	No treatment – an apparently benign effect
Drug interactions	Potentiate alcohol, other sedatives and narcotic analgesics	Avoid

Side effects. Commonly experienced side effects of tricyclic antidepressants are due to anticholinergic effects of the drug. These include dry mouth, blurred vision, constipation and urinary hesitancy. These and other side effects of tricyclics are shown in Table 5.

ANTIPSYCHOTIC DRUGS

The most commonly used antipsychotic drugs in the treatment of chronic pain are the phenothiazines and butyrophenones. These drugs are of particular value when pain is considered to be a delusional symptom. The majority of evidence for antipsychotic-induced pain relief comes from anecdotal single-patient examples. Groups studied have included diabetic neuropathy (Gade et al. 1980), cancer pain (Maltbie and Cavenar 1977), thalamic pain (Margolis and Gianascol 1956), postherpetic neuralgia (Sigwald et al. 1959; Taub 1973). Experimental studies have shown a distinct analgesic action for trimeprazine, chlorpromazine and promazine (Moore and Dundee 1961). Two controlled trials have shown single dose effectiveness of antipsychotics to be equivalent to that of usual analgesic doses of morphine in mixed groups of acute and chronic pain disorders (Montilla et al. 1963; Bloomfield et al. 1964).

Mode of action. Some antipsychotics are considered to have an analgesic action per se (Moore and Dundee 1961). Haloperidol, the most commonly used butyrophenone, is chemically related to pethidine. In animal models haloperidol has been shown to enhance morphine analgesia (Head et al. 1979) and to bind to opiate receptors (Clay and Brougham 1975). Little clinical data is currently available to support these effects in man. The efficacy of neuroleptics in the treatment of chronic pain has also been attributed to their antiemetic and sedative actions. This may be of particular value for patients with malignancy, especially those being treated with chemotherapy or DXRT.

Choice of drug. The antipsychotics show varying degrees of selectivity with relation to antipsychotic, sedative, antiemetic, extrapyramidal and peripheral activity. Choice of drug is determined by the desired pharmacological profile. Chlorpromazine is the drug of choice when sedation is required. The butyrophenones are potent dopamine antagonists and most effective antiemetics.

Side effects. Anticholinergic side effects such as dry mouth, blurred vision are common. Postural hypotension may be dose limiting. Parkinsonism is common with the more potent dopamine antagonists such as haloperidol and trifluoperazine. Prolonged treatment with

TABLE 6
Side effects of antipsychotic drugs.

Site of action	Effect	Management
Autonomic nervous system	Dry mouth, blurred vision, urinary hesitancy, constipation erectile dysfunction	Reassure patient and/or decrease dosage
Cardiovascular system	Postural hypotension	Advise patient to get up slowly. Decrease dosage
	Quinidine-like action	Cardiological examination. Avoid Type 1 anti-arrythmics
Endocrine system	Amenorrhoea, galactorrhoea	Reassurance
	Weight gain	Diet
Central nervous system	Acute dystonic reaction	Anticholinergic
	Akathisia	Lower dose
	Parkinsonism	Lower dose/anticholinergic
	Later onset tardive dyskinesia	Cease medication
	Convulsions	Lower dose
Ocular	Pigmentary retinopathy	Prevention – limit dose
	Pigment in lens/cornea	Benign
Dermatological system	Blue/gray pigmentation	
	Photosensitivity	Avoid exposure to sun
Haematological system	Agranulocytosis	Cease drug
Drug interactions	Potentiate alcohol, other sedatives and narcotic analgesics	Avoid

neuroleptics may result in the development of tardive dyskinesia. These and other side effects of neuroleptics are shown in Table 6.

Combined antipsychotic-antidepressant therapy

Anecdotal case reports and uncontrolled studies have suggested that combinations of tricyclic antidepressants and antipsychotics may be of particular value in the treatment of chronic pain (Merskey and Hester 1972; Taub 1973; Kocher 1976; Gade et al. 1980; Clarke 1981).

Many different drug combinations have been used. No clear conclusions regarding the combined use of these drugs can be drawn as controlled clinical trials comparing the use of antidepressants and antipsychotics alone and in combination are not available.

Lithium carbonate

Uncontrolled trials have demonstrated the value of lithium in the treatment of episodic and chronic cluster headaches (Ekbom 1974; Kudrow 1977; Pearce 1980). The mode of action is unknown.

Management and side effects. Lithium has been prescribed in a manner similar to that for the treatment of affective disorder. The usual dosage varies from 750 mg to 2.5 g daily, in divided doses. Estimation of plasma lithium levels is mandatory. The therapeutic range is 0.6 to 1.0 mmol/l. This is based on a standardised estimate 12 – 14 hours after the last lithium dosage. Common side effects include metallic taste, nausea, diarrhoea and fine digital tremor (Table 7). Lithium toxicity results in vomiting, diarrhoea, confusion and ataxia.

Benzodiazepines

Benzodiazepines are effective muscle relaxants and may be of value in the alleviation of pain due

TABLE 7
Common side effects of lithium therapy.

	Early treatment period	Long-term treatment	Toxicity
Nausea and loose motions	+		
Vomiting and severe diarrhoea			+
Fine tremor	+	+	
Coarse tremor			+
Metallic taste	+		
Polyurea and polydipsia	+	+	
Goitre and hypothyroidism		+	
Oedema		+	
Weight gain		+	
Skin rash	+		
Acne	+	+	
Sluggishness, drowsiness			+
Vertigo, unsteadiness		+	
Dysarthria			+

to or exacerbated by muscle tension. Anxiety, fear and insomnia commonly exacerbate pain and benzodiazepines are the treatment of choice in dealing with these problems.

Management and side effects. Many benzodiazepines are available for clinical use. Choice of drug is based on two aspects of the pharmacokinetics of benzodiazepines, namely, speed of onset of action and duration of action (Table 8) in order to minimise side effects. The choice of initial dosage should be conservative. The most common side effects are tiredness and drowsiness, other side effects include paradoxical behavioural responses such as increased aggression and hostility, uncharacteristic criminal offences and excessive emotional responses, excessive weight gain, skin rash, impairment of sexual function and menstrual irregularities. Tolerance, dependence and a definite withdrawal syndrome have been described.

ANTICONVULSANTS

Several anticonvulsants have been used in the management of chronic pain. These include carbamazepine, diphenylhydantoin, clonazepam and sodium valproate. Carbamazepine is chemically related to the tricyclic antidepressants and increases brain levels of 5-HT. Valproate may increase brain levels of the inhibitory neurotransmitter gamma-aminobutyric acid. Most often the anticonvulsants have been used in the treatment of 'stabbing' or 'shooting' pains such as trigeminal neuralgia or peripheral nerve damage (Hatangi et al. 1976; Swerdlow 1980).

Their efficacy has been attributed to suppression of abnormal hyperexcitability and discharge to other neuron pools. Dosages used have generally been less than those required for the treatment of epilepsy (Williams 1981). Clonazepam has the added advantage of being a benzodiazepine derivative and thus possesses anxiolytic and muscle relaxant properties. Thus its use

TABLE 8
The elimination half-life values of some benzodiazepines and their active metabolites, where this is known.

Parent drug (half-life range h)		Major active metabolites (half-life range h)	
Chlordiazepoxide	(5 – 30)	Desmethylchlordiazepoxide	(?)
		Demoxepam	(?)
		Desmethyldiazepam	(50 – 200)
Diazepam	(20 – 100)	Desmethyldiazepam	(50 – 200)
Clorazepate	(1 – 3)[a]	Desmethyldiazepam	(50 – 200)
Clobazam	(12 – 60)	Desmethylclobazam	(?)
Nitrazepam	(20 – 40)		
Bromazepam	(10 – 20)	3-Hydroxybromazepam[b]	(?)
Lorazepam	(10 – 20)		
Oxazepam	(4 – 15)		
Temazepam	(8 – 22)		
Alprazolam	(6 – 20)	α-Hydroxyalprazolam[b]	(?)
Flurazepam	(2 – 6)	Desalkylflurazepam	(40 – 250)
Flunitrazepam	(15 – 30)	Desmethylflunitrazepam	(?)

[a] Does not reach the systemic circulation in clinically important amounts.
[b] ? Active metabolites.
The values show wide interindividual variation and their magnitude depends on whether they were studied after a single or repeatedly administered dose of the drug.

should be considered in conditions such as chronic back pain where peripheral nerve damage or irritation and muscle spasm are co-existent.

Conclusions

In this brief chapter it is only possible to give a general overview of the psychiatrist's role in the assessment and management of chronic pain disorders. The psychiatrist is formally trained in the identification and management of patients in whom psychological and interpersonal factors strongly influence chronic pain. The psychiatrist should be a regular member of the pain clinic team and complements the other members of the team. Specific contributions to therapy include individual and group psychotherapy, family and marital therapy, cognitive therapy, behaviour modification, relaxation therapy, hypnosis, biofeedback and the prescription of psychotropic medication, and liaison with other clinicians and team members.

References

American Psychiatric Association (1980) Diagnostic and Statistical Manual of Mental Disorders, 3rd edn. A.P.A., Washington D.C.

Anderson, E. G. and Proudfit, H. K. (1981) The role of the bulbo-spinal serotonergic system. In: B. L. Jacobs and A. Gelperin (Eds.), Serotonin-Neurotransmission and Behavior. MIT Press, Cambridge, Mass. pp. 307 – 338.

Biegon, A. and Samuel, D. (1980) Interaction of tricyclic antidepressants with opiate receptors. Biochem. Pharmacol. 29, 460 – 462.

Black, R. G. (1976) The chronic pain syndrome. Clin. Med. 82, 17 – 20.

Bloomfield, S., Simard-Savoie, S., Bernier, J. and Tetreault, L. (1964) Comparative analgesic activity of levomepromazine and morphine in patients with chronic pain. Can. Med. Assoc. J. 90, 1156 – 1159.

Brena, S. F. and Chapman, S. L. (1981) The 'learned pain syndrome'. Postgrad. Med. 69, 53 – 62.

Bruhn, J. G. (1977) Effects of chronic illness on the family. J. Fam. Pract. 4, 1057 – 1060.

Chapman, C. R. (1977) Psychological aspects of pain treatment. Arch. Surg. 112, 767 – 772.

Clarke, I. M. C. (1981) Amitriptyline and perphenazine (Triptafen DA) in chronic pain. Anaesthesia 36, 210.

Clay, G. A. and Brougham, I. R. (1975) Haloperidol binding to an opiate receptor site. Biochem. Pharmacol. 24, 1363.

Couch, J. R. and Hassanein, R. S. (1979) Amitriptyline in migraine prophylaxis. Arch. Neurol. 36, 695 – 699.

Couch, J. R., Ziegler, D. K. and Hassanein, R. (1976) Amitriptyline in the prophylaxis of migraine. Neurology 26, 121 – 127.

Davis, J. L., Lewis, S. B., Gerich, J. E., Kaplan, R. A., Schultz, T. A. and Wallin, J. D. (1977) Peripheral diabetic neuropathy treated with amitriptyline and fluphenazine. J. Am. Med. Assoc. 238, 2291 – 2292.

Diamond, S. and Balter, B. J. (1971) Chronic tension headaches treated with amitriptyline. A double-blind study. Headache 11, 110 – 116.

Ekbom, K. (1974) Lithium vid kroniska symptom av cluster headache. Preliminark. Neddelande Opusc. Med. 19, 148 – 156.

Ellard, J. (1970) Psychological reactions to compensable injury. Med. J. Aust. 2, 349 – 355.

Elton, D., Stanley, G. V. and Burrows, G. D. (1983) Psychological Control of Pain. Grune & Stratton, Sydney, pp. 193 – 206.

Engel, G. (1959) 'Psychogenic' pain and the pain prone patient. Am. J. Med. 26, 899 – 918.

Feinmann, C., Harris, M. and Cawley, R. (1984) Psychogenic facial pain: presentation and treatment. Br. Med. J. 288, 436 – 438.

Fields, H. L. and Basbaum, A.I. (1978) Brainstem control of spinal pain transmission neurons. Ann. Rev. Physiol. 40, 217 – 248.

Flannery, J. G. (1978) Alexithymia. II. The association with unexplained physical distress. Psychother. Psychosom. 30, 193 – 197.

Fordyce, W. E. (1976) Behavioral Methods for Chronic Pain and Illness. C. V. Mosby, St Louis.

Gade, G. D., Hofeldt, F. D. and Treece, G. L. (1980) Diabetic neuropathic cachexia. J. Am. Med. Assoc. 243, 1160 – 1161.

Gebhardt, G. F. (1982) Opiate and opioid effects on brain stem neurons: relevance to nociception and anti-nociceptive mechansims. Pain 12, 93 – 140.

German, A. (1980) The shaping of a psychiatrist. Aust. N.Z. J. Psychiatry 14, 291 – 298.

Gerschman, J. A., Burrows, G. D., Reade, P. C., Wright, J. and Holwill, B. (1981) The burning tongue syndrome. In: G. D. Burrows (Ed.), Studies in Affective Disorders. Proceedings of The Scientific Meeting Accompanying the 47th Beattie-Smith Lecture. Department of Psychiatry, University of Melbourne. pp. 25 – 32.

Gessel, A. H. (1975) Electromyographic biofeedback and tricyclic antidepressants in myofascial pain-dysfunction syndrome. Psychological prediction of outcome. J. Am. Dent. Assoc. 91, 1048 – 1052.

Gomersall, J. D. and Stuart, A. (1973) Amitriptyline in migraine prophylaxis. J. Neurol. Neurosurg. Psychiatry 36, 684 – 690.

Gringas, M. (1976) A clinical trial of tofranil in rheumatic pain in general practice. J. Int. Med. Res. 4, 41 – 49.

Hameroff, S. R., Cork, R. C., Scherer, K., Crago, B. R., Neuman, C., Womble, J. R. and Davis, J. P. (1982) Doxepin effects on chronic pain, depression and plasma opioids. J. Clin. Psychiatry 43, 22 – 26.

Hatangi, V. S., Boas, R. A. and Richards, D. G. (1976) Post herpetic neuralgia: management with antiepileptic and tricyclic drugs. In: J. J. Bonica and V. Ventafridda (Eds.), Advances in Pain Research and Therapy, Vol. 1. Raven Press, New York, p. 583.

Head, M., Lal, H., Puri, S., Mantione, C. and Valentino, D. (1979) Enhancement of morphine analgesia after acute and chronic haloperidol. Life Sci. 24, 2037.

Hirschfeld, A. H. and Behan, L. C. (1967) The accident process – an overview. J. Rehabil. 4, 27 – 31.

Hökfelt, T., Ljungdahl, A., Terenius, L., Elde, R. and Nilsson, G. (1977) Immunohistochemical analysis of peptide pathways possibly related to pain and analgesia. Enkephalin and substance P. Proc. Natl. Acad. Sci. U.S.A. 74, 3081 – 3085.

Hughes, A., Chauvergne, J., Lisslour, J. and Lafgarde, C. (1963) L'imipramine utilisée comme antalgique majeur en carcinologie: étude de 118 cas. Presse Med. 71, 1073 – 1074.

Johansson, F. and Von Knorring, L. (1979) A double-blind controlled study of a serotonin uptake inhibitor (zimelidine) versus placebo in chronic pain patients. Pain 7, 69 – 78.

Kalucy, R. (1980) Commentary on 'Why psychiatry is a branch of medicine'. Aust. N.Z. J. Psychiatry 14, 279 – 290.

Katon, W. (1984) Panic disorder and somatization. Am. J. Med. 77, 101 – 106.

King, R. B. (1980) Pain and tryptophan. J. Neurosurg. 53, 44 – 52.

Klein, R. F., Dean, A. and Bogdanoff, M. D. (1967) The impact of illness upon the spouse. J. Chron. Dis. 20, 241 – 248.

Kocher, R. (1976) The use of psychotropic drugs in the treatment of chronic severe pain. Eur. Neurol. 14, 458.

Kudrow, L. (1977) Lithium prophylaxis for chronic cluster headache. Headache 17, 15 – 18.

Lance, J. W. and Curran, D. A. (1964) Treatment of chronic tension headache. Lancet 1, 1236 – 1239.

Lascelles, R. G. (1966) Atypical facial pain and depression. Br. J. Psychiatry 112, 651 – 659.

LeShan, L. (1964) The world of the patient in severe pain of long duration. J. Chron. Dis. 17, 119 – 126.

Lipowski, Z. J. (1974) Consultation-liaison psychiatry: an overview. Am. J. Psychiatry 131, 623 – 630.

Maltbie, A. A. and Cavenar, J. D. (1977) Haloperidol and analgesia; case reports. Military Med. 142, 946 – 948.

Margolis, L. H. and Gianascol, A. J. (1956) Chlorpromazine in thalamic pain syndrome. Neurology 6, 302 – 304.

McDonald Scott, W. A. (1969) The relief of pain with an antidepressant in arthritis. Practitioner 202, 802 – 807.

Mendelson, G. (1981) Persistent work disability following settlement of compensation claims. Law Inst. J. (Australia) 55, 342 – 345.

Merskey, H. and Hester, R. A. (1972) The treatment of pain with psychotropic drugs. Postgrad. Med. J. 48, 594 – 598.

Merskey, H. and Spear, E. G. (1967) Pain: Psychological and Psychiatric Aspects. Bailliere, Tindall & Cassell, London.

Montilla, E., Frederik, W. S. and Cass, L. J. (1963) Analgesic effect of methotrimeprazine and morphine. Arch. Int. Med. 111, 91 – 94.

Moore, J. and Dundee, J. W. (1961) Alterations in response to somatic pain with anaesthesia. VII. The effects of nine phenothiazine derivatives. Br. J. Anaesthesia 33, 422.

Noone, J. F. (1977) Psychotropic drugs and migraine. J. Int. Med. Res. 5, 66 – 71.

Pearce, J. M. S. (1980) Chronic migrainous neuralgia: a version of cluster headache. Brain 103, 149 – 159.

Pilowsky, I. (1976) The psychiatrist and the pain clinic. Am. J. Psychiatry 133, 752 – 755.

Pilowsky, I. and Spence, N. D. (1976) Illness behaviour syndromes associated with intractable pain. Pain 2, 61 – 71.

Pilowsky, I., Halletts, E. C., Bassett, D. L., Thomas, P. G. and Perhall, R. K. (1982) A controlled study of amitriptyline in the treatment of chronic pain. Pain 14, 169 – 179.

Sherwin, D. (1979) New method for treating 'headaches'. Am. J. Psychiatry 136, 1181 – 1183.

Sigwald, J., Bouttier, D. and Caille, F. (1959) Le traitement du zone et des algies zostériennes. Étude des resultats obtenus avec la levomepromazine. Thérapie 14, 818 – 824.

Stagoll, B. (1981) Work injuries and invalidism in migrant families. A systems view. Aust. J. Fam. Ther. 2, 63 – 75.

Steinglass, P., Temple, S., Lisman, S. A. and Reiss, D. (1982) Coping with spinal cord injury. The family perspective. Gen. Hosp. Psychiatry 4, 259 – 264.

Sternbach, R. A. (1974) Pain Patients. Traits and Treatments. Academic Press, New York.

Swerdlow, M. (1980) The treatment of shooting pain. Postgrad. Med. J. 56, 159.

Taub, A. (1973) Relief of post herpetic neuralgia with psychotropic drugs. J. Neurosurg. 39, 235 – 239.

Turkington, R. W. (1980) Depression masquerading as diabetic neuropathy. J. Am. Med. Assoc. 243, 1147 – 1150.

Tyrer, S. P. (1985) The role of the psychiatrist in the pain clinic. Bull. R. Coll. Psychiatr. 9, 135 – 136.

Walters, A. (1961) Psychogenic regional pain alias hysterical pain. Brain 84, 1 – 18.

Watson, C. P., Evans, R. J., Reed, K. et al. (1982) Amitriptyline versus placebo in post herpetic neuralgia. Neurology 32, 671 – 673.

Watson, G. D., Chandarane, P. C. and Merskey, H. (1981) Relationships between pain and schizophrenia. Br. J. Psychiatry 138, 33 – 36.

Williams, N. E. (1981) Current view of the pharmacological management of pain. In: M. Swerdlow (Ed.), The Therapy of Pain. MTP Press Ltd., pp. 87 – 110.

Woodeford, J. M., Dwyer, B., McElven, B. W. et al. (1965) Treatment of post herpetic neuralgia. Med. J. Aust. 2, 869 – 872.

Burrows/Elton/Stanley (eds.) Handbook of Chronic Pain Management
© *1987 Elsevier Science Publishers B.V. (Biomedical Division)*

29

Sexual adjustment and chronic pain

TOSHIHIKO MARUTA

Pain Management Center, Department of Psychiatry and Psychology, Mayo Clinic and Mayo Foundation and Mayo Medical School, Rochester, MN 55905, U.S.A.

Introduction

Before the decade of the 1970's, most medical publications about sexuality addressed disease and reproductive aspects of sexual function (Cole and Cole 1981). Now, sexual health has become an acceptable focus for physician-patient interaction and treatment (Cole et al. 1973; Maruta and Osborne 1978; Mohamed et al. 1978; Hamilton 1981; Sjögren and Fugl-Meyer 1981; Conine and Evans 1982; Elst et al. 1984). As could be easily predicted, the frequency with which sexual problems are identified in medical practice reflects the physician's initiative in seeking sexual information and his or her ease in discussing sexual material. Based on the data at the Mayo Clinic Pain Management Center (PMC) (Maruta et al. 1981), it can be anticipated that over half of the patients with chronic pain will have deterioration in the frequency and quality of sexual activity, a percentage equal to the highest rate of sexual problems seen in any group of nonpsychiatric patients (Burnap and Golden 1967). What follows are examples of sexual and marital aspects of the management of patients with chronic pain.

Illustrative cases and comment

Case 1: A 57-year-old factory worker had been a relaxed and loving husband before his low back pain began, 4 years previously. His wife, who now did everything for him, reported that he was not the same man she married. 'He is always upset and tense. He is critical of the kids and he won't do anything or go anywhere!' After 35 years of marriage, a divorce seemed imminent. When she reported he went to bed right after dinner, the question was asked about their sexual relationship. Although the patient had earlier stated 'All is well', his wife reported a dramatic deterioration in both frequency and quality of their sexual contact, adding that the patient had begun to have difficulty ejaculating. The wife was smouldering with resentment, yet she did not tell the patient that, when he had stopped working and had withdrawn from family and outside activities, she felt he was 'giving in to the pain'. He wanted to be taken care of as a 'sick person' but felt guilty and ashamed that he was making too many demands and was unable to do much in return. His wife felt obliged to care for him, but her frustration was growing daily. Their sexual problems were undiscussed and they began avoiding sexual contact to avoid any repeated failure. By the time they came to the PMC, the situation was covertly hostile and clearly deteriorating.

Partially because the patient was frightened by the threat to his marriage and the possible loss of his caregiver, he was willing to participate in the PMC program (Swanson et al. 1979) which was designed to help him cope more effectively with pain. The program, multidisciplinary in nature, utilized operant conditioning, physical rehabilitation, medication management, education, biofeedback and relaxation, and group discussion to guide him to a better acceptance of his chronic pain. The medical staff was neither sympathetic nor hostile when he complained of pain or limited his activities because of pain. He was encouraged and praised when he increased his physical activity, independent function, or social contact. This was the way his wife was later instructed to respond to him.

In the group discussion and in 3 days of therapy with the patient and his wife, an attempt was made to show them how much of the problem was due to their complex reactions to the pain. The patient gradually came to understand how his invalidism was affecting his wife, and she was finally able to express to him the growing resentment and frustration that had replaced the love she had for him. When they left the PMC, the patient was still in pain but they were committed to their relationship, their sexuality, and his rehabilitation.

Three months after dismissal, the patient reported that he had returned to his job, was continuing his exercises, and had joined the church choir. Their sexual problems were resolved and, although they were not having sex as often as before the back pain began, they were satisfied with their functioning.

COMMENT

Like the wife in this case, spouses of patients with chronic pain are placed in an ambiguous situation in which they must struggle with how much they believe is actually physical pain. While the spouse feels obliged to care for the medically ill patient, the couple often develops a superficial harmony, pseudomutuality (Maruta et al. 1981), or sick role homeostasis (Waring 1977) with ever increasing conflicts underneath. Society supports chronic pain behavior as a demonstration of the reality of the patient's physical disability. Workmen's Compensation and Social Security payments reward the chronic pain patient for withdrawing from active work instead of redirecting the patient into jobs that are less physically taxing. The effect is to encourage patients, as in this case, to assume the role of a disabled person whose reduced activity and greater dependency are proof of disability. The burden of this socially sanctioned pain behavior falls squarely on the healthy spouse. Therefore, the goal should be to reverse this sick role conditioning so that the patient can resume a full and active independent life.

Recently, 50 married patients referred to the PMC program were studied concerning their marital-sexual adjustment (Maruta et al. 1981). Identical but separate interviews were conducted with each patient and each spouse during the course of their participation in the program. In regard to the sexual relationship prior to the onset of pain, 80% said they were satisfied. After the onset of pain, however, approximately 50% of both patients and spouses expressed dissatisfaction in their sexual relationship. There was no statistically significant difference in how the patient and spouse groups rated their marriage before the onset of pain. However, in rating the 'last 6 months', a significantly higher number of spouses rated their marriages 'below average', whereas the majority of patients rated their marriage 'average' or 'above average'. The same applied to changes in marital adjustment as the result of pain; 75% of the patients rated it 'no changes', but the majority (65%) of the spouses rated it 'worse' or 'deteriorating'.

This discrepancy deserves careful attention. Between the tendency of the patient to minimize or to deny conflicts in marriage and the reluctance of the spouse to bring up anything 'irrelevant' or 'unimportant' or 'too personal', clinical information obtained only from the patient gives us a skewed view of the marital environment.

Fear of pain and lack of understanding about its true nature can also cause sexual difficulties in some patients with chronic pain.

Case 2: A 25-year-old office worker who had hip, leg, and groin pain after an operation for hernia repair developed difficulty in keeping an erection. His wife reported that he had attempted sexual activity with her nearly every night but generally had been unsuccessful. He was now working only part-time, and she had difficulty in expressing her anger and frustration about the added responsibilities she had acquired because of his pain and especially about his sexual dysfunction.

When interviewed at the PMC, the patient said that his major goal in seeking treatment was 'to have sex with my wife; to be a man again'. In this case, the sexual dysfunction and subsequent marital difficulties clearly seemed to have evolved out of chronic pain. Yet, on closer examination, it was discovered that the patient had morning erections. However, he was extremely anxious about both the level of his pain during sex and his ability to perform sexually after the hernia repair. The pain was real enough; but the sexual problem resulted from his fear and from his anger at the surgeons who had been unable to relieve the problem.

Once he understood that his pain need not affect his sexual performance, the patient was ready to discuss the problem openly with his wife and to deal with their frustration in a direct manner. Three months later they reported that they were again enjoying satisfactory intercourse and that he had returned to full-time work.

COMMENT

It would be dangerous to assume that all sexual problems of patients with chronic pain are merely the result of the pain. Chronic pain can also develop as an accompaniment to chronic marital discord in which sexual maladjustment is a consequence. Withdrawal from the sexual relationship can be a way of demonstrating the authenticity of the pain, of communicating anger toward a demanding spouse, and of expressing a need to be cared for.

Case 3: A 38-year-old housewife with chronic arm pain had been having marital conflict with her corporate executive husband well before the onset of her pain after a traumatic accident. Following the accident, which occurred not long after the announcement of her husband's promotion to a job in a distant community, the patient withdrew from her numerous community activities and took a leave of absence from her job.

After the move she sought no new job or outside contact and her daily activity decreased to almost exclusively self-care tasks. Her husband and children were forced to do the daily cooking and household cleaning.

Although clearly a bright person, the patient's self-confidence slipped dramatically and she became very resentful of her husband's career success. Complaining that her husband 'talked down to her', she became very aloof from her family and the couple's social activity dwindled to almost nothing. By the time the patient and her husband came to the PMC, she had become very irritable and at times was even physically abusive to her husband. The frequency of their sexual activity had decreased from more than three times a week to about once a month, he said, and his rating of the quality of their marriage had dropped from 'average' before the pain to 'below average' for the last 6 months. Interestingly, she rated both periods as 'above average'. After completing the PMC program the couple still needed marital counseling to resolve their long-standing difficulties.

Three months later, on a follow-up questionnaire, the patient said that she felt very well and was much more active than she had been before treatment. She was now doing housework and going to college and said that she was enjoying evening social activities. Her sexual activity with her husband was also restored.

COMMENT

This case shows an excellent example of 'sick role homeostasis' (Waring 1977) in marriage. The patient assumed the sick role and rejected any marital or family responsibilities. Increasingly resentful of the added demands placed upon him, the husband tried to maintain a calm surface in order to keep peace in the family and to continue their limited sexual relationship. The patient, on the other hand, tended to use sexuality to maintain her advantageous position; she was 'in too much pain even to have sex', let alone clean house and care for her family.

Unlike the case of definitive pain disorders such as with pain due to cancer or deforming arthritis, in the case of patients with chronic pain, the spouses are placed in ambiguous situations in which they have to struggle with how much they believe is actually physical pain. In spite of repeated negative medical and surgical work-ups, the patient complains of pain, takes massive amounts of analgesics, and causes financial hardship by not working. With the spouse's feeling of obligation and a need to care for the medically ill person, this condition often brings a couple to a superficial harmony.

Prescription drug use and dependency are major causes of sexual problems in patients with chronic pain. Abuse of sedatives and analgesics frequently compromises a patient's normal mental and sexual functioning (Buffum et al. 1981).

Case 4: A 34-year-old teacher was unable to teach because of severe facial and head pain. During his initial interview at the PMC, he reported that sexual activity was difficult due to his pain and said that his wife had been 'a saint' about the problem.

His wife's perception of the problem was quite different. She said that she felt frustrated and angry with the patient and that she was on the verge of leaving the marriage. They had been considering having children, but she had discarded the idea because of marital problems and their lack of sexual activity, which had decreased from two or three times a week to less than once every couple of months. In fact, the patient had begun sleeping in the guest room and she stayed away from home as much as possible to avoid being with him. As part of his treatment at the PMC, the patient went through a 10-day medication-reduction schedule to withdraw from his use of flurazepam, 60 mg at bedtime, oxycodone, 6 – 8 tablets a day, and diazepam, 10 mg four times a day. A few days after completion of the withdrawal schedule, he started noticing differences in his cognitive functioning, and his self-esteem improved markedly. During the last 3 days of the program, he and his wife had an overnight pass to a motel where they had a 'wonderful' sexual encounter.

COMMENT

This case is typical of chronic pain patients who abuse sedatives, hypnotics, analgesics, or tranquilizers. Unless these patients discontinue the medications, they continue to have the same problems in spite of their good intentions to make an adjustment.

Discussion

How far, then, should the physician inquire into the sexual problems of patients with chronic pain? It depends upon the priority of other medical conditions and the realistic limitations of time. However, it is clear that sexuality is no less important in medically ill patients than in healthy people. Even a brief empathetic interview with both the patient and spouse may help open the way to exploring and resolving this hidden problem. Along this line, a guideline suggested by Lief and Berman (1981) is of some help. The following are the basic principles of taking a sexual history as described by them.

1) The physician should be comfortable and at ease. Despite the intimate nature of the inquiry, the physician has society's sanction to ask his patient questions about matters usually kept private. If the patient does not raise concerns about sexual functioning, the physician should initiate discussion.

2) The physician should establish empathy with the patient and do so before launching into the details of the sexual history.

3) The physician's values must not have a negative effect on the interview.

4) The greater the physician's knowledge, the more skillful the interview, unless discomfort

or prejudice interferes. (For example, the simple omission of the sexual history can suggest to the patient that sex is unimportant or is a part of his life that does not matter to the physician.)

5) Questions should be as precise as possible within the limits imposed by tact.

References

Buffum, J., Smith, D. E., Moser, C., Apter, M., Buxton, M. and Davison, J. (1981) Drugs and sexual function. In: H. I. Lief (Ed.), Sexual Problems in Medical Practice. American Medical Association, Chicago, pp. 211 – 242.

Burnap, D. W. and Golden, J. S. (1967) Sexual problems in medical practice. J. Med. Educ. 42, 673 – 680.

Cole, T. M. and Cole, S. S. (1981) Sexual health and physical disability. In: H. I. Lief (Ed.), Sexual Problems in Medical Practice. American Medical Association, Chicago, pp. 191 – 198.

Cole, T. M., Chilgren, R. and Rosenberg, P. (1973) A new programme of sex education and counselling for spinal cord injured adults and health care professionals. Paraplegia 11, 111 – 124.

Conine, T. A. and Evans, J. H. (1982) Seuxal reactivation of chronically ill and disabled adults. J. Allied Health 11, 261 – 270.

Elst, P., Sybesma, T., van der Stadt, R. J., Prins, A. P. A., Muller, W. H. and den Butter, A. (1984) Sexual problems in rheumatoid arthritis and ankylosing spondylitis. Arthritis Rheum. 27, 217 – 220.

Hamilton, A. (1981) Sexual problems in arthritis and allied conditions. Int. Rehabil. Med. 3, 38 – 42.

Lief, H. I. and Berman, E. M. (1981) Sexual interviewing throughout the patient's cycle. In: H. I. Lief (Ed.), Sexual Problems in Medical Practice. American Medical Association, Chicago, pp. 119 – 129.

Maruta, T. and Osborne, D. (1978) Sexual activity in chronic pain patients. Psychosomatics 19, 531 – 537.

Maruta, T., Osborne, D., Swanson, D. W. and Halling, J. M. (1981) Chronic pain patients and spouses: marital and sexual adjustment. Mayo Clin. Proc. 56, 307 – 310.

Mohamed, S. N., Weisz, G. M. and Waring, E. M. (1978) The relationship of chronic pain to depression, marital adjustment, and family dynamics. Pain 5, 285 – 292.

Sjögren, K. and Fugl-Meyer, A. R. (1981) Chronic back pain and sexuality. Int. Rehabil. Med. 3, 19 – 25.

Swanson, D. W., Maruta, T. and Swenson, W. M. (1979) Results of behavior modification in the treatment of chronic pain. Psychosom. Med. 41, 55 – 61.

Waring, E. M. (1977) The role of the family in symptom selection and perpetuation in psychosomatic illness. Psychother. Psychosom. 28, 253 – 259.

Burrows/Elton/Stanley (eds.) Handbook of Chronic Pain Management
© *1987 Elsevier Science Publishers B.V. (Biomedical Division)*

30

Management of chronic oro-facial pain syndromes

J.A. GERSCHMAN and P.C. READE

Oro-Facial Pain Clinic, Department of Dental Medicine and Surgery, University of Melbourne, 711 Elizabeth Street, Melbourne, Victoria 3000, Australia

Introduction

Acute, intermittent or continuous pains in all parts of the head, face and neck are relatively common occurrences (Editorial 1984). Pain is the most common symptom of oro-facial disease. Other signs and symptoms include swelling, loss of function, haemorrhage, mucosal ulceration, loosening of teeth and changes in sensation (Gerschman and Reade 1984). Many organs and structures with diverse functions and innervation, as well as psychosocial factors, may have an influence on pain in the oro-facial area.

Benign chronic oro-facial pain syndromes have been described by Dworkin (1983) as being disorders in which mandibular and maxillo-facial pain is the central and often exclusive symptom. These disorders fall into three major groups:

1) pain stemming from musculo-skeletal disorders (e.g. temporomandibular joint disorders);
2) pain stemming from neuropathy (e.g. trigeminal neuralgia);
3) a miscellaneous category of pain syndromes including referred pain and psychogenic pain.

Pain in the oro-facial region may originate from many organs and structures including teeth, periodontium, muscles, ears, eyes, bones, paranasal sinuses, blood vessels, nerves or from remote sources.

Although pain of dental origin and that due to diseases of the paranasal sinuses are the most common oro-facial pains, it is not usual for them to be described as contributing to a chronic pain syndrome. Chronic periodontal disease (including chronic pericoronitis), chronic alveolar abscesses, exposed cementum and dentine, pulpal pathology, post-endodontic therapy, the supraerupted tooth pain-dysfunction syndrome and chronic sinusitis can be associated with either severe or minor pain which may be intermittent or continuous. Such pains are usually straightforward to identify and are managed by routine methods.

TABLE 1

Distribution of patients according to their main presenting complaints to the Oro-Facial Pain Clinic, Department of Dental Medicine and Surgery, University of Melbourne.

Presenting complaint	Number
Oro-facial pain	
TMJ disorders	47
Atypical facial pain	50
Trigeminal neuralgia	5
Trigeminal neuropathy	3
Dental causalgia (post-traumatic pain) (phantom tooth pain)	20
Mimo-causalgia	10
Metabolic neuropathy	3
Post-herpetic neuralgia	3
Vaso-dilating facial pain	4
Periodic migrainous neuralgia	6
Muscle tension headache	18
Migraine (and variants)	18
Pulpitis	6
Periodontitis	1
Idiopathic odontalgia	9
Idiopathic periodontalgia	5
CNS pathology (central pain)	2
Neoplastic pain	5
Hyperalgesia	2
Hypoalgesia	3
Other	2
Oral dysaesthesia	
Glossodynia/glossopyrosis	25
Stomatopyrosis	37
Persistent cacogeusia	7
Subjective xerostomia	8
Hyperaesthesia	2
Hypoaesthesia	2
Intolerance of prosthetic appliances	20
Cheek biting/chewing	3
Slimy coating on teeth	5
Bubbles in saliva	3
Particulate saliva	4
Sensation of swelling	4
Sensation of bone/wire in gums	2
Miscellaneous	
Self-mutilation	7
Desire to re-arrange occlusion	4
Pseudo-dislocated jaw	1
Hysterical sensory loss	9
Hysterical unilateral lingual protuberance	1
Sporadic nocturnal auto-hypno-exodontia	1
Other	1
Total	368

N.B.: Main complaint is indicated but many patients had multiple symptoms.

The findings of various pain clinics (Gregg and Ghia 1981) including our own (Gerschman et al. 1979) (Table 1) have reported chronic oro-facial pain conditions, including temporomandibular pain-dysfunction syndrome, atypical facial neuralgia, oral dysaesthesias (including glossodynia and glossopyrosis), migraine and its variants, muscle contraction headache, post-traumatic pain syndromes, trigeminal neuralgia and post-herpetic neuralgia. A number of these conditions will now be described in detail.

Temporomandibular joint pain-dysfunction syndrome (TMJPDS)

This pain-dysfunction syndrome is relatively common and has a number of synonyms including myofascial pain dysfunction. It has attracted much attention since first described by Costen in 1934. Many explanations have been suggested for the aetiology of this problem, but no consensus has been reached. Propositions as widely different as a functional aetiology on the one hand and a psychological aetiology on the other, currently have strong support. Although an impression is gained from clinical practice and from many reports that patients suffering from this problem are predominantly female, the work of Helkimo (1976) indicates that the sex distribution is equal. The apparent female predominance may result from females being more likely to seek attention for chronic pain and discomfort conditions.

An explanation based on a two-stage process is most appropriate (Reade 1984a). It seems most likely that the disturbance is precipitated by an injury of the order of a sprain to one or both temporomandibular joints. Approximately one half of patients diagnosed as suffering from a TMJPDS can recall the precipitating incident which may range from major trauma, such as from a head or neck injury in a motor car accident, to a minor incident such as a wide uncontrolled yawn. The joint injury sustained may resolve spontaneously; at other times the pain and dysfunction can persist and worsen over long periods of time sometimes to the point of psychological decompensation. At least one major reason for the pain-dysfunction syndrome persisting is related to occlusal factors (e.g. deep overbite, displacing contacts, lack of molar support) which up to the time of trauma had been adequately accommodated during function but which act to maintain the joint problems once incurred, because of joint overload. In an effort to limit joint function, muscle splinting occurs resulting in spasm and associated pain, sometimes intense and paroxysmal and sometimes less intense and persistent. Most of the symptoms listed in Table 2 and the signs listed in Table 3 are related to painful muscle spasm.

TABLE 2
The complex symptoms of TMJPDS.

Nature of pain:	acute or chronic, constant or intermittent, sharp or dull, tolerable to severe
Duration:	from days to years, on waking or later in day
Location:	any of the muscles of the head, neck, shoulders and arms, eyes, ears, tongue, larynx, teeth, temporomandibular joint(s)
Associated phenomena:	crepitus, locking, limited mandibular movement, occlusal changes, stuffy ears, tinnitus, vertigo, hyper or hypoacusis, nausea, blurred vision, husky voice, dysaesthesia

TABLE 3
The signs of TMJPDS.

Any age	Sometimes joint noises
Either sex, female: male 4:1	Sometimes mandibular jolting or deviation on opening
Usually pain on palpation of: – slightly open temporomandibular joint(s) – masseter muscle(s) – superior head of trapezius muscle(s) – medial pterygoid muscle(s)	Various aspects of malocclusion may be obvious including tooth loss or unsatisfactory dentures
	Various parafunctional habits may be noted
	Psychological signs may be observed

With an adequate history of symptoms and with at least some of the appropriate signs having been demonstrated, a diagnosis of TMJPDS is usually straightforward. Approximately two-thirds of the patients will respond to counselling and advice on managing the problem by rest from vigorous function. The remaining one-third usually require functional therapy in the form of a carefully adjusted occlusal splint, and sometimes relaxants or antidepressants. An occlusal splint is worn each night, often for several months, with an amount of opening up to 10 mm at the incisal edges. This distracts the mandibular condyles from their fossae on tooth-to-splint contact thus reducing the functional load on the joints and allowing resolution of the sprain, with consequent reduction of muscle spasm pain (Reade 1984b). The splint is used at night because long periods of tooth-to-tooth contact occur during sleeping but not waking hours. In TMJPDS, as in other chronic pain syndromes, psychological problems can complicate therapy. They should be managed concurrently with a team approach for satisfactory results.

Trigeminal neuralgia

The most important oro-facial neuralgias are varieties of trigeminal neuralgia (Dworkin 1983). True trigeminal neuralgia (tic douloureux) occurs in a relatively fixed pattern along one or more branches of the trigeminal nerve in middle-aged and elderly persons. Atypical trigeminal neuralgia is a more loosely defined collection of oro-facial neuralgias in which distribution of pain and age of onset are variable. Oro-facial neuralgias with specific causes include post-traumatic and post-herpetic trigeminal neuralgia.

Sweet (1968) has provided the most enduring classification of trigeminal neuralgia: 1) idiopathic (central, true trigeminal neuralgia, or tic douloureux); 2) symptomatic of some other specific neurological entity (i.e. post-herpetic, post-traumatic, neoplasms, multiple sclerosis) sometimes called secondary trigeminal neuralgia, and 3) atypical.

The aetiology of primary and atypical trigeminal neuralgia remains largely unknown, but opinion is divided between peripheral and central theories. Peripheral theories are most common and have been favoured historically. They ascribe the neuralgia either to compression of the dorsal root by exostoses of the petrous portion of temporal bone (Gardener et al. 1956), or to compression of the trigeminal nerve in the posterior fossa by vascular loops (Kerr and Miller 1966).

The diagnosis of primary trigeminal neuralgia is based principally on the criteria of White and Sweet (1955). Classical features are 1) excruciating, lancinating, searing, paroxysmal pain lasting seconds to minutes; 2) pain provoked by non-nociceptive stimuli to a trigger zone; 3) pain occurring along the anatomic distribution of the fifth cranial nerve; 4) unilateral pain in any one paroxysm and 5) no objective loss of sensation.

Less classical features, which distinguish atypical or secondary trigeminal neuralgia from primary trigeminal neuralgia, include 1) continuous or long-lasting burning or aching pain, 2) episodic pain not provoked or worsened by stimulation but spontaneously recurrent, 3) pain extending to the neck and posterior scalp, 4) pain remaining unilateral, and 5) spontaneous hyperaesthesia unrelated to therapy. Most investigators also report psychologic symptoms, notably depression.

When symptoms of trigeminal neuralgia, especially the less classic features, occur in patients less than 50 years of age, multiple sclerosis should be suspected (Dalesio 1980). Loeser (1977) suggested that the more a facial pain syndrome deviates from the classic criteria, the less likely is primary trigeminal neuralgia to be the correct diagnosis. As with most clinical pain states, whose aetiology is only imperfectly understood, treatment of trigeminal neuralgia is often based on the theoretical biases of clinicians.

The anticonvulsants, carbamazepine and phenytoin have proven especially useful, either as the sole therapy or as an adjunct preoperatively and postoperatively. Carbamazepine is the drug of choice, providing relief in 60–80% of cases, in doses of 400–1000 mg/day. Phenytoin is reported to be effective in 20% of cases in doses of 300–600 mg/day. Drug resistance and toxicity, especially to formed blood elements, are the major side effects.

Unfortunately, the optimistic early results reported with carbamazepine as the sole therapy have not been supported by later results. Good to excellent results have been reported for about 70% of patients in the first 3 months of therapy, but after 3–42 months, this is reduced to 50% of patients. Both carbamazepine and phenytoin depress synaptic transmission in the spinal trigeminal nucleus and drugs with a similar action, especially chlorphenesin and baclofen (Loeser 1977), have been used less extensively for the control of trigeminal neuralgia.

Tricyclic antidepressants (e.g. doxepin, 150 mg, daily) combined with a phenothiazine (e.g. trifluoperazine, 1 mg, t.i.d.) in addition to carbamazepine have proved useful for resistant cases (Sisk 1983).

Percutaneous radiofrequency trigeminal gangliolysis is one of the safest, most common, least expensive and most reliable surgical procedures for relief of tic douloureux. Patients retain nearly normal tactile-discriminatory sensory functions (Hakanson 1981). Long-term results show a cure rate of 80% with complications in less than 5% of cases. The procedure can be performed on the sedated, but not unconscious, patient and is particularly suited to the elderly, debilitated patient, who is a poor surgical risk.

Decompression of the trigeminal nerve, a more invasive surgical procedure, is used in the management of primary trigeminal neuralgia when other approaches, notably pharmacotherapeutic, have failed. Jannetta (1976) devised this microvascular technique to modify vascular structures compromising the trigeminal nerve.

Microvascular decompression results in relief of the pain of trigeminal neuralgia without the altered sensation and possibility of anaesthesia dolorosa and severe dysaesthesia associated with the thermocoagulation procedures. Follow-up studies of the microvascular decompression technique have indicated that the recurrence of pain may be less frequent than with the other commonly used methods of treatment.

When the previously described approaches have failed, trigeminal tractotomy can be performed. The descending trigeminal nerve tract is divided at the cervicomedullary junction. This procedure usually relieves primary trigeminal neuralgia but causes more general loss of pain and temperature sensations. It is not advocated as an initial procedure and is recommended only with reservation.

Alternative treatments for trigeminal neuralgia, especially for tic douloureux, include nerve blocks with local anaesthetics, cryosurgery and rarely alcohol injection, of the peripheral branches of the trigeminal nerve. These are usually viewed as temporary measures. Acupuncture has been attempted, but its effectiveness is largely unproven. Recently, trigeminal neuralgia has been successfully treated by retrogasserian glycerol injection, a fairly safe procedure with minimal risk of extensive nerve damage.

Post-traumatic pain syndromes

Terms for post-traumatic pain syndromes include the following: causalgia, major causalgia, minor causalgia, mimo-causalgia, post-traumatic sympathetic dystrophy, phantom limb phenomenon, post-traumatic trigeminal neuropathy and anaesthesia dolorosa.

Post-traumatic trigeminal neuropathy

Post-traumatic trigeminal pain has been characterized as the sustained, diffuse, spreading, and non-provocable pain often accompanied by sensations of burning, boring, pulling and intense pressures (Elfenbaum 1954). The pain may be continuous for hours, and it may develop a long time after trauma from external violence, cured local infection or local extracranial surgery. Goldstein et al. (1963) reviewed 61 cases in which pathologic trigeminal pain resulted from such diverse sources as accidental lacerations, removal of impacted third molars, denture trauma, lip biopsy, sinusitis treatments and inferior alveolar anaesthetic injections.

The pathogenesis of post-traumatic pain usually has been explained on the basis of faulty peripheral regeneration of nerve tissues, neuroma formation, excessive scar contractions, ischaemia from vasospasm, differences in remyelinization patterns, and failures in receptor regeneration (Visoso and Young 1948). An alternative theory stated that facial pain after peripheral trauma resulted from pathologic conditions and afferent imbalances in the central portions of the trigeminal system. It has also been postulated that post-traumatic facial pain may be analogous to phantom limb pain (Gregg 1971).

A psychogenic overlay is common in these syndromes (Elfenbaum 1954). Post-traumatic facial pain, causalgia and some cases of atypical facial pain have been postulated as having a similar pathogenesis (Bonica 1974). Without clear evidence of a lesion impinging on the nerve, exploratory surgery such as examination of the retromolar fossa or repeated curettage of an apparently well-healed tooth socket is rarely justified and may complicate diagnosis and treatment (Rees and Harris 1978). Many sensory abnormalities of this type gradually resolve. Slow disappearance of the pain and increased paraesthesia and tingling often signal return to normal sensation with only small areas of numbness remaining after several months have passed. Loss of sensation in the lower lip produces a functional abnormality similar to that seen following a mandibular block regional anaesthetic injection; loss of proprioceptive sensation prevents the lip being closely adapted to the teeth and apparent drooping of the lip may be mistakenly interpreted as a facial paralysis. Areas of diminished sensation to pinprick or graded von Frey hairs may be detected by comparing skin and mucous membrane on the affected and unaffected sides.

Post-traumatic pain, if mild, has been treated with analgesics in conjunction with electric or mechanical stimulation to the affected area, with hypnosis, acupuncture or with drugs such as carbamazepine, phenytoin, or tricyclic antidepressants if the pain is prolonged and accompanied by a noticeable depressive reaction (The Medical Letter 1975). In rare cases, section of the affected nerve proximal to the suspected painful focus may be attempted. Post-traumatic pain may arise from a lesion affecting neurons in the central nervous system that resulted from an original traumatic episode to a peripheral nerve. In such cases, section of the nerve may not completely remove the pain. Peripheral neurolysis is effective for some resistant patients.

CAUSALGIA

Causalgia has been defined as a sustained burning pain after a traumatic nerve lesion combined with vasomotor and sudomotor dysfunction and later trophic changes (Merskey 1983). Gregg (1971) claimed that although causalgia of the trigeminal distribution had been described as a sequel of peripheral trauma, its incidence and pathogenesis were unknown. Causalgia affecting the mouth and face has also been referred to as a minor reflex sympathetic dystrophy (Lynch 1977).

Bonica (1974) felt that although rare, dental causalgia was known to occur as a post-extraction (amputation) phenomenon. He further stated that causalgia is pre-eminently a result of penetrating wounds usually due to high-velocity missiles, and believed it to be caused by a 'stretch' injury of peripheral nerves. Formation of a neuroma may be part of the aetiology.

Behrman (1949) described a series of 10 cases of dental causalgia which occurred following the extraction of a molar. Elfenbaum (1954) found that it occurred after the extraction of maxillary first molars, maxillary anterior teeth (especially canine teeth) and mandibular premolars.

Elfenbaum (1954) in his review of over 30 cases of dental causalgia found that all patients admitted that the syndrome became intensified under emotional stress. Many of these patients were addicts of polysurgery. Cooper and Braceland (1950) felt that the well-adjusted individual could distract his attention from a toothache if the peripheral stimulus was not physically overpowering. Possibly they felt that the causalgia victim could not divert his attention from what would be subliminal impulses for most people. In Bonica's cases (Bonica 1974) psychogenic overlay was commonplace.

Psychotherapy, drug therapy, analgesic block (primarily sympathetic block) and surgery are possible forms of treatment (Gregg and Ghia 1980). Most authors are pessimistic on the subject of treatment. Analgesics and local anaesthetics to interrupt trigeminal or glossopharyngeal nerve function provide only partial relief. The majority of sufferers are middle-aged females. This diagnosis often is made by exclusion and confused with trigeminal neuralgia; it can be differentiated by its continuous nonparoxysmal quality. There is some suggestion that trigeminal neuralgia of many years' standing or after treatment with carbamazepine might gradually convert to a chronic, more nearly continuous, less intense pain. Other conditions which may be included in this category include idiopathic periodontalgia and idiopathic odontalgia (Harris 1974).

Atypical facial pain

Atypical facial pain has many synonyms such as facial neuralgia; sympathetic algia; neuralgic headache; cephalgia; pseudotrigeminal neuralgia; atypical odontalgia and psychalgia. Most commonly used are atypical facial pain, atypical facial neuralgia and psychogenic oro-facial pain (Gerschman and Reade 1984). The use of the last term appears preferable because many aspects of this pain are typical rather than atypical.

A multiplicity of signs and symptoms is attributed to this syndrome which features persistent or intermittent bouts of moderate to severe pain, sometimes described as burning, drawing, aching, stabbing or throbbing. There are unsubstantiated descriptions of swelling, ulceration or discharge which encourage surgical intervention such as extraction of teeth, removal of bone and sectioning of nerves. Patients describe other oral sensory problems such as burning, dryness and taste aberrations.

The pain is often experienced deep in the hard tissues of the affected area which is usually within that supplied by the trigeminal nerve. The distribution of pain is not anatomic, often radiating between division and across the midline. Few consistent precipitating or aggravating factors are evident, with the exception of stress in various forms.

According to the N.I.D.R. Classification of 1974 (Burket's Oral Medicine 1977), atypical oro-facial pain refers to pain that does not conform to recognized anatomic pathways in its distribution.

Included within this definition, therefore, are:

1) oro-facial pains that cannot be relieved by interruption of trigeminal or glossopharyngeal pathways;
2) oro-facial pains that have no identifiable neuropathic or non-neuropathic (extraneural or central) focus, and
3) oro-facial pains that are associated with a potential pain-producing focus but which are out of proportion to the nature of the focus, or not strictly related to it in terms of recognized anatomical pathways, and physioneurological mechanisms.

Since all of these features are negative, it follows that a diagnosis of psychogenic oro-facial pain is made by exclusion. Many studies have identified the syndrome as a manifestation of depressive illness and have specified its treatment with antidepressant medication and supportive psychotherapy, albeit at times in a covert form.

ORAL DYSAESTHESIA

Oral dysaesthesia and disordered oral sensations are terms used to describe patients who report ill-defined chronic oral sensory problems (usually of mixed symptomatology) and for whom specific anatomic diagnoses are hard to find (Harris 1974; Brightman 1977). Their complaints include chronic discomfort, disordered taste, localized and general burning, subjective xerostomia, 'lumpy', 'gritty' or particulate saliva, areas of numbness and abnormalities of textural sensation. Uncomfortable burning sensations, either localized to the tongue (glossodynia, glossopyrosis) or affecting other areas of the oral mucosa (stomatopyrosis), are the most common complaints. Description of the symptoms varies from pain, to burning, tingling or numbness.

Patients who complain of painful burning sensations can be classified in two groups.

1) Some patients have clinically observable changes to the tongue, e.g. erythema migrans or other identifiable physical causes. These include local irritants and systemic disease and deficiency states such as pernicious anaemia, iron deficiency anaemia, coeliac disease, sideropenic dysphagia, diabetes mellitus and associated oral candidosis and peripheral neuropathy, amyloidosis, multiple myeloma, malignant lesions metastasing to the tongue, neuropathy of the lingual nerve, glossopharyngeal neuralgia and TMJPDS.
2) Patients without observable clinical changes or identifiable causes often are middle-aged and female, but can be of any age and either sex. The complaint usually is of a painful burning

sensation which gradually increases in severity and frequency until it is constant. It may be present on waking, building to maximum intensity during the day, and can be unilateral, bilateral or involve only the tip of the tongue. There can be associated burning sensations in the mucosa of the palate and lips together with facial pain (which is not necessarily related to a distinct anatomical region).

Many of these patients have a fear of cancer. Multiple consultations, ineffective investigations including biopsies and other surgical procedures, multiple medications and many sets of dentures are characteristic features. Various authors conclude that the primary disorder in these patients is depressive illness, often in an 'atypical' or 'masked' form.

Usually the patients have hypochondriasis with distortions and excessive concern about normal sensations, which they interpret as abnormal and associate with an impending life-threatening disease.

Antidepressant therapy clonazepam and supportive, often covert, psychotherapy have been found to be extremely effective for many.

Summary

Oro-facial pain is often acute and has a recognizable cause. Less commonly the aetiology is more obscure and the condition may be relatively intractable. More commonly occurring benign chronic oro-facial pain syndromes include TMJPDS, trigeminal neuralgia, post-traumatic pain, dental causalgia, atypical facial pain and oral dysaesthesia. Chronic oro-facial pain syndromes are best managed through a multidisciplinary approach.

References

Behrman, S. (1949) Facial neuralgias. Br. Dent. J. 86, 197 – 201.
Blumer, D. and Heilbronn, M. (1982) Chronic pain as a variant of depressive disease: the pain prone disorder. J. Nerv. Ment. Dis. 170, 381 – 406.
Bonica, J. J. (1974) Organization and function of a pain clinic. In: J. J. Bonica (Ed.), Advances in Neurology, Vol. 4. Raven Press, New York, pp. 433 – 443.
Brightman, J. J. (1977) Disordered oral sensation and appetite. In: The Chemical Senses and Nutrition. Academic Press, New York, pp. 363 – 380.
Cooper, I. S. and Braceland, F. I. (1950) Psychosomatic aspects of pain. Med. Clin. North Am. 34, 981 – 984.
Costen, J. B. (1934) A syndrome of ear and sinus symptoms dependent upon disturbed function of the temporomandibular joint. Ann. Otol. Rhinol. Laryngol. 43, 1 – 15.
Crue, B. L. (Ed.) (1979) Chronic Pain: Further Observations from City of Hope National Medical Centre. MacMillan, New York, pp. 13 – 27.
Dalessio, D. J. (Ed.) (1980) Wolff's Headache and Other Head Pain, 4th edn. Oxford University Press, New York.
Diagnostic and Statistical Manual of Mental Disorders (3rd edn.) (1980) American Psychiatric Association, Washington D.C.
Dworkin, S. F. (1983) Benign chronic orofacial pain. Postgrad. Med. 74, 239 – 248.
Editorial (1984) Head and face pain management. Br. Dent. J. 156, 5, 155.
Elfenbaum, A. (1954) Causalgia in dentistry: an abandoned pain syndrome. Oral Surg. Oral Med. Oral Path. 7, 594 – 597.
Gardener, W. J., Todd, E. M. and Pinto, J. P. (1956) Roentgenographic findings in trigeminal neuralgia. A.J.R. 76, 346 – 350.

Gerschman, J. A. and Reade, P. C. (1984) Orofacial pain. Aust. Fam. Phys. 13, 1, 14–24.

Gerschman, J. A., Burrows, G. D. and Reade, P. C. (1977) Orofacial pain. Aust. Fam. Phys. 6, 1219–1225.

Gerschman, J. A., Burrows, G. D. and Reade, P. C. (1979) Chronic orofacial pain. In: J. J. Bonica, J. C. Liebeskind and D. G. Albe-Fessard (Eds.), Advances in Pain Research and Therapy. Raven Press, New York, pp. 317–323.

Goldstein, N. P., Gibilsco, J. A. and Rushton, J. G. (1963) Trigeminal neuralgia, J. Am. Med. Assoc. 184, 458–462.

Gregg, J. M. (1971) Post-traumatic pain: experimental trigeminal neuropathy. J. Oral Surg. 29, 260–263.

Gregg, J. M. and Ghia, J. N. (1980) Comparative aspects of chronic pain in the head and neck versus trunk and appendages: experiences of the Multidisciplinary University of North Carolina Pain Clinic. National Institute of Drug Abuse Research Monograph Series, 1980, 36, 112–117.

Hakanson, S. (1981) Trigeminal neuralgia treated by the injection of glycerol into the trigeminal cistern. Neurosurgery 9, 638–646.

Harris, M. (1974) Psychogenic aspects of facial pain. Br. Dent. J. 136, 199–205.

Helkimo, M. (1976) Epidemiological surveys of dysfunction of the masticatory system. Oral Sci. Res. 7, 54–57.

International Classification of Disease, 9th revision (1978) WHO, Geneva.

Jannetta, R. (1976) Microsurgical approach to the trigeminal nerve for tic douloureux. Prog. Neurol. Surg. 7, 180–200.

Kerr, F. W. and Miller, R. H. (1966) The pathology of trigeminal neuralgia. Electron microscopic studies. Arch. Neurol. 15, 308–319.

Kruger, L. K. (1984) Introduction to mechanisms of acute and chronic pain. In: L. Kruger and J. C. Liebeskind (Eds.), Advances in Pain Research and Therapy, Vol. 6. Raven Press, New York, pp. 95–104.

Little, T. F. (1981) Chronic pain: modern concepts in management. Aust. Fam. Phys. 10, 265–270.

Loeser, J. D. (1977) The management of tic douloureux. Pain 3, 155–162.

Lynch, M. A. (Ed.) (1977) Burket's Oral Medicine, 7th edn. J. B. Lippincott & Co., Philadelphia.

Merskey, H. (1983) Universal language of pain syndromes. In: J. J. Bonica, U. Lindblohm and A. Iggo (Eds.), Advances in Pain Research and Therapy, Vol. 5. Raven Press, New York, pp. 37–52.

Moulton, R. E. (1955) Oral and dental manifestations of anxiety. Psychiatry 18, 261–265.

Ratner, E. J. Person, P., Kleinman, D. J. et al. (1979) Jaw bone cavities and trigeminal and atypical facial neuralgia. Oral Surg. Oral Med. Oral Path. 48, 3–20.

Reade, P. C. (1984a) An approach to the management of temporomandibular joint-pain dysfunction syndrome. J. Pros. Dent. 51, 91–96.

Reade, P. C. (1984b) An alternative view of temporomandibular joint-pain dysfunction syndrome. Aust. J. Ortho. 8, 77–81.

Rees, R. T. and Harris, M. (1978) Atypical odontalgia. Br. J. Oral Surg. 16, 212–218.

Sisk, A. L. (1983) Surgical treatment of chronic orofacial pain. Anaesth. Prog. 180–184.

Sweet, W. H. (1968) Trigeminal neuralgias. In: C. C. Alling (Ed.), Facial Pain, 3rd edn. Lea and Febiger, Philadelphia, pp. 89–106.

The Medical Letter on Drugs and Therapeutics (1975) 3.

Visoso, A. D. and Young, J. Z. (1948) Internode length and fibre diameter in developing and regenerating nerves. J. Anat. 82, 110–114.

Wall, P. D. (1984) Mechanisms of acute and chronic pain. In: L. Kruger and J. C. Liebeskind (Eds.), Advances in Research and Therapy, Vol. 6. Raven Press, New York. pp. 95–99.

White, J. G. and Sweet, W. H. (1955) Pain, Its Mechanism and Neurological Control. Thomas Springfield, Ill.

Williams, J. B. and Spitzer, R. L. (1982) Idiopathic pain disorder: a critique of pain-prone disorder and a proposal for a revision of the DSM-III category psychogenic pain disorder. J. Nerv. Ment. Dis. 170, 415–417.

Burrows/Elton/Stanley (eds.) Handbook of Chronic Pain Management
© *1987 Elsevier Science Publishers B.V. (Biomedical Division)*

31

Management of pain in the rheumatic diseases

F. McKENNA and V. WRIGHT

Rheumatism Research Unit, 36 Clarendon Road, Leeds LS2 9PJ, U.K.

Epidemiology

The rheumatic diseases are a major cause of morbidity in most countries. A survey in general practice in England and Wales several years ago showed that the chronic rheumatic diseases are the commonest cause of all patients consulting their GP – over 10% of patients seeking help for rheumatic disease (Logan and Cushion 1958). The commonest problems in patients under the age of 45 years are muscular rheumatism and prolapsed intravertebral disc. Osteoarthritis predominates after the age of 65. The number of consultations per patient per year varies between two and three for muscular rheumatism and osteoarthritis to about nine for rheumatoid arthritis. The rheumatic diseases are also an important cause of absenteeism at work (Sze 1963). Between 7 and 10% of working days lost is due to arthritis and rheumatism. This accounts for on average approximately one working day lost per year for every person in employment.

Among rheumatic diseases, the greatest problem numerically is degenerative joint disease. Osteoarthritis, as determined radiologically is common. Forty per cent of males and 37% of females show evidence of disc degeneration of the cervical spine, the prevalence rising from 1% before the age of 24 years to 87% of males and 74% of females over the age of 65 years (Lawrence et al. 1963). Approximately half of these patients have moderate or severe disease. The relationship between cervical disc degeneration and cervico-brachial pain is debatable (Heller et al. 1983) although there appears to be a relationship between the radiological changes and symptoms in patients up to the age of 45 years. Disc degeneration in the lumbar spine however does appear to be associated with low back pain. The prevalence of peripheral osteoarthritis varies with the different joints, the majority of patients over the age of 65 years having some evidence of osteoarthritis in the hand. Fifty per cent will have some osteoarthritis of the knee and 10% will have osteoarthritis of the hip.

Although osteoarthritis numerically is the most common of the rheumatic diseases, rheumatoid arthritis causes the worst disabilities. Definite rheumatoid arthritis is found in 2–3% of all populations studied. Probable disease varies more widely but is of similar prevalence. Of the other rheumatic diseases, ankylosing spondylitis and psoriatic arthritis both have a prevalence in the region of 1%. The remaining rheumatic diseases are less common.

Neuroanatomy of the joint (Wyke 1981)

All the synovial joints including the apophyseal, costo-vertebral and costo-transverse joints of the spine have similar receptor nerve endings. These can be categorised into four different types. Type 1 are found in the superficial layers of the fibrous capsules of joints, their parent nerve fibres being small myelinated fibres, 6–9 μm in diameter. They have a low threshold, are slow in adapting, and are static and dynamic mechanoreceptors. Type 2 are found in deeper sub-synovial layers in the fibrous capsules of joints and also in the articular fat pads. These have medium myelinated parent nerve fibres from 9 to 12 μm in diameter. These are also low threshold receptors but are rapidly adapting dynamic mechanoreceptors. Type 3 receptors are applied to the surfaces of joint ligaments, both collateral and intrinsic, and have large myelinated parent nerve fibres between 13 and 17 μm in diameter. These are also dynamic mechanoreceptors but have a high threshold and are slowly adapting. Type 4 receptors are of two types. Type a are tri-dimensional plexuses of the myelinated nerve fibres which are found in fibrous capsules of joints, articular fat pads and adventitial sheaths of articular blood vessels. Type b are free un-myelinated nerve endings which are found in both collateral and intrinsic joint ligaments. Both types of receptors have very small myelinated parent nerve fibres between 2 and 5 μm in diameter and some unmyelinated parent nerve fibres less than 2 μm in diameter. These are nociceptive mechanoreceptors with a very high threshold and are non-adapting. They are also chemo-sensitive to abnormal tissue metabolites. There are no nerve fibres found in articular cartilage.

The innervation of each individual synovial joint is provided from varying arrays of articular nerves that fall into two categories, primary and accessory. Each nerve contains a mixture of myelinated and unmyelinated nerve fibres that vary in diameter from a maximum of 17 μm diameter to less than 1 μm, although around 50% are less than 5 μm in diameter, those less than 2 μm being unmyelinated. Most of the myelinated fibres less than 5 μm in diameter represent the afferent fibres innervating the type 4 receptors in the related joint capsules, ligaments and fat pads, and are responsible for the slow transmission of impulses that give rise to joint pain. The unmyelinated fibres in the articular nerves are post-ganglionic sympathetic adrenergic fibres, the afferent activity in which controls the diameter of the articular blood vessels and thus in-fluences the blood flow rate through the joint tissues. Approximately 40–45% of articular nerve fibres have a diameter from 6 to 12 μm and consist of medium sized myelinated afferent fibres innervating type 1 and type 2 mechanoreceptors in the fibrous capsules. The smallest proportion of fibres in the articular nerves are between 13 and 17 μm and represent afferent fibres inner-vating the type 3 receptors in the collateral and intrinsic ligaments of the joints (although these are not present in all joints).

No joint in the body, whether in the limbs or the vertebral column, is innervated by afferent fibres entering just a single segment, but rather there is a plurisegmental innervation and this varies widely from joint to joint. Even a single apophyseal joint in the spinal column is inner-vated from several segments of the spinal cord. This plurisegmental innervation is greatest in the cervical spine and least in the lumbar spine although even the lumbar apophyseal joints are inner-vated from at least three contiguous dorsal nerve roots.

Primary articular nerves are independent branches of adjacent peripheral nerves and often ac-company blood vessels supplying the joint tissues in neurovascular bundles. They traverse the connective tissue planes between their originating nerve trunk and the joint capsule that they in-nervate, and some become embedded in the periosteum covering the bones adjacent to the at-tachments of the joint capsule. The accessory articular nerves are branches of intramuscular nerves traversing some, but not all, of the muscles that are attached to or pass over the joint capsules. They run to the joint through the intervascular connective tissue within the muscles and then into and through the fascial sheaths of the muscles. In the ankle, knee and elbow joint the sparse additional accessory innervation may be provided through smaller twigs that come off the cutaneous nerves which innervate part of the skin overlying the joint. It can therefore be seen that the innervation of the joints is a complex pattern and it is not possible to identify a single nerve in any joint which is responsible for all the afferent impulses from that joint.

The essential prerequisite for the experience of joint pain is irritation of the type 4 nociceptive receptor system distributed throughout the fibrous capsules, ligaments and fat pads of the joints. Such irritation may develop from either abnormal mechanical stresses within the joints or from the accumulation in the tissue fluid within joint capsules of sufficiently high concentrations of abnormal tissue metabolites. Joint pain may be therefore either mechanical or chemical, or a combination of the two.

MECHANICAL JOINT PAIN

Articular nociceptive receptor irritation may be caused or enhanced by changes in the pressure gradient between the atmosphere and the interior of the joint, if this was sufficient to produce increases in the tension in the joint capsules. Such a change may arise from the development of a joint effusion or haemarthrosis or alternatively consequent on a marked decrease in atmospheric pressure. Some patients with chronic joint pain experience an increase in symptoms when the barometric pressure falls relatively quickly. Dislocation or subluxation of joints, or internal distortion of a joint capsule from a meniscal tear also distort the joint capsule and produce pain.

A less direct cause of mechanical articular pain particularly in the spinal apophyseal joints producing neck and back pain arises when there is a decrease in the vertical height of intervertebral discs from degenerative disc disease or prolapsed intervertebral disc, or also following collapse of the vertebral bodies such as crush fractures in osteoporosis. There is a subsequent increase in the tension of the capsules of the apophyseal joints producing diffuse back pain and neck pain.

CHEMICAL JOINT PAIN

The unmyelinated nerve fibres of type 4 receptors are stimulated by exposure to a variety of chemical substances. Lactic acid, potassium ions, polypeptide kinins, 5-hydroxytryptamine, prostaglandin E and histamine are all substances which are released from the cells of ischaemic or injured tissue and from acute or chronic inflammation of the tissues. Since the chemical composition of the tissue fluid in the capsules of joints is in equilibrium with that of the synovial fluid, the accumulation of any of these substances in synovial fluid in various forms of synovitis results in a similar rise in their concentration in the capsular tissue fluid and thus in irritation of the type 4 receptors. Synovial tissue itself does not contain such receptors.

MODULATION OF JOINT PAIN

It has become clear that afferent discharges from a variety of tissue mechanoreceptors (type 1 and 2) may exert a central pain suppressive effect. The probability that an incoming nociceptive input from mechanically or chemically irritated nociceptive receptors in joint tissues would traverse the gateway synapses in the basal spinal nuclei and thus be transmitted into the brain to produce the experience of joint pain, is inversely related to the ongoing frequency of discharge from joints, cutaneous and muscle mechanoreceptors since afferents from these receptors converge on the same inhibitory interneurons in the dorsal horns of the spinal gray matter. This is a likely explanation of the benefit many patients derive from physiotherapy and manipulation. In addition, transcutaneous nerve stimulators stimulate the afferent nerve fibres as they traverse the mass of nerves beneath the skin flooding the neuronal system of the dorsal horns in the spinal gray matter. The benefit patients find from the use of a rocking chair may be explained by the rhythmic stimulation of mechanoreceptors producing a massive presynaptic inhibitory blockade of ongoing nociceptive impulse.

Symptoms

Pain is the most significant and troublesome symptom of most patients with chronic rheumatic disease. The cause of pain in arthritis is complex. Environmental and psychological factors are superimposed on local inflammatory and/or mechanical factors.

The importance of pain to the patients is reflected in the results of a survey of 240 patients attending our clinic (McKenna and Wright 1985b). Half of these patients had rheumatoid arthritis, the majority of the remainder had degenerative joint disease. The patients were asked to rank in order of severity over the course of their disease the symptoms of pain, swelling, stiffness and disability. Sixty-six per cent of the patients with rheumatoid arthritis considered that pain had been their worst symptom, whereas 22% thought the disability caused by the disease had been their worst problem. The patients ranking disability as the worst symptom, however, in general had end stage disease. Twelve per cent of patients ranked stiffness as the worst symptom. Less than 2% of patients found that the swelling of the joints had been the most problematic. Swelling of the joints was usually ranked last by nearly all the patients. Seventy-five per cent of the patients with degenerative joint disease classed pain as their worst symptom, whilst 17% thought the disability produced by the disease outweighed the pain. Only 6% thought stiffness to be the worst symptom and only one patient (2%) thought the swelling of the joints was the worst part of the disease. However, patients with degenerative joint disease tended to find it more difficult to differentiate between pain and other symptoms compared to patients with rheumatoid arthritis. A similar survey (Gibson and Clark 1985) in patients with rheumatoid arthritis also found that the majority of patients ranked pain relief as the most desirable objective of their treatment, although this was a smaller proportion than in our study. This may have been due to their sampling more patients with end stage disease.

The quality of pain experienced in patients with arthritis has been examined recently (Charter et al. 1985). The affective component of the pain was found to be more intense than the sensory component, indicating the importance of emotional factors, and this did not alter with the duration of disease. The sensory aspects of the pain were more complex than the affective ones, reflecting the varied sources and combinations of somatic pathology. No differences were found in the overall pain experience between rheumatoid and degenerative disease.

Assessment of pain

Pain, being a subjective symptom, is difficult to evaluate. It is, however, of importance, not only in evaluating treatment in any individual, but also in comparing different treatment regimes in drug trials. Laboratory studies have shown that there are no reliable physiological indices of pain. Measurement of galvanic skin responses, heart rate and respiration rate cannot be specifically correlated with the experience of pain. There are, however, many problems in recording the verbal reports of patients. It is often difficult for some patients to remember previous experiences of pain and to rank them with their current symptoms. The level of depression is likely to alter the experience of pain. A 4-point scale has been described and is a useful method, particularly in view of its simplicity, describing pain as slight, moderate, severe or agonising. Another method may be to evaluate pain compared with the patient's last visit as being either worse, better or unchanged. Expressing pain on a visual analogue scale has received much attention, particularly since the work of Huskisson (1974). The visual analogue scale has been studied in our group by Dixon and colleagues (Dixon and Bird 1981). The reproduceability has been found to vary along the length of the scale with a tendency to estimate too high and there is a greater variation towards the centre rather than at the edges of the scale. However, significantly different values were recorded by patients when repeated even after one hour, indicating the inaccuracy of the assessment (Hinchliffe et al. 1985). Different methods of evaluating pain have been compared. One study evaluated a 5-point scale, a visual analogue scale and a 9-point scale using pictures (Frank et al. 1982). There was an acceptable correlation between all three scales in measurement of changes in degree of pain. It remains to be determined whether one method is preferable to any other.

Treatment — general principles

The control of pain from rheumatic disease is approached in two ways. Firstly, the pain is treated with analgesics, augmented if necessary with physical treatment. The mainstay of treatment for all patients with rheumatic disease is mild analgesia such as paracetamol. This is a peripherally acting analgesic and is given either alone or often in combination preparations with other, centrally acting, analgesic drugs such as dextropropoxyphene, codeine, dihydrocodeine or pentazocine. Paracetamol alone is remarkably well tolerated, as in general are the mild centrally acting analgesics, except for problems of nausea and constipation. In addition, the non-steroidal anti-inflammatory drugs (NSAIDs) discussed later have a direct analgesic effect as well as being anti-inflammatory, and may therefore be useful in treating pain even when this is not a direct result of inflammation. It has been suggested that simple analgesics are not useful in inflammatory arthritis such as rheumatoid arthritis and some studies have shown the simple analgesics to be less effective than the anti-inflammatory drugs given alone. We believe that both the NSAIDs and the mild analgesics deserve a therapeutic trial, and there is usually a place for both classes of drugs either given alone or in combination, or as supplements to other treatment.

The second approach to treatment is the use of physical treatment and exercises. Simple methods are preferred so that patients can then continue with the application of heat or ice at home. Teaching patients to improve muscle tone with regular exercises has been shown to relieve pain, and patients are encouraged to persist with their regime of exercises at home indefinitely. The use of aids to daily living is important in the management of most patients. The use of a walking stick (in the contralateral hand) of patients with disease of weight bearing joints often reduces symptoms. A raised toilet seat, bath board and bath seat may allow patients with hip or knee disease to be independent. Other aids such as a pick-up stick, or devices to open doors or sink taps may ease the burden of disability and pain caused by arthritis.

The third approach is the treatment, if possible, of the underlying pathogenic mechanism of the disease leading to pain. One good example of this is the treatment of septic arthritis. The offending aetiologic agent, i.e. the bacterium, is isolated and specific anti-bacterial drugs are then prescribed. The treatment of gout with the xanthine-oxidase inhibitor allopurinol is another disease where specific therapy is used in correcting, in this case, a metabolic defect of uric acid metabolism. The treatment of polymyalgia rheumatica with corticosteroids, although not curative, is so effective in producing a complete remission as to be considered as specific treatment. The so-called disease modifying drugs or slow acting anti-rheumatoid drugs used in rheumatoid arthritis can be regarded as being specific treatment aimed at controlling the disease process and so reducing the symptoms of pain and stiffness. Gold salts, D-penicillamine, anti-malarials, sulphasalazine and the cytotoxic drugs cyclophosphamide, chlorambucil, methotrexate and azathioprine have all been shown to have the properties of disease modifying drugs. These are discussed later. Corticosteroids in high dosage in rheumatoid arthritis may also be considered similarly.

NON-STEROIDAL ANTI-INFLAMMATORY DRUGS

NSAIDs, as mentioned, can be considered as both analgesic and also anti-inflammatory, inhibiting the pain producing mechanisms. The first NSAID was aspirin, and this is the most widely used drug of all time. Several theories have been considered as to the possible mode of action of NSAIDs. These have included the release of an endogenous anti-inflammatory substance, the depression of general metabolism in inflamed tissues, the reduction of leukocyte migration and the inhibition of lysozomal enzyme release from phagocytosing leukocytes. However, no endogenous anti-inflammatory substance has been isolated, the drugs do not reduce exogenously applied inflammatory mediators, thus they do not antagonise mediator activity at the receptor level, the doses required to reduce leucocyte migration are much higher than those which prevent oedema, erythema and hyperalgesia, and the rank order of potency of NSAIDs on the inhibition of lysozomal enzyme release does not correlate with the anti-inflammatory activity. The most convincing explanation of the mechanism of action of NSAIDs, however, was first proposed in 1971 by Vane and his colleagues, who won the Nobel Prize for their work. They demonstrated that aspirin and related drugs selectively inhibit the synthesis of prostaglandins (see Higgs et al. 1980). It is useful to review this area.

Prostaglandins are generated when living tissue is mechanically or chemically stimulated and they are always present following injury. They have potent inflammatory properties which cause the well-known features of calor, dolor, rubor and tumor of inflammation. Prostaglandins are derived from polyunsaturated fatty acids such as arachidonic acid, which in turn is released from membrane phosphilipids by the activity of phospholipase A2. Corticosteroids inhibit the release of arachidonic acid and prevent any subsequent production of prostaglandins. Arachidonic acid is metabolised into three groups of substances: the prostaglandins produced following the enzymatic action of cyclo-oxygenase, the 5-HPETE products and the leukotrienes resulting from the action of lipoxygenase and the 15-HPETE products also as a result of lipoxygenase activity (Fig. 1). Inhibitors of leukotrienes are an active field of current investigation but will not be considered further here. The cyclo-oxygenase products of interest in inflammation include prostacyclin (PGI_2), thromboxane A_2, PGE_2 and PGF_2 alpha. The inflammatory properties of these products include vascular effects, effect on leukocyte migration and the production of pain, hyperalgesia and fever. Prostacyclin and PGE_2 have a potent action on vascular smooth muscle, producing vasodilatation and erythema. The concentrations of PGE_2 and prostacyclin in inflammatory exudates are sufficient to contribute to the erythema of acute inflammation.

Oedema formation is the result of an interaction between mediators which separately cause vasodilatation and increase vascular permeability. When prostaglandins are given in combination with bradykinin or histamine, there is an augmentation of plasma exudation. Prostaglandin concentrations in inflammatory exudates increase in parallel with the accumulation of leukocytes during the early stages of inflammation, although inhibition of prostaglandin production does not correlate with the reduction of leukocyte migration. (The effect of the lipoxygenase products on leukocyte migration, however, is probably more important.)

It has been demonstrated that PGE produces hyperalgesia and pain. However, subdermal infusions in animals of prostaglandins, bradykinin or histamine have been shown not to produce pain unless PGE_1 was given before histamine or bradykinin. Prostaglandins of the E series have also been shown to enhance the pain-producing effects of bradykinin in dog knee joints, suggesting that the inflammatory mediators with the direct pain-producing action are enhanced when afferent pain endings are sensitised by prostaglandins. PGE_2 and other stable prostaglandins produce a hyperalgesic effect which is cumulative and long-lasting. The other effect of prostaglandins of the E series is that of fever. PGE_1 is the most potent pyretic agent known when given centrally, although the importance of prostaglandins in the regulation of body temperature is debatable.

Interestingly, certain prostaglandins may have both pro-inflammatory and anti-inflammatory effects. Exogenous PGE has been shown to reduce inflammation in adjuvant arthritis in the rat, an effect which is mediated via cyclic AMP (Kunkel et al. 1981). In view of this potential anti-

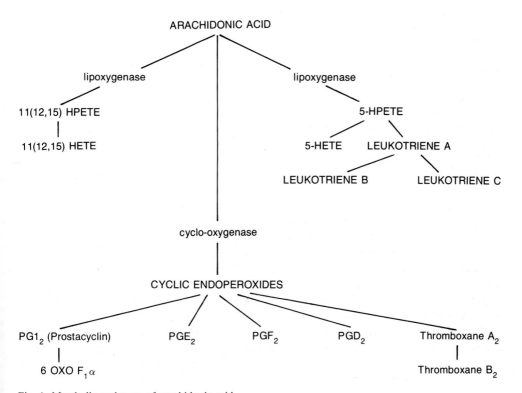

Fig. 1. Metabolic pathways of arachidonic acid.

inflammatory effect of cyclic AMP, we undertook a pilot study evaluating the phosphodiesterase inhibitor aminophylline (which inhibits the breakdown of cAMP) in the treatment of patients with active rheumatoid arthritis. Six patients who had failed to respond to penicillamine were followed monthly for 3 months with evaluation of pain score, duration of morning stiffness, articular index, grip strength, haemoglobin, erythrocyte sedimentation rate, C-reactive protein, plasma viscosity, histidine and sulphydryl concentrations, whilst receiving 450 mg slow release aminophylline daily in divided doses. The penicillamine was continued without alteration of the dose. None of the patients showed any improvement. It seems unlikely therefore that such an approach to treatment is tenable, although the additional treatment with NSAIDs in all the patients may possibly have prevented a therapeutic effect.

All the NSAIDs inhibit the synthesis of the prostaglandins mentioned above, and the evidence suggests that this accounts for their therapeutic effects. In addition, however, the NSAIDs also have a central analgesic effect; the relief of pain following the use of these drugs does not therefore imply an inflammatory component in the disease. Conversely, the NSAIDs do not have a profound effect in relieving the chronic inflammation of rheumatoid arthritis, although their effect in relieving the symptoms of this disease is unquestioned.

The major problem encountered in the use of oral NSAIDs is the high incidence of dyspepsia and peptic ulceration. The likely reason for this is the inhibition of prostaglandins which are important in maintaining the mucus-gel barrier of the gastric mucosa. With the breakdown of this protective barrier, the mucosa is subject to direct damage from the low gastric pH (see also Chapter 19).

Treatment of specific pain syndromes

LOW BACK PAIN

Low back pain is estimated to affect approximately 65% of population samples. It is usually felt over the lumbar spine or sacro-iliac joints. The pain frequently radiates to the buttocks and may refer down the leg. Patients commonly complain of pain in the hips when this arises from pain in the low back radiating into the iliac region. Pain radiating down the leg may be anterior or lateral, or in a sciatic distribution radiating posteriorly to the heel. A wide variety of conditions produce pain in the back. Disc herniations account for only 5% of back disorders. Lumbar spondylosis and intervertebral disc degeneration are much more common and may be more symptomatic when associated with spinal stenosis. Spondylolisthesis may be secondary to degenerative disc disease, may be traumatic or may be congenital in origin. Inflammatory disease of the lower back is not uncommon. Ankylosing spondylitis has a prevalence in some studies approaching 1%. This should be suspected in patients presenting at an early age with low back pain without a history of preceding trauma, and with a history of prolonged morning stiffness. Pyogenic vertebral osteomyelitis producing back pain should not be overlooked. Tuberculosis of the spine is a rare cause of low back pain in the West although it is common in Third World countries and must be remembered among immigrants.

Plane radiographs of the lumbar spine and sacro-iliac joints are likely to help in diagnosis in the majority of patients. A raised erythrocyte sedimentation rate (ESR) is suggestive of inflammatory or infectious disease of the spine, although a normal ESR does not exclude ankylosing spondylitis. Myelography is considered only if there is thought to be a surgically correctable lesion.

Patients with acute prolapsed disc should be treated with complete bed rest for at least 2 weeks. This may mean admission to hospital. Traction may be helpful (although this may simply help by keeping the patient in bed!). In addition to bed rest, patients are treated with analgesics and benzodiazepines to relieve muscle spasm. If signs of nerve root entrapment do not resolve, then a discectomy or laminectomy may be necessary. The treatment of lumbar spondylosis and degenerative disc disease is, in general, unrewarding. Patients are encouraged to lose weight if obese and to have a trial with a lumbar support corset. Simple analgesics are the mainstay of treatment. In addition, patients should have a therapeutic trial of NSAIDs. Physiotherapy is useful but may have little more than a placebo effect. For patients who fail to respond to these measures, transcutaneous nerve stimulation may be helpful. In addition, patients should have regard for correct posture, care with lifting and carrying, and ensure their bed has a well-supported mattress.

The treatment of ankylosing spondylitis consists of a daily regime of exercises for the patient in addition to NSAIDs and simple analgesics. Indomethacin in large doses is often effective. Patients who are resistant to other NSAIDs may however respond to phenylbutazone, which is prescribable from hospital only in the U.K. All patients need to be encouraged to continue with exercises. Severe relapse is treated with in-patient physiotherapy. We have adopted a regime of admitting the most severely affected patients on an annual basis for physiotherapy in a spondylitis 'class' of similar patients. This appears to offer some degree of prophylaxis as well as psychological support for certain patients. Patients are also encouraged to participate in the National Ankylosing Spondylitis Society — a self-help organisation which offers support and useful advice. Such a regime has now made treatment with radiotherapy redundant.

Neck pain

In addition to pain localised in the neck, patients with disease of the cervical spine often complain of pain radiating to the occiput, scapular area, shoulders and arms. The differential diagnosis is similar to that considered for the lumbar spine. Cervical spondylosis is the commonest problem. Although radiologically this appears in most of the population above 50 years of age, it is only symptomatic in a proportion. Treatment is aimed at reducing the risk of nerve root irritation, avoiding lifting and carrying, wearing a support collar for any activities that involve flexing the neck, and wearing a soft collar to sleep in order to support the lordosis of the cervical spine whilst supine.

Analgesics are useful, and patients should have a therapeutic trial of NSAIDs. Benzodiazepines, baclofen and dantrolene may be helpful in patients with apparent muscle spasm, and physical treatment with gentle exercises or traction may help. Patients with ankylosing spondylitis are treated as described above. Collars in general are only used as a last resort, although a soft collar to support the neck in bed at night may be useful.

Painful shoulder

This is a common problem. In addition to synovitis of the shoulder, patients with cervical spondylosis often complain of pain radiating into the shoulder, and may develop a secondary adhesive capsulitis of the joint. This produces pain and restriction of movement. Supraspinatus tendonitis produces pain on resisted abduction of the shoulder, whereas bicipital tendonitis produces pain with resisted flexion and supination of the elbow. Tendons of the supraspinatus, infraspinatus, teres minor and subscapularis combine to produce the rotator cuff. A tear in this structure from trauma produces a painful arc — with painless abduction of the arm to 45°, pain with abduction from 45° to 90°, pain with assisted abduction from 90° to 110° and painless abduction from 110° to 180°. Such a lesion may lead to an adhesive capsulitis. Treatment of all of the above conditions is with intralesional steroids and physiotherapy. This is useful in relieving pain, although the full range of movement may not recover for 2 years.

OSTEOARTHRITIS

Hip joint. Degenerative disease of the hip joint produces pain which initially occurs with standing and walking. The pain usually occurs in the groin and radiates to the upper thigh and occasionally to the buttock. Progression of the disease produces symptoms at rest which may disturb sleep. Articular gelling — stiffness occurring after sitting or resting — may be particularly disabling. Treatment is initially with analgesics and a trial of NSAIDs; obese patients are encouraged to lose weight. Physiotherapy usually offers only temporary relief but patients are encouraged to continue mobilisation exercises preferably in a pool when possible. When the disease interferes with the patient's lifestyle with restricted mobility or uncontrolled pain (particularly when disturbing sleep), arthroplasty of the joint is usually curative. The introduction of successful hip arthroplasty is probably the greatest ever single advance in the treatment of arthritis.

Knee joint. Osteoarthritis of the knee joint is a common cause of disability in the elderly. It is usually bilateral and may produce instability with resultant deformity. The inevitable wasting of the quadriceps muscle group which accompanies the disease causes difficulty in walking, rising from a chair and climbing stairs, and is a common cause of falls in the elderly with the knee 'giving way'. Treatment is similar to treatment of the hip with analgesia, trial of NSAIDs, and weight reduction in obese patients. Exercises aimed at strengthening the quadriceps decrease the pain and improve disability, but need to be constantly encouraged. A study in our unit demonstrated that patients tend to persist with such exercises, and have a better response, if they are given a follow-up appointment by the physiotherapist, rather than discharged. However, patients instructed to exercise at home fared as well as patients receiving treatment in the physiotherapy department, demonstrating the value of home-based treatment (Chamberlain et al. 1982).

Intra-articular steroid injection offers benefit in most patients, but is usually short lived, and in view of the potential risk of steroid arthropathy is best avoided except as a last resort. Arthroplasty of the knee joint is not yet as successful as the hip, but is recommended particularly when there is instability of the joint associated with intractable pain and disability.

RHEUMATOID ARTHRITIS (RA)

RA affects approximately 3% of the population in the Western world. It may present at any age, but reaches a peak in the fourth decade, and is twice as common in women as men. It is an illness characterised by relapse and remission, and produces synovitis in common with systemic features (McKenna and Wright 1985a). The commonest onset is of generalised stiffness with a polyarthritis developing over days or weeks. There is pain and swelling, particularly in the small joints of the hands, wrists and feet. Except for the hip joint, the large joints are commonly affected early in the disease. RA may present as an acute monoarthritis or an asymetric oligoarthritis, but within a few months 95% of patients will develop synovitis of the small joints in the hands or feet. Diagnosis rests on the clinical picture, the detection of circulating rheumatoid factor (present in up to 70% of patients) and the presence of erosions on X-ray. Pain is the predominant symptom in RA, and effective relief of symptoms can only be obtained by a comprehensive approach to treatment. It should be remembered that pain in rheumatoid arthritis may be caused either from synovitis in the joint, or through the resultant joint deformity causing secondary osteoarthritis. The most effective approach to pain relief in patients with synovitis in the joints is to direct treatment towards the inflammatory process. When pain arises from the result of joint deformity, pain relief is attempted by standard analgesic drugs in addition to physical treatment and other measures.

TREATMENT OF RHEUMATOID SYNOVITIS

The initial advice for patients is to rest. Bed rest reduces all the manifestations of the inflammatory process with reduction in pain and stiffness, and improvement in the haemoglobin, ESR and acute phase reactants. Localised rest from splintage of the hand, wrist or knee joints may offer significant symptomatic relief if there is active synovitis in these joints. Physical treatments are useful in all patients and many simple measures may be used at home. The application of heat from a hot water bottle, heat pad or lamp often offers pain relief, even if only temporarily. Hot wax baths for the hands and feet may be used routinely in the patient's home, as well as in the hospital physiotherapy department. Some patients find the application of ice packs offers symptomatic relief when heat does not. Other more sophisticated methods of heat, e.g. short wave diathermy are often beneficial. A study in our unit comparing different methods of physical treatment of the hand (Hawkes et al. 1985), however, demonstrated no difference between the use of wax baths and exercises when compared with either ultrasound and exercises, or the combination of ultrasound, faradic hand baths and exercises. Significant improvement in grip strength, joint size, and articular index, the range of joint movement and the duration of a timed task was seen in all treatment groups. In addition to physical therapy, patients are instructed in exercises. Passive exercises followed by active exercises whent the disease is responding may not only improve muscle tone, but appears to augment pain relief.

Most patients with RA will require treatment with NSAIDs during the course of their illness, and many will remain on one or other of these drugs indefinitely. They all offer some degree of symptomatic relief in patients with active disease, and there is little difference in efficacy between any of the drugs when compared in clinical trials. There is, however, a variability in response between individual patients, which may in part be explained by inequality in dosage. The use of drugs with a longer half-life reduces the frequency of dosage and thus may secure better compliance (e.g. naproxen, piroxicam). A similar schedule can be achieved by slow release formulations, although the danger of longer half-lives is accumulation, and this has to be watched, particularly in the elderly in whom a reduced dose is often advisable. It is sensible to 'ring the changes' with the drugs if there is toxicity or poor response with any one drug after a trial period of 3 weeks. The logical choice is to use a drug from a different chemical group if a drug from one group is unsuccessful (see Table 1). Aspirin is often as effective as newer NSAIDs if used in sufficient dosage, but the newer drugs enjoy a reduced incidence of toxicity, particularly on the upper gastrointestinal tract, and therefore are usually preferred, particularly for long-term treatment. If salicylates are used, the enteric coated preparations obviate some gastric toxicity. An alternative is the pro-drug, benorylate, which is only metabolised to aspirin and paracetamol from its chemical combination after absorption. It is not unusual for patients to take more than one NSAID, although this may increase the risk of peptic ulceration. A second NSAID may be added at night for example to relieve early morning stiffness. A survey in our

TABLE 1
Classification of NSAIDs.

Salicylic acids	Indole, indene acetic acids	Enolic acids
Aspirin	Indomethacin	Phenylbutazone
Benorylate	Sulindac	Oxyphenbutazone
Salsalate		Azapropazone
Diflunisal		Feprazone
Aloxipirin		
Anthranilic acids	Arylpropionic acids	Arylacetic acids
Mefenamic	Ibuprofen	Diclofenac
Flufenamic	Flurbiprofen	Fenclofenac
	Ketoprofen	
	Naproxen	
	Fenoprofen	
	Indoprofen	
	Carprofen	
	Fenbufen	
	Heteroaryl acetic acids	Oxicams
	Tolmetin	Piroxicam
		Isoxicam

clinic has shown that 38% of patients with RA were taking two or more NSAIDs in addition to other drugs.

Additional analgesia with a simple analgesic is usual, and a sensible approach is to prescribe paracetamol and evaluate the response. Further benefit may be obtained with the use of the compound tablets of paracetamol with dextropropoxyphine, pentazocine, codeine or dihydrocodeine, if paracetamol alone is insufficient. Occasionally, patients may require a higher dosage of the mild/moderate opiate derivative analgesics, but their use is complicated by an increased incidence of side effects.

Corticosteroids are in widespread usage in various forms. Intra-articular steroids are useful in treating synovitis when this is prominent in a small number of joints. Of concern, however, is the potential risk of a steroid arthropathy following intra-articular steroids particularly in weight bearing joints. It is wise therefore to restrict such treatment to a minimum. Large boluses of pulsed intravenous methyl prednisolone induce a remission which may last for up to 8 weeks, and are particularly useful in obtaining an earlier remission when commencing treatment with an anti-rheumatoid drug (Neumann et al. 1985). Oral corticosteroids are very effective in relieving symptoms in RA, but the difficulties in weaning patients off the drug and the problem of side effects with long-term use tend to lead to restriction of their use in young patients, except when other therapy has failed. All steroids are used with less restriction in elderly patients, and in this group are often remarkably effective particularly in relieving joint stiffness resistant to other drug therapy.

With the possible exception of high dose steroids, the drugs mentioned above only have an effect in reducing the symptoms of disease, but do not inhibit the progression of the disease with resultant deformity. The slow acting anti-rheumatoid drugs induce a remission of disease reflected in an improvement in all parameters of disease activity, e.g. joint pain, stiffness, swelling and tenderness, with correction of anaemia and reduction in acute phase proteins (Bird and Wright 1982). These drugs include chloroquine, sulphasalazine, D-penicillamine, gold salts and the cytotoxic drugs, azathioprine, cyclophosphamide, chlorambucil and methotrexate. The hope with treatment is that these drugs will inhibit or slow the development of erosions and joint deformity. Although this has not been proven in clinical trial, the anti-rheumatoid drugs, through the reduction in synovitis, offer a greater symptomatic relief than other drugs, and are indicated for this alone. Because of potential toxicity, the anti-rheumatoid drugs are reserved for patients with moderate or severely active synovitis affecting several joints, usually with concomitant anaemia and raised ESR, C-reactive protein and other acute phase reactants. Improvement is rarely seen before 8 weeks of treatment, but in responders there is then gradual improvement in parameters of disease activity up to 6 months of treatment. Once a response is achieved, treatment is continued indefinitely, unless there is a relapse or signs of toxicity. The choice of drugs tends to depend on previous drug history and severity of disease, e.g. anti-malarials are less effective but also better tolerated than the other drugs. When treatment with a single anti-rheumatoid drug has failed, the combination of treatment with a second drug may offer some advantage.

TREATMENT OF END-STAGE RHEUMATOID DISEASE

Most patients enter a long-lasting remission late in the disease – so-called 'burnt out' disease. Problems then are not of synovitis, as much as of pain resulting from joint deformity with resultant secondary osteoarthritis. Pain relief centres on physical treatment, mild/moderate analgesia, and a therapeutic trial with NSAIDs. Other measures which are employed include weight loss in obese patients, the use of splints, support of deformed feet in handmade shoes, and exercises to maintain muscle tone and joint function. Exercises to improve the tone of the quadriceps muscles are particularly useful in reducing knee instability and pain arising from this. Slow acting anti-rheumatoid drugs are usually ineffective, but oral steroids may be useful in relieving stiffness.

GOUT

Gout may be classified as either primary or secondary. Primary gout occurs only in males and post-menopausal females, whereas secondary gout may be precipitated by a number of conditions that affect uric acid. The commonest cause is probably that secondary to the use of diuretics, particularly thiazides, to renal failure, and in patients with a rapid cell turnover following treatment with cytotoxic drugs. The clinical presentation of gout may be as an acute monoarthritis, which may be recurrent, as chronic tophaceous deposits, or a polyarthritis.

Acute monoarthritis from gout most commonly affects the first metatarso-phalangeal joint, although it may affect other joints, particularly the large joints. The treatment is high doses of a NSAID. Indomethacin is commonly used, with a dose of 100 mg repeated 4-hourly until symptoms decrease, when it is rapidly reduced. Colchicine is effective, but usually produces gastrointestinal disturbance, which is dose-related and NSAIDs are therefore preferred. It does remain a useful diagnostic tool, however, as a positive response to a therapeutic trial of colchicine is seen only in gout. Patients with recurrent acute attacks of gout will have a reduced frequency of attacks with the use of uricosuric agents, such as probenecid or sulphinpyrazone, or the xanthine oxidase inhibitor, allopurinol, on a long-term basis. A low purine diet and reduction in alcohol consumption may also be helpful.

Patients with chronic tophaceous gout and polyarticular gout are treated with NSAIDs for symptomatic improvement and long-term allopurinol. Patients who fail to obtain an adequate response are also prescribed a low purine diet and advised to restrict alcohol. Alternatively, uricosuric agents may be helpful, although they are not used if there is evidence of urate calculi or renal impairment. Azapropazone is a useful NSAID in the treatment of gout, as it has a significant uricosuric effect, which acts synergistically with allopurinol in lowering serum concentrations of uric acid (although care needs to be exercised in elderly patients because of its fluid retaining propensity). As in other areas of medical practice the patient's treatment is tailored to the clinical response rather than to any biochemical abnormality. However, it is thought that maintaining a low serum uric acid should reduce the risk of renal failure consequent on the deposition of urate crystals in the kidney, hence patients with a persistently high serum uric acid may be recommended to have long-term allopurinol despite infrequent symptoms.

SERONEGATIVE SPONDARTHRITIS

Ankylosing spondylitis, psoriatic arthritis, Reiter's syndrome, and enteropathic arthritis are associated by the increased frequency of the presence of HLA-B27 antigen, in addition to a number of overlapping clinical features − particularly the presence of bilateral sacro-iliitis (Wright and Moll 1976). The management of inflammatory disease of the spine has been discussed earlier. The peripheral joint synovitis is managed with analgesics, NSAIDs, physical treatment and exercises similar to the management of RA. An oligoarthritis is usual and intra-articular steroids may therefore be helpful but systemic steroids are rarely indicated. A total colectomy when indicated for the treatment of ulcerative colitis will usually cause a remission in the peripheral joint arthritis, but has no effect on any spondylitis. Gold salts may be beneficial in severe active psoriatic arthritis, but penicillamine and anti-malarials should probably be avoided, although the risk of exfoliative dermatitis may have been overstated. Treatment with either PUVA therapy or methotrexate may however relieve both the skin and joint disease. Etretinate has recently been evaluated (Hopkins et al. 1985), but its side effects on mucosal surfaces are likely to restrict its use.

SYSTEMIC LUPUS ERYTHEMATOSUS

This is an uncommon disease, usually presenting in young women. It produces a mild polyarthritis, which is usually non-erosive and non-deforming. Systemic features may predominate, including malaise, skin rash, photosensitivity, alopecia, mouth ulcers, serositis and, less commonly, renal and neurological disease. The symptoms of joint disease can usually be managed with physical treatment and NSAIDs, with additional mild analgesia when required. Patients with frank synovitis in one or two joints may benefit from intra-articular steroids. Anti-malarials are indicated for skin disease unresponsive to topical therapy, and for persistent low grade synovitis. Corticosteroids are used for more active joint disease or for vital organ involvement. Life-threatening disease is treated with high dose steroids and cyclophosphamide.

Summary

The rheumatic diseases are a major cause of pain and disability throughout the world. The management of pain can be separated into general, and specific treatment. The use of physical treatment (including the application of heat), and a regime of exercises are likely to benefit most patients. Simple analgesia and a therapeutic trial of non-steroidal anti-inflammatory drugs can also be considered for most patients. Specific therapy includes anti-bacterial chemotherapy for septic arthritis, xanthine oxidase inhibitors for gout, corticosteroids for polymyalgia rheumatica, and the slow acting anti-rheumatoid drugs for RA. Despite such treatment most patients will need to adapt to living with chronic pain.

References

Bird, H. A. and Wright, V. (1982) Applied Drug Therapy of the Rheumatic Diseases. Wright PSG, Bristol.

Chamberlain, M. A., Care, G. and Harfield, B. (1982) Physiotherapy in osteoarthritis of the knees. A controlled trial of hospital versus home exercises. Int. Rehab. Med. 4, 101 – 106.

Charter, R. A., Nehemkis, A. M., Keenan, A., Person, D. and Prete, P. E. (1985) The nature of arthritis pain. Br. J. Rheumatol. 24, 53 – 60.

Dixon, J. S. and Bird, H. A. (1981) Reproduceability along a 10 cm vertical visual analogue scale. Ann. Rheum. Dis. 40, 87 – 89.

Frank, A. J. M., Moll, J. M. H. and Hort, J. F. (1982) A comparison of three ways of measuring pain. Rheumatol. Rehab. 21, 211 – 217.

Gibson, T. and Clark, B. (1985) Use of simple analgesics in rheumatoid arthritis. Ann. Rheum. Dis. 44, 27 – 29.

Hawkes, J., Care, G., Dixon, J.S., Bird, H. A. and Wright, V. (1985) Comparison of three physiotherapy regimes for hands with rheumatoid arthritis. Br. Med. J. 291, 101 – 106.

Heller, C. A., Stanley P., Lewis-Jones, B. and Heller, R. F. (1983) Value of X-ray examination of the cervical spine. Br. Med. J. 287, 1276 – 1278.

Higgs, G. A., Moncada, S. and Vane, J. R. (1980) The mode of action of anti-inflammatory drugs which prevent the peroxidation of arachidonic acid. In: E. C. Huskisson (Ed.), Clinics in Rheumatoid Diseases. Anti-Rheumatic Drugs II, Vol. 6, W. B. Saunders Co. Ltd., London – Philadelphia – Toronto, pp. 675 – 693.

Hinchliffe, K. P., Surrall, K. E. and Dixon, J. S. (1985) Reproduceability of pain measurements by patients with rheumatoid arthritis using visual analogue scales. Pharmaceut. Med. 1, 99 – 103.

Hopkins, R., Bird, H. A., Jones, H., Hill, J., Surrall, K. E., Astbury, C., Miller, A. and Wright, V. (1985) A double blind controlled trial of etretinate (Tigason) and ibuprofen in psoriatic arthritis. Ann. Rheum. Dis. 44, 189 – 193.

Huskisson, E. C. (1974) The measurement of pain. Lancet 2, 1127 – 1131.

Kunkel, S. L., Ogawa, H., Conran, P. B., Ward, P. A. and Zurier, R. B. (1981) Suppression of acute and chronic inflammation by orally administered prostaglandins. Arth. Rheum. 24, 1151 – 1158.

Lawrence, J. S., de Graaff, R. and Laine, V. A. I. (1963) Degenerative joint disease in random samples and occupational groups. In: M. R. Jeffry and J. Ball (Eds.), The Epidemiology of Chronic Rheumatism, Vol. I. Blackwell Scientific Publications, Oxford, pp. 98 – 120.

Logan, W. P. D. and Cushion, A. A. (1958) Morbidity Statistics From General Practice, Vol I (general). General Register Office, Studies on Medical and Population Subjects No. 14.

McKenna, F. and Wright, V. (1985a) Clinical manifestations. In: P. D. Utsinger, N. J. Zweifler and G. E. Ehrlich (Eds.), Rheumatoid Arthritis. J. B. Lippincott Co., Philadelphia, pp. 283 – 307.

McKenna, F. and Wright, V. (1985b) Pain in rheumatoid arthritis. Ann. Rheum. Dis. 44, 805.

Neumann, V., Hopkins, R., Dixon, J., Watkins, A., Bird, H. and Wright, V. (1985) Combination therapy using pulsed methyl prednisolone in rheumatoid arthritis. Ann. Rheum. Dis. 44, 747 – 751.

Sze, T. A. (1963) Mortality and morbidity from chronic rheumatic diseases in the U.K. and Western Europe. In: M. R. Jeffrey and J. Ball (Eds.), The Epidemiology of Chronic Rheumatism, Vol. I. Blackwell Scientific Publications, Oxford, pp. 1 – 9.

Wright, V. and Moll, J. M. H. (1976) Seronegative Polyarthritis. Elsevier/North-Holland Publ. Co., Amsterdam – New York – Oxford.

Wyke, B. (1981) The neurology of the joints: a review of general principles. In: P. Hasselbacher (Ed.), Clinics in Rheumatic Diseases: The Biology of the Joint. W. B. Saunders Co. Ltd, London – Philadelphia – Toronto, pp. 223 – 239.

Burrows/Elton/Stanley (eds.) Handbook of Chronic Pain Management
© *1987 Elsevier Science Publishers B.V. (Biomedical Division)*

32

Management of cancer pain by the oncologist

T. D. WALSH*

Department of Developmental Chemotherapy, Memorial Sloan Kettering Cancer Center, 1275 York Avenue, New York, NY 10021, U.S.A.

Cancer pain

Improvements in active, i.e. curative care of cancer, have probably contributed to the problem because patients live longer although long-term survival for many of the common primary sites is low. A substantial proportion of pain in cancer patients is due to the therapy directed at the cancer. This is doubly disturbing in that many patients with common malignancies have widespread disease, i.e. are beyond cure by available techniques at the time of presentation. Much modern cancer therapy is investigational in nature. Unfortunately, chemotherapy and other regimes are often applied uncritically to those who have no hope of cure, even when there is no evidence of symptom palliation from such therapy and indeed when it may substantially contribute to a patient's symptoms.

Provided simple principles are followed the majority of patients can have their pain controlled most of the time. About 10% of patients have 'pain problems' which require specialist (e.g. hospice, pain clinic) management or advice. It is important to remember that the disease (and the pain) changes with time (implying regular re-evaluation) that a significant minority of patients (up to 10%) have pain unrelated to the cancer, and that some cancer patients die of their disease without ever having any pain. The same logical approach to pain management and therapy should be adopted as would be employed in any other medical problem. In therapeutic terms the greatest rewards in terms of patient benefit lie in ensuring that analgesics are taken regularly and in adequate dosage; the specific drug used is often less important but drug therapy is the mainstay of cancer pain management.

* *Formerly:* Research Fellow, St Christophers Hospice, Sydenham, London, U.K.

PREVALENCE

The prevalence of pain in the cancer patient varies according to the stage of the disease becoming more common as the disease progresses. The incidence in individual diseases is substantially affected by the primary (and secondary) sites of disease. Amongst those dying from cancer and in pain up to 20% do not have their pain satisfactorily relieved. In a major cancer center amongst 36,800 admissions, 9% were referred to a Pain Service (Foley 1979) for consultation. An evaluation of inpatients over a one week period in the same institution showed that of 540 patients, 29% (excluding the postoperative) had pain which required the use of analgesics. In a mixed group of general hospital inpatients and outpatients (Daut and Cleeland 1982) suffering from six common cancers, amongst 667 patients up to 75% reported pain in the month preceding the study. In a retrospective study (Oster et al. 1978) of 122 deaths at Columbia Presbyterian Medical Center, 70% of the cancer patients had pain the week before death. Those dying from non-malignant causes were twice as likely to be free of pain at this time. Amongst 324 patients with advanced cancer (Pannuti et al. 1979) 88% had tumor-related pain at some stage for more than 15 days and the prevalence of pain was little affected by therapeutic intervention. Pain is not an inevitable part of the illness as a significant minority never have any pain. In hospice practice (Walsh and Saunders 1984) pain is the commonest symptom (69%) in terminal cancer patients. The prevalence of pain is also a reflection of the efficacy of the measures used to combat it and indeed of the degree of recognition of the problem. Failure to do this has resulted in inappropriate management (Marks and Sachar 1973) by medical and nursing staff. Given that 20% of all deaths in Western Europe and North America are due to cancer, the issue of cancer pain is a substantial social and medical problem. Whilst it seems clear that the prevalence of pain increases as the disease progresses, the use of such terms as 'early' to describe this is meaningless. It would be preferable for future descriptions of these problems to be related to accepted international cancer staging and classification systems. In summary, pain is common in cancer patients, increases in prevalence as the disease progresses, and is often badly managed.

INCIDENCE

The incidence varies according to the type of malignancy and is determined by the pathophysiology and natural history of the disease process (particularly metastatic spread), the anatomical location of the primary site, e.g. head and neck, and likely secondary sites, e.g. bone metastases. These factors determine not only the pain syndromes produced, but also the frequency of associated symptoms and relative difficulties in therapy. The efficacy of available curative therapy (and the vigor with which it is applied) earlier in the disease affects the frequency and complexity of subsequent pain syndromes. Clinical observation confirms that there are large variations in the frequency of pain associated with lesions which appear pathologically and clinically similar. It is noteworthy that cancer of the cervix was the single most common primary site associated with pain requiring admission to a Pain Relief Unit (Lloyd et al. 1978) 2 – 3 times more often than other common problem primary sites such as bladder, rectum, lung and breast. The single most important determinant of the incidence and severity of pain is the presence or absence of bone metastases.

SEVERITY AND DURATION

These are the two characteristics (acute/chronic; continuous/intermittent) which determine the clinical challenge posed by pain associated with cancer. Pain which is chronic may still be episodic, e.g. occurring only on movement. This is easier to tolerate (although not easier to treat) than continuous pain and has important implications insofar as choice of treatment is concerned. Both of these characteristics also determine the secondary effects of chronic pain on the personality, level of activity, psychological status and interpersonal relationships – which in turn influence pain threshold and the response to therapy. Persistent pain is a common feature of advanced disease (Lloyd et al. 1978; Pannuti 1979) being reported as present for more than 2 weeks in 75% or more of those with carcinoma of the cervix, ovary, rectum, breast, lung, colon and stomach; this includes all those with cancer of the ovary and cervix. Pain in advanced cancer is associated too with relapse of disease. Median time from diagnosis to the onset of pain varies from 2 to 20 months, and of survival with pain from 1.3 to 7 months depending on the primary site (Lloyd et al. 1978). Bone metastases cause the most frequent persistent pain, followed by visceral and soft tissue deposits. Hospital admission does not guarantee relief from pain as a retrospective study (Oster et al. 1978) showed that 75% of inpatients dying from cancer had some pain during the last week of life. In general, those with metastatic disease have more severe pain.

Curiously the chronic benign pain patients report more pain than do terminal cancer patients whose pain level is similar to that seen with rheumatoid arthritis (Daut and Cleeland 1982). This has been confirmed using objective measures of pain sensation. Knowledge that the pain is due to cancer has a significant impact on the perceived severity of the pain and on its impact on daily activities.

SOCIAL, FAMILY AND SPIRITUAL INFLUENCES

Pain in the cancer patient is an amalgam of physical, psychological, social and spiritual distress (Walsh and Saunders 1984). An awareness of the individual in the context of the family, work, social life and religious beliefs is an integral part of management. The relative contribution of these components varies from individual to individual. Younger patients with continuing family responsibilities present great difficulties as do those who have been lied to, misdiagnosed or mismanaged in some way at an earlier point in the illness. It is not always possible or appropriate to intervene in these areas but they should at least be explored with the aim of eliminating sources of distress.

ORGANIZATION OF CARE

Patients with pain due to early disease will usually be managed by a radiotherapist and/or medical oncologist – hopefully by one who believes that caring and curing are not incompatible objectives. It is appropriate for such specialists to continue care in the advanced or terminal stages and/or share care with a family physician. The latter is ideally placed to deliver such care but in practice many feel uncomfortable with such problems (although this is changing). A conflicting feature is the unwillingness of many oncology or radiotherapy units to consider palliative care as being of equal importance to earlier attempts to eradicate the disease. The objective should be to keep the patient functioning at home as much as possible and in many cases to die there rather than in hospital. It is common for those with advanced disease to enter a situation where no one individual assumes responsibility for their care and/or those who are involved have no interest or expertise in symptom relief. This gap has been partly filled in some countries by the development of hospice and similar units devoted to symptom control in advanced cancer (Walsh and Saunders 1984) with consequent improvements in the treatment of pain.

Drugs

Analgesics

The greatest single problem in chronic pain therapy concerns analgesics: to ensure that adequate doses of analgesics are prescribed, to get nursing staff to administer the required dosage at the time specified, and occasionally to persuade patients to take the drugs particularly if they are well-known opiates or familiar proprietary names. Regular giving prevents pain returning, reducing anxiety and the pain threshold. Provided dosage is titrated against the pain, it is possible to deliver adequate (and on occasion substantive) doses of analgesics without clouding the sensorium. Individualization of dosage increases therapeutic flexibility, allows for variations in drug metabolism and reduces side-effects. Flexibility is increased by provision of a 'breakthrough' analgesic, e.g. Tylenol which a patient can take or nursing staff administer if pain should intervene between regular drug rounds. It is important to instruct patients/staff on an appropriate scheme to reduce drug dosages if side-effects appear. Flexible dosing is also worthwhile, e.g. allowing a dose increment, and/or additional medication in the event a change in the pain pattern is anticipated.

In common with most areas of therapeutics, it is wise to know the use of a small number of drugs well. In the case of analgesics approximate equianalgesic dosage schemes allow rational changes in drug/dosage (Table 1). Some claim that when opiates are given at equianalgesic dosages side-effects are indistinguishable – in clinical practice this is not true and there are qualitative and quantitative differences in side effects, i.e. if a patient is intolerant of one opiate it is worthwhile trying another.

One important practical point is to avoid drugs which because of their pharmacological characteristics or formulation have to be given too frequently, need too many tablets, or are in an unpalatable formulation. A good way of ensuring the last is for the prescribing physician to examine and/or taste the medications! Fixed drug combinations may be convenient in stable situations, but they should be avoided where dosage is being adjusted or altered – both benefits and side-effects are predetermined. Four hours is a reasonable minimum duration of action, otherwise the day becomes a constant round of medication. The aim is to relieve pain whilst allowing as normal a life as possible.

When opiates are used, agonist drugs, e.g. morphine, methadone are best; the mixed agonist/antagonist group have unpleasant psychotomimetic and other side-effects and are best avoided as they have no advantages in analgesic efficacy over agonist or partial agonist drugs. The agonist drugs are more flexible, effective and less toxic.

TABLE 1
Equianalgesic doses of opiates*

Drug	Route	Dose (mg)
Morphine	p.o.	30
	I.M.	10
Codeine	p.o.	120
Dihydrocodeine	p.o.	60
Oxycodone	p.r.	30
Phenazocine	p.o.	5

* Refers to doses during repeated administration.

Most cancer patients do not have severe or continuous pain and can be managed for much of the time by intermittent use of a variety of opiate and non-opiate analgesics. Classification of such analgesics into minor and major is outmoded and misleading, e.g. non-steroidal anti-inflammatory drugs (NSAIDs) used alone are capable of relieving some moderate/severe pain. Distinctions of efficacy are relevant to the use of opiates for chronic severe pain when they need to be given repeatedly; clinical experience (Walsh and Saunders 1984) has shown that pethidine, pentazocine and dipipanone are unsuitable when given orally. Acetaminophen, NSAIDs (various), buprenorphine, codeine and agonist opiates such as methadone and morphine are useful. The suitability of a drug is determined by:

a) incidence of side-effects
b) route of administration
c) efficacy during oral administration
d) formulation (liquid, sublingual tablet)
e) frequency of administration.

Choice of particular medications is therefore not solely dependent on analgesic efficacy but on a number of considerations, including practicality.

When assessing the suitability of analgesic drugs for use in cancer, it is helpful to consider them from the viewpoint of:

a) those suitable for intermittent or 'as required'
b) those useful for repeated administration either orally or parenterally
c) those appropriate for novel routes of administration or specific actions, e.g. inhibition of prostaglandin synthesis.

The aspirin-codeine-morphine 'stepladder' concept is outdated but valuable in drawing our attention to the fact that 'old' drugs dominate pain therapy, and that it is necessary to have a systematic approach to therapy.

For intermittent use acetaminophen, aspirin or one of its relatives may be tried for mild/moderate pain, and pethidine, dextromoramide for moderate/severe pain. In repeated use for chronic persistent pain codeine, oxycodone, dihydrocodeine are efficacious orally (pethidine, pentazocine and dextromoramide are best avoided) for mild/moderate pain; for moderate/severe pain morphine, heroin, phenazocine and methadone are appropriate. High-potency drugs, e.g. buprenorphine are attractive for intrathecal administration. Corticosteroids, NSAIDs, antidepressants all have adjuvant analgesic actions useful in particular situations.

OPIATE ANALGESICS

Brompton cocktail. This term is used to describe a series of strong analgesic mixtures which until recently were in common use in hospitals in the U.K. and Ireland. The title is derived from the Brompton Chest Hospital London and used in a generic sense to describe mixtures containing an opiate, cocaine, alcohol, flavoring and water, and sometimes other ingredients. The opiate was usually morphine or heroin, the alcohol gin, whiskey or brandy; in recent years a phenothiazine was often added. The exact composition varied from hospital to hospital and the mixtures did not even appear in the British National Formulary until the last decade. The use of such mixtures was based on early reports of benefit in advanced malignancy (Snow 1896).

They were widely used as post-thoracotomy analgesics and in the terminal care of those dying of cancer or tuberculosis. It is unclear whether the cocaine was included because of its local anesthetic qualities, as an antiemetic or because it combats the sedative effects of opiates (Snow 1896). Such mixtures have been given wide publicity (Gever 1980) in recent years because of the desire to improve the treatment of cancer pain. Controlled evaluation has shown no benefit over simpler mixtures of morphine alone in aqueous solution (Mount et al. 1976; Melzack et al. 1976, 1979). The use of Brompton mixtures and the clinical evaluations quoted have been of value in focusing attention on the relief of pain by oral (rather than parenteral) opiate (Hillier 1983) using individualization of dosage. The traditional mixtures may be outdated but there is still a role for combinations of drugs particularly for the multisymptomatic patient with advanced disease.

Morphine. Amongst units experienced in symptom control in advanced cancer, morphine is favored for pain control (Walsh 1984b). Its use is derived from the Brompton cocktail. Most physicians prefer to use morphine in aqueous solution. This is given in individual doses (2.5 – 180.0 mg of morphine sulfate), repeated regular 4-hourly administration being best. It is possible to control severe pain provided dosage is flexible. It is usual to start with a low dose, e.g. 5 mg every 4 hours and increase at 24 – 48 hour-intervals if pain persists (Walsh 1983). Some have fixed increments (e.g. 2.5 – 5.0 to 10.0 – 15.0); others use percentage increases, e.g. 10%. Dosage is increased until the patient is pain-free or pain-controlled. It is important to emphasize that adjuvant drugs are very important in achieving optimal pain control and that morphine alone cannot be relied on, e.g. neuropathic pain responds poorly to morphine. In most cases, five doses per 24 hours are sufficient. A sixth is added if sleep is disturbed by pain or if the patient awakes in pain in the morning (or alternatively a double dose may be given last thing at night).

Most patients do not need > 20.0 mg every 4 hours (provided adjuvant drugs are employed appropriately) irrespective of the duration of use of morphine. The liquid formulation is very flexible for changing dosage, is easily swallowed and the bitter taste can be disguised by adding orange juice or other beverage. After an initial titration period, most doses plateau for some time. If it is necessary to reduce the dose this can be done in the same stepwise fashion and provided this is done withdrawal symptoms are not a problem.

The majority of patients with pain can be managed for most of their illness using morphine. It is always worthwhile to advise patients to have a breakthrough analgesic available. The same principles apply to the use of other opiates although few offer any substantive advantages over morphine. It is reasonable for a non-specialist who has followed a logical diagnostic approach to pain to titrate to morphine sulfate 20 mg every 4 hours (100 mg/24 hours). If pain is unrelieved, diagnosis and therapy should be reviewed before increasing the dose further. Once 60 mg every 4 hours is reached (300 mg/24 hours) referral for specialist evaluation, e.g. pain clinic, hospice is indicated.

Side-effects are uncommon other than nausea, sedation and constipation. It is common practice to start an antiemetic (48 – 72 hours) with the morphine by which time the nausea has usually subsided but some require long-term use. If sedation does not subside after a few days, two approaches may be used:

a) addition of a suitable agent to combat the drowsiness, e.g. amphetamine, methylphenidate;
b) 'fine-tuning' of morphine dosage to achieve a satisfactory balance of pain control versus sedation.

Most patients prefer to be in a little pain but to be clear-headed. It is important to review all drugs and exclude non-essential ones which might contribute to sedation, e.g. benzodiazepines. Constipation is universal but can be avoided by regular, i.e. daily laxative use; always prescribe these when starting a patient on any regular opiate regime. Provided the guidelines above are followed respiratory depression is rare (Mount 1980, Walsh 1984a). Addiction (as distinct from some element of physical dependence) is also rare. Provided a correct diagnostic approach is employed, appropriate adjuvant drugs are used and sufficient doses of morphine are prescribed, tolerance, i.e. poor pain control despite rapidly increasing dosage, is uncommon. It is noteworthy that this general approach also makes intramuscular injections unnecessary in most. Dyspnea, cough and diarrhea are common in the cancer patient and all respond favorably to morphine (see also Chapter 19).

Slow-release morphine. Two new sustained release morphine preparations available for 12-hourly use are satisfactory once pain-control has been achieved. They are not suitable for dosage titration or for those whose analgesic requirements are changing rapidly. Clinical study (Walsh 1985) has shown them to be comparable to liquid morphine in analgesic efficacy and side-effects. A minority require them to be given 8-hourly for satisfactory control. For unknown reasons, some patients tolerate the 4-hourly liquid better than the 12-hourly tablets or vice versa and if side-effects, e.g. nausea, are a problem it is always worthwhile switching from one to the other. The tablets must be swallowed whole for them to retain their sustained release action.

Buprenorphine. Amongst those with pain due to cancer, about 2/3 appear to obtain satisfactory relief with either oral or parenteral administration if given repeatedly. Continuous use for several months has been reported but in the ambulant nausea and vomiting may be a problem. Constipation is not a common side-effect (Robbie 1979) – an important benefit in the cancer population. Side-effects were less common in those confined to bed. The usual dose is 1 – 4 mg I.M./I.V./S.C. 3 – 4 hourly; 2 mg is equianalgesic to 10 mg morphine. The parenteral route and pentazocine like side-effects are serious disadvantages in the cancer patient. Buprenorphine has much the same problems and indications as other opiates.

Dextromoramide. Analgesia lasts up to 6 hours after a dose of 5 – 20 mg (Matts 1962). During repeated administration (although it has a rapid onset and peak effect) the duration of analgesia appears to be short requiring 2 or 3 hourly administration (Saunders 1982). It is unsuitable for chronic cancer pain but valuable for acute intermittent pain, e.g. painful dressings, or for breakthrough pain intervening between regular doses of more long-lasting drugs.

Dextropropoxyphene. This is usually combined with acetaminophen, although it is controversial whether the combination has any advantage over acetaminophen used alone. Dextropropoxyphene is effective orally and seems to perform better in clinical use than in analgesic drug studies. No controlled study of its efficacy during repeated administration has been done (Drugs and Therapeutics Bulletin 1983).

Codeine and dihydrocodeine. Both drugs are useful orally active analgesics. Codeine retains about 50% of its potency when given orally. They may also be given intramuscularly (Beaver 1978a). Codeine is often combined with acetaminophen, aspirin, caffeine, etc. in various formulations. Neither drug has any advantage over morphine for parenteral use. Their main disadvantage is constipation which may be severe and seems more prominent than with morphine.

Drowsiness, nausea and vomiting may also occur. Codeine 60 mg is equivalent to 10 mg morphine; side-effects are more common with codeine than dihydrocodeine.

Oxycodone. Oxycodone is structurally related to codeine and also retains about 50% of its parenteral potency when given orally (Beaver et al. 1978a). It is also very effective as a suppository given 8-hourly. Oxycodone 10 mg orally is calculated to be comparable to methadone 10 mg or 100 mg codeine p.o. (Beaver et al. 1978b). It is an excellent oral analgesic and better tolerated than codeine.

Pethidine. Pethidine is the most widely used (Chan 1979) analgesic for parenteral administration in hospital practice. It is commonly prescribed '50 – 100 mg 4 – 6 hourly p.r.n. I.M.'. Although suitable for intermittent postoperative pain pethidine is not satisfactory in the cancer patient, principally because it is ineffective orally. Given parenterally it is associated with too many peaks and troughs in analgesia and side-effects – continuous infusions are better (Austin et al. 1980). Pethidine may also be associated with significant neurotoxicity due to its active metabolite norpethidine (Kaiko 1983).

Pentazocine. Pentazocine is associated with an unacceptably high incidence of psychotomimetic side-effects during repeated administration. The commonest side-effects are sweating, sedation, and changes (fall or rise) in blood pressure.

Methadone. Pharmacokinetic evaluation (Ettinger et al. 1979) has shown a long terminal half-life which varies from 13 to 58 hours and varies between single dose and repeated administration. Because of this and due to its pharmacologically active metabolites, there is a tendency to serious side-effects particularly in the elderly or those with impaired liver/kidney function.

Titration of the dose of methadone against the pain (Maxwell 1980) as described for morphine is effective. Doses of oral methadone begin at 2.5 – 5.0 mg every 6 or 8 hours; the longer dose interval is employed once pain is relieved. Those who had received opiates previously without relief would start on the higher dose. An alternative approach is to begin with a loading dose and then continue the titration dosage at a lower level. Using this method, the cumulative actions of methadone are obvious at 48 hours and reliable analgesia obtained between 96 and 120 hours.

It has been suggested (Sawe et al. 1981) that patients be allowed to self-regulate their methadone dosage – 10 mg p.r.n. at not less than 4-hour intervals for 3 – 5 days followed by a fixed 8 to 12-hour interval. This is based on an interesting and valuable study of patient-controlled dosage amongst 14 patients with advanced cancer. Patients on the fixed 10 mg dosage showed an increase in the dosage intervals over one week and a decrease in the daily dose at which point they were stabilized at their chosen 8 – 12 hourly interval.

Phenazocine. Phenazocine is a synthetic opiate of the benzomorphan group. One tablet every 4 – 6 hours using up to 20 mg as a single dose, gives pain relief within 20 minutes and lasts 5 – 6 hours, although pain relief falls off rapidly after 4 hours (Blair 1967). It is said to produce relatively less spasm of the sphincter of Oddi and this may be advantageous in biliary and pancreatic disease.

PSYCHOTROPIC DRUGS

Many major tranquilizers and antidepressants have been reported (Walsh 1983) to be beneficial in treatment of cancer pain either used alone or in conjunction with opiates (Sadove et al. 1954). There is no doubt that some have an analgesic effect used alone (Beaver 1966). No satisfactory controlled study has been done in chronic cancer pain although psychotropic drugs are widely used in practice. Evaluation as analgesics is made difficult by the complexity of diagnosing depression or other psychiatric illness in the context of severe physical illness. Certainly in a 'pain problem' situation, a trial of antidepressants is indicated – sometimes with gratifying results. It is best to start with lower doses than would be used otherwise if the patient is also receiving regular opiates otherwise side-effects (particularly dry mouth and sedation) may be a problem. Antidepressants have also been reported to be effective in neuropathic pain and amitriptyline in conventional doses, e.g. 150 mg/day is usually used. There are many reports of an opiate-sparing effect from psychotropic drugs particularly antidepressants. This is not an indication for their use. It is usual to give antidepressants in a single dose last thing at night.

Phenothiazines, e.g. chlorpromazine 25 mg every 6 hours p.o. have sedative and antiemetic as well as analgesic actions. They have powerful calming effects and may usefully be combined with opiates particularly in terminal agitation. Any patient showing evidence of anxiety unresponsive to conventional management should have a trial of a phenothiazine as should anyone with a 'pain problem' unresponsive to conventional approaches. Pain which is neuralgic in nature often responds to phenytoin or carbamazepine in similar doses to that used for trigeminal neuralgia. Other drugs acting on the nervous system including cocaine and tetrahydrocannabinol may have some analgesic effects but there is insufficient data to recommend introduction into routine practice.

CORTICOSTEROIDS AND NON-STEROIDAL ANTI-INFLAMMATORY DRUGS

Corticosteroids (CS) have many indications in advanced cancer (Walsh 1983b) associated with pain relief, e.g. successful treatment of superior vena caval compression. Two areas where specific pain relief is obtained are that due to nerve compression/infiltration and that from bone metastases. NSAIDs share the latter indication. The basis on which the drugs are recommended for treatment of bone pain is thought to be interference with prostaglandin (PG) synthesis – CS do this less selectively than NSAIDs. The supposed benefits of CS in pain due to nerve compression/infiltration may be reduction in perineural edema and inflammation; this type of pain is however often due to bone collapse compressing the nerve so the basic mechanism is probably modification of bone disease. More recently, attention has focused on the analgesic benefits to be derived from NSAIDs in the management of other types of pain, e.g. postoperative (Martens 1982) and chronic cancer (Romeu 1982).

The early literature on NSAIDs included benefit in bone metastases from indomethacin (Hart and Boardman 1963) and phenylbutazone (Mampel 1958). The hypercalcemia associated with some tumors may respond to NSAIDs (Brereton et al. 1974); it is usually associated with bone metastases (Fisken et al. 1981). Hypercalcemia and bone resorption appear to be related to PGE production by the tumor (Seybearth et al. 1975).

The side-effects of NSAIDs and CS are well-known and will not be described here. It is important to emphasize that given current knowledge there is no evidence that any one drug is superior to another in terms of efficacy for bone pain. It seems best to choose first a drug with fewest side-effects, and only later – if this is ineffective – use a better established but (usually) more toxic drug e.g. indomethacin.

The greatest experience in the use of NSAIDs is derived from rheumatology; some principles have emerged which are useful to consider in the cancer patient. There are two major groups and seven chemical classes of NSAIDs; there are currently 24 proprietary preparations available in the U.K. (see also Chapter 31).

1) Side-effects are consistent within a group.
2) Actions and side-effects are similar between groups which are nevertheless chemically distinct.
3) There is wide interindividual variation in their effects even within a group.
4) The effects of most increase with dosage.
5) It is best to use one drug at a time over the dose range available.
6) Small increases in dosage may cause large increases in side-effects.
7) Individualize drugs by switching within and between groups.
8) Drugs given twice daily will take a week to show full effect.
9) Drugs given once daily will take 2 – 3 weeks for full effect.

If rapid control of bone pain is desired it may be better to achieve it with aspirin 4-hourly and then switch to a long-action aspirin or other NSAID preparation.

Insofar as CS are concerned, prednisone is a pro-drug for prednisolone and this or dexamethasone given orally should be used. Sometimes the combination of CS and NSAIDs is necessary. Some believe that cimetidine or ranitidine should be given as well to prevent gastric bleeding and/or ulceration – although this is expensive and seems unjustifiable unless there is a specific clinical problem – particularly in view of the documented drug interactions associated with cimetidine.

NSAIDs used correctly may relieve severe pain even when used alone. They are particularly useful in widespread bone metastases where more specific therapy is impossible, has failed or is impractical because of extensive disease. In those with advanced disease receiving morphine, about 30% also require NSAIDs – morphine alone will not relieve bone pain. It is also true that NSAIDs have a central analgesic effect independent of their anti-inflammatory effect (Kantor 1979) and so they are useful all-purpose adjuvant drugs. There is evidence recently of their benefit in somatic visceral and soft tissue pain postoperatively (Reasbeck et al. 1982) and further investigation of their use in cancer patients is likely to be rewarding.

In the most extensive experience of NSAIDs in cancer pain (Ventafridda et al. 1980), it is clear they are ineffective for pain of neural origin. Amongst those (58%) who get effective pain relief (50% relief for one week) this falls over the ensuing weeks to 20% at 5 weeks, i.e. approximately 10% of total patients treated. There is no doubt that in clinical analgesic studies combinations of aspirin (or acetaminophen) with opiates like codeine or oxycodone increase analgesia more than can be obtained by doubling the dose of either agent (Beaver 1981) and may reduce side-effects compared to comparable doses of single constituents.

Hormonal and cytotoxic chemotherapy

The types of tumors which show a good response to chemotherapy (with complete remissions and associated prolonged survival) are not those in which pain is a prominent feature, nor do they constitute the common cancers. However, even in advanced disease, if a tumor has known sensitivity to chemotherapy, e.g. Hodgkins, then aggressive chemotherapy may be indicated as a cure may still be possible and symptoms palliated. Soft tissue lesions respond best and bone metastases least well. Performance status is important (Glick 1982) because poor status reduces the likelihood of response, and in general severe or moderate side-effects are unacceptable in terminal disease. In addition to cytotoxic drugs, hormonal manipulation using drugs such as tamoxifen, aminoglutethimide and calcitonin is possible. Hormonal therapy is favored in advanced disease because it can often be given orally, shows good efficacy and low toxicity.

A decision to employ cytotoxic or hormonal chemotherapy to relieve pain must take into account the considerations listed in Table 2. Chemotherapy (Table 3) is most appropriate if there is:

1) disseminated disease
2) known sensitivity to chemotherapy
3) low toxicity
4) more than 2 months to live
5) pain not amenable to radiotherapy or nerve blocks
6) poor response to analgesics
7) pain associated with other intractable symptoms, e.g. dyspnea which may respond too.

It must be remembered that the onset of pain relief may be slow, is often unpredictable, may be at the expense of serious toxicity, and involve the patient in no little discomfort and considerable inconvenience. Criteria for cytotoxic chemotherapy use in advanced cancer have been suggested (Bates and Vanier 1978). The drugs should be active orally, need little specialist supervision and have minimum controllable side-effects, e.g. chlorambucil, cyclophosphamide; both may be given orally, and are active against cancer of the ovary and breast and lymphomas. If intravenous regimens are needed they should be kept simple, the frequency of injections kept

TABLE 2
Considerations in the use of chemotherapy for pain relief in advanced cancer.

Symptoms	Rate of progression
Natural history	Responsiveness to chemotherapy
Age	Nutritional status
General health	Psychological status
Toxicity	Objectives
Performance status	Clinical research
Single-agent therapy?	Benefits of no therapy, e.g. bone marrow

TABLE 3
Cytotoxic drug use in a hospice (Bates and Vanier 1978).

%	Tumors treated by primary site
20.0	Melanoma
16.0	Ovary
6.8	Breast
3.0	CIT
2.5	Head and neck
2.0	CNS
1.0	Bronchus
3.3	Total

to a minimum, and the dosage monitored to reduce side-effects. Up to 10% of admissions to hospice units may benefit from continuation or start of hormonal (10%) (Table 4) or cytotoxic (3%) chemotherapy.

CYTOTOXIC DRUGS

Breast. Pain palliation is often seen with chemotherapy (2 – 3 weeks) or hormones (4 – 5 weeks) or both used together (Bates and Vanier 1978). Single agent therapy is very useful. Cyclophosphamide 100 mg/day p.o. may give a worthwhile response in 30%. 5-Fluorouracil 500 mg I.V. every 7 days is a useful alternative. Overall adriamycin is the most active single drug but unsuitable in terminal disease because of hair loss.

Cancer of the ovary. Chlorambucil 5 mg p.o. b.d. may be helpful in recurrent ascites. Cyclophosphamide 100 mg/day p.o., intraperitoneal thiotepa 60 mg are alternatives. Melphelan may be helpful (Brule 1979).

Leukaemia. Bone pain is common and responds to chemotherapy. Methotrexate may relieve pain due to meningeal and cerebral deposits (Brule 1979).

Myeloma. Diffuse bone pain is common and responds well to chemotherapy.

Bone metastases. Adriamycin relieves pain in 65% with pain due to metastatic breast cancer.

Liver metastases. 5-Fluorouracil is useful in colonic metastases producing pain (Brule 1979) especially in rapidly developing lesions.

Bronchus. Cyclophosphamide alone or combined with other drugs produces good palliation of pain (and dyspnea) in oat-cell cancer (Brule 1979).

Brain metastases. Nitrousureas are ineffective; radiotherapy or corticosteroids are superior for relief of headache.

Pancoast. It is best to combine chemotherapy and radiotherapy. The response to chemotherapy unfortunately does not always include pain relief.

TABLE 4
Sex hormone use in a hospice (Bates and Vanier 1978).

%	Tumors treated by primary site
87.0	Prostate
29.0	Breast
18.0	Kidney
6.0	Endometrium
3.6	Cervix
7.0	Total

Head and neck cancer. Regional perfusion of drugs may have dramatic pain relieving effects (Bonadonna and Molinari 1979) irrespective of the effect on the disease, but as local complications are common intra-arterial chemotherapy can only continue for 15 – 30 days. Intramuscular bleomycin 15 mg twice a week for 3 – 4 weeks may help advanced squamous cell cancer. Side-effects may be a problem; the dose should be limited to avoid pulmonary fibrosis (Bates and Vanier 1978).

Cancer of the cervix. Pelvic pain may respond to adriamycin 50 mg, and methotrexate 20 mg I.V. on day 1, and methotrexate 20 mg, I.V. on day 8.

HORMONES

A welcome advance in cancer therapy has been the gradual replacement of surgical ablation of endocrine organs by hormonal manipulation. When pain breakthrough occurs after an initial response or while therapy is in progress, further benefit may be obtained by endocrine ablative surgery (Mathews et al. 1973). The number of patients suitable for surgery at this point is likely to be small. In general, beneficial subjective responses occur in the absence of objective evidence of disease regression.

Cervix. Adenocarcinoma of the cervix (but not squamous cell) may respond to progestagens.

Renal adenocarcinoma. Progesterone has been reported to produce good pain relief in 25% (Brule 1979) and medroxy progesterone in 42%.

Prostate. Pain remissions of 48 – 100% have been described with estrogens (diethylstilbestrol diphosphate), cyproterone acetate, and medroxyprogesterone acetate. Buserelin, a potent gonadotrophin-releasing hormone analogue which can be given intranasally has been reported to relieve bone pain (Waxman 1983) and other symptoms of advanced prostatic cancer.

Cancer of the breast. Androgens produce objective remissions of 8 – 27%, and subjective remissions 22 – 28%. Little data is available on the specific effect of androgens on pain. Worthwhile pain relief is obtained with antiestrogens (tamoxifen 33%), L-dopa (33%), progestagens (61%), and CS (61%). It has been claimed (Pannuti 1979b) that the best (44%) results appeared to be attained with androgens. Fluoxymesterone is the least virilizing androgen and given 10 mg t.d.s. is useful in both pre- and postmenopausal women for painful bone metastases (Bates and Vanier 1978). Locally advanced breast disease shows remissions in 50 – 70% of those treated (cytotoxics and/or hormonal chemotherapy) with good pain relief.

Calcitonin and diphosphonates. A controlled study of salmon calcitonin (Hindley et al. 1982) amongst 32 patients has shown analgesic benefit. The majority had bone metastases from various primary sites including rectum, cervix, breast, prostate, myeloma, kidney, colon and bronchus.

MAP. Extensive clinical experience with this drug in advanced breast cancer has been reported (Pannuti 1979). Better results were obtained with high dose (1500 mg/day) than low doses (500 mg/day) with relief rates of 83% and 21%, respectively. Pain remissions of 57 – 100% have been claimed but intramuscular administration is commonly (15%) associated with abscess formation.

Tamoxifen and aminoglutethimide. In a randomized study Smith et al. (1981), compared tamoxifen and aminoglutethimide patients. Aminoglutethimide was ineffective in premenopausal women (unlike tamoxifen). It was superior to tamoxifen for painful bone metastases but at the expense of more side-effects (lethargy, drowsiness, and rash frequently). Tamoxifen is useful in both pre- and postmenopausal women (Bates and Vanier 1978) can be given orally, and used alone or combined with cyclophosphamide 10 – 20 mg b.d.

Radiotherapy

Radiotherapy (RT) has an important role (Table 5) in palliation of pain and other symptoms (Richter 1982) and a substantial proportion of the work of a department may be devoted to this. There is a dose-response relationship between RT and cell-death but not of a dose-response relationship between radiation dose and pain relief (Hunter 1981). There is probably little point exceeding doses of 3000 rads given in a small number of sessions. Success can be achieved by single doses which are below the limits of tissue tolerance to radiation. This implies that sophisticated approaches are unnecessary in the majority (Hunter 1981) and megavoltage photon therapy satisfactory for most purposes. Radiation may of course itself produce pain and other side-effects (Ricci 1979). The size and location of the area treated partly determines side-effects, e.g. half-body irradiation in metastatic bone disease may produce severe vomiting. Because of this it is important to ensure insofar as possible that the area or lesion treated is the one actually producing the pain (Richter 1982).

In general, RT is most effective when the tumor is well localized, sensitive to irradiation, and given in adequate dosage to a defined area of the central nervous system, lung, mediastinum, or retroperitoneum. There is disagreement over whether RT will control pain from tumors of low mitotic activity but it is effective in many tumors even those classically considered to be insensitive to radiation. The number of tumors which commonly present with pain problems is fairly small. Another interesting feature is that relief is not necessarily related to disease regression as pain relief is often very rapid, e.g. within 24 hours in bone metastases. Whilst the number

TABLE 5
Common pain indications for palliative radiotherapy (modified from Richter 1982).

Primary	Clinical problem
Lung	Chest pain
	Bone metastases
	Brain metastases
Breast	Chest wall recurrence
	Inoperable cancer
	Bone metastases
	Central nervous system metastases
Genitourinary	Bone metastases
	Tissue and nodal involvement
Gastrointestinal	Pelvic/perineal pain
	Esophageal obstruction
	Bone, brain and liver metastases
Head and neck	
Gynecological	Pelvic pain

of histological types associated with cancer is large the final common pathways of pain are few. RT probably relieves pain by several mechanisms including reducing pressure and tumor infiltration, promotion of ulcer healing, resolution of peri-tumor inflammation and promoting capillary hemostasis. Most painful tumors show some response and irradiation of small areas, e.g. scalp, eyelids, axilla, or distended organs (liver/spleen) is effective with low morbidity (Parker 1974). RT is less suitable for extensive disease particularly in the very ill; nevertheless, because its effects on pain are rapid it may still be contemplated in those with days/weeks to live. Fractionation schedules should be determined by the clinical situation (Richter 1982). Conventional fractionation doses ($<$ 200 rads) over long periods of time are appropriate if there is long (months/years) life expectancy, quiescent disease, a large tumor mass (e.g. 10×10 cm) a solitary metastasis associated with a controlled primary site, or where palliative and curative regimes are similar, e.g. $4000-5000$ rads over $3-6$ weeks for palliation of head and neck, male and female genitourinary cancers. Short courses (Richter 1982) at a higher daily dosage ($>$ 200 rads) are appropriate when there is short (days/weeks) life expectancy, rapid progression of tumor or early recurrence following definitive therapy. Even if fractions $>$ 400 rads are used radiation-induced fibrosis and vascular damage will not be apparent for several months (Richter 1982) by which time the patient will often be dead.

The commonest cause of referral for pain to a radiotherapy department is bone metastases (Hunter 1981) with or without pathological fractures. These are usually associated with carcinomas of the breast, lung, prostate, colon, thyroid, bladder and kidney (Parker 1974). Pelvic pain due to recurrent rectal or cervical cancer is another problem. One study (Bolund 1982) reported that nearly complete relief was obtained in 75%. Metastatic tumors of breast, bronchus and lymphoma nearly always responded immediately; responses were delayed in cancer of the kidney and prostate (Hendrickson et al. 1976) and one-third did not respond at all. Bolund (1982) reported that 2000 rads in 4 doses over 2 weeks was as effective as 4000 rads in 20 doses. Repeated small doses over several weeks are thus unnecessary and inappropriate for palliation.

RT provides pain relief in bone metastases $-$ 70% overall 4 weeks postradiation (Hendrickson and Sheinkop 1975; Hendrikson and Pagano 1981) and promotes recalcification. A single dose of 1000 rads is effective and well tolerated provided the area treated is of reasonable size (Boland 1969). Bone pain is usually due to metastases not all of which are painful $-$ the reason for this is unclear (Hendrickson and Sheinkop 1975). Primary tumors vary in their responsiveness $-$ Ewings and lymphomas respond well, whereas osteosarcomas and chondrosarcomas do not (Parker 1974). Megavoltage RT relieves 90% of pain due to bone metastases and is long-lasting even in tumors not noted for their radiosensitivity (Jensen and Roesdam 1976) so this concept should not inhibit the use of RT if otherwise indicated. Whilst 80% of those with bone metastases get relief, and this is complete in $65-70\%$ of breast cancers, it is less effective in pain due to bone erosion by soft tissue tumors or in pelvic pain.

Central nervous system. Palliative cranial irradiation can completely relieve headache; the overall response rate is 60% with a median survival of $4-6$ months (Borget 1980).

Head and neck. Metastatic disease or infiltration in the neck or base of the skull gives good relief due to RT, although there is little improvement in motor function. Tumors not previously irradiated respond well (Ricci 1979a) particularly advanced paranasal sinus tumors (unless blood supply is reduced).

Chest. RT (Haas 1957) improves pain (as well as cough, dysphagia and dyspnea) whether the tumor is primary or secondary. It is particularly valuable in infiltration of the brachial plexus and intercostal nerves or rib metastases. The irradiated lung area must be restricted to avoid (where possible) uninvolved lung and reduce radiation fibrosis and pneumonitis. Doses over 5000 rads are unnecessary (Richter 1982).

Abdomen, pelvis, genitalia. Amongst the pelvic malignancies, RT is more effective in cervical and endometrial lesions; results in prostatic, colorectal and bladder lesions are unpredictable although some report good results (Ricci 1979b). Pelvic pain usually needs 4000 – 5000 rads using a shrinking field technique (Richter 1982). RT for pain due to carcinoma of the uterus is moderately effective (Ricci 1979b) and is of variable value for lymphedema due to enlarged inguinal lymph nodes.

Prostate. In advanced disease with involvement of endopelvic tissues and organs, RT provides good pain relief (Hazra 1974). When there is progressive or persistent pain unresponsive to oral analgesics or hormonal manipulation, 3000 rads in 10 fractions is adequate (Haferman 1983).

Nerve blocks

The historical development of nerve blocks is reviewed elsewhere (Bonica 1979); it is estimated that 5 – 10% of patients with advanced cancer may benefit (Levy 1982) from such procedures. The techniques are well described elsewhere (Brown 1981). Some blocks may be done repeatedly, e.g. local anesthetic and sympathetic blocks and form a useful part of the overall treatment plan for patients with cancer (Loeser 1980). Some blocks, e.g. diagnostic may be done as an outpatient procedure (Table 6), and although the majority require fluoroscopic control, it is possible in extreme circumstances to do them as a bedside procedure. Local anesthetics are useful for sympathetic blocks, and have low morbidity. Neurolytic blocks (using alcohol or phenol) have higher morbidity; small volumes are injected (which may be increased according to the response) into the cranial nerves, sympathetic ganglia and intrathecally (see also Chapter 18).

Nerve blocks are usually performed by anesthetists or others with special training and skill in the field. Consideration of patients should treat such interventions with the same gravity and clarity of purpose as any surgical procedure (Table 7). Patients should be fully informed of the nature and purpose, the expected benefits and possible unwanted effects. They should not be done as routine service procedures but only as part of a therapeutic program. It is important to remember that they are frequently unsuccessful and may be associated with significant morbidity (and occasional mortality). Resultant functional impairment may cause more difficulties than the original pain. Unwanted effects include unintended sympathetic block, paraesthesiae, dysaesthesias, incontinence, motor weakness, paralysis and loss of protective functional sensa-

TABLE 6
Role of diagnostic nerve blocks.

1) Can distinguish somatic from visceral pain
2) Helps decide the anatomical or neural (e.g. autonomic) origin of pain
3) May define the psychological component of pain sensation
4) Allow a decision to be made concerning the value of a neurolytic block
5) Can demonstrate (temporarily) what the loss of sensation (permanent) after neurolytic block is like

tions, e.g. pressure (Levy 1982). Because of progression of disease, pain often recurs outside the blocked area (Arner 1982); despite this, they may still be appropriate to consider in those with a short life expectancy as benefit is immediate. In general, they tend to be done too late in the illness and some favor a more interventionist approach (Lund 1982). Successful blocks may allow discontinuation of opiates; pain itself is a stimulus to respiration and its sudden removal may produce ventilatory failure in those on opiates, so appropriate care should be taken. Reduction of opiate dosage in itself is not an indication for nerve block procedures. Continuous pain (non-meylinated C fibres) may be more easily treated (Arner 1982) than intermittent.

Neurosurgery

The role of neurosurgery in pain relief is affected by many of the same considerations which affect nerve blocks. Many procedures are available which are technically feasible; this does not imply that they are therapeutically useful or that they are superior to other methods of pain control. They are often associated with significant morbidity and some mortality and (in general) their relative efficacy has not been subjected to controlled clinical trial. The role of the surgeon in the general care of advanced cancer is admirably described elsewhere (Williams 1978).

There are about 15 neurosurgical procedures available for pain relief, all introduced since the beginning of this century (Pagni 1974). Good results may be obtained provided patients are carefully selected. There is no consensus on the best approach to the use of neurosurgical techniques for cancer pain (Portlock and Goffinet 1980). For example, it can be argued that procedures with serious side-effects should be reserved (Hitchcock 1981) for those with severe disease; this is not necessarily true as often the procedure-related morbidity may make the end of a patient's life worse than it might otherwise have been.

Modern techniques have improved some aspects of the procedures, e.g. the use of local anesthetic blocks to try and predict the efficacy of a given procedure. Some believe that in advanced disease neurosurgery should be restricted to those techniques which can be done percutaneously (Levy 1982). There is no doubt that percutaneous stereotactic procedures are replacing the older approaches (Hitchcock 1981) because they do not require general anesthesia, need shorter hospitalization and have fewer complications. Even procedures such as thalamotomy are possible using stereotactic techniques (Pagni 1974). Others believe that neurosurgery has only a

TABLE 7
Selection of patients for nerve blocks.

---

1) What is the response to other therapy, e.g. drugs?
2) Have non-interventionist measures been given adequate trial, e.g. have sufficient dosages of opiates been used?
3) What is the physical and psychological condition of the patient?
4) What is the likely prognosis (days/weeks/months)?
5) What is the site of the painful lesion?
6) What are the characteristics of the pain?
7) What is the likely morbidity and is it acceptable (to the patient)?
8) Are there any contraindications (physical or psychological) to nerve block?
9) Is a block technically possible?
10) Is appropriate expertise available?
11) Are there any alternatives, e.g. radiotherapy?

---

limited role (Abrahm 1982) in cancer pain because of its morbidity and relatively low efficacy. Excellent pain relief is obtained in only 50% of those treated (a selected population anyway) and none in 25%. The procedures are used in complex disease and the aims of therapy should be clearly defined. In recent years, neurosurgical techniques are less popular because of more successful use of nerve blocks and medical therapy (Shapshay 1980). Neurosurgical intervention is probably only appropriate if prognosis is in excess of 4 months.

Cryosurgery

When a peripheral block is needed, cryosurgery or cryoanalgesia may be preferable to avoid the neuromas which complicate the use of phenol. The minimum tissue temperature for a cryolesion is $-20°C$. There is no scarring or neuroma formation and effects last about a month. Cryoanalgesia can be used to block peripheral nerves or destroy nerve endings. One technique uses nitrous oxide gas delivered under high pressure to the tissues. This extracts heat and in peripheral nerves causes complete loss of function for 3 weeks. Sensory and motor recovery return thereafter but pain may be relieved for several months.

Miscellaneous

STIMULATION TECHNIQUES

Brain stimulation to produce relief of pain was first done 25 years ago, during subsequent years there has been intense research interest in the technique and it is technically well established. An interesting feature is that there is some dissociation of the components of pain sensation and all aspects of pain are not relieved equally.

Electrodes may be implanted in both thalamic and hypothalamic nuclei with benefit in chronic cancer pain. Stimulation of the spinal cord is also possible. This requires a laminectomy under general anesthesia, and use of the stimulators is associated with significant morbidity (Loeser 1980). Intracerebral stimulation is effective in about half the patients treated (Meyerson 1982) but is primarily a research technique. Such techniques are difficult and expensive to use in everyday practice but continue to be of interest because of the insight given into pain mechanisms (see Chapter 5). In common with many other special techniques patient selection is a problem.

ACUPUNCTURE

Beneficial effects of electro-acupuncture in cancer patients (Rico and Trudnowski 1982) have been reported amongst those with no experience of acupuncture. Relief is often immediate and gives good quality pain relief including reduction in analgesic requirements. A wide variety of techniques are used making analysis of results difficult (Loeser 1980). Detailed descriptions of the techniques are available (Mehta 1981). There is no doubt that effective analgesia is possible although it is of short duration.

HYPNOSIS

Hypnosis has been used as adjunctive treatment in advanced cancer patients with apparent benefit in some. It is thought by some to be ineffective when there is a substantive organic basis for chronic pain (Merskey 1971). Reports of benefit in cancer pain are available including an opiate-sparing effect, although no controlled studies have been conducted (Noyes 1981). Hypnotherapy has the advantage of relative simplicity, does not prevent the use of other modalities, and may have beneficial effects on mood and appetite; its main disadvantage is unpredictable efficacy. Hypnosis is most effective in stable, well-motivated individuals (Abrahm 1982) (see also Chapter 27).

TRANSCUTANEOUS NERVE STIMULATION

This technique involves the delivery of electrical impulses through the skin; the type of impulse is individually adjusted (Avellanosa and West 1982). Sixty-five percent achieved an initial good response at 2 weeks but this fell to 33% at 3 months. Pain in the trunk and limbs gave the best response while pelvic and perineal pain responded badly. Some believe the mechanism is the same as acupuncture (Orne 1980). Long-term benefit varies from 15 to 50%. To be effective, the sensation from the electricity must be appreciated, i.e. it is of no value for pain in anesthetic areas, and best results are obtained when the stimulus is perceived in the area where the pain is. The advantages are freedom from side-effects and a patient-controlled therapy (Orne 1980). The consensus is that it is useful as an adjunctive technique in well-selected patients (Mehta 1981). It is particularly useful for peripheral nerve, amputation stump, and phantom limb pain (see also Chapter 25).

BIOFEEDBACK

In general, biofeedback has been assessed in situations, e.g. migraine where psychological components are important and organic disease difficult to measure. It is influenced by the availability of therapists, and dependent on the patient's cooperation and concentration. Compliance may be affected by opiates, sedatives etc. and it is impractical in advanced disease.

Summary

In the management of pain in the cancer patient, the following points merit reiteration. The efficacy of available curative therapy, and the vigor with which it is applied earlier in the disease, affect the frequency and complexity of subsequent pain syndromes. Pain therapy needs to be delivered in the context of a therapeutic relationship, preferably in an environment supportive of the individual and his family. The role of the oncologist in cancer pain management should be to protect the patient from overenthusiastic technological intervention, while ensuring that simple time-proven principles of pain management are put into effect. There is nowadays no need for any cancer patient to die in unrelieved pain. The oncology specialist must realize the limitations of chemotherapy in providing control of pain and other symptoms, and accord control of pain (particularly in advanced disease) the same importance and diligence of effort as would be given to chemotherapy or any other therapeutic intervention at earlier stages of the disease.

References

Abrahm, J. L. (1982) Psychophysiology of pain. In: B. R. and P. A. Cassileth (Eds.), Clinical Care of the Terminal Cancer Patient. Lea & Febiger, Philadelphia, pp. 76–90.

Austin, K. L., Stapleton, J. V. and Mather, L. E. (1980) Multiple intramuscular injections: a major source of variability in analgesic response to meperidine. Pain 8, 47–62.

Arner, S. (1982) The role of nerve blocks in the treatment of cancer pain. Acta Anaesth. Scand. (Suppl. 74) 104–108.

Avellanosa, A. M. and West, C. R. (1982) Experience with transcutaneous electrical nerve stimulation for relief of intractable pain in cancer patients. J. Med. 13, 203–213.

Bates, T. D. and Vanier, T. (1978) Palliation by cytotoxic chemotherapy and hormone therapy. In: C. M. Saunders (Ed.), The Management of Terminal Disease. Edward Arnold, London, pp. 125–133.

Beaver, W. T. (1981) Aspirin and acetaminophen as constituents of analgesic combinations. Arch. Int. Med. 141, 293–300.

Beaver, W. T., Wallenstein, S. L., Houde, R. W. and Rogers, A. (1966) A comparison of the analgesic effects of methotrimeprazine and morphine in patients with cancer. Clin. Pharm. Ther. 7, 436–446.

Beaver, W. T., Wallenstein, S. L., Rogers, A. and Houde, R. W. (1978a) Analgesic studies of codeine and oxycodone in patients with cancer. 1. Comparisons of oral with intramuscular codeine and of oral with intramuscular oxycodone. J. Pharm. Exp. Ther. 207, 92–100.

Beaver, W. T., Wallenstein, S. L., Rogers, A. and Houde, R. W. (1978b) Analgesic studies of codeine and oxycodone in patients with cancer. J. Pharm. Exp. Ther. 207, 92–100.

Blair, J. S. G. (1967) Phenazocine hydrobromide BPC in the management of incurable malignant disease. Br. J. Clin. Pract. 21, 124–126.

Boland, J., Glicksman, A. and Vargha, A. (1969) Single dose radiation therapy in the palliation of metastatic disease. Radiology 93, 1181–1184.

Bolund, C. (1982) Pain relief through radiotherapy and chemotherapy. Acta Anaesth. Scand. (Suppl. 74) 114–116.

Bonadonna, G. and Molinari, R. (1979) Role and limits of anticancer drugs in the treatment of advanced cancer pain, pp. 131–138.*

Bonica, J. J. (1979) Introduction to nerve blocks, pp. 303–310.*

Bonica, J.J. (1974) Current role of nerve blocks in diagnosis and therapy of pain. In: J. J. Bonica (Ed.), Advances in Neurology, Vol. 4, International Symposium on Pain. Raven Press, New York, pp. 445–453.

Bonica, J. J. and Ventafridda, V. (Eds.) (1979) Advances in Pain Research and Therapy, Vol. 2. International Symposium on Pain of Advanced Cancer. Raven Press, New York.

Borget, B. (1980) The palliation of brain metastases: final results of the first two studies by the Radiation Therapy Oncology Group. Int. J. Radiat. Oncol. Biol. Phys. 6, 1–9.

Brereton, H. D., Halushka, P. V., Alexander, R. W., Mason, D. M., Keiser, H. R. and Devita, V. T. (1974) Indomethacin-responsive hypercalcemia in a patient with renal-cell adenocarcinoma. N. Engl. J. Med. 102, 83–85.

Brown, A. S. (1981) Current views on the use of nerve blocking in the relief of chronic pain. In: M. Swerdlow (Ed.), The Therapy of Pain. Current Status of Modern Therapy, Vol. 6. MTP Press, England, pp. 111–134.

Brule, G. (1979) Role and limits of oncologic chemotherapy of advanced cancer pain, pp. 139–144.*

Chan, K. (1979) The current use of narcotic analgesics in hospital practice. Br. J. Clin. Pharm. 438P–439P.

Daut, R. L. and Cleeland, C. S. (1982) The prevalence and severity of pain in cancer. Cancer 50, 1913–1918.

Ettinger, R. S., Vitale, P. J. and Trump, D. L. (1979) Important clinical pharmacologic considerations in the use of methadone in cancer patients. Cancer Treat. Rep. 63, 457–459.

Fiskin, R. A., Heath, D. A., Somers, S. and Bold, A. M. (1981) Hypercalcaemia in hospital patients. Lancet 24, 202–207.

Foley, K. M. (1979) Pain syndromes in patients with cancer. In: J. J. Bonica and V. Ventafridda (Eds.), Advances in Pain Research and Therapy, Vol. 2. Raven Press, New York, pp. 59–75.

---

* See Bonica and Ventafridda (1979) for full reference.

Gever, L. N. (1980) Brompton's mixture; how it relieves the pain of terminal cancer. Nursing 80, May, 57.

Glick, J. H. (1982) Palliative chemotherapy: risk/benefit ratio. In: B. R. and P. A. Cassileth (Eds.), Clinical Care of the Terminal Cancer Patient. Lea and Febiger, Philadelphia, pp. 53 – 64.

Haas, L. L. (1957) The place of the betatron in radiotherapy. Arch. Intern. Med. 100, 190 – 195.

Hafermann, M. D. (1983) Cancer of the prostate – external radiotherapy. In: G. P. Murphy (Ed.), Clinics in Oncology, Vol. 2, No. 2. W. B. Saunders Co. Ltd., pp. 371 – 405.

Hart, F. D. and Boardman, P. L. (1963) Indomethacin: a new non-steroid anti-inflammatory agent. Br. Med. J. 955 – 970.

Hazra, T. A. (1974) The role of radiotherapy in management of carcinoma of the prostate. Maryland Med J. 23, 48 – 49.

Hendrickson, F. R. and Pagano, M. (1981) Palliation of osseous metastases; preliminary report. In: L. Weiss and H. A. Gilbert (Eds.), Bone Metastases. C. J. Hall Boston.

Hendrickson, F. R. and Sheinkop, M. B. (1975) Management of osseous metastases. Semin. Oncol. 2, 4 – 10.

Hendrickson, F. R., Shehata, W. and Kirchner, A. (1976) Radiation therapy for osseous metastases. Int. J. Radiat. Oncol. Biol. Phys. 1, 275 – 278.

Hillier, E. R. (1983) Oral narcotic mixtures. Br. Med. J. 287, 701 – 702.

Hindley, A. C., Hill, E. B., Leyland, M. J. and Wiles, A. E. (1982) A double-blind controlled trial of salmon calcitonin in pain due to malignancy. Cancer Chemother. Pharmacol. 9, 71 – 74.

Hitchcock, E. (1981) Current views on the role of neurosurgery for pain relief. In: M. Swerdlow (Ed.), The Therapy of Pain. Current Status of Modern Therapy. Vol. 6. MTP Press, England, pp. 135 – 170.

Hunter, R. D. (1981) Current views on the management of pain in the cancer patient. In: M. Swerdlow (Ed.), The Therapy of Pain. Current Status of Modern Therapy, Vol. 6. MTP Press Ltd., England, pp. 191 – 214.

Jensen, N. H. and Roesdam, K. (1976) Single dose irradiation of bone metastases. Acta Radiol. Ther. Phys. Biol. 15, 337.

Kaiko, R. F. (1983) Central nervous system excitatory effects of meperidine in cancer patients. Ann. Neurol. 13, 180 – 185.

Kantor, T. G. (1979) Ibuprofen. Ann. Int. Med. 91, 877 – 882.

Levy, M.H. (1982) Symptom control manual. In: B. R. and P. A. Cassileth (Ed.), Clinical Care of the Terminal Cancer Patient. Lea & Febiger, Philadelphia, pp. 214 – 261.

Lloyd, J. W., Glynn, C. J., Adams, C. B. T. and Durrant, K. R. (1978) The pain of cancer. Practitioner 220, 453 – 456.

Loeser, J. D. (1980) Nonpharmacologic approaches to pain relief. In: L. K. Y. Ng and J. J. Bonica (Eds.), Pain, Discomfort and Humanitarian Care. Developments in Neurology, Vol. 4. Elsevier/North-Holland Inc., New York, pp. 275 – 292.

Lund, P. C. (1982) The role of analgesic blocking in the management of cancer pain: current trends. J. Med. 13, 161 – 182.

Mampel, E. (1958) Butazclidin. Ther. D. Gegenw. 97, 230 – 233.

Marks, R. M. and Sachar, E. J. (1973) Undertreatment of medical inpatients with narcotic analgesics. Ann. Intern. Med. 173 – 181.

Martens, M. (1982) A significant decrease of narcotic drug dosage after orthopaedic surgery. A double-blind study with naproxen. Acta Othop. Belg. 48, 900 – 906.

Mathews, G. J., Zarro, V. and Osterholm, J. L. (1973) Cancer pain and its treatment. Semin. Drug Treat. 3, 45 – 53.

Matts, S. G. Flavell (1962) Dextromoramide analgesia in the acute general medical patient. Practitioner 188, 524.

Maxwell, M. B. (1980) How to use methadone for the cancer patient's pain. Am. J. Nurs. 80, 1606 – 1608.

Mehta, M. (1981) Current views on non-invasive methods in pain relief. In: M. Swerdlow (Ed.), The Therapy of Pain. Current Status of Modern Therapy, Vol. 6. MTP Press, England, pp. 171 – 189.

Melzack, R., Ofiesh, J. G. and Mount, B. M. (1976) The Brompton mixture: effects on pain in cancer patients. Can. Med. Assoc. J. 115, 125 – 129.

Melzack, R., Mount, B. M. and Gordon, J. M. (1979) The Brompton mixture versus morphine solution given orally: effects on pain. Can. Med. Assoc. J. 120, 435 – 438.

Merskey, H. (1971) An appraisal of hypnosis. Postgrad. Med. J. 47, 572.

Meyerson, B. A. (1982) The role of neurosurgery in the treatment of cancer pain. Acta Anaesth. Scand. 74, 109 – 113.

Mount, B. M. (1980) Narcotic analgesics. In: R. G. Twycross and V. Ventafridda (Eds.), The Continuing Care of Terminal Cancer Patients, Milan 19 – 20 October 1979. Pergamon Press, Oxford, pp. 97 – 116.

Mount, B. M., Ajemian, I. and Scott, J. F. (1976) Use of the Brompton mixture in treating the chronic pain of malignant disease. Can. Med. Assoc. J. 115, 122 – 124.

Noyes, R., Jr. (1981) Treatment of cancer pain. Psychosom. Med. 43, 57 – 70.

Orne, M. T. (1980) Nonpharmacological approaches to pain relief: hypnosis, biofeedback, placebo effects. In: L. K. Y. Ng and J. J. Bonica (Eds.), Pain, Discomfort and Humanitarian Care. Developments in Neurology, Vol. 4. Elsevier/North-Holland, Amsterdam, pp. 253 – 274.

Oster, M. W., Vizel, M. and Turgeon, L. V. (1978) Pain of terminal cancer patients. Arch. Intern. Med. 138, 1801 – 1802.

Pagni, C. A. (1979) Cancer pain in the head and neck: role of neurosurgery. pp. 543 – 552.*

Pannuti, F., Rossi, A. P., Marraro, D., Strocchi, E., Cricca, A., Piana, E. and Pollutri, E. (1979a) The natural history of cancer pain. In: R. G. Twycross and V. Ventafridda (Eds.), The Continuing Care of Terminal Cancer Patients. Pergamon Press, Oxford, pp. 75 – 78.

Pannuti, F., Martoni, A., Rossi, A. P. and Piana, E. (1979b) The role of endocrine therapy for relief of pain due to advanced cancer. pp. 145 – 165.*

Parker, R. G. (1974) Selective use of radiation therapy for the cancer patient with pain. In: J. J. Bonica (Ed.), Advances in Neurology, Vol. 4. Raven Press, New York, pp. 491 – 493.

Portlock, C. S. and Goffinet, D. R. (1980) Manual of Clinical Problems in Oncology. Little, Brown & Co., Boston, pp. 262 – 265.

Reasbeck, P. G., Rice, M. L. and Reasbeck, J. C. (1982) Double-blind controlled trial of indomethacin as an adjunct to narcotic analgesia after major abdominal surgery. Lancet 2, 115 – 117.

Ricci, S. B. (1979a) Radiation therapy. In: J. J. Bonica and V. Ventafridda (Eds.), Advances in Pain Research and Therapy, Vol 2. Raven Press, New York, pp. 167 – 174.

Ricci, S. B. (1979b) Radiation therapy. In: R. G. Twycross and V. Ventafridda (Eds.), The Continuing Care of Terminal Cancer Patients. Proceedings of an International Seminar on Continuing Care of Terminal Cancer Patients. Milan. Pergamon Press, Milan, pp. 91 – 95.

Richter, M. P. (1982) Palliative radiation therapy. In: B. R. and P. A. Cassileth (Eds.), Clinical Care of the Terminal Cancer Patient. Lea & Febiger, Philadelphia, pp. 65 – 75.

Rico, R. C. and Trudnowski, R. J. (1982) Studies with electro-acupuncture. In: R. J. Trudnowski (Ed.), J. Med. PJD Publications, New York, pp. 247 – 252.

Robbie, D. S. (1979) A trial of sublingual buprenorphine in cancer pain Br. J. Clin. Pharm. 7, 315s – 317s.

Romeu, J. (1982) Indomethacin therapy in symptomatic hepatic neoplasms. Am. J. Gastroenterol. 77, 655 – 659.

Sadove, M. S., Levin, J. M., Rose, R. F., Schwartz, L. and Witt, F. W. (1954) Chlorpromazine and narcotics in the management of pain of malignant lesions. J. Am. Med. Assoc. 12, 626 – 628.

Saunders, C. (1982) Principles of symptom control in terminal care. Med. Clin. North. Am. 66, 1169 – 1183.

Sawe, J., Hansen, J., Ginman, C., Hartvig, P., Jakobsson, P. A., Nilsson, M. I., Rane, A. and Anggard, E. (1981) Patient-controlled dose regimen of methadone for chronic cancer pain. Br. Med. J. 282, 771 – 773.

Seybearth, H. W., Sergre, G. V., Morgan, J. L., Sweetman, B. J., Potts, J. T. and Oates, J. A. (1975) Prostaglandins as mediators of hypercalcemia associated with certain types of cancer. N. Engl. J. Med. 293, 1278 – 1283.

Shapshay, S. M., Scott, R. M., McCann, C. F. and Stoelting, I. (1980) Pain control in advanced and recurrent head and neck cancer. Otolaryng. Clin. North. Am. 13, 551 – 560.

Smith, I. E., Harris, A. L. and Morgan, M. (1981) Tamoxifen versus aminoglutethimide in advanced breast carcinoma: a randomised cross-over trial. Br. Med. J. 283, 1432 – 1434.

Snow, H. (1896) Opium and cocaine in the treatment of cancerous disease. Br. Med. J. September, 718 – 719.

---

* See Bonica and Ventafridda (1979) for full reference.

Ventafridda, V., Fochi, C., De Conno, D. and Sganzeria, E. (1980) Use of non-steroidal anti-inflammatory drugs in the treatment of pain in cancer. Br. J. Clin. Pharmacol. (Suppl 2) 343S–346S.

Walsh, T. D. (1983) Antidepressants in chronic pain. Clin. Neuropharm. 6, 271–295.

Walsh, T. D. (1984a) Opiates and respiratory function in advanced cancer. In: Recent Results in Cancer Research, Vol. 89. Springer-Verlag, Berlin, pp. 115–117.

Walsh, T. D. (1984b) Oral morphine in chronic cancer pain. Pain 18, 1–11.

Walsh, T. D. (1985) Clinical evaluation of slow-release morphine tablets. In: Fields (Ed.), Advances in Pain Research, Vol 9. pp. 727–730.

Walsh, T. D. and Cheater, F. M. (1983) Use of morphine for cancer pain. Pharm. J. October, 525–527.

Walsh, T. D. and Saunders, C. M. (1984) Hospice care: The treatment of pain in advanced cancer. In: M. Zimmermann, P. Drings and G. Wagner (Eds.), Recent Results in Cancer Research. Pain in the Cancer Patient, Pathogenesis, Diagnosis and Therapy, Vol 89. Springer-Verlag, Berlin, pp. 201–211.

Waxman, J. H., Wass, J. A. H., Hendry, W. F., Whitfield, H. N., Besser, G. M., Malpas, J. S. and Oliver, R. T. D. (1983) Treatment with gonadotrophin releasing hormone analogue in advanced prostatic cancer. Br. Med. J. 286, 1309–1312.

Williams, M. R. (1978) The place of surgery in terminal care. In: C. M. Saunders (Ed.), The Management of Terminal Disease. Edward Arnold, London, pp. 134–138.

Burrows/Elton/Stanley (eds.) Handbook of Chronic Pain Management
© *1987 Elsevier Science Publishers B.V. (Biomedical Division)*

33

The gynecologist's approach to chronic pelvic pain

ALLAN CHAMBERLAIN[1] and JOHN J. LaFERLA[2]

[1]*Department of Obstetrics-Gynecology, University of West Virginia Medical School, Morgantown, WV 26505, and* [2]*Department of Obstetrics-Gynecology, Hutzel Hospital, The Detroit Medical Center, 4707 St. Antoine Boulevard, Detroit, MI 48201, U.S.A.*

Introduction

Pain is a frequently expressed symptom at gynecologic outpatient visits. Fortunately, most painful symptoms have a readily recognizable pattern and treatment is both prompt and effective. When pelvic pain becomes chronic and is resistant to standard therapeutic efforts, both the patient and the gynecologist may become frustrated, angry and demoralized. To avoid this, it should be made clear from the onset that the physician will help the patient to deal with her problem, but that he or she can not guarantee a cure. In fact, the doctor should not become too invested in seeing the pain relieved. To do so risks overtreatment and worsening of the problem. Nevertheless, the majority of chronic pelvic patients will improve significantly with accurate diagnosis and appropriate treatment, especially if adequate resources can be devoted to their care.

This chapter is in three parts. First, pelvic pain mechanisms are reviewed, then a plan for evaluating patients who present with this problem is presented, and finally the pathogenesis and treatment of several chronic pain syndromes are discussed.

Pelvic pain mechanisms

The pelvis is innervated by a complex network of fibers that is not completely understood (Malinak 1984). There is considerable cross-innervation and impulses from a given organ may enter at several spinal segments. Nevertheless, a fundamental knowledge of the pelvic nerves is necessary to understand and treat pelvic pain. The pelvis is supplied by both somatic and autonomic fibers. The pudendal nerves carry well-localized sensation from the perineum and lower vagina to the sacral segments while somatic afferents from the lumbar segmental nerves supply the surrounding areas. There are four principal pelvic autonomic plexuses: the vesical, rectal, ovarian and vaginal-uterine-tubal plexuses. This last network coalesces to form the presacral plexus and ultimately contributes to the lumbar sympathetic chains and hypogastric plexuses. Thus, pelvic sensation is carried to segments as high as the lower thoracics and as low as the distal sacral segments. These pathways are diagrammed in Fig. 1.

Pain localized to superficial pelvic structures may be due to stimulation of somatic afferents, to referral of sensation carried in autonomic fibers to similar segments, or to events at higher levels interpreted as representing nociceptive inputs from these structures. Trauma, inflammation, ischemia or infiltrating neoplasms of the skin, fat, muscles, nerves or vasculature of superficial tissues may produce pain (Chorowski 1984). Deeper in the pelvis, the upper vagina and external cervical os are relatively less sensitive to minor irritation. Pregnancy or neoplasia may slowly stretch the uterus and ovaries to very large proportions without pain. Nevertheless, the cervix may be exquisitely sensitive when inflamed and rapid dilation of the internal os or torsion of an ovarian mass can produce excruciating pain.

Patients tend to describe pain from any pelvic organ in similar terms. Renaer and Guzinski (1978) have defined dorsal and ventral pelvic pain zones: the ventral zone extends across the lower abdomen below the anterior superior iliac spines and the dorsal zone covers the upper sacrum and medial gluteal areas. There may or may not be relative localization within these boundaries. Cul de sac pain may be described as somewhat lower and ovarian pain as more epigastric. The relative similarity of pelvic pain from a variety of sources can lead to diagnostic errors. Therefore, results of examinations, laboratory and diagnostic tests and other historical features must be considered carefully before a definitive diagnosis is made.

Whatever the impulses from the peripheral organs, it is the central processing of these impulses which defines pain. Pelvic pain without peripheral stimulation is not only possible, but is indistinguishable by the patient. Patients are reluctant to accept this idea, since it conjures up images of unreality, insanity or malingering. Owing to the perjorative connotations of functional

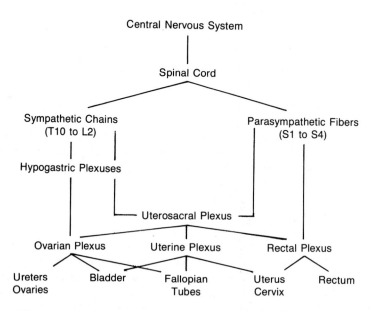

Fig. 1. The innervation of the pelvic viscera.

or non-organic pain patients may react very negatively if they are told 'It is all in your head'. Clinicians must, nonetheless, be cognizant of the capacity of higher centers to originate, to augment and to diminish perception of pain.

Evaluation of the patient

The diagnosis and treatment of chronic pelvic pain can not be entirely separated. Often several sessions are required to collect historical information and records, perform physical examinations and diagnostic procedures and administer and explain the results of laboratory and psychometric tests. Over the course of this process the physician can develop rapport with the patient and the patient may come to a clearer understanding of the causes of her problem.

Evaluation of women with pelvic pain can begin with a questionnaire that the woman completes at home prior to the first visit. The questionnaire helps the patient review her problem in an unpressured setting, saves time in office or clinic and provides an historical record of her pre-treatment condition. This questionnaire can be modeled after the McGill Pain Questionnaire (Melzack 1975). The duration, location, character and intensity of the pain and its association with the menstrual cycle, intercourse, activity and gastrointestinal and urinary functioning is sought. The questionnaire also seeks a more general pain history, including memories of early pain experiences and her and her caretakers' responses to them. She is asked about family members who have suffered from chronic pain and about child abuse, rape and incest. Her recollections of her first menstrual period and first sexual intercourse and any subsequent problems are collected. Finally, the patient is asked to map her pain on a human figure, to answer a psychometric/pain inventory describing her present condition and to list the activities she would be able to undertake if she were free of pain. This document is mailed back to the doctor and reviewed prior to the patient's first visit.

THE PELVIC EXAMINATION IN CHRONIC PELVIC PAIN

The objective of the pelvic examination in chronic pelvic pain is to discover as much as possible about the patient's anatomy and sensitivity. An attempt is made to isolate each pelvic structure from the others and to examine it independently. A contract can be made with the patient that if the examination becomes painful, the physician will persist only as long as a slow count to three, repeating the same part of the examination, if necessary, only after the patient has rested (Steege 1984). After performing a general screening physical examination, the patient is asked to assume a semi-upright modified lithotomy position. This facilitates the patient's involvement in the exam and helps her to relax her abdominal muscles. She is then asked to point to the area of greatest pain, and then other painful areas. This information is used to plan the remainder of the procedure.

On examination of the vulva, evidence of lesions, abrasions, discharges, and inadequately repaired perineal lesions or trauma may be seen. A lubricated speculum is inserted and samples taken as may be indicated for Pap smear, wet preparations and cultures for chlamydia and gonorrhea. Mycoplasma and herpes cultures may also be obtained if the history is suggestive. The bimanual examination begins by touching first the patient's thigh and then the area around and within the introitus, looking for muscle belly tenderness, open lesions and perineal muscle spasm. Next the bladder and urethra are examined using the internal hand only, to avoid confusion with abdominal wall tenderness. This may elicit an urge to void but is not painful unless the urinary tract is inflamed or the patient is histrionic. The cervix is then gently examined, and degree of tenderness noted. The size, shape, mobility and any tenderness of the adnexal structures are evaluated, as are the same features of the uterine fundus. Usually it is necessary to change examining hands to best study the opposite adnexa. Finally, a rectovaginal examination may reveal point tenderness consistent with appendiceal or other abscesses, uterosacral nodularity suggesting endometriosis, or occult fetal blood. Immediately after the examination it may be helpful to remind the patient of the poor correlation between examination findings, pathology and pain.

LABORATORY STUDIES AND CONSULTATIONS

The laboratory work-up of pelvic pain patients must be highly individualized. In addition to microbiologic tests, a complete blood count, sedimentation rate and urinalysis are usually indicated. Screening studies for liver, gall bladder and pancreatic problems may be collected as well. If necessary, diagnostic studies and consultations to rule out urologic, gastrointestinal and orthopedic disorders should be obtained. Psychological assessment and treatment should parallel other investigations at every step. Most patients will accept referral for psychologic evaluation if it is seen as a routine part of the total evaluation of chronic pelvic pain. If psychological counselling is not part of the routine work-up, patients who seem to suffer from emotional complications of their illness may be less amenable to referral when this is viewed as a last resort.

Although ultrasound is often less helpful than one might hope, this technique can detect adnexal masses, uterine enlargement, hydrosalpinx, and a variety of other pathological conditions. A strong point favoring the use of ultrasound is its non-invasiveness. On the other hand, patients may misinterpret ultrasound images or reports of small functional cysts as indicating serious organic pathology. Ultrasound must be used and interpreted carefully therefore, in patients with chronic pelvic pain.

Laparoscopy, anesthetic procedures and psychometric studies are often required to accurately diagnose pelvic pain. As with the history and physical examination, these procedures are frequently therapeutic as well as diagnostic.

LAPAROSCOPY

The superiority of laparoscopy over the diagnostic modalities in chronic pelvic pain has been demonstrated repeatedly. Laparoscopy often reveals unsuspected lesions or confirms their absence (Cunanan 1983). It may allow for staging or definitive treatment of disease. Specific indications include pain of long duration, or where there is suspicion of a pelvic mass, distortion of the rectovaginal septum or uterosacral ligaments, dysmenorrhea unresponsive to three cycles of non-steroidal anti-inflammatory agents, and moliminal gastrointestinal or urinary symptoms (after gastrointestinal and urinary tract evaluation). When endometriosis is suspected laparoscopy must be performed before definitive therapy is undertaken.

Laparoscopy may ultimately be necessary in the evaluation of almost all patients with chronic pelvic pain, but it is such a simple procedure that gynecologists are sometimes tempted to 'take a peek' prematurely, before a thorough history, physical and laboratory evaluation are complete. One should not be too hasty to perform laparoscopy since some pain, expense and morbidity is involved. Furthermore, if no pathology is identified, it is important to have already developed some rapport with the patient to help her cope with this disappointment or to augment her sense of relief.

The issue of whether or not specific laparoscopic findings are etiologically involved in pelvic pain poses one of the principal dilemmas in the management of these patients. Approximately one third of pelvic pain patients have normal laparoscopic studies; on the other hand, adhesions and endometriosis are frequently found in asymptomatic women. Kresch et al. (1984) report a qualitative difference between the adhesions seen in symptomatic and asymptomatic patients. They feel that adhesions associated with pain are much more likely to restrict the motion or distensibility of involved organs. These authors also found an interaction between a history of pelvic surgery or inflammatory disease and the report of pain in patients with adhesions. A discussion of techniques for preventing and lysing adhesions is beyond the scope of this chapter, but remains an area of active research interest (Stangel 1984). Patients whose pain is 'grossly in excess of what would be expected from the physical findings' meet one of the criteria for diagnosis of the 'Psychogenic Pain Disorder' (Engel 1959) and deserve complete evaluation for this syndrome.

ANESTHETIC TECHNIQUES

One area of increasing research interest is the application of anesthetic block techniques to chronic pelvic pain. Slocumb (1984) has reported successful injection of abdominal and pelvic 'trigger points' with local anesthetics and steroids. These injections presumably block peripheral stimulation of central pain mechanisms. They may permanently relieve pelvic pain and dyspareunia clinically reminiscent of myofascial pain syndrome, levator syndrome, and pelvic floor myalgia.

Paracervical block anesthesia may be helpful in localizing pelvic pain and may help predict whether simple hysterectomy will offer relief. Paracervical anesthesia blocks sensation from the uterus and tubes but not from the bladder, ovaries or rectum. The block is placed in the usual fashion and the patient is asked to record the extent and duration of relief, but she is not told how long the block will last. A response of greater than 50% relief for 1 – 2 hours is consistent with the pharmacologic effect of 1% Lidocaine. Patients who report either weeks of relief or no relief are felt to be less likely to respond to hysterectomy than those whose relief parallels the interval expected from the pharmacodynamics of the drug.

Patients who complain of persistent burning pelvic pain may respond clinically to repeated selective lumbar epidural as though they suffered from a reflex sympathetic dystrophy as described by Bonica et al. (1984). These patients may sustain longer and longer relief, ultimately requiring no further treatment. No definitive series of patients who have been managed in this way has been published. Nevertheless, patients who do not respond to traditional techniques may profit from referral to a physician experienced in placing and monitoring epidural anesthetics.

HYSTERECTOMY

The role of hysterectomy in the treatment of patients with chronic pelvic pain remains controversial, particularly when no pathology is noted at laparoscopy. Judgement regarding surgery must be tempered with the total evaluation of the patient, but from time to time hysterectomy may be seen as a last resort when other therapies have been given an adequate trial.

Many experienced clinicians report excellent response to hysterectomy in patients with chronic pelvic pain, even when the pathology report reveals no diagnostic abnormalities. On the other hand, about one third of patients referred to specialized chronic pelvic pain clinics have already undergone hysterectomy without relief. It may be that not all pathological conditions which cause pelvic pain are visible under the pathologist's microscope. It is equally plausible that removal of a woman's uterus may resolve unconscious conflict, apply sufficient punishment to assuage subconscious guilt, or act as a potent placebo. In any event, hysterectomies continue to be performed on occasion for chronic pelvic pain and many, though not all, women seem to benefit.

Specific syndromes seen in chronic pelvic pain clinics

DYSMENORRHEA

Dysmenorrhea is a symptom complex comprising menstrual pain or uterine cramping and often nausea, vomiting, fatigue, diarrhea, backache and headache (Dawood 1984). Dysmenorrhea has been an immense public health problem: 50% of women may suffer from dysmenorrhea at one time or another, and it has been the greatest single cause of lost work and school days among women (Chan 1983). Primary dysmenorrhea, in which no disease is detectable, is much more common than dysmenorrhea secondary to another disorder.

With primary dysmenorrhea, pain usually starts simultaneously with flow and lasts for the first 24 – 72 hours of menstruation, closely following prostaglandin levels in menstrual effluent. One study found that dysmenorrheic women produced 8 – 13 times as much prostaglandin F as did normal women (Pickles et al. 1965). There is considerable evidence that prostaglandins induce intense uterine contractions that result in uterine ischemia and thus the pain of primary dysmenorrhea.

Oral contraceptives reduce the elevated menstrual prostaglandin release of dysmenorrheic patients to levels below that of normal controls (Chan and Dawood 1980). For this reason, at least three fourths of women taking oral contraceptives show improvement. Non-steroidal anti-inflammatory drugs (NSAIDs) like mefenamic acid, ibuprofen and indomethacin effectively block the formation of prostaglandins by inhibiting the cyclo-oxygenase enzyme. Double-blinded studies reveal that 56 – 87% of subjects are relieved by these agents (Owen 1984). An additional 10 – 25% will respond to higher dosages or a different NSAID. Oral contraceptives and NSAIDs are so effective that patients who do not respond to three cycles of treatment probably should undergo evaluation to rule out secondary dysmenorrhea.

Secondary dysmenorrhea may be caused by endometriosis, pelvic inflammatory disease, an intrauterine device (IUD) or an anatomic abnormality. It usually begins more than 2 years after menarche, but may start with the first period if it is caused by a congenital malformation. Treatment is directed at the underlying cause. Prostaglandin inhibiting agents tend to be less effective in secondary dysmenorrhea but an exception to this rule applies to IUDs. Treatment with NSAIDs may correct IUD associated menorrhagia as well as dysmenorrhea.

The discovery of the role of increased production of prostaglandins in dysmenorrhea has dramatically changed the way that we think of this problem. Years ago dysmenorrhea was felt to be a largely psychosomatic complaint. However, prostaglandin inhibiting drugs are so effective that it is now held to be a minor biochemical aberration. In spite of this, the question must still be raised why some women have dysmenorrhea and the pattern of elevated prostaglandins that is presumed to cause it, while others do not. Furthermore, there is evidence that sleep, hypnosis and biofeedback can reduce uterine contractions and prostaglandin levels. Primary dysmenorrhea thus remains an important area for future research in psychoneuroendocrinology (Chan 1983).

ENDOMETRIOSIS

Endometriosis, or functioning endometrium outside its usual location, is found in about one third of women undergoing laparoscopy for pelvic pain or infertility. After 80 years of study its cause is not known and therapy is controversial (Ranney 1980). Even with optimal management about one tenth to one third suffer recurrences within one year. Endometriosis may be silent but at least two thirds of patients report dyspareunia, dysmenorrhea, dysuria and/or dyschesia. Pain, infertility and hormonal therapy may place a seemingly unbearable emotional burden on the patient and her family.

Ectopic endometriosis islands proliferate with estrogen stimulation and tend to 'menstruate' when hormones are withdrawn. Surrounding tissue is irritated and becomes inflamed. Ultimately, dense puckering scars, cystic masses and solid nodules are found. Scar retraction tends to retrovert the uterus, imposing the tender organ between the sacrum and the penetrating penis. Pelvic examination conducted during menstruation may reveal abnormal tenderness, fixed retroversion, adnexal masses and, by rectovaginal examination, tender uterosacral nodules. Laparoscopy should be performed if history and physical examination are suggestive of endometriosis.

The objective of endometriosis treatment is to relieve pain and restore fertility. Medical therapy seeks to inactivate implants with oral contraceptives or androgens, especially Danazol. Danazol treatment is superior but costly (Barbieri et al. 1982). In the future, an analog of gonadotropin-releasing hormone (GRH) may become the treatment of choice. Therapy should continue for 6 – 12 months and may be repeated. More than 80% of patients achieve subjective improvement, often beginning early in treatment. One third to one half will become pregnant after treatment.

Surgical approaches to endometriosis are varied according to the extent of disease and desire for fertility. Minimal endometriosis may be treated through the laparoscope. Cautery of implants and fulguration of the nerve plexuses in the uterosacral ligaments may relieve pain. Conservative laparotomy to maximize fertility has four goals: removal of implants, lysis of adhesions, presacral neurectomy and uterine suspension (to relieve dyspareunia). Surgery is at least comparable to medical therapy in relieving pain and restoring fertility. If fertility is not desired, hysterectomy with or without oophorectomy may be performed.

Psychological therapy for patients with endometriosis is similar to that provided for other chronic pain states. Support groups for patients and their spouses may be particularly useful since dyspareunia and infertility are shared stresses. Couples may be able to view their own difficulties more constructively if they are exposed to others with similar concerns. Endometriosis may contribute to a chain reaction of sexual dysfunction even after therapy has been successful. Decreased libido, vaginismus, arousal phase dysfunction and male performance anxiety that began when endometriosis was active may require active treatment even after pain has been relieved.

DYSPAREUNIA

Dyspareunia, difficult, painful intercourse, is a symptom that may be associated with a combination of emotional and physical findings. The most important historical feature is whether the pain is superficial or deep, as this will direct the subsequent work-up and treatment. Physical abnormalities such as painful episiotomy site, urethral diverticulum, vaginitis or deep pelvic pathology may cause anxiety, inhibit arousal and result in dyspareunia. Poor psychosexual adjustment may also impair arousal and lead to painful intercourse and perineal and pelvic trauma.

Vaginismus, the spastic contraction of the vaginal outlet in response to perceived attempts at penetration, is probably more common than has been appreciated (Steege 1984). It may exist alone or in association with other sources of pain. One review found that organic and anatomic lesions were found in 56% of vulvar dyspareunia patients in a private practice (Huffman 1983). Abnormalities included anomalies and ambiguous genitalia, scars from perineal surgery and inflammation, cysts and tumors. Inadequate lubrication due to individual variation and climacteric changes as well as to psychogenic factors may be found. Relaxing surgery, including 'hymenotomy', is contraindicated in the presence of normal anatomy and when indicated should always be accompanied by psychosexual counselling. Systematic desensitization and retraining form the basis of therapy for vaginismus. Success levels are higher if the patient and her partner are motivated to achieve relief.

Reamy (1982) recommends the following approach to the patient with vaginismus. Treatment begins with education during the pelvic examination. The normal size and structure of the patient's anatomy is stressed. Vaginospasm is observed by the physician and patient (with the aid of a small mirror) and assurance is given that it can be overcome. During the examination, the patient is instructed in intermittent contraction and relaxation of her perivaginal and other pelvic floor muscles (Kegel exercises) and is encouraged to practice at home. These exercises increase body awareness and voluntary control over the pelvic musculature. Intercourse is proscribed at first and weekly visits are scheduled to monitor progress. After a week of Kegel exercises alone, the patient is given gradually progressive desensitization tasks. First one finger is placed at the introitus, then inside. Later two or three fingers, the partner's fingers and ultimately his penis is used. Passive containment and ultimately thrusting are recommended. Conjoint counselling is always preferable, but the woman may be treated alone if necessary.

Pelvic inflammatory disease

One million women receive treatment for pelvic inflammatory disease in the United States annually (Shafer et al. 1982). The rate of antibiotic failure is recognized to be 20 – 30% (Thomason 1984). Furthermore, many more cases are never recognized or treated. All the classic signs: pain, fever, elevated WBC count and adnexal tenderness, are present in only 20% of laparoscopicly proven cases. Predeliction to recurrence, tubo-ovarian abscess, infertility and chronic pain are common sequelae (Roberts and Dockery 1984).

The key to controlling the morbidity of chronic pelvic infection is to insure adequate diagnosis and treatment of acute disease and recurrences. Endogenous flora carried into the genital tract, probably by sperm, may produce relapsing infection. The antibiotic regimens recommended by the Center for Disease Control reflect the polymicrobial nature of the disease and the importance of anaerobes and Chlamydia trachomatis. Compliant, afebrile patients without pelvic masses or IUDs may receive a trial of outpatient treatment. All other patients and those who fail outpatient treatment should be admitted. Chronic pelvic pain due to extensive and recurrent pelvic infection may be resistant to antibiotic treatment. Thus, surgery may be indicated in selected cases to remove chronically infected tissue.

Psychological disorders presenting with chronic pelvic pain

The Diagnostic and Statistical Manual of Mental Disorders, 3rd edition, of the American Psychiatric Association (1980) lists three syndromes within the somatoform disorders group that may present with pain: Somatization Disorder, Psychogenic Pain Disorder and Hypochondriasis. These processes are frequently seen in combined forms in clinical settings and can often serve to exacerbate pain from physical abnormalities. Other emotional disorders are frequently associated with pain. For example, at least 50% of depressed patients complain of pain. Chronic pain itself induces a syndrome virtually indistinguishable from major depression (Reuler et al. 1980). Several authors have noted very high levels of personality disorder among pelvic pain patients whether or not organic pathology is found (Castelnuovo-Tedesco and Krout 1970; Gross et al. 1980). Rarely, psychotic patients may suffer from bizarre delusional pain. Careful early psychological evaluation is a cornerstone of chronic pelvic pain management.

With somatization disorder, formerly known as Briquet's syndrome or hysteria, patients present with exaggerated complaints, often on an emergency basis. Multisystem problems requiring self-medication or physician attendance are the rule, but characteristically there is poor documentation of physical abnormality. The present doctor may be glorified while previous physicians are vilified. Social, sexual and personal lives are typically chaotic. Polypharmacy, polysurgery and substance abuse disorders are common. Differential diagnosis includes systemic diseases that present with vague symptoms (e.g. porphyria, hypothyroidism), and also other forms of psychopathology. This disorder is chronic, with intermittent exacerbations and remissions. Care must be supportive. When medical work-up is required, the least invasive studies should be chosen.

The patient with hypochondriasis is pre-occupied by an unrealistic conviction that she suffers from a serious illness. She resists reassurance and her functioning is impaired. In contrast to somatization disorder, the patient is concerned about underlying disease rather than with the symptoms themselves. Hypochondriasis is commonly a symptom of other disturbances, such as depression, dysthymic disorder or generalized anxiety disorder. Psychiatric referral is indicated if the concern over an undocumented disease becomes a fixed delusion.

Two features are necessary for the diagnosis of psychogenic pain disorder: pain grossly in excess of what would be expected from physical findings and the presence of psychological precipitating factors. The patient is not indifferent to the pain but refuses to consider the importance of psychological factors in its origin. Pain may allow her to avoid a noxious obligation or may have symbolic importance, a conversion reaction. Psychological treatment is indicated

TABLE 1
Overview of the evaluation of the patient with chronic pelvic pain: Pain Questionnaire (e.g. Melzack 1975).

Interview:	General medical history
	Pain history
	Family and social history
	Psychometric testing
Examination:	General examination
	Pelvic examination
Laboratory studies:	Microbiologic
	Biochemical (WBC, sedimentation rate, amylase, etc.)
	X-rays (genitourinary, gastrointestinal)
	Ultrasound
Nerve blocks:	Paracervical block
	Abdominal wall 'trigger points'
	Epidural/spinal
Surgical:	Laparoscopy

and hypnosis may be a useful adjunct. An overview of the evaluation of the patient with chronic pelvic pain is presented in outline form in Table 1.

CHRONIC PELVIC PAIN WITHOUT OBVIOUS PATHOLOGY

Patients with pelvic pain for which no cause can be found are among the most challenging. All series of pelvic pain patients include a group accounting for 10 – 50% of all pelvic pain patients who have no obvious pathology. Two possibilities exist: organic pathology is present but not demonstrated, or it is absent.

Pathology may be missed if it acts without distorting pelvic anatomy of if it is only intermittently present. Neurologic, orthopedic, gastrointestinal and urologic processes may meet this criterion, as may gynecologic infections, adenomyosis and even tumors. In 1952, Taylor (1961) made recordings of the thermal conduction of the vaginal wall and concluded that chronic pelvic pain could be caused by 'pelvic congestion' that occurred with arousal or stress. Other authors believed that pelvic varicose veins were an important cause of pain (Schaupp 1962). Allen and Masters (1955) proposed, in turn, that enigmatic broad ligament lacerations caused pain. Although such lesions are indeed sometimes discovered their pathophysiology remains obscure.

The term Chronic Pelvic Pain Without Obvious Pathology has been used to describe a subgroup of patients with a predictable pattern of emotional and physical findings (Renaer 1980). The patients are usually parous women in their 20's or 30's. Their pain waxes and wanes, often with pre-menstrural exacerbations. It is localized to the lower abdomen and back and is frequently associated with deep dyspareunia. Other symptoms in the reproductive, neurologic, gastrointestinal and cardiovascular systems are usually present and are reminiscent of the somatization disorder. Gynecologic examination reveals diffuse tenderness. The uterus may be minimally enlarged and boggy, but diagnostic studies are non-productive.

There is a very high incidence of emotional and psychosexual pathology in this group. Massive and fundamental difficulties in relating to others is seen (Castelnuovo-Tedesco and Krout 1970). Markedly abnormal dependency needs and poor role adjustment are very common. One third have been victims of incest. Family backgrounds commonly include divorce, abandonment, violence, alcoholism and prostitution. Psychometric evaluation sometimes reveals hysterical, depressive and hypochondriacal tendencies, but may be normal. As a group these patients are resistant to psychiatric referral and seem to be eager for hysterectomy.

Treatment is similar to that for other chronic pain states. Supportive counselling is provided and substance abuse disorders are treated. Tricyclic antidepressants and NSAIDs are the pharmacologic agents of choice. Antidepressants have been found by some to be effective for chronic pain conditions even if depression is not an overtly obvious component. Patients may respond at lower doses and with shorter latency intervals than typically noted for patients experiencing endogenous depression.

Biofeedback therapy is sometimes useful, frequently producing beneficial effects even if the pain is not completely relieved. Through biofeedback and related relaxation exercises, patients gain a greater sense of mastery of their bodies, and may find relief from related problems like headache, low back pain and sleep disturbance.

The patient should be encouraged to gradually resume healthful activity. The course of this disorder is characterized by advances and declines but approximately half of patients will remit spontaneously during evaluation or within one year of treatment. This syndrome is uncommon after the age of 40. An overview of treatment modalities for patients with chronic pelvic pain is presented in Table 2.

TABLE 2
Treatment of the patient with chronic pelvic pain* (a list of possibly useful therapeutic modalities).

General:	Exercise/nutrition
	Rapport between doctor and patient
Medications:	Analgesics
	Antibiotics
	Antidepressants
Psychological:	Relaxation training
	Biofeedback
	Hypnosis
	Psychotherapy
Surgical:	Anesthetic blocks
	Laparoscopy
	Hysterectomy
	Presacral neurectomy
Other:	Transcutaneous electronic nerve stimulation
	Acupuncture

* Treatment must obviously be individualized.

Conclusion

Patients with chronic pelvic pain represent a diverse group of individuals who suffer from a wide range of psychological and physical illnesses. The innervation of the pelvis is complex, and history and physical findings are often misleading. Laparoscopy, anesthetic blocks and appropriate consultation may improve diagnostic accuracy. Treatment depends on the nature of both organic and psychologic pathology and must be individualized. Psychological features commonly seen in this patient group make them challenging to care for, but awareness of these factors can be used to plan more effective therapy. Much more research is needed to better define which diagnostic and therapeutic modalities are most effective. In the interim, empiric treatment offers best long-term outcomes.

References

Allen, W. M. and Masters, W. H. (1955) Traumatic laceration of uterine support. Am. J. Obstet. Gynecol. 70, 500 – 513.

American Psychiatric Association (1980) Diagnostic and Statistical Manual of Mental Disorders, 3rd edn. American Psychiatric Association, Washington, D.C., pp. 241 – 252.

Barbieri, R. L., Evans, S. and Kistner, R. W. (1982) Danazol in the treatment of endometriosis: analysis of 100 cases with a four year follow-up. Fertil. Steril. 27, 737 – 746.

Blumer, D. (1982) Psychiatric aspects of chronic pain: nature, identification, and treatment of the pain-prone disorder. In: S. Rothman and A. Simeone (Eds.), The Spine. W. B. Saunders, Philadelphia, pp. 1090 – 1117.

Bonica, J. J. (1984) Sympathetic nerve blocks for diagnosis and therapy. In: Fundamental Considerations and Clinical Applications, Vol. 1. Winthrop-Breon Laboratories, New York, pp. 1 – 16.

Castelnuovo-Tedesco, P. and Krout, B. M. (1970) Psychosomatic aspects of chronic pelvic pain. Int. J. Psychiatr. Med. 1, 109 – 126.

Chan, W. Y. (1983) Prostaglandins and non-steroidal anti-inflammatory drugs in dysmenorrhea. Ann. Rev. Pharmacol. Toxicol. 23, 131 – 149.

Chan, W. Y. and Dawood, M. Y. (1980) Prostaglandin levels in menstrual fluid of non-dysmenorrheic and dysmenorrheic subjects with and without oral contraceptive or ibuprofen therapy. Adv. Prostaglandin Thromb. Leukotriene Res. 8, 1445 – 1448.

Chorowski, M. (1984) Pelvic pain. In: D. H. Nichols and J. R. Evrard (Eds.), Ambulatory Gynecology. W. B. Saunders, Philadelphia, pp. 175 – 192.

Cunanan, R. G., Jr., Courey, N. G. and Lippes, J. (1983) Laparoscopic findings in patients with pelvic pain (Review). Am. J. Obstet. Gynecol. 146, 589 – 591.

Dawood, M. Y. (1984) An update on dysmenorrhea. Contemp. Obstet. Gynecol. June, 73 – 94.

Engel, G. L. (1959) 'Psychogenic' pain and the pain-prone patient. Am. J. Med. 36, 899 – 918.

Gross, R. J., Doerr, H. et al. (1980) Borderline syndrome and incest in chronic pelvic pain patients. Int. J. Psychiatr. Med. 10, 79 – 96.

Huffman, J. W. (1983) Dyspareunia of vulvo-vaginal origin: causes and management. Postgrad. Med. 73, 287 – 295.

Kresch, A. J., Seifer, D. B. et al. (1984) Laparoscopy in 100 women with chronic pelvic pain. Obstet. Gynecol. 64, 672 – 674.

Malinak, R. L. (1984) Operative management of pelvic pain. In: J. J. Sciarra (Ed.), Gynecology and Obstetrics, Vol. 1, revised edition. Harper and Row, Philadelphia.

Melzack, R. (1975) The McGill Pain Questionnaire: major properties and scoring methods. Pain 1, 277 – 290.

Owen, P. R. (1984) Prostaglandin synthetase inhibitors in the treatment of primary dysmenorrhea: outcome trials reviewed. Am. J. Obstet. Gynecol. 148, 96 – 103.

Pickles, V. R., Hall, W. J., Best, F. A. et al. (1965) Prostaglandin levels in endometrium and menstrual fluid from normal and dysmenorrheic subjects. Br. J. Obstet. Gynaecol. 72, 185 – 195.

Ranney, B. (1980) Endometriosis: pathogenesis, symptoms and findings. Clin. Obstet. Gynecol. 23, 865 – 874.

Reamy, K. J. (1982) The treatment of vaginismus by the gynecologist: an eclectic approach. Obstet. Gynecol. 59, 58 – 62.

Renaer, M. (1980) Chronic pelvic pain without obvious pathology in women: personal observations and a review of the problem. Eur. J. Obstet., Gynecol. Reprod. Biol. 10, 415 – 463.

Renaer, M. and Guzinski, G. M. (1978) Pain in gynecologic practice. Pain 5, 305 – 331.

Reuler, J. B., Girard, D. E. and Nardone D. A. (1980) The chronic pain syndrome, misconceptions and management. Ann. Intern. Med. 93, 558 – 596.

Roberts, W. and Dockery, J. L. (1984) Operative and conservative treatment of tubo-ovarian abscess due to pelvic inflammatory disease. South. Med. J. 77, 860 – 863.

Schaupp, J. B. (1962) Pelvic varicose veins and varicocele. Surg. Clin. North Am. 42, 975 – 984.

Shafer, M. B., Irwin, C. E. and Sweet, R. L. (1982) Acute salpingitis in the adolescent female (review). J. Pediatr. 100, 339 – 350.

Slocumb, J. C. (1984) Neurological factors in chronic pelvic pain: trigger points and the abdominal-pelvic pain syndrome. Am. J. Obstet. Gynecol. 149, 536 – 543.

Stangel, J. J. and Kwon, T. H. (1984) Pelvic adhesions. II. Management and prevention. The Female Patient 9, 25 – 32.

Steege, J. F. (1984) The evaluation and treatment of women with pelvic pain. In: J. J. Sciarra (Ed.), Obstetrics and Gynecology, Vol. 6. Harper and Row, Philadelphia, pp. 1 – 11.

Taylor, H. C. (1961) The syndrome of pelvic pain in women. Aust. N.Z. J. Obstet. Gynaecol. 1, 5 – 16.

Thomason, J. L. (1984) Pelvic inflammatory disease: diagnosis and management. The Female Patient 9, 38 – 56.

Burrows/Elton/Stanley (eds.) Handbook of Chronic Pain Management
© *1987 Elsevier Science Publishers B.V. (Biomedical Divison)*

34

The neurosurgeon and chronic pain

B. S. NASHOLD, Jr.[1] and BRIAN P. BROPHY[2]

[1]*Department of Neurological Surgery, Duke University Medical Center, Durham, North Carolina, U.S.A. and* [2]*Department of Surgery, Flinders Medical Centre, Bedford Park, South Australia 5042, Australia*

> '*Chronic pain in man is sustained by central mechanisms which differ significantly from that signalling and providing awareness of acute noxious stimuli.*'

Sweet 1980

Introduction

The treatment of the chronic pain syndrome is one of the most challenging aspects of neurosurgery as well as its greatest frustration. Historically, neurosurgery has had a direct commitment to the treatment of pain beginning with the development of the spinal cordotomy with surgical section of the lateral spinothalamic tract. The spinothalamic cordotomy was based on the neuroanatomical fact that this tract is known to carry noxious stimuli to the brain. Recent neuroanatomical studies have revealed additional pain pathways, some very old such as the paleothalamic or spinoreticular pathways. The multiplicity of these pain pathways probably explains the recurrence of pain after a cordotomy and why failure can occur if the neurosurgeon considers only a unitary approach to the treatment of pain.

Patients and physicians are often perplexed by pain which is referred to anesthetic regions of the body, and phantom pain still remains an enigma. Many kinds of chronic pain are the result of deafferentation. The resulting pain is due to a partial or complete interruption of sensory input into the central nervous system. Thalamic pain and pain of brachial plexus avulsion are prime examples of deafferentation pain, one due to a lesion in the sensory thalamus and the other to a disturbance of secondary neurons in the dorsal horn which have lost their connections with their peripheral receptors. The patients with these pain disorders often suffer intense, burning pain in a region of the body where sensation may be absent or greatly disturbed.

Evaluation of the patient with chronic pain

The most difficult decision the neurosurgeon must make is at what point to intervene with a patient with chronic pain. Most of the time the cause of the painful syndrome is self evident from the clinical history and examination. The time to think of neurosurgical treatment is at that point when addictive drugs are being considered. Unfortunately, some of these patients are already taking addictive drugs, and it may be necessary to begin a drug withdrawal program, usually in the setting of a Pain Clinic. A psychological profile in each chronic pain patient is important and necessary, along with a psychiatric evaluation, since half of the patients with chronic pain have an associated depression requiring psychiatric treatment. It should be remembered, even with the relief of the patient's depression the pain syndrome may not be relieved and that this problem will then have to be dealt with. An anesthesiologist skilled in the use of nerve blocks is also important, particularly where the pain originates from injured peripheral nerves. It should be remembered that following traumatic injuries to the peripheral and/or central nervous system, multiple components of the sensory system may be involved in the pain syndrome. It then becomes a 'detective' story to sort out each culprit associated with the pain syndrome so that appropriate neurosurgical treatment can be planned.

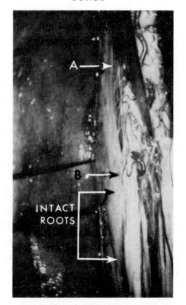

Dorsal root avulsion
Operative photos

Cervical   Conus

INTACT ROOTS

A →

B →

A →

B →

INTACT ROOTS

Dorsal roots avulsed   Dorsal roots avulsed
C 6 - T 1   L 4 - S 1

Fig. 1. Operative exposure of cervical cord (left) and conus medullaris (right). Shows avulsed roots A to B.

Treatment of pain in cervical and conus medullaris avulsion injuries

Disconnection of the dorsal roots from their central spinal cord connection occurs with avulsion injury in the cervical cord and conus medullaris. Until recently, the deafferentation pain that resulted was difficult to relieve until the introduction of the dorsal root entry zone (DREZ) operation in 1976 (Nashold et al. 1976).

Severe long-term pain from avulsion injury occurs in 10% of patients (Nashold et al. 1976). Parry (1980) points out that avulsion injuries are more commonplace and cervical dorsal roots may be avulsed (Fig. 1). The onset of the pain syndrome occurs early after the trauma and may last the lifetime of the patient. The injuries occur in young individuals so that long-term treatment strategies are needed. The neurophysiologic basis for this type of pain still remains speculative, although laboratory experiments in animals suggest a type of deafferentation hypersensitivity involving the secondary neurons of the Rexed layers I and V. Certainly pain represents a central disturbance of sensory integration, the exact nature of which still eludes us.

The recognition of avulsion injury is not difficult, although, due to the multiple injuries these persons sustain, the avulsion injury may not be initially recognized. The patient exhibits a flaccid, senseless arm with pain usually localized to the hand and fingers, especially the thumb and index fingers. Two kinds of pain occur – one, a diffuse aching, crushing sensation in the involved limb and a second more episodic, explosive pain with electrical shooting qualities. Once the pain syndrome becomes evident, corrective and medical treatment may not be successful. All patients should be treated conservatively at first (first 3 months) and the rehabilitation methods of Parry instituted. If this fails and the pain continues, a DREZ operation should be considered along with an intercostal nerve transplant to innervate the biceps muscle, facilitating elbow flexion. We usually carry out the DREZ operation first, closely followed by the reinnervation procedure. Clinical diagnosis can be confirmed by a cervical myelogram which will show various types of traumatic meningomyeloceles (Fig. 2). The technique of the DREZ operation has

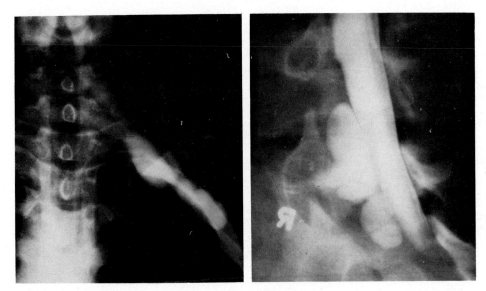

Fig. 2. Myelogram of cervical and lumbar area showing the traumatic meningomyelocele due to avulsion injury.

386

already been reported and the therapeutic lesions are made in the spinal cord with either a thermal electrode (Radionics) or with a laser (Cosman et al. 1984) (Fig. 3).

An avulsion injury in the brachial region is readily recognizable by most physicians familiar with the problem. Less familiar are the avulsion injuries of the dorsal roots of the conus medullaris usually involving L5 or S1 (Nashold and Bullitt 1981). The injury producing this avulsion is a severe fracture dislocation of the pelvic bones associated with trauma. We have seen this type of avulsion also following gunshot wounds in the lower thoracic spine and in one young motorcyclist, a complete avulsion from L1 through the conus was produced by a traumatic hemipelvectomy. The onset of pain in the conus injury is early, as with brachial injury, and the character of the pain similar to that described in the arm. The physician may be thrown off the track, thinking the pain is due to a peripheral nerve injury in the pelvis, but a lumbar meylogram will often reveal a traumatic meningomyelocele as seen in the cervical region, comfirming the diagnosis of an avulsion injury. The combination of pain associated with severe pelvic injury and a myelographic defect should alert the physician to the possibility of a conus medullaris avulsion, and a DREZ operation will also successfully relieve the pain in this group of patients, as it does in the brachial avulsions.

Phantom limb pain

Following amputation, a patient may develop pain in the stump or in the phantom limb. Phantom pain is present associated with root avulsion, the DREZ operation may be satisfactory in relieving the pain. On the other hand, stump pain alone does not respond to this procedure and should not be carried out. Stump pain is best treated by the use of either transcutaneous electrical stimulation or direct nerve stimulation (Saris et al. 1985).

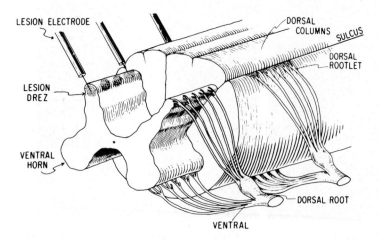

Fig. 3. Schematic drawing of spinal cord showing method of producing DREZ lesions.

Paraplegia and chronic pain

One does not usually associate paraplegia with chronic pain. The spinal cord is permanently interrupted at some level, and the patient suffers from paralysis of the limbs, loss of sensation and sexual function. Unfortunately, 10% of paraplegics suffer from a major pain problem (Nashold and Bullitt 1981). Historically, two patterns of chronic pain occur. The first pattern is the early onset of pain referred to the paralyzed limbs, and it is usually aggravated by touching or rubbing the skin in the dermatomes just above the level of the spinal injury: overfilling of the bladder or bowel may activate the pain. We believe the pain originates from the spinal cord segments just above the level of the complete spinal transection. Trauma is the leading cause of paralysis and the pathological changes in the traumatized cord may extend above the transection. The neural mechanism responsible for the pain may be some form of deafferentation of the secondary sensory spinal cord neurons in the spinal cord segments just above the trauma. On physical examination, a cutaneous zone usually extending just above the level of the spinal injury can be found where various types of tactile stimulation will activate the patient's pain. We call this the dermatomal transition zone, and it may be very narrow or extend over 3 or 4 inches until one reaches the normal cutaneous sensation. These cutaneous changes reflect disturbance in the segment of the cord just above the level of the injury and the DREZ procedure is carried out at this level, usually extending bilaterally over 2 to 3 spinal segments. The second type of pain experienced by paraplegics is one that comes on some years after the spinal injury. The patient may begin to complain of pains radiating to one or both legs and may also exhibit the same hypersensitivity in the dermatome just above the level of the transection, or they may notice that their spinal level is ascending. In our group of patients with this delayed onset of pain, 60% have been found to have an associated intraspinal cord cyst. This can only be discovered with myelographic and/or CT examinations of the area of the spinal cord just above the transection (Fig. 4). The cyst may extend for varying lengths above the level and/or below the level of spinal transection, but it is the spinal segments above the trauma responsible for the genesis of the intractable pain. At the time of the surgical exploration of the spinal cord, evacuation of the cyst should be carried

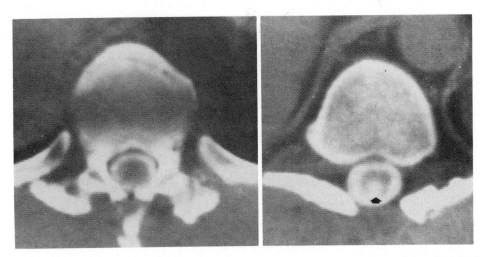

Fig. 4. Thoracic myelogram in traumatic paraplegia combined with CT examination, on left outline of spinal cord, 6 hours later, cyst (arrow) filled with contrast.

388

out with an attempt to establish a permanent type of drainage to prevent its reaccumulation, at the same time a bilateral DREZ operation through the upper three spinal segments above the level of transection is done. Although drainage of the cyst may temporarily reduce the patient's pain, in the long run the pain will return and will require a DREZ procedure later.

Post-herpetic neuralgia

The development of post-herpetic infection in elderly persons is not uncommon; however, a small percentage of these patients develop intractable pain in the distribution of the herpetic cutaneous involvement. This occurs most often in thoracic dermatomes, but it may also appear in cervico-lumbar and in some cases the first division of the trigeminal nerve. Two types of pain are often described in this group of patients. One, a rather deep aching, diffuse type of pain and a second rather sharp, electrical, shooting quality which spreads over the involved dermatome. In the case of the patient with involvement of the ophthalmic division of the trigeminal nerve, there may be a deep aching pain behind the eye and shooting electrical types of shocks over the surface of the scalp, forehead and top of the head. The DREZ operation is almost specific for the shooting type of pain (Friedman et al. 1985). The DREZ operation is done in the dorsal roots involved in the pain. This may include from 3 to 6 dorsal roots. In the case of herpes ophthalmicus, the DREZ coagulations are carried out on the ipsilateral nucleus caudalis from the level of the obex down to the dorsal origins of the C2 dorsal root (Fig. 5). In both cases, approximately three fourths of the patients will get good pain relief sustained for at least periods up to and over 2 years.

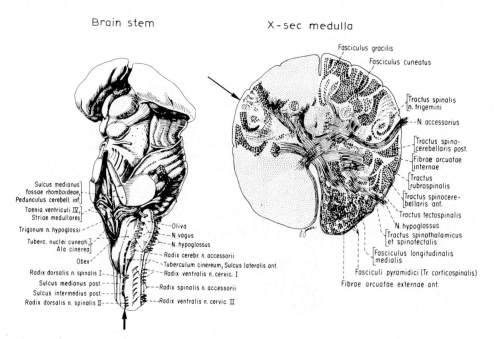

Fig. 5. Arrow indicates DREZ lesion area for caudalis nucleus lesion for facial pain.

Chronic incisional pain

Why a healed surgical incision may become painful is puzzling; if it were a commonplace occurrence, general surgery would soon become a lost art. As a general rule, it is rare for an incision to become painful over the long term. There are three areas of the body, however, in which chronic pain may originate after surgery incisions – the posterior cervical triangle, the thoracic area and the lower abdominal-inguinal area. Surgical exploration of the posterior cervical triangle is often carried out to remove an enlarged lymph node for diagnosis. On rare occasions, the surgery may result in injury to the branch of the spinal accessory nerve to the trapezius muscle (Woodhall 1957). Persistent chronic pain is a consequence of this along with partial or incomplete paralysis of the trapezius and drooping of the shoulder. The patients complain bitterly of localized pain in the neck in the area of the incision, plus diffuse pain around the shoulder joint. It is important for the operating surgeon to recognize the syndrome early and refer patients to a neurosurgeon for re-exploration. At the time of re-exploration, it may be necessary to resuture the nerve or there may be a constricting suture found around the nerve itself, and this must be removed and a decision made as to whether to carry out end-to-end anastomosis. If the condition is not recognized early (within 3 months), then chronic changes occur with atrophy of the trapezius muscle, scar tissue around the shoulder joint, and at that time only a selective dorsal rhizotomy or a DREZ operation may be successful in reducing the pain. It will not, of course, correct the weakness of the trapezius muscle. So the key here is early diagnosis and treatment of this condition.

Thoracotomy incisions also become painful and the pain difficult to treat. Indeed, prevention may be the answer to this chronic pain syndrome (White and Kjellberg 1973). The incision usually parallels one of the upper ribs and may extend from the posterior axillary line anteriorly to the anterior chest wall. Localized peripheral nerve blocks, either at the level of the dorsal ganglion or the intercostal nerve, do not result in pain relief in these individuals. The patient's description of the pain may give us a clue to the etiology. They often describe it as occurring deep within the chest wall over a much larger area than the incision. The pain may be described as burning, cutting with electrical shooting quality radiating into the anterior thoracic region. I believe that the pain is of central origin due to stretching of the intercostal nerves when the chest cavity is open. It might be prevented by relaxing the tension on the retractor during the operation. Most surgical treatments are unsuccessful, and our attempts to control thoracotomy pain with a DREZ operation have not been successful. So the answer as far as the etiology and treatment of this painful condition is still unclear. It is probably best prevented by being very careful not to produce a wide gap in the rib cage at the time of the surgery, or perhaps to release the retractors during the surgical procedure for a few minutes to allow structures to regain their normal configuration and blood supply.

The lower abdominal region is another area prone to develop chronic incisional pain, particularly following incisions into the inguinal area. The etiology may be very similar to the pain after surgery in the posterior cervical triangle, in that the ilioinguinal nerve becomes entrapped in a suture or the nerve is injured during the surgical procedure. Again, prevention is probably the best way to cure in these individuals whereas attempts at nerve anastomosis or neurolysis or dorsal rhizotomy are unsuccessful in relieving the pain. Transcutaneous electrical stimulation may be helpful in ameliorating the pain from an incision and can be used for long periods without complication.

Coccygeal pain

Chronic coccygeal pain can occur following localized trauma to the coccyx due to a fall or after an abdominal-peroneal resection for carcinoma (Loeser 1972). Post-traumatic coccygeal pain due to a fall may be aggravated by surgical removal of the tip of the coccyx, not a recommended surgical operation. The pain is localized to the buttocks and may radiate into the perineum. Tenderness can be elicited by palpation over the sacral bone, particularly at its lower end. The patient has difficulty sitting for any length of time and even prolonged walking may be uncomfortable. Localized nerve blocks using anesthetic agents are helpful in the diagnosis and may indicate which dorsal roots must be sectioned to produce relief of pain.

As a general rule, surgical section of S3,4 and 5 will relieve the post-traumatic pain; however, if the S2 dorsal root is also involved, as determined by nerve blocks, section of this root can be

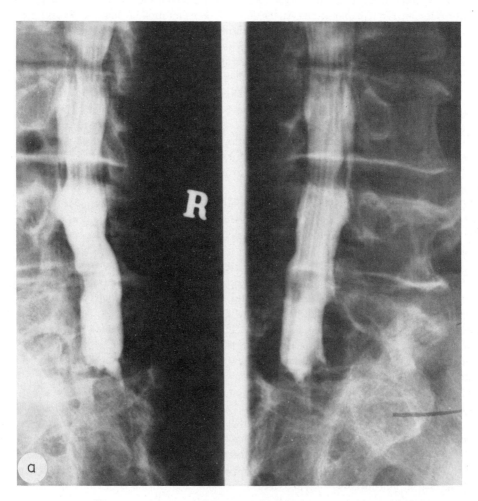

Fig. 6. A 69-year-old male. Two previous laminectomies. Recurrent left sciatica. (a) Myelogram – non-filling of left L5 nerve root. (b) CAT scan – mass ventral to theca on left side separated from scar posteriorly by low density epidural fat. Diagnosis: disc prolapse

done without serious consequence to bladder function (Bohm and Franksson 1958/1959; Bohm 1962).

The pain in the coccygeal region after abdominal-peroneal resection for carcinoma may be of two types. In one, the pain experienced is sharp in nature and localized to the coccygeal tip with reference into the rectal region. This usually occurs immediately following the surgical procedure and one can think of it as a phantom rectal pain. The pain is not related to metastasis or localized invasion of the tissue by the carcinoma.

The pain associated with carcinomatous involvement of the peroneal and coccygeal region is more diffuse in nature and may spread into the upper thigh, and the pain may be referred into the upper thighs and into the anterior peroneal region. Examination will reveal a diffuse tenderness over the tip of the coccyx, the perineum and perirectal region. A body CT scan of the lower pelvis will show the extent of recurrent tumor, usually anterior to the coccygeal bone. It is often necessary to section the dorsal roots from S1 to S5 to relieve pain from carcinomatous invasion. Some bladder dysfunction will occur, but can be minimized by leaving one dorsal S1 root intact. It is important for the neurosurgeon to use the operating microscope to identify the

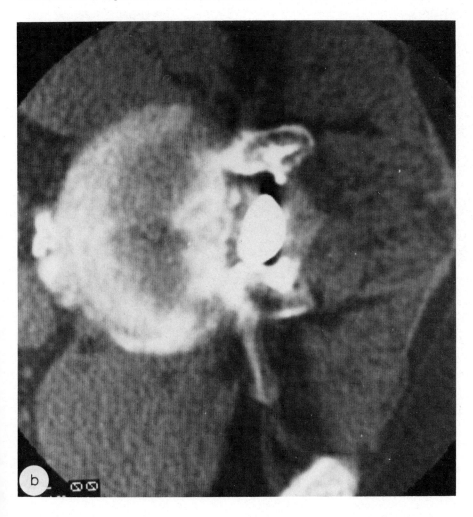

dorsal and ventral roots after he exposes the caudal sac of the sacrum by unroofing the coccyx. If the S1 dorsal root is to be sectioned, and this should be determined by previous localized nerve blocks, the removal of the L5 lamina will facilitate the surgical exposure of the S1 dorsal root. The neurosurgeon can distinguish the dorsal and ventral roots under the operative microscope, we always electrically stimulate the dorsal and ventral roots to confirm the motor root localization and to spare it from the surgical section. Over half of the patients will experience good pain reduction following dorsal root section carried out in this manner.

Failed spinal surgery

The patient with persisting pain following multiple low back operations is a daunting prospect for further management. A specific diagnosis is frequently wanting and further surgery statistically has little chance of success (Waddell et al. 1979). The treating physician is often

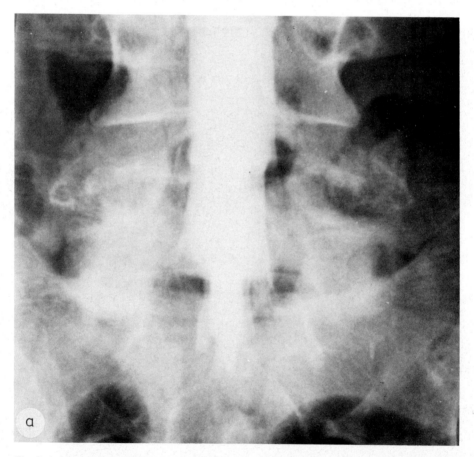

Fig. 7. A 46-year-old male. Two previous right lumbosacral discectomies. Acute right sciatica with S1 signs (a) Myelogram – non-filling of S1 nerve root on right side. (b) CAT scan – non-filling of S1 nerve root due to a homogeneous mass of tissue sited extradurally and contiguous with the laminal defect and the extraspinal scar. Diagnosis: root fibrosis.

reduced to using methods designed to help the patient understand and cope with his pain and modifying factors commonly psychosocial in nature which are aggravating the situation. These patients frequently have had a large number of treating doctors and records and radiology are often misplaced. The original indication for the surgery is difficult at times to establish. Workman's compensation and other third party insurers are or have been involved in a high proportion of cases. Assessment is further complicated by the fact that standard investigations such as plain radiographs, myelography and CT scanning can only provide limited insight into the problem.

Examination of such patients must be meticulous and is particularly directed at the identification of abnormal neurological signs and hysterical features. The presence of neurological signs indicates a wide range of possible causes (persisting compression, root injury or arachnoiditis) and the possibility that the pain may be deafferent (Tasker et al. 1980) or neurogenic in nature. Overt hysterical features are frequently present in pending compensation cases and not uncommonly persist following settlement. Such features make assessment extremely difficult and in general should make one wary of the use of invasive techniques in the further management of

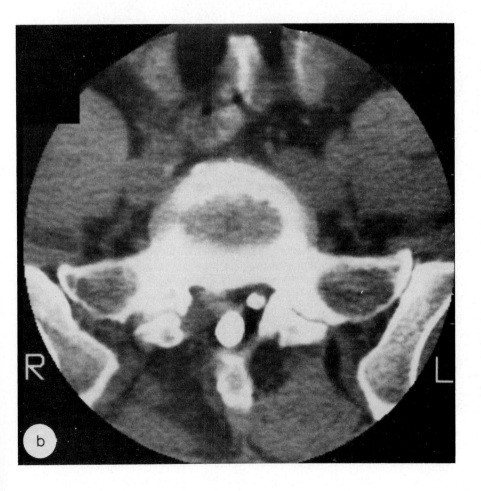

the patient. Psychiatric evaluation is important and pain neurosis (Engel 1959; Blumer 1978), should be readily identified by neurosurgeons practicing in this area. It must be remembered that pain is a symptom and psychological factors play a major part in its perception. Depression either as a primary disorder or as a secondary feature of chronic pain may be an important factor in the presentation of the patient.

CAUSES OF FAILED SURGERY

Recurrent prolapse or prolapse at another level is an important cause of persisting pain following spinal surgery. It is important however when considering the question of recurrent disc prolapse to establish that the patient in fact had a disc excision (Fig. 6). The term laminectomy is at times a true description of the procedure, meaning that the nerve root was simply decompressed, but more commonly indicates that the patient had a discectomy. If the patient had a previous discec-

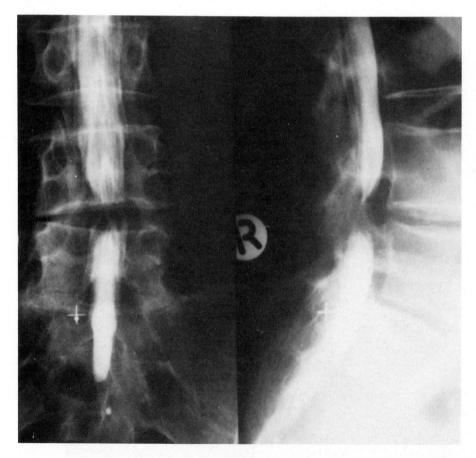

Fig. 8. A 55-year-old female. Two previous explorations of the L4-5 space. Second exploration of L4-5 performed bilaterally via an interlaminar extradural approach with difficulty due to scar. No disc prolapse detected. No pain relief. Diagnosis: central disc rupture treated by laminectomy and transdural excision.

tomy recurrent disc prolapse is less likely. Exploration on these occasions is frequently negative apart from the finding of dense scar in relation to the nerve root (Fig. 7). The clinical picture of root fibrosis can mimic that due to recurrent disc prolapse and myelography cannot differentiate these two conditions (Irstam 1984). The CT scan appearances can also be very similar. However, if the abnormality deforming the nerve root or in the vicinity of the nerve root is contiguous with the operative scar posteriorly it is more likely to be root fibrosis. Likewise if it is separated from the operative scar by epidural fat it is more likely to be disc material (Figs. 6 and 7). A ventral abnormality is of course more likely to be prolapsed disc than scar if the previous surgery was laminectomy alone. Intravenous contrast may be useful in differentiating scar from prolapse (Schubiger et al. 1983).

Re-exploration of a disc space is difficult and carries a greatly increased risk of damage to the nerve root and must be done with great care. Magnification will be helpful. Because of this, when the abnormality extends medially consideration should be given to a transdural approach. At times a transdural approach is mandatory (Fig. 8).

Persisting pain may also be due to an incorrect primary diagnosis or inadequate treatment of a primary disorder. All too frequently it is apparent that the initial surgery was performed for back pain alone. In this respect it is important to remember the admonition of Sternbach (Sternbach 1977): the spinal surgeon . . . 'who keeps firmly in mind that his primary task is not to relieve pain but to treat pathology will avoid being coerced into inappropriate intervention by the patient's insistence on relief'. Specific diagnosis in this group of patients with back pain alone remains difficult and requires careful consideration of a wide range of possibilities (Bogduk and Long 1980). It is not surprising that spinal surgery frequently fails. There has been increasing emphasis on the role of the apophyseal joints as a cause of back pain and this needs consideration (Fig. 9). Neurosurgeons in general have not accepted the concept of discogenic pain or that disc degeneration as characterised by discography is a likely cause of pain. It is possible however that central disc ruptures can cause intractable back pain without neurological signs (Fig. 10).

In the area of inadequate treatment of the primary disorder laminectomy performed for canal stenosis may fail to produce complete relief of pain because of failure to relieve lateral canal stenosis or foramenal stenosis. Laminectomy for spondylolisthesis and spondylolysis may not succeed because of failure to remove the pseudoarthrosis associated with the spondylolysis (Jayson 1984).

Arachnoiditis (Burton 1978; Shaw et al. 1978), may be one of the factors in persisting pain following spinal surgery but this disorder has most frequently been associated with the use of oil based contrast media. The condition varies in severity from a relatively focal involvement of several roots of the cauda equina to a more extensive involvement of the whole of the lumbar theca and finally a progressive disorder involving the spinal cord as well. The incidence of this problem is declining due to the more widespread use of water soluble contrast media. Intrathecal steroids and neurolysis of the cauda equina have been advocated but management of this disorder remains difficult. A percentage of cases may obtain relief from epidural stimulation (Urban and Nashold 1978).

Finally, it should be stated that persisting pain and disability may be the result of pending compensation or other third party claims. In this group in particular surgery should only be performed for the most clearcut indications. Even then results will at times be disappointing. Great care needs to be taken in the assessment and management of such individuals.

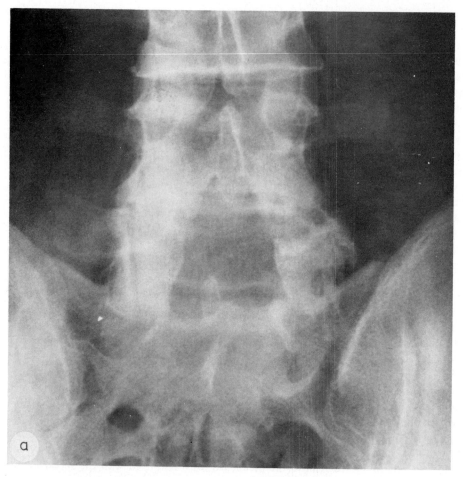

Fig. 9. A 63-year-old male. Laminectomy for low back and left leg pain. No signs. No relief of pain. (a) Plain X-ray reveals gross osteoarthritis of the left L5-S1 apophyseal joint. (b) Needle positioned for facet arthrography and injection of local anesthetic and corticosteroid. Short-term pain relief provided.

MANAGEMENT

Further surgery will be advisable in only a small percentage of cases who have had multiple low back operations. The most reliable indicator of success will be careful clinical assessment supported by a review of all the available information combined with carefully selected additional investigations. Differential epidural blocks may be helpful (Cherry et al. 1985).

Psychiatric help and involvement of a variety of social agencies will at times be important in helping the majority of these patients to live with an untreatable problem. Indiscriminate use of narcotics is to be deprecated and provision of medication should be under the supervision of a clinic well versed in the assessment and management of chronic pain patients.

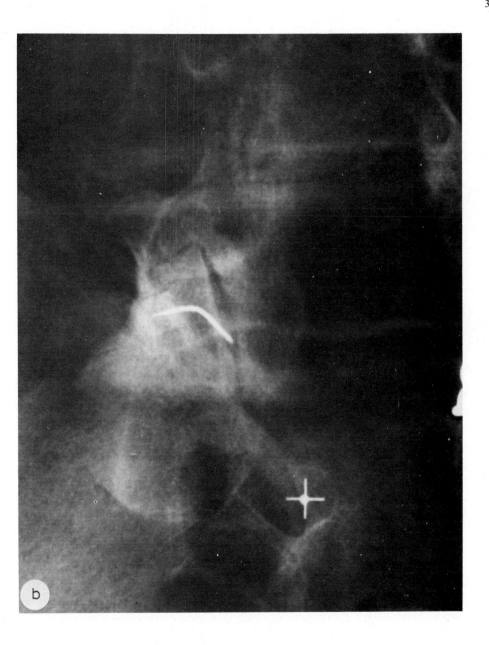

b

With the multidisciplined support provided by a Pain Clinic the patient will be helped to gain insight into his problem. Transcutaneous stimulation will give symptomatic relief in a percentage of cases and when all conservative measures have been exhausted, consideration may be given to dorsal column stimulation. Approximately 30% of unselected back patients with low back pain following multiple operations will obtain significant pain relief for a period with this technique (Urban and Nashold 1978).

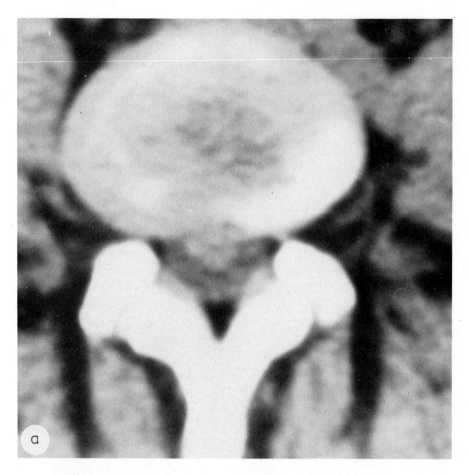

Fig. 10. A 64-year-old female. Intractable back and leg pain. CAT scans (a, b) reveal a central disc prolapse at the L4-5 interspace.

The gains achieved in management of this group of patients are likely to be small and in a significant percentage of such cases the support of the Pain Clinic is all that can be offered. This highlights the need for greater care in the assessment of patients for spinal surgery and in the performance of that surgery. Ideally surgeons involved in spinal surgery should have an ongoing association or commitment to a Pain Clinic dealing with failed spinal surgery so as to be aware of the many problems associated with this difficult group of patients.

References

Blumer, D. (1978) Psychiatric and psychological aspects of chronic pain. Clin. Neurosurg. 25, 276 – 283.
Bogduk, N. and Long, D. M. (1980) Percutaneous lumbar medial branch neurotomy. Spine 5, 193 – 197.
Bohm, E. (1962) Late results of sacral rhizotomy in coccygodynia. Acta Chir. Scand. 123, 6 – 8.

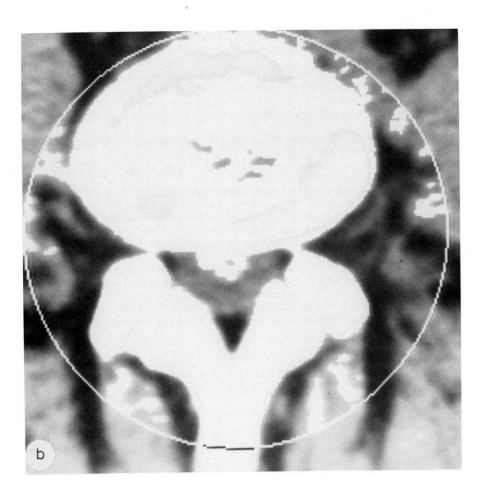

b

Bohm, E. and Franksson, C. (1958/1959) Coccygodynia and sacral rhizotomy. Acta Chir. Scand. 116, 268–274.

Burton, C. (1978) Lumbosacral arachnoiditis. Spine 3, 24–30.

Cherry, D. A., Gourlay, G. K., McLachlan, M. and Cousins, M. J. (1985) Diagnostic epidural opioid blockade and chronic pain: preliminary report. Pain 21, 143–152.

Cosman, E. R., Nashold, B. S. and Ovelmen-Levitt, J. (1984) Theoretical aspects of radiofrequency lesions in the dorsal root entry zone. Neurosurgery 15, 945–950.

Engel, G. L. (1959) Psychogenic pain and the pain-prone patient. Am. J. Med. 26, 899–918.

Friedman, A. H., Nashold, B. S. and Ovelmen-Levitt, J. (1985) Dorsal root entry zone lesions for the treatment of post-herpetic neuralgia. J. Neurosurg. 62, 72–76.

Gill, G. G., Manning, J. C. and White, H. L. (1955) Surgical treatment of spondylolisthesis without spine fusion. J. Bone Joint Surg. 37A, 493–518.

Irstam, L. (1984) Differential diagnosis of recurrent lumbar disc herniation and postoperative deformation by myelography. Spine 9, 759–763.

Jayson, M. I. V. (1984) Difficult diagnoses in back pain. Br. Med. J. 288, 740–741.

Loeser, J. (1972) Dorsal rhizotomy for relief of chronic pain. J. Neurosurg. 36, 745–750.

Nashold, B. S., Jr. and Bullitt, E. (1981) Dorsal root entry zone lesions to control pain in paraplegics. J. Neurosurg. 55, 414–419.

Nashold, B. S. and Ostdahl, R. H. (1979) Dorsal root entry zone lesions for pain relief. J. Neurosurg. 51, 59–69.

Nashold, B. S., Urban, B. and Zorub, D. S. (1976) Pain relief by focal destruction of the substantia gelatinosa of Rolando. In: J. J. Bonica et al. (Eds.), Advances in Pain Research and Therapy, Vol. 1. Raven Press, New York, pp. 959 – 963.

Parry, W. C. B. (1980) Pain in avulsion lesions of the brachial plexus. Pain 9, 41 – 53.

Saris, S. C., Iacono, R. P. and Nashold, B. S. (1985) Dorsal root entry zone lesions for post-amputation pain. J. Neurosurg. 62, 72 – 76.

Schubiger, O. and Valavanis, A. (1983) Post-operative lumbar C.T. technique. Results and indications. AJNR 4, 595 – 597.

Shaw, M. D. M., Russell, J. A. and Grossart, K. W. (1978) The changing pattern of spinal arachnoiditis. J. Neurol. Neurosurg. Psychiatry 41, 97 – 107.

Sternbach, R. A. (1977) Psychological aspects of chronic pain. Clin. Orthopaed. Relat. Res. 129, 150 – 155.

Sweet, W. H. (1980) Central mechanisms of chronic pain (neuralgias and certain other neurogenic pains). In: J. J. Bonica et al. (Eds.), Pain, Vol. 58. Raven Press, New York, pp. 287 – 305.

Tasker, R. R., Organ, L. W. and Hawrylyshyn, P. (1980) Deafferentation and causalgia. In: J. J. Bonica et al. (Eds.), Pain, Vol. 58. Raven Press, New York, pp. 305 – 329.

Urban, B. J. and Nashold, B. S. (1978) Percutaneous epidural stimulation of the spinal cord for relief of pain. J. Neurosurg. 48, 323 – 328.

Waddell, G., Kummel, E. G., Lotto, W. N., Graham, J. D., Hall, H. and McCulloch, J. A. (1979) Failed lumbar disc surgery and repeat surgery following industrial injuries. J. Bone Joint Surg. 61A, 201 – 206.

White, J. C. and Kjellberg, R. N. (1973) Posterior spinal rhizotomy: a substitute for cordotomy in the relief of localized pain in patients with normal life expectancy. Neurochir. 16, 141 – 170.

Woodhall, B. (1957) Operative injury to the accessory nerve in the posterior cervical triangle. AMA Arch. Surg. 74, 122 – 127.

Burrows/Elton/Stanley (eds.) Handbook of Chronic Pain Management
© *1987 Elsevier Science Publishers B.V. (Biomedical Division)*

35

Sports activity for patients with chronic pain problems

R. PETER WELSH

*Sports Medicine Clinic, Orthopaedic and Arthritic Hospital, 43 Wellesley Street East, Room 319,
Toronto, Ontario M4Y 1H1, Canada*

Introduction

Regular sport and recreational activity brings to the healthy individual certain undisputed benefits, both physical and psychological. To the sufferer from chronic pain, these advantages become even more important as they may be the only positive features in the daily routine otherwise dominated by their malady. To many such individuals the overwhelming influence in their life in day to day activity is their disease and the pain state that dictates, indeed controls, their whole pattern of living.

If however, a favourable alteration can be effected in their activity level a whole chain of events can be initiated and an overall enhancement of the day to day standard of living achieved. The single most important factor contributing to this turn around has to be one of attitude. Beaten down, as it were, by their illness both physically and emotionally, an individual must perceive that continuing pain is not an indicator of continuing harm, that the presence of pain does not necessarily indicate an advancement of the disease process and that aggravation of their pain in the course of activity is not necessarily harmful. In order to make this quantum step in living with their pain problem, an individual has to accept that with any increase in the tempo of activity, there must necessarily be an alteration in the sensations that they experience. Some of these can be painful as in any athlete undertaking a conditioning programme. A period of adjustment has to be experienced as the body accommodates to a new level of activity. Some of these sensations are distressing to the sufferer from chronic pain; and the development of new pain can in itself be a threat. This must at the outset be countered with positive reassurance that such experience is not harmful, is not an indicator of further disease problem, that an exercise programme can be embarked upon with confidence and that real benefits will accrue from such activity.

Therefore, at the very outset, if a major physical or recreational programme is to be undertaken, it is important that the patient be totally reassured by appropriate physical and laboratory check-up, determining that the individual is indeed fit to undertake such a programme and that the programme itself will be nonharmful. Indeed, it is most important that any programme be tailored to the individual needs of the participant. Support through the initial weeks is vital as these physical discomforts which naturally arise and, with them, the anxieties they evoke must be handled sympathetically but yet encouragingly in order to have the subject continue with the programme. It is through this make and break phase that support must be sustained until measureable benefit with lessening discomfort can be perceived by the participant.

Here the benefits of 'group' therapy are undoubted as like 'sufferers' struggle with similar difficulties. Thus exercise undertaken in a group setting can be most beneficial, but care must be taken that invidious comparisons are not drawn by an individual who perceives that his or her individual progress is less than that of a peer. Truly does the individuality of each participant's problem have to be emphasized.

Advantages of an activity programme

There are essentially four beneficial aspects to any activity programme:

1) Physical benefits – improved overall physical fitness: cardiorespiratory and musculoskeletal.
2) Psychological – improved self-esteem and body image.
3) Better handling of anxiety and stress
4) Reduction of depression

PHYSICAL BENEFITS

Enhanced cardiorespiratory and musculoskeletal fitness brings distinct benefits to all bodily function. At the cellular level an accelerated level of metabolism only enhances the overall efficiency of the body unit, and as a consequence of improved oxygenation of the tissues, one sees an improvement in the general body processes.

From a systems viewpoint, digestive, urological, and neurological benefits are obvious with enhanced appetite, regular bowel habits, improved renal function and healthy sleep patterns. Musculoskeletal improvement is shown in improved muscle strength, durability and flexibility.

This combination of advantages combines to support the patient with a chronic pain problem. The obvious physical improvement in form and function particularly enhances the patient's sense of self-worth, or overall sense of body image. Such physical reinforcement of the perceived benefit is so vital to the sustainment of the physical exercise programme. Thus a programme of physical exercise must emphasize general body conditioning and be combined with dietary measures for weight control, as well as attention to correct dress and deportment. Changes in these areas can be so vital to reinforcing the overall sense of improvement.

Physical benefits and pain control. Pain is essentially a perceived 'response' to peripherally mediated stimuli of an obnoxious type. These stimuli and the response are subject to modification at different levels in the pain pathway. This may be either peripherally where the pain is evoked, or at an intermediate level in the course of its transmission, or centrally at the level of the cerebral cortex.

Physical activity stimulates muscle and joint proprioceptors and the central projection of this information through the spinothalamic pathways increases activity within the reticular neuronal loops (Shephard 1974; Phillips and Porter 1977). This competes as it were, with other peripheral-ly mediated stimuli as from a source of chronic pain, the gate being blocked and the intensity of the pain stimuli reaching the cerebral cortex modified. This effect is maximal during the period of intense activity – indeed, all noxious stimuli may be blocked out completely under times of great stress. For example, in the heat of battle, extremely valiant deeds are undertaken despite major painful wounds having been sustained, it not being until the action is complete that the 'hero' becomes aware of his injuries. It is under situations such as these of intense pro-vocation that great feats of superhuman character may be performed without the slightest inhibi-tion, or even recognition of pain or discomfort. Similarly, the patient suffering from a chronic pain syndrome may undertake vigorous physical activity and during the course of that activity the chronic pain which previously dominated their perceptions is completely overshadowed.

Unfortunately, the pain will return following discontinuance of the activity, but the benefit is by no means confined to the period of that activity. For it is most important in the manage-ment of any chronic pain problem that the pattern of regular pain be broken. If the pattern of pain can be broken in a routine manner it may be possible to desensitize the individual by a regular programme of sports activity. Over a period of time, the strength of the chronic pain syndrome and its disabling features are gradually ameliorated and the level of intensity of the pain stimulus may subside.

Chemical responses.   Chemical factors may further enhance this process. The stimulant action of drugs such as amphetamines is well recognized, and with increasing evidence that some disorders of affect are due to disturbance of catecholamine metabolism (Maas 1972; Schildkraut 1973) the effect upon a chronic pain sufferer becomes very important.

Vigorous physical activity leads to a release of both norepinephrine and epinephrine partly in the active regions of the brain but also at the sympathetic nerve endings which secrete norepinephrine plus small amounts of epinephrine. The adrenal medulla is a further source of catecholamine production with increased production of epinephrine with any stressful activity, or indeed with any fall in the blood glucose level below $2.8 - 3.9$ mmol/l (Shephard 1982).

For prolonged activity, that is constant exercise for longer than an hour, or exercise at an in-tensity level exceeding 70% of maximal oxygen uptake, or with the superadded stimulus of com-petition, measureable elevation of catecholamine levels definitely occurs (Shephard 1982). It is tempting therefore, to suggest that physical activity increases arousal much as if one had taken a shot of Dexedrine (Dextroamphetamine sulphate). Indeed, the internal secretion of chemicals may contribute to the 'runner's high', although quantitative elevation is difficult to establish during moderate exercise. Our inability though to measure elevated levels of these chemicals may well be a reflection of our inability to measure the substances accurately with the techniques cur-rently available as well as being a consequence of their extremely rapid breakdown.

The interaction of these mechanisms undoubtedly plays a role in the processes that modify pain, but so too does the activity of a hypothalamic centre. Just as electric stimulation of these regions of the brain can persuade animals to run to exhaustion and even death (Anend 1961), humans also seem to engage in physical activity until the hypothalamic centre is somewhat satiated. The mechanism of activation of this system is still uncertain but includes impulses such as the hypothalamic temperature as well as information from glucose receptors and feedback loops from the limb proprioceptors. This 'normally' regulated mechanism can be modified, that is, reset depending on the nature of the combined input. Elevation of the threshold may bestow great benefits to the overall system by blocking out noxious stimuli thus protecting the individual from these otherwise aversive influences.

These physical and chemical responses therefore may be extremely important in the mediation of the process whereby physical activity can exercise a positive benefit upon the individual by interfering with the normal pain processes.

PSYCHOLOGICAL BENEFITS

Physical activity exerts a very positive benefit upon the chronic pain sufferer by improving the sense of self-esteem and body image, reduces anxiety levels and modifies unfavourably depressive tendencies.

Self-esteem and body image. Adequate self-esteem is an important facet of mental health. With a state of chronic pain self-worth is often at a low ebb but this may be reversed to some extent by regular physical activity. The improved capacity of an individual to undertake physical or mental work as well as the physical improvement in form and physique are seen as visible confirmation of improvement and a definite enhancement of self-esteem accrues. These improvements in body image encourage compliance with an exercise programme and the combining process further assists in breaking the pain cycle. With reduction in pain and with improved self-esteem, the cloud of negativism which enshrouds the pain sufferer begins to lift.

Anxiety. Anxiety surrounding the illness and the impact such illness has on lifestyle, career ambitions and recreational programmes may be modified by a regular exercise programme. The fact that activity, previously not considered as possible is now regularly undertaken, is associated with improvement in the level of overall health and is attended by an improvement in self-image, assists greatly in alleviating anxieties and makes easier goals set in other areas.

Perceived health. A whole new perception of a chronic illness may thus be presented by the ability to participate in a regular exercise programme previously not considered possible. The illness is no longer perceived as all pervasive and restricting but rather something than can be lived with, and not just lived around.

Depression. The overwhelming all pervasive nature of a chronic pain state and the underlying disease with which it is associated is inevitably associated with a state of reactive depression. It has been shown that regular physical activity can be particularly helpful in countering the reactive depression seen in conditions such as myocardial infarction (Kavanagh et al. 1975). It is only reasonable to suggest that positive benefits will accrue in the chronic pain sufferer who has also suffered the same difficulties with regard to sexual problems, feelings of inadequacy in the work place, or interactional difficulties with family and workmates, combined with the associated loss of personal confidence.

A turn around in this state of mind may be effected by regular sports participation. The arousal and improvement of body image associated with such regular exercise programme bring welcome relief from all these natural reactions.

THE NATURE OF THE INDIVIDUAL RECREATIONAL PROGRAMME

The actual programme undertaken for any particular individual will necessarily need to be modified by several factors. These include the nature of the pain pattern, its location, duration, intensity, and the nature of provocative factors. The underlying disease process itself will affect the outcome, as will the system involved and the pathologic process, particularly whether it is benign or malignant. Associated problems in other systems such as within the cardiorespiratory or musculoskeletal system will modify the type of programme that can be undertaken. Finally, and perhaps most importantly, the individual and his or her personality type has to be considered together with their particular reaction to the chronic pain state and underlying disease.

Objectives. Goals must be realistic, that is, attainable. Subjective benefits must be felt early and must necessarily be reinforced by objective measureable gain in some tangible form.

This may be in some instances simple, in that regular exercise is associated with less dependence on medication. That is a reduction in both dose and frequency of analgesic or sedative pharmaceuticals. With such early gains, compliance is encouraged and continuance much easier to maintain.

The nature of the pain. The more constant the pain stimulus, the more important does it become to have recourse to a means of relief outside the use of habit forming medications. To break the pain cycle with physical activity, any provocative influences should be minimized and the activity should not induce a rebound phenomenon of intensified pain post-activity. Programmes do indeed have to be tailored to the needs of each individual. Especially is this so if systemic disease otherwise affects the individual's overall capability. Furthermore, the psychological needs of each individual have to be met and any programme must ensure that this aspect be fulfilled as adequately as possible if compliance to continue is to be achieved.

The disease process. Chronic pain is often associated with chronic disease. Painful diseases involving the musculoskeletal system, such as arthritis, are associated with physical limitations because of joint involvement producing not only pain but limitation of motion and function. Involvement of peripheral joints of the upper or lower extremity may preclude running, jumping, or throwing sports such as jogging, tennis, and squash. Swimming, however, becomes an ideal substitute with the body supported in the water and joint stress minimized unless the shoulder is significantly involved.

Those with spine dysfunction, chronic neck and back pain, should be maintained on a regular programme which emphasizes postural corrective exercises, abdominal strengthening and flexibility routines. Sudden explosive effort is to be avoided as in the racquet sports, but cycling, swimming and running can all be incorporated into a programme.

Difficulties en route. A sense of realism has to be instilled in the participant in any regular physical fitness programme. For such activity is in its own right attended by problems commonly known as overuse syndromes. Such conditions as bursitis of the shoulder, tendinitis of the elbow, knee or ankle produce a morbidity and discouragement factor of their own. These must be managed effectively as they arise lest they interfere with the goals of the overall programme.

An increase in the level of pain may be experienced both during and following exercise. It is essential that the underlying disease state be so defined that no possibility of increased damage or harm can accrue from the sports programme undertaken. Thus, sufferers from chronic arthritis of the knees would have increased pain of the 'harmful' kind were they to embark on a jogging programme, whereas muscle soreness and aching seen after a programme of aerobics and cycle training would be an indicator of increased workload but of a 'nonharmful' type.

For those of hypochondriacal disposition, the sensations regarding cardiorespiratory function associated with an aerobic exercise are enough in their own right to discourage continuance of an active programme. A programme of lesser intensity must be planned for such individuals with supportive encouragement as well as guidance in the activity itself.

Physical programmes can thus be planned for each individual based on his or her own particular physical limitations, the genesis of their pain process, and the nature of the underlying disease. Specific requirements of the individual must also be met. So planned, a gratifying response can be seen in the improved quality of life which these individuals may enjoy.

Conclusion

While the obvious management of any chronic pain syndrome lies in control of the underlying disease process, such control unfortunately is often not available. Furthermore, the pain pattern may be so firmly established that conventional treatments with medication and physical remedies lose their efficacy. Supportive benefit is often achieved in the management of the pain state by redirecting the patient's energies, interrupting the pain mechanics and boosting psychologic support by the involvement of the chronic pain sufferer in a regular programme of physical exercise and activity.

References

Anend, B. K. (1961) Nervous regulation of food intake. Physiol. Rev. 41, 677 – 708.

Horvath, S. M. (1967) The physiological stimuli to training in a normal climate. Can. Med. Assoc. J. 96, 791 – 793.

Kavanagh, T., Shephard, R. J. and Tuck, J. A. (1975) Depression after myocardial infarction. Can. Med. Assoc. J. 113, 23 – 27.

Maas, J. W., Fawcett, J. A. and Dekirmenjian, H. (1972) Catecholamine metabolism, depressive illness and drug response. Arch. Gen. Psychiatry 26, 252 – 262.

Phillips, C. G. and Porter, R. (1977) Cortico-Spinal Neurones. Their Role in Movement. Academic Press, New York.

Schildkraut, J. J. (1973) Norepinephrine metabolites as biochemical criteria for classifying depressive disorders and predicting responses to treatment: preliminary findings. Am. J. Psychiatry 130, 695 – 698.

Shephard, R. J. (1974) Men at Work. Applications of Ergonomics to Performance and Design. C. C. Thomas, Springfield, Ill.

Shephard, R. J. (1982) Exercise Physiology and Biochemistry. Praeger, New York.

Burrows/Elton/Stanley (eds.) Handbook of Chronic Pain Management
© *1987 Elsevier Science Publishers B.V. (Biomedical Division)*

36

The pain center: Development, structure, and dynamics

GERALD M. ARONOFF and JEFFREY M. WAGNER

Boston Pain Center, Spaulding Rehabilitation Hospital, Boston, MA, U.S.A.

Introduction

Pain is so compelling that its experience leads inexorably towards development of methods to alleviate it. Its treatment throughout the ages may have been the best that clinicians could offer at the time, based on the limitations of knowledge, theory, diagnostics, and therapeutics in the variety of disciplines that address the problem of pain. Thus, the multidisciplinary pain center (MPC) may well represent a clinical 'state of the art' for a certain subset of chronic pain patients.

While much has been written on the MPC, most articles are descriptions of individual programs. What is lacking in this body of literature is an overall view of the MPC. This chapter is an attempt to fill that void and will address the MPC as a treatment for chronic pain syndromes. Included in this chapter is a discussion of the theoretical underpinnings and development of MPCs and the similarities and goals of pain centers, in general. We will present a section on the effectiveness of pain centers and the problems inherent in assessing outcome. Finally, we will discuss future trends in pain treatment and how the MPC may fit into these trends. First, however, it is necessary to describe what we mean when we refer to a pain center.

Many types of pain facilities exist: modality-oriented unidisciplinary clinics (TENS, nerve blocks); syndrome-oriented unidisciplinary or multidisciplinary clinics (low back pain, headache); and MPCs. It is this last category that will be the focus of this chapter. While the MPC can be either in-patient or out-patient, we will limit our focus to structured in-patient treatment settings that address problems of chronic non-malignant pain. Crue and Pinsky (1981) have referred to this type of pain problem as the Chronic Intractable Benign Pain Syndrome (CIBPS). Aronoff (1983) has described such a pain center as one which offers 'multidisciplinary evaluation, treatment, and a cohesive pain team approach, directed toward both modification of pain and drug-seeking behavior and the interruption of the disability process' (p. 378).

It is important to remember that not every organized group is a 'pain center' as described above. A comprehensive pain center must be multidisciplinary, must address the medical, psychological and social contributions to the pain problem, and must be staffed by a group of health professionals with interest and experience in managing pain.

Theoretical underpinnings of the multidisciplinary pain center

While it would be impossible to credit all of the individuals who contributed to the theoretical understanding of pain, the observations and insights of Beecher (1959) focused attention on the crucial importance of psychosocial factors in the pain experience. His observations of soldiers wounded in battle led him to conclude that factors of context and meaning of any injury influence the perception of pain and modify drug-seeking behavior (injured soldiers' requests for fewer analgesics than one would have anticipated based on extent of tissue damage). His conclusion that no direct relationship exists between extent of tissue damage or organicity and experienced pain is a major tenet of the MPC.

The role of psychological factors in the experience of pain, achieved theoretical importance in Melzack and Wall's (1965) gate control theory of pain. This theory postulates that somatic input is subjected to a modulating influence of a theoretical 'gate' in the dorsal horn of the spinal cord before pain perception and response are evoked. Psychological factors of attention, affect, motivation, and cognition modify the action of the gate via efferent fibers. In a summary of research on gate control theory, Wall (1978) states that while some of the 'wiring diagram' has been modified, 'an essential feature of the gate control hypothesis was that the cord cells which received nociceptive afferents would be under descending control, and this has proved to be the case in all cells so far examined' (p. 11).

Weisenberg (1976) states that gate control theory has 'legitimized behavioral and psychological procedures by its view of pain as a complex sensory and motivational phenomenon' (p. 7). This complex multidimensional view of pain has been further explicated by Melzack (1973) who discusses the sensory-discriminative, affective-motivational, and cognitive-evaluative dimensions of pain.

Giving theoretical credit to Melzack and Wall, Heinrich et al. (1982) have stated that both Sternbach (1974) and Fordyce (1976) 'expanded that (Melzack and Wall 1965) model of pain into a broader, more complex behavioral and interpersonal concept' (p. 119). It is this theoretical view of pain as a complex multidimensional experience that underlies the development of the MPC.

Development of the multidisciplinary pain center

Although the development of MPCs is the result of numerous contributions, including attitudes towards health care and advances in behavioral medicine, credit must be given to J. J. Bonica for both conceptualizing the form, function, and structure of the pain center and persevering in its growth and development (Bonica and Black 1974). The pain center that was developed by Bonica at the University of Washington and that at the New Hope Pain Center directed by Ben Crue, are both approaching their silver anniversaries. At this review there are approximately 1000 facilities listing themselves as MPCs in the U.S.A. (Aronoff et al. 1983a). According to Zeicher (1984), there were 17 MPCs in Europe. Obtaining a precise count of MPCs is made difficult by the lack of standards that would separate these types of pain centers from other types of pain facilities. Estimates of the number of pain centers range from Zeicher's count of 126

MPCs to the over 1000 pain centers previously mentioned. A discussion of standardizations for MPCs will be presented later in this chapter.

CHANGES IN THE NATURE OF PAIN PROGRAM

Through the past 25 years, there have been changes in the nature of MPCs. Some of these changes are due to practical considerations (e.g. third party reimbursement). Some parallel the emergence and development of the field of behavioral medicine, and follow shifts in the orientation in psychology. Development/maturation of the MPC has also seen changes in the relationship to a more traditional medical model. There has been an increase in complexity as well as a focus on organization, and an increased attention to the role of psychosocial factors in pain.

RELATIONSHIP OF THE MULTIDISCIPLINARY PAIN CENTER TO THE TRADITIONAL MEDICAL MODEL

The traditional medical approach to pain is one that may be applicable to acute pain, but is inappropriate in dealing with chronic pain. Throughout the development of the MPC there has been a movement away from the medical model and its treatment of chronic pain as an extension of acute pain. In the traditional medical intervention for pain, 'most treatments are directed at the patient alone and seek to discover and alleviate the source of the presumed nociceptive stimulation' (Aronoff 1983). This approach is characteristic of what Crue (1983) would call the peripheralist approach to pain. In fact, this treatment approach would be consistent with the specificity theory of pain (Sweet 1959) – a direct relationship between stimulus and psychological percept. Just as, from a theoretical standpoint, specificity theory is unable to satisfactorily account for pain phenomena, treatments that emphasize only alleviation of nociception and do not take into account psychosocial factors are inappropriate with chronic pain patients.

In the development of the MPC, there has been increased recognition of the importance of these 'central' factors and movement away from peripherally oriented treatments. Hallett and Pilowsky (1982) state 'early clinics, while recognizing the importance of psychosocial aspects, tended to be concerned with the anesthetic and surgical methods for pain relief' (p. 365).

Bonica, himself an anesthesiologist, has emphasized differences between nerve block clinics and pain clinics with more comprehensive approaches (Bonica and Black 1974). A pain center described by Cairns et al. (1976) describes a two-stage approach that can be seen as representing a type of 'midpoint' on this development away from the traditional medical model. The first stage of their program includes medical evaluation, and identification and treatment of structural (peripheral) sources of pain using nerve blocks primarily. Evaluations by psychology, occupational therapy, and physical therapy are also conducted, and patients are placed on an interval schedule of narcotic analgesic medications rather than on an as needed (p.r.n.) basis. If a patient's pain complaints persist and activity levels continue to be low, they are transferred to phase II, where no medical-surgical procedures will be given. Thus, the opposite orientation from phase I is stressed. The authors state, 'any injections or nerve blocks during phase II would shift the focus away from well behavior back to concern over pain sources' (pp. 303, 304). The psychologist becomes the program manager.

This program thus emphasizes traditional medical management in the first phase with diagnostics and evaluations, peripheral nociceptive interventions (when necessary) and narcotic analgesic administration. In phase II, psychological factors are given precedence, with the psychologist as team leader, operant conditioning of pain behaviors, a treatment strategy, goal setting, group therapy, family conferences, and medication reduction. In essence, the second phase of this program represents the direction that most MPCs have continued to take.

While this two-stage program addresses the role of psychological factors in pain, the message that psychological and central factors are considered only if medical-surgical interventions are unsuccessful, seems unavoidable. In fact, perceiving the pain center as a 'second best' alternative is a consistent bias of patients who present to pain centers and one which needs to be addressed and challenged early in a patient's admission.

The MPC at the New Hope Pain Center, directed by Dr. Ben Crue, is one designed around a 'centralist concept of chronic pain' (Crue 1983). Crue defines the centralist as one who 'questions the need for any presumed continued peripheral input . . . as an explanation for chronic pain . . .' (p. 5). The in-patient pain unit, directed by a psychiatrist, emphasizes narcotic analgesic reduction, subjective pain reduction, changes in attitude and life outlook, and changes in use of the health care system in terms of further medical and/or surgical treatment (Crue and Pinsky 1981).

One does not have to accept wholeheartedly Crue's position as a centralist to emphasize the multidimensional nature of pain and its bio-psychosocial determinants, and to de-emphasize unidimensional, peripherally oriented treatment strategies for pain problems. While description of the many MPCs sharing this orientation is beyond the scope of this paper, descriptions of several of these programs are available in a monograph published by The National Institute on Drug Abuse (1981).

SHIFTS IN PSYCHOLOGICAL ORIENTATION

As MPCs have developed in the direction of increased emphasis on psychosocial factors, they have changed in accordance with changes in the orientation within the field of psychology and behavioral medicine. Within psychology, this change has been from a focus on operant conditioning and the 'radical behaviorism' of B. F. Skinner (Skinner 1974) to a cognitive-behavioral approach represented by theorists and clinicians such as Meichenbaum (1977) and Turk et al. (1983).

The pain program at the University of Washington was one of the first purely behaviorally oriented treatment programs for chronic pain patients. Fordyce and his colleagues (1973) deserve credit for applying principles of operant conditioning and behavior modification to the treatment of chronic pain patients. Principles including modification of pain behavior, drug-seeking behavior, increase in 'up time' and general activity level, developed by Fordyce and his group, constitute a mainstay of most MPCs, even though principles explaining the mechanisms by which such pain related behaviors are maintained have evolved beyond a purely operant approach.

Fordyce (1978) discusses several aspects of a behavioral approach to pain that continued to be crucial to the function of MPCs. One is that the behavior of an individual has significance in its own right and is not to be understood only as an expression of something else (e.g. pain within the individual). Behavior is subject to influence by a variety of environmental conditions. Second, an emphasis is placed on observations, operationalizations, and measurements of behavior, and criteria for 'success or failure' in a treatment program depend on changes in those behaviors. Taken together, these principles can account for a large aspect of treatment of pain patients in MPCs. For example, the conditioning of pain behaviors through reinforcement by family members necessitates family intervention. In addition, reinforcement by the medical community in the form of drugs leads to methods of medication reduction. Furthermore, a behavioral approach to chronic pain, with its emphasis on observable and measurable events, makes establishment of criteria for change easier to approach. The well known difficulty in measuring pain itself is circumvented (but by no means solved) by focussing on and modifying observable 'illness behavior' (cf. Pilowsky and Spence 1976).

Along with a general movement in psychology away from a purely operant approach and toward a more cognitive one, treatment in an MPC has, in general, become more cognitive-behavioral. While this cognitive-behavioral approach is not a unitary one, there are similarities among various approaches, such as cognitive therapy (Beck 1976), rational emotive therapy (Ellis and Harper 1961), multimodal behavior therapy (Lazarus 1976), and stress inoculation (Meichenbaum 1977). Turk et al. (1983) state that commonalities across approaches appear to be 'an interest in the nature and modification of patients' cognitions and feelings, as well as behaviors, and some commitment to the use of behavior therapy procedures in promoting change' (p. 5).

Processes and strategies by which cognitions and feelings are modified include (according to Turk et al. 1983) reconceptualization of patient's perspective on the problem (e.g. pain) monitoring 'automatic' dysfunctional thinking patterns (e.g 'I have no control over my pain') and learning and rehearsing new coping strategies (e.g. 'I can get through this pain episode by using relaxation').

Cognitive-behavioral approaches to pain began making their appearance in the early to mid-1970's. Gottlieb et al. (1977) describe a cognitive-social learning program for low back pain patients that includes a therapeutic milieu, educational lectures, self-regulated medication reduction program (in consultation with a physician) and psychotherapy emphasizing assertiveness, problem-solving, and self-control skills.

Khatami and Rush (1978) describe an out-patient program emphasizing 'symptom control, stimulus control, and social system intervention' that lean heavily on the cognitive modification techniques of Aaron Beck who, in turn, was instrumental in developing cognitive therapy of depression. An overview of the cognitive approach to pain in behavioral medicine is perhaps best illustrated in a recent book entitled *Pain and Behavioral Medicine: A Cognitive-Behavioral Perspective,* by Turk et al. (1983).

As in much of psychology, the developmental process may be viewed as a pendulum, with, perhaps, moves towards the outer limits of a conceptualization (e.g. rigid emphasis on self-regulation) supplying a necessary corrective for another (e.g. rigid emphasis on environmentally based operant conditioning). Operant conditioning may also be viewed as a 'corrective' for exclusive reliance on a disease-based medical model. Most MPCs today offer a flexible hybrid of orientations that include evaluation and diagnosis, medical treatments, (perhaps) nerve blocks, operant conditioning, coping skills training, insight-oriented psychotherapy, confrontation, systematic relaxation training, biofeedback, and family therapy.

In addition to a natural developmental process, it also seems likely that staff in MPCs have become increasingly sophisticated in knowledge and more comfortable in its clinical application. In essence, it is no longer heretic to view 'medical' problems as having psychosocial dimensions. With this change, more rigid adherence to doctrine (whether operant or medical) can be supplanted by 'style'. As an example, the senior author of this paper uses confrontation as a means of overcoming resistance and promoting change in chronic pain patients. Clinicians for whom this is not a comfortable style may not meet with as much success using this technique. Despite the fact that most MPC programs have become shorter over time, perhaps to conform to changes in policies on third-party payers, accountability and insurance considerations, increased staff expertise and expansion of 'working hours' to include evenings and weekends assure quality care.

Commonalities among multidisciplinary pain centers

Despite the myriad of approaches and treatment strategies offered in the range of MPCs, there are similarities and assumptions common to most. This section will discuss fundamental assumptions of clinicians working in MPCs, how these fundamental assumptions get operationalized in terms of treatment approaches, and a range of techniques that are employed.

First, mention must be made of a difference between an MPC, as has been discussed, and a pain facility that may have separate components. One primary difference is that the MPC is integrated and organized in addition to being differentiated. Thus, staff within a program presents a consistent message to patients. It is important to recognize that a pain facility that offers several disciplines (often by interconsultation only) does not necessarily mean that these disciplines are integrated in a team approach. Bonica and Black (1974) state 'to achieve maximum results, it is essential that the activities of the members of the clinic be finely coordinated so that the group functions as an efficient team, working on the common goal of making the correct diagnosis and formulating the most effective therapeutic strategy' (p. 116). In essence, while mention is often made of the therapeutic nature of the patient's milieu, it is just as important to consider the milieu of staff of a MPC as possessing therapeutic (or not) qualities. This subject requires more research.

ASSUMPTIONS UNDERLYING TREATMENT AT A MULTIDISCIPLINARY PAIN CENTER

A universal assumption underlying all MPCs is that a pain problem always involves psychological and social factors in addition to physiological ones. This assumption, inherent in gate control theory, in Melzack's (1973) treatise on the multidisciplinary nature of pain and in Sternbach's (1974) discussion of pain patients has led pain clinicians to focus on the non-medical systems that impinge on patients. Systems and factors such as family, social disability or worker's compensation, medical-legal, social developmental, psychological (emotions, cognitions, and behaviors) become, by definition, appropriate and necessary points of focus for clinicians at MPCs. Brena (1981) has referred to chronic pain as 'often a conditioned socio-economic disease' (p. 76). Aronoff (1981) stresses that 'any treatment program designed for pain patients must be holistic in its orientation if it is to be effective' (p. 34).

Along similar lines, MPCs view the pain syndrome itself as the focus of treatment. Crue and Pinsky (1981) state that, 'chronic pain and its attendant epiphenomena threaten to or actually become the central focus of the sufferer's existence' (p. 139). This view is one that is also consistent with the distinction between acute and chronic pain (cf. Hendler and Fenton 1979).

A second assumption underlying the philosophy of MPCs is that patients benefit from taking an active role in the management of their pain problems. There are several different theoretical underpinnings for this view − ranging from Seligman's learned helplessness (1975) to an object relations concept of mature dependency (Guntrip 1961).

Research is equivocal regarding the extent to which belief in one's ability to influence events (e.g. internal locus of control) effects treatment and/or outcome in an MPC (cf. Tait et al. 1982). However, this equivocation may reflect difficulties in the operationalization of the concept of active responsibility rather than the concept itself. A review of the research of internal/external locus of control (cf. Weisenberg 1977) is beyond the scope of this chapter, suffice it to say that taking a more active role in one's pain management is a necessary part of a shared reconceptualization of the pain problem between patient and the staff of a pain center.

There are at least two aspects of the concept of active responsibility and control. One is the more limited belief that individual active control over pain diminishes its intensity. Another more general concept, consistent with behavioral medicine, is that an individual can improve functional abilities, quality of life, and reduce the effect of 'the problem' on his or her life. Aronoff (1981) discusses the issue in terms of 'a handicap versus disability'. A handicap is a disadvantage that makes achievement of certain goals unusually difficult. A disability is what someone does with the handicap and is greatly influenced by attitude and motivation. It is an assumption of all MPCs, indeed of all rehabilitative medicine, that patients can, through taking a more active responsibility in their own recovery, often prevent a handicap from becoming a disability.

Closely related to this aspect of active responsibility is the assumption of MPCs that 'cure' of pain in the sense of alleviation of the source of nociception, may not be possible but that pain complaints and behaviors need not be the focal point of the patient's life. Of course, from what has been said previously about the multidimensional nature of pain, the lack of direct relationship correlation between stimulus and percept, and the inadequacy of the acute pain disease model in accounting for chronic pain, 'cure' is not possible in the commonly accepted sense of the word. Patients must have some concept of this view if MPC treatment is to be effective. This becomes part of the shared reconceptualization of the problem. Most MPCs have educational lectures to assist in this process (e.g. Gottlieb et al. 1977). Once cure in the passive sense is not seen as a focus of treatment, a patient can be more easily recruited as a 'member' of the treatment team and begin to plan for ways of getting on with life despite pain. It is important that the patient not assume this view is a 'second best, learn to live with it' resignation, but a chance to influence one's life in a more healthy and productive manner (e.g. pain becomes a challenge, not a threat).

OPERATIONALIZATION OF ASSUMPTIONS

Just as there are commonalities among pain centers regarding assumptions underlying treatment and views of pain and pain problems, these assumptions, in general, are operationalized in more or less similar ways. Most important, these assumptions must be shared with the patient at the level of assumptions. Much energy is devoted from each discipline into promoting this shared conceptualization of pain. It must be realized that some of the problems encountered in comparing one MPC with another are that these comparisons are made only at the lowest level of abstraction. Thus, pain centers have been compared on choices of particular measures, goals, and so forth, without much regard to the similarity of the assumptions that generate these particular measures.

A recognition of the multifaceted nature of the pain experience leads to treatment programs designed to address these diverse issues in an organized way. Thus, group and/or individual psychotherapy is a mainstay in all multidisciplinary pain centers, although the precise form of psychotherapy may differ. Some offer a more directed group approach such as assertiveness (e.g. Gottlieb et al. 1977), cognitive therapy (Khatami and Rush 1978), while others are more dynamically oriented (e.g. Aronoff and Rutrick 1985). In one MPC (Finer 1982), the fact that the psychologist has a chronic pain problem is used therapeutically. Important issues addressed in psychotherapy include depression (cf. Aronoff et al. 1984), pain 'games' (Sternbach 1974b), early developmental history and pain proneness (Blumer and Heilbronn 1982) and inappropriate demands for care (Aronoff 1985). Group therapy is used extensively (although not exclusively) to combat the isolation and withdrawal common in pain patients and to give the patients the sense that they are not alone in their difficulties. Also, patients often listen to other patients as they would not listen to staff. Thus, resistance and defensiveness are decreased. Family therapy and social services are also common and necessary treatment interventions. Again, the precise form of these interventions will reflect the therapeutic orientation of the therapist or that of the center. For instance, Fordyce (1981), a proponent of operant conditioning in pain treatment, states, 'Significant family members . . . are trained in how to identify pain and well behaviors, to become aware of their own responses to these, and, as needed, to acquire and practice more effective alternatives' (p. 69).

MPCs also utilize psychological evaluations and testing to clarify diagnosis and prognosis. These evaluations are either in the form of paper and pencil tests such as the MMPI, POMS, or MPQ, or in behavioral analyses (Fordyce 1976) or psychiatric interviews (Finer 1982; Aronoff and Rutrick 1984). The area of psychological evaluation is one of those that is most subject to the lack of standardization mentioned throughout MPCs. While pain centers are unanimous in their belief in the psychological dimension of pain, the way this assumption becomes operationalized is vastly different in each pain center. Needs for standardization have repeatedly been discussed (cf. Aronoff and Evans 1982; Aronoff et al. 1983b) since results of treatment and psychological correlates of other pain related variables become difficult to compare. It is important to realize that lack of correlates at the operationalized level does not negate the relationship at the level of assumption.

A necessary focus also is the secondary gain aspect of the pain problem. Over the years, pain-related behavior has become part of a patient's repertoire. Some programs (e.g. Fordyce et al. 1973) see secondary gain as learned pain behavior and take steps to extinguish these behaviors and supplant with 'well behaviors'. While all MPCs employ a variant of reduction of pain behaviors, some use a more confrontative approach in dealing with secondary gain (e.g. Sternbach 1974b; Aronoff 1985). Closely related to the secondary gain aspect is litigation. Some programs will not accept patients until all litigation is settled. This itself indicates its importance. The programs that do accept patients on litigation must address this issue, whether by confrontation, education, or interpretation.

Physical therapy is present in one form or another, at most MPCs. Again, specific approaches vary as a function of the orientation of the program. For example, at the Northwest Pain Center, no passive physical therapy modalities such as heat, massage, or manipulation are offered (Seres et al. 1981). The program described by Gottlieb et al. (1977) has a similar approach to physical therapy. Other programs (Finer 1982; Hallett and Pilowsky 1982; Aronoff 1985) include modality-oriented physical therapy treatments as well as active exercise programs. Some programs offer medical evaluation and diagnostic services, consultations, and/or medically-oriented interventions such as nerve blocks or surgery (Cairns et al. 1976; Aronoff 1981; Hallett and Pilowsky 1982). In the experience of the authors, most patients who are referred to an MPC expect this aspect of a treatment approach to be either the only service offered or at least the one that is most stressed. This belief not only represents an 'external' approach common to many pain patients, but is also fostered by the traditional medical model and disease-based orientations. It is a belief or expectation that must be acknowledged and addressed — since 'failed expectations' can accrue to a core of deprivation that is common to many pain patients (cf. Blumer and Heilbronn 1982) and increased resistance to treatment. In addition, patients expecting primarily 'medical' treatments may view the presence of psychosocial treatments to imply that their pain is 'all in their head' and imaginary. Formal educational presentations can be of great benefit in this reorientation. One of us (J. M. Wagner) has developed a workshop series on psychophysiology that is an aid in letting patients know that their pain is accepted as real, while educating them to the psychosocial factors that influence their pain experience.

Systematic relaxation training and biofeedback training are also offered in most pain centers.

The precise nature of these treatments is also approached based on the orientation of the program. Originally, biofeedback training was thought of as falling within the rubric of operant conditioning of a physiological process such as muscle tension (Budzynski et al. 1973). Biofeedback training as well as relaxation training can be viewed as a counterconditioning procedure such as in systematic desensitization (Wolpe 1959). For discussion of the application of the counterconditioning aspect of relaxation training in pain patients, see Evans (1985). Also, biofeedback training can be seen within a cognitive attention diversion paradigm, or as a self-control coping skill (Turk et al. 1983). For a review of the use of relaxation training and biofeedback in pain, see Turner and Chapman (1982).

Within each structural modality, treatment approaches emphasize the rehabilitative role of active responsibility of the patient. The presence of a modality does not necessarily ensure appropriate interpretation of its message. The approach taken by clinicians within the modality can greatly influence its interpretation. Thus, while systematic relaxation training and biofeedback can be presented as skills and tools that a patient can use for the self-management of pain and physiological processes, this is not the only interpretation possible. Turner and Chapman (1982) state, 'the therapist eager to find problems suitable for biofeedback therapy may unwittingly collude in the process of somatization by delivering a physiologically focussed treatment that legitimates the patient's denial of life problems' (p. 17). On a similar note, hypnosis as a method of pain control can too often be attributed solely to the expertise of the operator with little acknowledgment of the role the patient himself plays in the process (cf. Barber 1982).

Narcotic medication reduction, a feature in most MPCs, is also a modality with a message. The patient can easily interpret medication reduction as something being taken away from him by staff and thus become fearful or angry (or both). Some programs (e.g. Gottlieb et al. 1977) rely on a self-administered medication reduction program (in consultation with a physician) to circumvent this possibility and emphasize the active responsibility of the patient in decreasing his or her own medications. Most programs have a staff administered medications reduction program where medications are changed from a p.r.n. schedule to an interval schedule (to decrease the reinforcement value for pain in the form of a pill). Then, after some time to allow the patient to become familiar with the program and to begin learning alternative pain control techniques, such as relaxation, the amount of narcotic medication is tapered in a variant of the 'pain cocktail'. It is important to emphasize, through education and support, the negative effects of medication and side effects as well as their limited utility in chronic pain syndromes. In addition, much reinforcement is given for active use of alternatives, and attention is paid to the new found 'independence' from substance use/abuse.

The physical therapies, such as TENS, whirlpool, High Volt Direct Current (HVDC), or ultrasound (the modality-oriented physical therapies) or procedures like nerve blocks, can be especially susceptible to reinforcing the passivity of chronic pain patients. Again, some programs (e.g. Gottlieb et al. 1977; Seres et al. 1981) do not employ passive modalities for this reason. Where these modalities are employed, emphasis is (or should be) placed on what a patient can take with them when they leave the program, thus increasing independence and self-management skills. At the Boston Pain Center, TENS is interpreted to the patient in this way, and ice massage is presented as an inexpensive, effective and portable means of pain control. Patients are taught to be independent with ice massage as soon as possible. We have found that provision of passive treatments such as massage, whirlpool, hot packs, etc. can also be used to enhance a patient's feeling that their needs are being taken care of so that they are less resistant to other approaches like medication reduction and assertiveness training. In the review by these authors, pain centers outside of the United States seem to employ more invasive procedures such as nerve blocks or surgeries than those programs within the United States. With the more invasive procedures, it becomes especially important to emphasize the function desired rather than the passive nature of the treatments. Thus, the message delivered is that the staff at the MPC is helping to increase functional ability so that the patient can make further changes in life quality, environmental stressors, and the psychosocial factors such as self-esteem and mood, all of which will assist in pain control and management. Emphasis is taken off the view that staff is 'repairing' the patient to a previously acceptable level of functioning using solely medical-surgical interventions. Clearly, the extent to which a patient receives this message depends on the integration, consistency, and 'fine tuning' of the MPC staff. Staff 'dynamics' − least studied − may be most important in promoting the concept of active responsibility of the patient in his or her own recovery.

Finally, the focus on quality of life rather than on 'cure' leads to emphasis on psychological and physical functioning of the patient. Within this area, one urges the development of active coping strategies, learning to understand the previously discussed difference between a handicap and a disability, utilizing principles of goal setting. Here, return to work, frequently an issue, becomes of paramount importance. Some programs have in-house vocational counselors (e.g. Gottlieb et al. 1977), others refer to state or private patient agencies. In the area of work, the approach to a patient is of crucial importance, since many patients may view the MPC as an agent of their employer (or their insurance company) whose sole function is to get the patient back to a job that the patient detested and would like to avoid (perhaps throught continued pain complaints). Many patients, realizing they get no gain out of continuing pain complaints, resist improvements in *functioning,* for this reason. These problems transcend specific modalities in a pain center and need to be addressed by a variety of staff. The importance of openly acknowledging the issue of work and incorporating it in a return-to-work program in a MPC is discussed by Catchlove and Cohen (1982).

Outside the realm of work specifically, but within the quality of life orientation, is emphasis on leisure time activity and for the retired, perhaps volunteer work. In all cases, referral to appropriate aftercare facilities is an essential but often neglected aspect of treatment in a pain center. At the Boston Pain Center, we offer out-patient pain groups and opportunity for continued participation in an out-patient program following a patient's in-patient stay, as well as referral to psychotherapists, physical therapists and family therapists as needed. The impact of appropriate aftercare placement on maintenance of gains following therapy has not been adequately investigated.

Evaluation of effectiveness

A detailed review of the effectiveness of a MPC is beyond the scope of this chapter (see Turner and Chapman 1982; Tan 1982; Turk et al. 1983). However, a brief discussion will be presented. When evaluating the effectiveness of pain centers, there are several points to keep in mind. First, there is no general agreement on the definition of success or effectiveness across pain centers. Treatment facilities differ in their definitions and criteria as well as their measuring instruments. These problems will be further addressed in a separate section. Second, regardless of the criteria for success or failure, it is difficult to understand who the comparison groups are. Are patients treated in a MPC being compared with patients who have surgery for a similar condition or those who have had non-surgical conservative treatment such as traction or physical therapy? It is common for patients who come to a MPC to have already had many surgical or other medically oriented treatments, and thus the MPC is for many their 'last hope'. Thus, some patients treated in a MPC are implicitly being compared with patients who have had similar problems, but who are currently receiving no treatment. As several authors have indicated (e.g. Tan 1982; Turner and Chapman 1982), there are very few control studies of pain center treatment. These issues must be given some consideration when evaluating effectiveness. Nonetheless, there is some support for the conclusion that MPCs are effective in treating a segment of pain patients who have been highly refractory to other forms of intervention.

MPCs generally report successes in the areas addressed in treatment. These areas generally include report of pain reduction, increased activity level, and decreased analgesic intake (cf. Roy 1984). Studies of pain centers reporting outcome results (Turner and Chapman 1982) all reported success in at least one of these areas as measured by individual instruments. Some programs also include measures of employment, restoration and mood changes.

In one study comparing patients treated surgically with those participating in a pain center, Ignelzi et al. (1977) revealed that at 2 and 3 year follow-up there were no differences between surgical and non-surgical patients in activity levels, reported pain levels, or analgesic intake, with all patients reporting significantly decreased pain, decreased analgesic intake and increased activity level. An interesting finding in this study is that patients receiving surgery were more likely to be readmitted to the hospital for pain problems while patients treated in a MPC were more likely to be readmitted for some non-pain related medical problem. When assessing the utilization of health care facilities following treatment, it is important to keep these results in mind. Hallett and Pilowsky (1982) reported that 37% of treated patients demonstrated either 'complete or partial' pain relief while 59% were unchanged, and 4% reported worse pain. Khatami and Ruh (1978) report significant reductions in pain, depression, and drug intake in five patients treated in a MPC. These results were maintained at 6 months and one year follow-up (Khatami and Rush 1982). Sternbach (1974b) indicated that 67% of program completers noted pain reduction, increased activity levels, and decreased analgesic intake at program completion, although some increased pain and decreased activity levels were noted immediately following discharge. Aronoff (1981) notes 95% of all patients who entered the MPC taking narcotics or sedative-hypnotics are free from these medications at discharge. Two-thirds of these patients maintain these gains at one year follow-up. Cairns et al. (1976) report that 70% of 90 patients treated at their pain center demonstrated decreased pain and 58% demonstrated decreased analgesic intake at discharge. Roberts and Reinhart (1980) stated that 77 of their treated patients were leading normal lives without medications for pain. Gottlieb et al. (1977) indicate 79% of 72 treated patients with low back pain had normal physical functioning levels while on follow-up 82% of those contacted (23 patients) were either employed or in training programs. Rosonoff et al. (1981) report 86% of their low back pain patients returned to full activity, 70% are 'fully occupied' and another 16% are able to work but are not placed due to 'prejudice against their medical history of low back disorder' (p. 109). Seres and Newman (1976) report meaningful gains in 75% of patients in the areas of objective physical measures, medication reduction, and decreased medical contacts. Finer (1982), in Sweden, reports, of 34 patients, 12.9% had increased symptoms, 49.7% were unchanged and 37.4% had decreased symptoms. Areas of evaluation were pain medications and mood. Keefe et al. (1981) report a pain reduction of 29% in their patients. Also, 49.2% of their patients decreased narcotic analgesic usage and 63.2% reported increased activity levels.

While these results are encouraging, they should be considered preliminary, and ones that demand further evaluation. Tan (1982) states that studies ' . . . provide some support, albeit tentative for the efficacy of multifaceted cognitive behavioral treatment regimens for the control of clinical pain . . .' (p. 215).

DIFFICULTIES IN EVALUATING EFFECTIVENESS

There are many reasons underlying the tentative and preliminary nature of the evaluation of the effectiveness of MPCs. One is that very few MPCs report outcome data. Turk et al. (1983) indicate that of the approximately 800 pain programs in the U.S.A. alone, only 21 have provided outcome data 'no matter how meager' (p. 129).

In addition to the paucity of data, that which has been reported is subject to numerous methodological difficulties inherent in outcome research. One of those difficulties, discussed by Crue and Pinsky (1981) involves defining the population in question. Some effort in this direction is made with distinctions between chronic and acute pain, benign and malignant pain, and some further definition is gained with the concept of the CIBPS patient (Crue and Pinsky 1981). However, even within this latter category, there are many different salient variables including compensation and litigation, presence of psychopathology, ambulatory status, and age, to name just a few, that effect treatment outcome and prevent direct comparison of MPCs as well as prohibiting wide ranging statements regarding the effectiveness of pain centers.

A major methodological problem that plagues outcome research including that of MPCs, is the lack of adequate or appropriate control groups. So great is this problem that several reviewers of treatment strategies for pain (e.g. Merskey et al. 1980; Tan 1982; Turner and Chapman 1982; Aronoff et al. 1983) have used phrases like 'no definitive statements supporting the consistent efficacy' (Tan 1982) are made. One exceptional study is that of Roberts and Reinhart (1980) who reported an outcome study with control groups that indicated a 77% success rate.

The groups of this study included 26 treated patients, 20 patients rejected by the clinic, and 12 patients who had refused treatment. While it seems likely that these groups were not equivalent prior to entering treatment, and thus conclusions are still equivocal, the use of control groups makes this study an exception within the genre of outcome research in MPCs. Aronoff et al. (1983b) state 'the possibility of finding patients who are acceptable for treatment and probably would successfully participate in a pain unit program but do not, seems almost impossible' (p. 10). Obviously, many more control studies are needed as well as creativity in establishing equivalence of groups.

Another major problem in evaluating outcome is the lack of standardization of measures. Although most MPCs evaluate and set goals for increased activity, decreased pain, decreased medications, increased mood, and, for some, return to work, the measurement instruments and tests are quite different and probably, with some exceptions, not even cohesive and unitary within the category. Thus, pain as measured on the MPQ and a visual analogue scale is not necessarily correlated, and mood as assessed by the POMS, BSI, and MMPI is not necessarily highly correlated. A multimode, multitrait analysis whereby measures of one category (e.g. mood) are measured by a variety of methods (question their observer ratings and patient behaviors) would decrease this problem while at the same time effect another problem, the over-reliance on self-report. For the present, the lack of standardization and the lack of cohesiveness in measures ostensibly designed to measure the same thing, decreased reliability and validity and thus will further call into question the evaluation of treatment results. The problems of follow-up of results are even more difficult, due to increased time spans, and are reviewed by Aronoff et al. (1983b). In summarizing problems of evaluation of outcome research, Turner and Chapman (1982) state 'the problems are extremely complex . . . large numbers of variables need to be measured over a number of time periods since the issue in question is one of pain chronicity. Researchers are thus plagued with missing data, difficulties of compliance and even ethical problems in the assignment of patients to convincing control conditions' (p. 42).

Prediction

With so many problems inherent in assessing effectiveness, discussion about predictions seems almost gratuitous. Nonetheless, predicting who will succeed in any treatment approach seems almost irresistable and also may be seen as a way of addressing the construct validity of the assumptions underlying treatment at MPCs (Meehl 1977). In addition, prediction at any given pain center may not only increase our knowledge of pain centers and their effect, but causes us to ask ourselves more questions about assumptions underlying our treatment.

At the Mayo Clinic, Maruta et al. (1979) compared a group of patients who were considered successes with those who were deemed failures. Items evaluated were: 1) modification of attitude; 2) decrease in pain medications; and, 3) increase in physical functioning. In studying 172 patients, 35 (20.3%) were considered failures with no improvement in any category, while 34 (19.8%) were successes, with strong or moderate improvement in all three categories. From this comparison. Maruta et al. found that the two groups differed significantly on five variables: 1) prior duration of pain; 2) work time lost; 3) number of operations related to pain; 4) subjective pain level; and, 5) drug dependency. There were no significant differences on MMPI profiles. A 7-item rating scale was developed.

This rating scale was employed by Aronoff and Evans (1982) at the Boston Pain Center, where 104 consecutive admissions to the program were evaluated according to: 1) staff judgment of improvement; 2) patient judgment of improvement; 3) pain change; and, 4) mood change. In a multiple linear regression analysis, the 7-item 'Maruta Index' did not predict treatment outcome at the Boston Pain Center. In fact, none of the myriad of variables examined was useful in predicting outcome, with the exception of age, which was negatively correlated with improvement.

However, in support of Maruta et al.'s result, Keefe et al. (1981) found, in comparing 28 patients with the greatest pain reduction with 28 patients showing least pain improvement, that the patients with most improvement demonstrated fewer years of continuous pain, rated their pain initially as more severe, were more likely to have had multiple surgeries. A greater percentage of patients with the least improvement were on disability. Age did not differ between the two groups and no MMPI scale differentiated between the 15 'best' and 10 'worst' patients. Regarding the MMPI, it is interesting to note that despite the ubiquity of this instrument in the psychological evaluation of chronic pain patients, its predictive power is extremely limited. In fact, a recent study has indicated that the MMPI cannot differentiate chronic pain population from a chronic illness population (Naliboff et al. 1982).

In comparing 'satisfied' with 'dissatisfied' patients, Swanson et al. (1978) showed that dissatisfied patients were more likely females with longer pain duration, increased previous hospitalizations, and more operations for pain.

Block et al. (1980), found that the presence of disability (state workers' compensation) was related to a lesser degree of improvement in a pain center than for those not on disability. These authors found that while all study patients referred to their pain center improved in pain report, affect, and feelings of control, the disability patients demonstrated less improvement, were hospitalized longer, and were less compliant. These results could not be explained on the basis of increased psychopathology in the disability group. No effect was found for depression, locus of control, or asssertiveness. However, no difference was found between disability and non-disability patients at the Boston Pain Center (Aronoff and Evans 1982).

Hallett and Pilowsky (1982) also found no relation between occupational or motor vehicle accident and improvement and no demographic or other descriptive data predicted outcome in their program. While results seem equivocal regarding the variables predicting success in MPCs, and these variables do not seem to be consistent with the assumptions underlying treatment, evaluation of reasons why patients regress following treatment is a bit more consistent with underlying assumptions. Painter et al. (1980) evaluated 25 most successful patients with an equal number of patients who had initially succeeded, then regressed following treatment. These authors found that those who regressed were more likely to demonstrate incentive for maintaining pain, such as disability compensation. Also, those in the failure group were more likely to hold a dependent, passive attitude as well as exhibit more depression. Finally, these authors state, 'the most striking differences were that those in the failure group showed little alteration in their environment state, communication, or reinforcement patterns, while the success group showed many environmental changes.'

It seems as though those who not only learned, but continued to employ the concepts underlying treatment at MPCs are the 'winners'. Consistent with these results, Lutz et al. (1983) report that, 'patient regression to pretreatment levels may well be due to insufficient follow-through of the skills and treatments learned and performed while participating in pain programs' (p. 308). In this study relating compliance with therapeutic regimens with long-term follow-up, they found first, that overall compliance was low and compliance in separate regimens was a better predictor than overall compliance measures. Separate measures included progressive ambulation, PT and OT exercises, home treatments such as ice, relaxation and self-hypnosis, and use of proper body mechanics. Of these, only 'use of proper body mechanics' was related to subjective pain, while this measure, relaxation, and overall compliance were related to overall improvement.

These results, while certainly preliminary, are heartening, since they are consistent with the use of treatment modalities that emphasize active participation of the patient and those that address the multidimensional nature of pain and pain problems. Perhaps more studies that compare pre-treatment measures with long-term follow-up will help explicate these complex and multidetermined relationships.

Future directions in pain management

Viewing pain syndromes as multidimensional phenomena necessitating collaborative team management has revolutionized treatment in pain centers. Similarly, the future of pain treatment, and the MPC will be largely determined by a multitude of factors working within a system. Thus, while traditional, basic research, increasing knowledge and clinical advances will undoubtedly contribute improved treatment of pain, so will the policies of legislation of third-party payers, accreditation, and public attitudes towards the health care system.

In recent years, there has been an increasing public awareness of health and wellness. This awareness has led to better understanding of preventative medicine and the influence of behavioral and lifestyle factors on health. This attitude is consistent with that of the MPC, and hopefully will continue to influence legislation and policies of third-party payers. It was not too long ago that MPCs were considered to be on the 'fringes' of acceptability in medicine. Luckily, this situation is no longer quite as prevalent, as third-party payers are educated in current theory and treatment concerning multidisciplinary approaches to pain.

This trend toward the 'mainstreaming' of MPCs is represented by the growth of the field of behavioral medicine. We expect that this growth will continue. There are now professional organizations and journals in this field. In 1985, a new journal, *Clinical Journal of Pain,* made its debut. This journal is designed to focus primarily on clinical aspects of treating chronic pain patients as opposed to the more experimental focus of the journal, *Pain*. In addition to professional organizations and journals, there are now graduate training programs in behavioral medicine. Many psychology doctoral internship programs include rotations in behavioral medicine and health psychology, and several are devoted exclusively to behavioral medicine. This trend will certainly influence pain treatment, for students of today will not have to be 'persuaded' to reconceptualize the nature of pain or the nature of health care.

A general reconceptualization of the nature of health care is important, for the way services are reimbursed is largely dependent on what is considered to be acceptable treatment. There has been a gap between current thinking on the nature of pain and pain treatment and what is reimbursed by third-party payers. Aronoff and Sweet (1985) have pointed out that physicians in pain management have found that diagnostic evaluations and invasive procedures have been reimbursed while conservative treatment in MPCs have not been.

As much as those of us concerned with clinical treatment of pain want third-party payers to recognize our point of view, we also need to recognize theirs — acceptable use of health care system, appropriate selection of patients, quality control, and acceptable guidelines for treatment. In the future, there will be increased accountability, necessitating guidelines and some form of internal quality control.

Currently there are no universally accepted guidelines for MPCs. Without guidelines, there is always the potential for abuse. As Vasudevan (1984), among others, has said, there is a need for some type of accreditation procedure. In the United States, the Commission for Accreditation of Rehabilitation Facilities (CARF), a non-profit organization founded in 1966, has begun an accreditation process for MPCs according to certain standards approved by the American Pain Society. Since July, 1983, 66 MPCs in the United States have been accredited according to these guidelines. Currently, these standards apply to MPCs, although in the future they will likely be expanded to cover syndrome and perhaps modality-oriented pain programs as well. This accreditation process is voluntary and is an attempt to provide a mechanism by which competent delivery of services can be assessed.

In the future, the practice of accreditation should become more widespread. As clinicians dedicated to providing the best services available for our patients, it is our obligation to encourage guidelines for responsible care. As multidisciplinary concepts are becoming concretized, more sophisticated diagnostic systems will be developed. Reich et al. (1983) have discussed the use of the American Psychiatric Association's Diagnostic and Statistical Manual, 3rd edn. to classify various types of chronic pain patients — taking into account the psychosocial components. Aronoff (1984) suggests guidelines for expanding and refining this diagnostic system for use in chronic pain patients.

Finally, the future may see a spirit of cooperation among MPCs and clinicians dealing with pain. The popularity and ubiquity of computers will enable data sharing, increased subject pool, and rapid transmission of information that will increase communication among professionals and begin to address some methodological research concerns. If the pain center is to remain on the cutting edge of multidimensional treatment of chronic pain, we need continuously developing models to integrate new discoveries with clinical methods.

References

Aronoff, G. M. (1981) A holistic approach to pain rehabilitation: the Boston Pain Unit. In: Lorenz K. Y. Ng (Ed.), New Approaches to Treatment of Chronic Pain: A Review of Multidisciplinary Pain Clinics and Pain Centers. National Institute of Drug Abuse, Research Monograph Series 36, May 1981.

Aronoff, G. M. (1983) The role of the pain center in the treatment for intractable suffering and disability resulting from chronic pain. Semin. Neurol. 3.

Aronoff, G. M. (1985) Psychological aspects of non-malignant chronic pain: a new nosology. In: Evaluation and Treatment of Chronic Pain. Urban & Schwarzenberg, Baltimore.

Aronoff, G. M. and Evans, W. O. (1982) The prediction of treatment outcome at a multidisciplinary pain center. Pain 14, 67 – 73.

Aronoff, G. M. and Sweet, W. S. (1985) Future of pain management. In: Gerald M. Aronoff (Ed.), Evaluation and Treatment of Chronic Pain. Urban & Schwarzenberg, Baltimore.

Aronoff, G. M., Crue, B. L. and Seres, J. (1983a) Pain centers: help for the chronic pain patient. Med. Pain 4, 1 – 5.

Aronoff, G. M., Evans, W. O. and Enders, P. O. (1983b) A review of follow-up studies of multidisciplinary pain units. Pain 16, 1 – 11.

Aronoff, G. M., Wagner, J. and Kleinke, C. (1984) Pain and depression. Med. Pain, 5, 1 – 5.

Aronoff, G. M., Rutrick, D. and Evans, W. O. (1985) Psychodynamics and psychotherapy of the chronic pain syndrome. In: Gerald M. Aronoff (Ed.), Evaluation and Treatment of Chronic Pain. Urban & Schwarzenberg, Baltimore.

Barber, J. (1982) Incorporating hypnosis in the management of chronic pain. In: Joseph Barber and Cheri Adrian (Eds.), Psychological Approaches to the Management of Pain. Brunner Mazel, New York.

Beck, A.T. (1976) Cognitive Therapy and the Emotional Disorders. International Universities Press, New York.

Beecher, H. K. (1959) Measurement of Subjective Responses. Oxford University Press, London.

Block, A. R., Kremer, E. and Gaylord, M. (1980) Behavioral treatment of chronic pain: variables affecting treatment efficacy. Pain, 8, 367 – 375.

Blumer, D. and Heilbronn, M. (1982) Chronic pain as a variant of depressive disease: the pain prone disorder. J. Nerv. Ment. Dis. 170.

Bonica, J. J. and Black, R. G. (1974) The management of a pain clinic. In: M. Swerdlow (Ed.), Relief of Intractable Pain. Excerpta Medica, Amsterdam, pp. 116 – 129.

Brena, S. F., Chapman, S. L. and Decker (1981) Chronic pain as a learned experience: Emory University Pain Control Center. In: Lorenz K. Y. Ng (Ed.), New Approaches to Treatment of Chronic Pain: A Review of Multidisciplinary Pain Clinics and Pain Centers. National Institute of Drug Abuse, Research, Monograph Series 36, May 1981.

Budzynski, T. H., Stoyva, J. M., Adler, C. S. and Mullaney, D. J. (1973) EMG, biofeedback and tension headache: a controlled outcome study. Semin. Psychiatry 5, 397 – 410.

Cairns, D., Thomas, L., Mooney, V. and Pace, J. B. (1976) A comprehensive treatment approach to chronic low back pain. Pain 2, 301 – 308.

Catchlove, R. and Cohen, K. (1982) Effects of a directive return to work approach in the treatment of workman's compensation patients with chronic pain. Pain 14, 181 – 191.

Crue, B. L. and Pinsky, J. J. (1981) Chronic pain syndrome: four aspects of the problem. In: Lorenz K. Y. Ng (Ed.), New Approaches to Treatment of Chronic Pain: A Review of Multidisciplinary Pain Clinics and Pain Centers. National Institute of Drug Abuse, Research Monograph Series 36, May 1981.

Ellis, A. and Harper, R. A. (1961) A guide to rational living. Institute for Rational Living.

Evans, W. O. (1985) A cognitive-behavioral approach to chronic pain. In: Gerald M. Aronoff (Ed.), Evaluation and Treatment of Chronic Pain. Urban & Schwarzenberg, Baltimore.

Finer, B. (1982) Treatment in an interdisciplinary pain clinic. In: Joseph Barber and Cheri Adrian (Eds.), Psychological Approaches to the Management of Pain. Brunner Mazel, New York, pp. 186 – 204.

Fordyce, W. E. (1976) Behavioral Methods for Control of Chronic Pain. C. V. Mosby, St. Louis.

Fordyce, W. E. (1978) Learning Processes in Pain. The Psychology of Pain. Raven Press, New York.

Fordyce, W. E., Fowler, R. S., Jr., Lehmann, J. F., Delateur, B. J., Sand, P. L. and Trieschmann, R. B. (1973) Operant conditioning in the treatment of chronic pain. Arch. Phys. Med. Rehab. 54, 399 – 408.

Gottlieb, H., Strite, L., Koller, R., Madorsky, A., Hockersmith, V., Kleeman, M. and Wagner, J. (1977) Comprehensive rehabilitation of patients having chronic low back pain. Arch. Phys. Med. Rehab. 58, 101 – 108.

Guntrip, H. (1961) Personality Structure and Human Interaction. Hogarth, London.

Hallett, E. C. and Pilowsky, I. (1982) The response to treatment in a multidisciplinary pain clinic. Pain 12, 365 – 374.

Heinrich, R. L., Cohen, M. J. and Naliboff, B. D. (1982) Coping in interpersonal contexts. In: Psychological Approaches to the Management of Pain. Brunner-Mazel, New York.

Hendler, N. and Fenton, J. A. (1979) Coping with Chronic Pain. Potter, New York.

Ignelzi, R. J., Sternbach, R. A. and Timmerman, G. (1977) The pain ward follow-up analyses. Pain 3, 277 – 280.

Keefe, F. J., Block, A. R., Williams, R. B., Jr. and Surwit, R. S. (1981) Behavioral treatment of chronic low back pain: clinical outcome and individual differences in pain relief. Pain 11, 221 – 231.

Khatami, M. and Rush, A. J. (1978) A pilot study of the treatment of outpatients with chronic pain: symptom control, stimulus control and social system intervention. Pain 5, 163 – 172.

Khatami, M. and Rush, A. J. (1982) A one-year follow-up of the multi-modal treatment for chronic pain. Pain 14, 45 – 52.

Lazarus, A. A. (1976) Multi-modal Behavior Therapy. Springer, New York.

Lutz, R. W., Silbert, M. and Olshan, N. (1983) Treatment outcome and compliance with therapeutic regimens: long-term follow-up of a multidisciplinary pain program. Pain 17, 301 – 308.

Maruta, T., Swanson, D. W. and Swenson, W. M. (1979) Chronic pain: which patients may a pain management program help? Pain 7, 321 – 329.

Meehl, P. E. (1977) Construct validity in psychological tests. In: Psychodiagnosis, Selected Papers. W. W. Norton & Co Inc., New York, pp. 3 – 31. First published in Psychological Bulletin (1954) L. J. Cronbach and P. E. Meehl (authors).

Meichenbaum, D. (1977) Cognitive-Behavior Modification. Plenum Press, New York.

Melzack, R. (1973) The Puzzle of Pain. Baric Books, New York.

Melzack, R. and Wall, P. (1965) Pain mechanisms: a new theory. Science 50, 971 – 979.

Merskey, H., Engelhardt, H. T., Eriksson, M. B., Houde, R. W. et al. (1980) The principles of pain management, group report. In: H. W. Kosterlitz and L. Y. Terenius (Eds.), Pain and Society, Dahlem Conference 1980. Weinheim Verlag Chemie Gnbh., pp. 483 – 500.

Naliboff, B. D., Cohen, M. J. and Yellen, A. N. (1982) Does the MMPI differentiate chronic illness from chronic pain? Pain 13, 333 – 341.

Ng, Lorenz K. Y. (Ed.) (1981) New Approaches to Treatment of Chronic Pain: A Review of Multidisciplinary Pain Clinics and Pain Centers. National Institute of Drug Abuse, Research Monograph Series 36, May 1981.

Painter, J. R., Seres, J. L. and Newman, R. I. (1980) Assessing benefits of the pain center: why some patients regress. Pain 8, 101 – 113.

Pilowsky, I. and Spence, N. D. (1976) Illness behavior syndromes associated with intractable pain. Pain 2, 61 – 71.

Reich, J., Rosenblatt, R. M. and Tupin, J. (1983) DSM-III: a new nomenclature for classifying patients with chronic pain. Pain 16, 201 – 206.

Roberts, A. H. and Reinhardt, L. (1980) The behavioral management of chronic pain: long-term follow-up with comparison groups. Pain 8, 151 – 162.

Rosomoff, H. L., Green, C., Silbert, M. and Steele, R. (1981) Pain and low back rehabilitation program at the University of Miami School of Medicine. In: Lorenz K. Y. Ng (Ed.), New Approaches to Treatment of Chronic Pain. A Review of Multidisciplinary Pain Clinics and Pain Centers. National Institute of Drug Abuse, Research Monograph Series 36, May 1981.

Roy, R. (1984) Pain clinics: reassessment of objectives and outcomes. Arch. Phys. Med. Rehab. 65, 448 – 451.

Seligman, M. E. P. (1975) Helplessness: on Depression, Development, and Death, W. H. Freeman, San Francisco.

Seres, J. L. and Newman, R. I. (1976) Results of treatment of chronic low back pain at the Portland Pain Center. J. Neurosurg. 45, 32 – 36.

Seres, J. L., Painter, J. R. and Newman, R. I. (1981) Multidisciplinary treatment of chronic pain at the Northwest Pain Center. In: Lorenz K. Y. Ng (Ed.), New Approaches to Treatment of Chronic Pain: A Review of Multidisciplinary Pain Clinics and Pain Centers. National Institute of Drug Abuse, Research Monograph Series 36, May 1981.

Skinner, B. F. (1974) About Behaviorism. Knopf, New York.

Sternbach, R. A. (1974a) Pain Patients: Traits and Treatment. Academic Press, New York.

Sternbach, R. A. (1974b) Varieties of pain games. In: J. J. Bonica (Ed.), Advances in Neurology. Raven Press, New York.

Swanson, D. W., Swenson, W. M., Maruta, T. and Floreen, A. C. (1978) The dissatisfied patient with chronic pain. Pain 4, 367 – 378.

Sweet, W. H. (1959) Pain. In: J. Field, H. W. Magoon and V. E. Hall (Eds.), Handbook of Physiology, Vol. 1. American Physiological Society, Washington, DC.

Tan, S. Y. (1982) Cognitive and cognitive-behavioral methods for pain control: a selective review. Pain 12, 201 – 228.

Tait, R., DeGood, D. and Carron, H. (1982) A comparison of health of control beliefs in low back patients from the U.S. and New Zealand. Pain 14, 53 – 61.

Turk, D., Meichenbaum, D. and Genest, M. (1983) Pain and Behavioral Medicine: A Cognitive-Behavioral Perspective. Guilford, New York.

Turner, J. A. and Chapman, C. R. (1982) Psychological interventions for chronic pain: a critical review. I. Relaxation training and biofeedback. Pain 12, 1 – 21.

Vasudevan, S. V. (1984) Is there a need for uniform guidelines for pain clinics/centers? What is being done in the United States of America? People to People International.

Wall, P. (1978) The gate control theory of pain mechanisms: a re-examination and re-statement. Brain 101, 1 – 18.

Weisenberg, M. (1976) Teaching behavioral pain control to health professionals. In: M. Weisenberg and B. Tursky (Eds.), Pain: New Perspectives in Therapy and Research. Plenum Press, New York.

Weisenberg, M. (1977) Pain and pain control. Psychol. Bull. 84, 1008 – 1044.

Wolpe, J. (1959) Psychotherapy by Reciprocal Inhibition. Stanford University Press, Stanford, CA.

Zeicher, M. (1984) Evaluation of pain facilities in Europe. People to People International.

Index